Handbook of
Experimental Pharmacology

Continuation of Handbuch der experimentellen Pharmakologie

Vol. 53

Pharmacology of Ganglionic Transmission

Contributors

D. M. Aviado · D. A. Brown · A. A. Bunatian · E. V. Erina
L. Gyermek · W. E. Haefely · D. A. Kharkevich
G. I. Klingman · J. D. Klingman · D. F. J. Mason
A. V. Meshcherjakov · A. Nistri · D. T. Organisciak
J. P. Quilliam · V. I. Skok · V. Trčka · R. L. Volle

Editor

D. A. Kharkevich

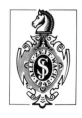

Springer-Verlag Berlin Heidelberg New York 1980

Professor Dr. DIMITRY A. KHARKEVICH, Department of Pharmacology, First Medical Institute, 2/6, B. Pirogovskaja St., USSR Moscow, 119435

With 72 Figures

ISBN 3-540-09592-6 Springer-Verlag Berlin Heidelberg New York
ISBN 0-387-09592-6 Springer-Verlag New York Heidelberg Berlin

Library of Congress Cataloging in Publication Data. Main entry under title: Pharmacology of ganglionic transmission. (Handbook of experimental pharmacology; v. 53) 1. Ganglionic blocking agents. 2. Ganglia, Autonomic. 3. Neural transmission. I. Aviado, Domingo M. II. Kharkevich, Dimitry Aleksandrovich. III. Series: Handbuch der experimentellen Pharmakologie: New Series; v. 53. QP905.H3 vol. 53 [RM323]. 615′.1′08s. [615′.78] 79–9406.

Printed in Germany.

The use of registered names, trademarks, etc. in this publication does not imply, even in the absence of a specific statement, that such names are exempt from the relevant protective laws and regulations and therefore free for general use.

Typesetting, printing, and bookbinding: Brühlsche Universitätsdruckerei, Gießen. 2122/3130-543210

Contents

CHAPTER 3

Methods for the Examination of Ganglion-Blocking Activity. L. GYERMEK.
With 16 Figures

CHAPTER 4a

**Relationship Between Chemical Structure and Ganglion-Blocking Activity.
a) Quaternary Ammonium Compounds.**V. TRČKA. With 1 Figure

CHAPTER 4b

**Relationship Between Chemical Structure and Ganglion-Blocking Activity.
b) Tertiary and Secondary Amines.** V. TRČKA

CHAPTER 5

Locus and Mechanism of Action of Ganglion-Blocking Agents. D. A. BROWN.
With 7 Figures

CHAPTER 6

Action of Ganglion-Blocking Agents on the Cardiovascular System. D. M. AVIADO

CHAPTER 7

Action of Ganglion-Blocking Agents on the Gastrointestinal Tract.
D. F. J. MASON

CHAPTER 8

Absorption, Distribution, Fate, and Excretion of Ganglion-Blocking Compounds.
D. F. J. MASON.

CHAPTER 9

Nicotinic Ganglion-Stimulating Agents. R. L. VOLLE. With 12 Figures

CHAPTER 10

Non-Nicotinic Chemical Stimulation of Autonomic Ganglia. W. E. HAEFELY.
With 3 Figures

Contents

CHAPTER 11

Ganglion Activity of Centrally Acting Neurotropic Agents.
A. NISTRI and J. P. QUILLIAM. With 1 Figure

CHAPTER 12

Ganglionic Actions of Anticholinesterase Agents, Catecholamines, Neuro-Muscular Blocking Agents, and Local Anaesthetics. R. L. VOLLE. With 10 Figures

CHAPTER 13

Ganglionic Activity of Cardiovascular Drugs. D. M. AVIADO

CHAPTER 14

Ganglion-Blocking Agents in Internal Medicine. E. V. ERINA. With 4 Figures

CHAPTER 15

Ganglion-Blocking Agents in Anaesthesiology. A. A. BUNATIAN and
A. V. MESHCHERJAKOV. With 6 Figures

List of Contributors

D. M. Aviado, Dr., Biomedical Research, Allied Chemical Corporate Headquarters, P.O. Box 102 1R, Morristown, NJ 07960/USA

D. A. Brown, Professor Dr., Department of Pharmacology, The School of Pharmacy, University of London, 29/39, Brunswick Square, GB London, WCIN IAX

A. A. Bunatian, Professor Dr., Institute of Clinical and Experimental Surgery, 2/6, B. Pirogovskaja Street, USSR Moscow, 119435

E. V. Erina, Dr., Institute of Cardiology, USSR Academy of Medical Sciences, 10, Petroverigska per., USSR Moscow, 101837

L. Gyermek, Professor Dr., University of California, Department of Anesthesiology, School of Medicine, Davis, CA 95020/USA (present affiliation: Wheeler Hospital, Gilroy, CA 95020/USA)

W. E. Haefely, Dr., Forschung Pharma, Abt. I (FP/I, Bau 69), Fa. Hoffmann-La Roche & Co AG, Grenzacherstraße 124, CH 4002 Basel

D. A. Kharkevich, Professor Dr., Department of Pharmacology, First Medical Institute, 2/6, B. Pirogovskaja Street, USSR Moscow, 119435

G. I. Klingman, Dr., Department of Biochemical Pharmacology, School of Pharmacy, SUNY at Buffalo, Buffalo, NY 14214/USA

J. D. Klingman, Professor Dr., Department of Biochemistry, Schools of Medicine and Dentistry, Faculty of Health Sciences, State University of New York at Buffalo, 102 Cary Hall, Buffalo, NY 14214/USA

D. F. J. Mason, Dr., Department of Pharmacology, The Medical College of Saint Bartholomew's Hospital, Charterhouse Square, GB London, EC1M 6BQ

A. V. Meshcherjakov, Dr., Institute of Clinical and Experimental Surgery, 2/6, B. Pirogovskaja Street, USSR Moscow, 119435

A. Nistri, Dr., Department of Pharmacology, The Medical College of Saint Bartholomew's Hospital, Charterhouse Square, GB London, EC1M 6BQ

D. T. Organisciak, Dr., Department of Biochemistry, School of Medicine, Wright State University, Dayton, OH/USA

J. P. Quilliam, Professor Dr., Department of Pharmacology, The Medical College of Saint Bartholomew's Hospital, Charterhouse Square, GB London, EC1M 6BQ

V. I. Skok, Professor Dr., Institute of Physiology, Academy of Sciences of UKR.SSR, 4, Bogomoletz Street, USSR Kiev 24

V. Trčka, Professor Dr., Pharmaceutical and Biochemical Research Institute, 17, Kouřimská, CSSR 13000 Praha 3

R. L. Volle, Professor Dr., UCONN Health Center, Preclinical and Graduate Education, The University of Connecticut, Farmington, CT 06032/USA

Introduction

D.A. KHARKEVICH

The history of the study of ganglionic substances begins with the paper of LANGLEY and DICKINSON (1889), who established the ability of nicotine to block the neurones in the superior cervical ganglion. This was a considerable discovery as the authors ascertained that impulses were transmitted from pre- to postganglionic neurones in the autonomic ganglia. Simultaneously they indicated the possibility of pharmacological influence upon interneuronal transmission in autonomic ganglia. The idea of ganglionic receptors specifically sensitive to nicotine followed logically.

Later, LANGLEY (1905, 1906) considered the problem of receptors with respect to neuro-effector synapses. It is remarkable that he was one of the first to put forward the theory of chemical mediation of excitation ("... the nervous impulse should not pass from nerve to muscle by an electric discharge, but by the secretion of a special substance at the end of the nerve": LANGLEY, 1906, p. 183). In addition, LANGLEY

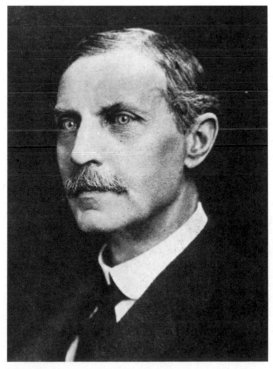

JOHN N. LANGLEY (1852–1926)

and his collaborators managed to define the topography of autonomic ganglia more precisely by means of nicotine. It should be mentioned that it was he who introduced the terms "autonomic nervous system" and "parasympathetic nervous system". Many of LANGLEY's papers were summarised in his well-known monograph "*The Autonomic Nervous System*" (1921). Thus, LANGLEY's contribution to the study of the morphology, physiology, and pharmacology of autonomic ganglia and the autonomic nervous system in general is considerable, as it has also stimulated further research in this field that is so important in biology and medicine.

Interest in autonomic ganglia can be explained first of all by the fact that they participate in the regulation of visceral organ functions. In addition, autonomic ganglia are a favourite object of study when the main modes of regulation of interneuronal transmission are being considered. BIKOV wrote on this point that a superior cervical ganglion "is like a piece of brain transmitted to periphery, but preserving, though in a low degree, all those qualitative peculiarities characteristic of the complicated construction of the central nervous system" (1942, p. 330).

Physiological investigations of autonomic ganglia developed in different directions. One of them followed the study of synthesis, storage, release, and inactivation of acetylcholine, which plays the leading role in ganglionic transmission, as was ascertained by FELDBERG and GADDUM (1934). A great deal of attention was paid to the elucidation of the principles of interaction between acetylcholine and ganglionic receptors, to the mechanism of generation of postsynaptic potential and action potential, and also to the origin of different components of action potential. In addition, the convergence of excitation, postactivating processes, and other peculiarities of neuronal activity has been carefully investigated.

Much attention was paid to research revealing the existence in the autonomic ganglia of not only nicotinic but also non-nicotinic receptors sensitive to different biogenic substances. Various types of receptors on the membrane of ganglionic neurones were revealed by means of different stimulants of autonomic ganglia and their antagonists. According to the data obtained, there are grounds for suggesting that the transmission of impulses in the autonomic ganglia is regulated not only by the main mediator, acetylcholine, but also by other physiologically active compounds acting as modulators of interneuronal transmission.

The discovery of different types of receptors in the autonomic ganglia is important for our appreciation of the principles of interneuronal transmission as well as for our understanding of complicated neurohumoral mechanisms that may affect the ganglionic transmission in the whole organism in normal and pathological conditions. In fact, many compounds formed in the organism are known to stimulate non-nicotinic receptors of autonomic ganglia. Thus, acetylcholine stimulates not only nicotinic but also muscarinic receptors in ganglia. Histamine, serotonin, angiotensin II, bradykinin, potassium ions, and other endogenous substances also possess a stimulating effect on the ganglia. For the majority of these stimulants there are special antagonists, which do not influence nicotinic receptors. For example, it is possible to use picrotoxin, propranolol, and cocaine to abolish the effect of serotonin, while the action of histamine is neutralised by antihistamines blocking H_1 receptors. The effect of angiotensin II is inhibited by the agents blocking H_1 receptors, morphine, cocaine, etc. Still, classic ganglion-blocking angents (of the hexamethonium or the pempidine type) selectively blocking nicotinic receptors reduce the sensi-

tivity of autonomic ganglia only to efferent nervous impulses and to nicotinomimet-
ics, without preventing the effects of other non-nicotinic stimulating compounds
formed in the ganglia or arriving with the blood flow. In this respect, the integration
of humoral influences in the autonomic ganglia with nervous stimuli entering the
ganglia both from the central nervous system and through afferent neurones of so-
called local reflexes is of much interest. Various aspects of the physiology of autonomic ganglia have been considered in detail in monographs and reviews by ECCLES
(1953, 1957), VOLLE (1966, 1969), TRENDELENBURG (1967), SKOK (1970, 1973), and
HAEFELY (1972), and are discussed in Chaps. 1, 9, and 10 of the present volume.

The study of metabolism in autonomic ganglia is of great importance, as the
function of ganglionic neurones and, consequently, the innervation of effector cells
depend on the state of metabolism. In addition, autonomic ganglia are used as a
biological model for the study of factors regulating the relationships between the
structure, function, and metabolism of neurones. Investigations of pre- and postsynaptic processes, of peculiarities of metabolism of neurones in the case of excitation of
different receptors (nicotinic and non-nicotinic), and other aspects are also of great
importance. But autonomic ganglia possess a rather complicated structure consisting of different types of nervous cells and of various receptors. Therefore it is often
quite difficult to differentiate what cells and what structures are responsible for the
events that occur.

Pharmacological substances are most often used for analysis of the causes of
definite metabolic changes. But the necessity of investigating the effects of different
substances possessing ganglionic activity upon metabolism in the ganglia persists.
This is important for a more precise understanding of the mechanism of action of
substances affecting transmission in the autonomic ganglia.

The above-mentioned aspects are presented in the publications of LARRABEE
(1958, 1961, 1968), VYSOTSKAYA (1957, 1960, 1963), BIRKS and MACINTOSH (1961),
DOLIVO and ROUTILLER (1969), DOLIVO (1974), MCBRIDE and KLINGMAN (1974),
MACINTOSH and COLLIER (1976), and many others.

The data dealing with the relationship between chemical structure of substances
and their ganglionic activity are worthy of special attention (see PATON and ZAIMIS,
1952; NÁDOR, 1960; KHARKEVICH, 1962, 1967; GYERMEK, 1967; BARLOW, 1968).
Formerly these investigations were of great importance for the synthesis of many
ganglion-blocking agents for medical practice. In addition, such studies are valuable
in that they reveal the organisation of ganglionic receptors. The principle of defining
how substances and the receptors complement each other (according to the maximum activity in the different series of compounds) has made it possible to form some
idea (albeit rather approximate) of the structural organisation of nicotinic receptors
of autonomic ganglia. On the other hand, a lot of problems remain unsolved. They
include space configuration of receptor structure, real topography of anionic centres,
and localisation of hydrophobic zones. As for the substance-receptor interaction, it is
necessary to investigate the role of ion-dipolic, dipole-dipolic, hydrophobic, and
dispersion interactions. From these points of view, the pooling and analysis of the
(rather extensive) data obtained can make a valuable contribution to improved
understanding of the organisation of nicotinic receptors and of their interaction with
gangliotropic substances of different structures (including asymmetrical bis-quaternary ammonium compounds, tertiary and secondary amines). But ideally, for all

these problems to be solved it is necessary to isolate nicotinic receptors of ganglia and to reveal their structural organisation in detail.

In addition to basic research, applied studies directed at the synthesis of selectively acting ganglion-blocking agents were carried out. The search for such agents supported by the fact that in many cases of pathology the block of efferent pathways at the level of autonomic ganglia is one mode of pathogenetic therapy.

As is known, the first ganglion-blocking substance used in practical medicine was tetraethylammonium, a mono-quaternary ammonium compound, which was thoroughly studied by ACHESON et al., (1946a,b). Then symmetrical and asymmetrical bis-quaternary ammonium salts such as hexamethonium (PATON and ZAIMIS, 1948, 1952), Pendiomid (BEIN and MEIER, 1950), Ecolid (PLUMMER et al., 1955), Camphidonium (KLUPP, 1957), dicolinum and dimecolinum (SHARAPOV, 1958, 1962), hygronium (KHARKEVICH, 1963) etc., appeared. The number of ganglion-blocking agents was enlarged by secondary and tertiary amines, such as nanophynum (SYRNEVA, 1950), pachycharpinum (MASHKOVSKY and RABKINA, 1952), mecamylamine (STONE et al., 1956), pempidine (SPINKS et al., 1958), and penbutamine (TRČKA and VANĚČEK, 1959). The structures of some ganglion-blocking agents are presented in Table 1, together with their synonyms.

Table 1. Ganglion-blocking agents

I. Bis-onium compounds

  a) Symmetrical

Hexamethonium
$$(CH_3)_3\overset{+}{N}CH_2CH_2CH_2CH_2CH_2CH_2\overset{+}{N}(CH_3)_3 \cdot 2I^-$$

Pendiomid
$$(CH_3)_2C_2H_5\overset{+}{N}CH_2CH_2NCH_2CH_2\overset{+}{N}C_2H_5(CH_3)_2 \cdot 2Br^-$$
$$\underset{\overset{|}{CH_3}}{}$$

Pentolinium
$$\left[\overset{+}{N}CH_2CH_2CH_2CH_2CH_2\overset{+}{N}\right] \cdot 2C_4H_5O_6^-$$
with CH_3 groups

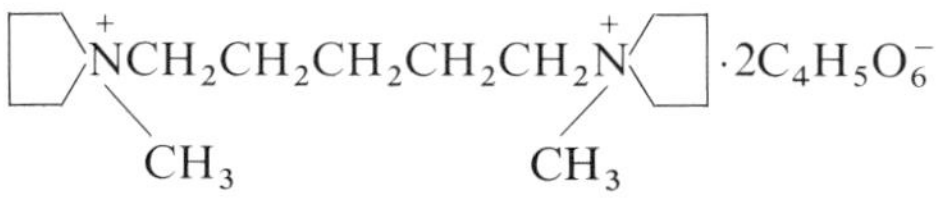

  b) Asymmetrical

Hygronium
(Trepirium iodide)
$$\overset{+}{N}-OCOCH_2CH_2\overset{+}{N}(CH_3)_3 \cdot 2I^-$$
$$H_3C \quad CH_3$$

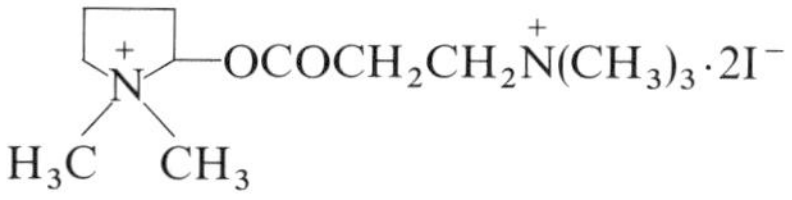

Dimecolinum
$$H_3C-\overset{+}{N}-OCOCH_2CH_2\overset{+}{N}(CH_3)_3 \cdot 2I^-$$
$$H_3C \quad CH_3$$

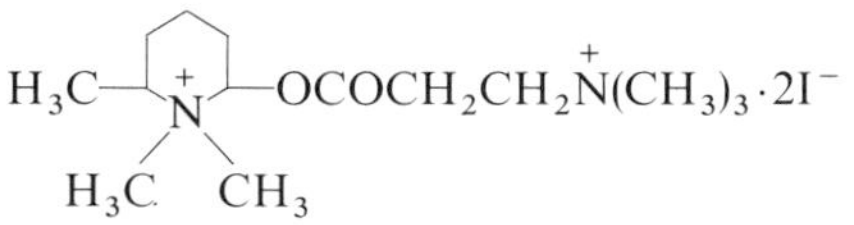

Camphidonium
$$CH_3$$
$$H_3C-CH_3\overset{+}{N}CH_2CH_2CH_2\overset{+}{N}(CH_3)_3 \cdot 2(CH_3SO_4)^-$$
$$CH_3$$

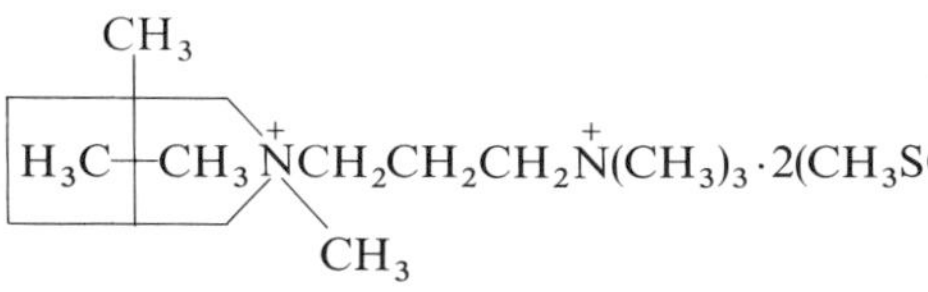

Table 1 (continued)

II. Mono-onium compounds

Quateronum
(Cvaterone)

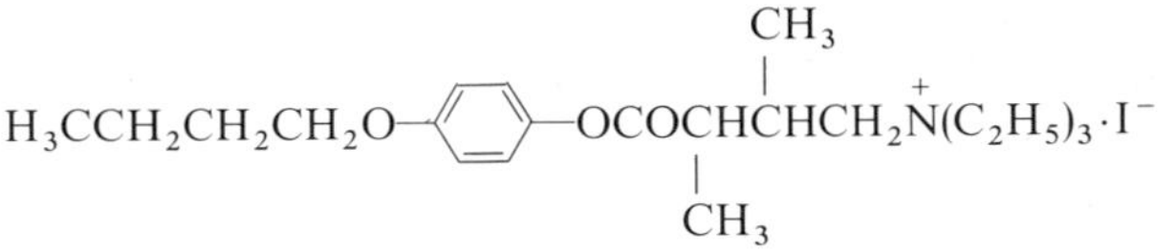

$$H_3CCH_2CH_2CH_2O-\langle\rangle-OCOCHCHCH_2\overset{+}{N}(C_2H_5)_3\cdot I^-$$

with CH_3 above and CH_3 below

Trophenium

$$H_3C-\overset{+}{N}-CH_2-CO-\langle\rangle-OCOCH-\langle\rangle\cdot Cl^-$$

with OH above

Imechinum

$$\begin{matrix}H_3C\\H_3C\end{matrix}\underset{\underset{CH_3}{|}}{\overset{+}{N}}\begin{matrix}CH_3\\CH_3\end{matrix}\cdot I^-$$

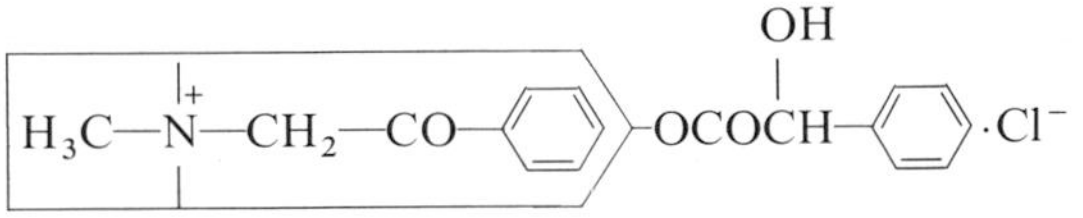

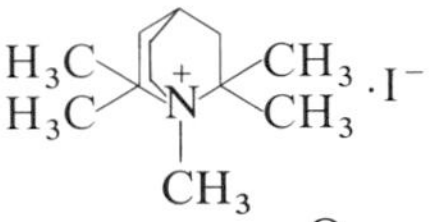

Trimetaphan

$$\langle\rangle-CH_2-N \quad N-CH_2-\langle\rangle$$

with O above, S below; $\cdot\bar{S}O_3-CH_2-$ with a camphor-like structure CH_3, CH_3, O

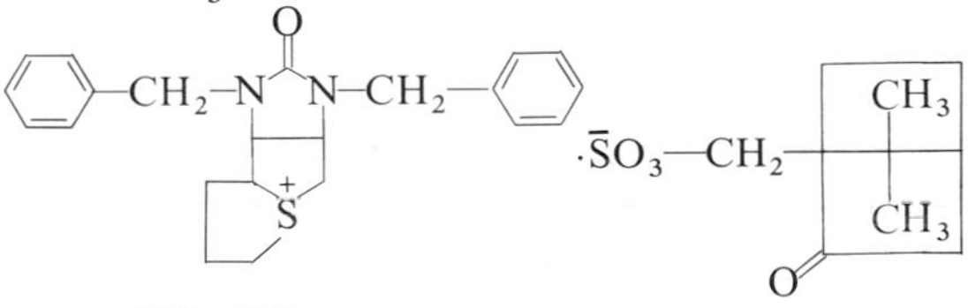

III. Tertiary amines

Penbutamine
(Heptamin)

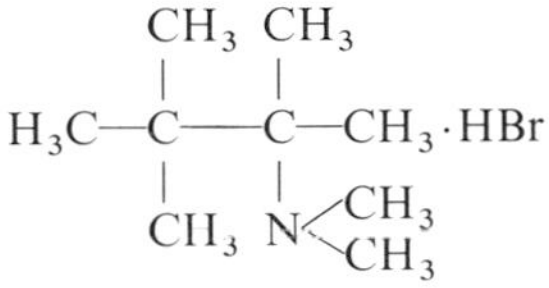

$$H_3C-\underset{\underset{CH_3}{|}}{\overset{\overset{CH_3}{|}}{C}}-\underset{N\langle^{CH_3}_{CH_3}}{\overset{\overset{CH_3}{|}}{C}}-CH_3\cdot HBr$$

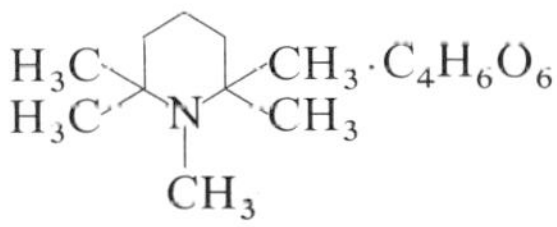

Pempidine

$$\begin{matrix}H_3C\\H_3C\end{matrix}\underset{\underset{CH_3}{|}}{N}\begin{matrix}CH_3\\CH_3\end{matrix}\cdot C_4H_6O_6$$

Temechinum
(Temechin)

$$\begin{matrix}H_3C\\H_3C\end{matrix}N\begin{matrix}CH_3\\CH_3\end{matrix}\cdot HBr$$

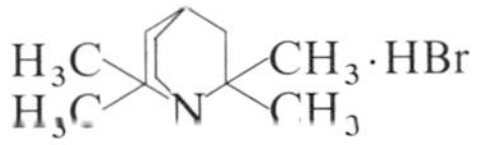

Pachycarpinum
hydroiodide
(Pachycarpin)

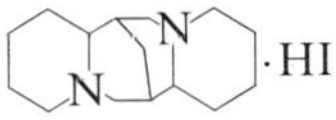

$\cdot HI$

IV. Secondary amines

Spherophysinum
(Sphaerophysin)

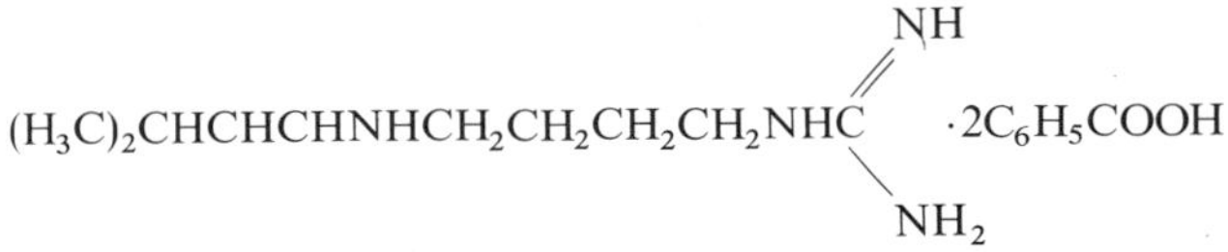

$$(H_3C)_2CHCHCHNHCH_2CH_2CH_2CH_2NHC \quad \cdot 2C_6H_5COOH$$

with NH (double bond) above and NH$_2$ below

Nanophynum
(Nanofin)

$$H_3C-\underset{\underset{H}{|}}{N}-CH_3\cdot HCl$$

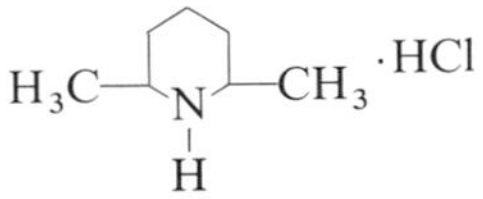

Mecamylamine

$$\begin{matrix}CH_3\\NHCH_3\cdot HCl\\CH_3\\CH_3\end{matrix}$$

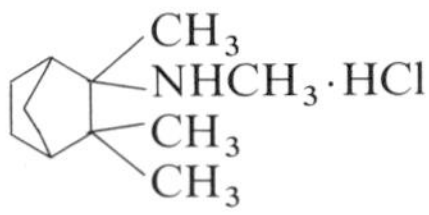

The introduction of ganglion-blocking agents into practical medicine was of great value in the treatment of a number of diseases, especially hypertension. For about 15 years ganglion-blocking substances remained the basic hypotensive agents. Owing to the emergence of better hypotensive agents, such as guanethidine, reserpine, methyldopa, a series of saluretics, antagonists of aldosterone, and other drugs, ganglion-blocking agents have considerably declined in popularity for the treatment of hypertension, and are now indicated rather rarely.

However, short-acting ganglion-blocking agents are quite extensively used for controlled hypotension (LITTLE, 1956; OSIPOV, 1967). The short-acting agents include such drugs as trimetaphan (RANDALL et al., 1949) and hygronium (KHARKEVICH, 1963, 1970). Besides blocking sympathetic ganglia, trimetaphan reduces arterial blood pressure to some extent, due to histamine release and a direct myotropic effect. Hygronium possesses a more selective ganglion-blocking action and, in addition, its toxicity is much lower than that of trimetaphan.

Controlled hypotension is widely used in cardiovascular surgery. It is of special importance that during the action of ganglion-blocking agents the impaired blood-flow in the peripheral tissues is improved, due to the elimination of arteriolar spasm. Neurosurgeons use ganglion-blocking agents for the prevention and treatment of brain oedema. In addition, the use of ganglion-blocking agents provides some protection against possible undesirable reflexes in the heart, vessels, and other visceral organs, which can occur during operations. A further reason for using controlled hypotension is because it can make performance of a number of operations easier, as the decrease in arterial pressure reduces bleeding from the vessels in the operational field. Controlled hypotension is also used in the treatment of lung oedema and in pregnancy complications followed by an increase in arterial pressure.

Thus a certain sphere of practical use of ganglion-blocking agents remains up to the present. In the present volume the importance of ganglion-blocking agents in internal medicine (Chap. 14) and in anaesthesiology (Chap. 15) is discussed.

More detailed information about the effect of ganglion-blocking agents on the cardiovascular system and the gastrointestinal tract and also some data on pharmacokinetics can be found in Chaps. 6, 7, and 8. Useful material dealing with the methods of experimental and clinical research on ganglion-blocking agents is presented in Chap. 3.

Clinicians as well as pharmacologists are greatly interested not only in the data on selectively acting ganglion-blocking agents but also in information about the ganglion-blocking properties of substances of different pharmacological groups. Thus, ganglion-blocking activity is clearly pronounced in procaine, amobarbitalum natricum, magnesium sulphate, fluothane, tubarine, benadrile, and other drugs. No doubt this should be taken into account when they are used in medical practice or in experiments. In addition, the presence of a ganglion-stimulating component in the action of a number of drugs (e.g., cardiac glycosides, anticholinesterase agents, psychostimulants of the phenylalkylamine group etc.) is also of great importance. These questions are discussed in detail in monographs by KHARKEVICH (1962, 1967) and in the present volume in Chapts. 11–13.

Thus, autonomic ganglia are still attracting the attention of scientists. As already mentioned, their main concerns are the revelation of the morphophysiological and biochemical bases of interneuronal transmission and the principle of its regulation by means of pharmacological substances. In addition, practical aspects concerning the continuing use of ganglion-blocking agents in medicine are still being investigated. The present volume presents the results of pure and applied research in this field and considers the perspectives of its development.

References

Acheson, G.H., Moe, G.K.: The action of tetraethylammonium ion on the mammalian circulation. J. Pharmac. exp. Ther., 87, 220–236 (1946a)

Acheson, G.H., Pereira, S.A.: The blocking effect of tetraethylammonium ion on the superior cervical ganglion of the cat. J. Pharmac. exp. Ther., 87, 273–280 (1946b)

Barlow, R.B.: Introduction to chemical pharmacology, 2nd ed. England: Methuen 1968

Bein, H.J., Meier, R.: Zur Pharmakologie des N,N,N', N'-3-pentamethyl-N-N'-diäthyl-3-azapentan-1,5-diammonium dibromid (CrBa 9295), ein ganglionär hemmende Substanz. Experientia, 6, 351–356 (1950)

Bikov, K.M.: Brain cortex and visceral organs. p. 330. Kirov: VMMA 1942 (Russ.)

Birks, R.J., McIntosh, F.C.: Acetylcholine metabolism of a sympathetic ganglion. Canad. J. Biochem., 39, 787–827 (1961)

Dolivo, M.: Metabolism of mammalian sympathetic ganglia. Fed. Proc., 33, 1043–1048 (1974)

Dolivo, M., Routiller, C.: Changes in ultrastructure and synaptic transmission in the sympathetic ganglion during various metabolic condition. In: Mechanisms of synaptic transmission. Progr. Brain Res., 31, 111–123 (1969)

Eccles, J.C.: The neurophysiological basis of mind. Oxford: Clarendon press 1953

Eccles, J.C.: The physiology of nerve cells. Baltimore: The John Hopkins press 1957

Feldberg, W., Gaddum, J.H.: The chemical transmission at synapses in a sympathetic ganglion. J. Physiol., 81, 305–319 (1934)

Gyermek, L.: Ganglionic stimulant and depressant agents. In: Drugs affecting the peripheral nervous system, 1, 149–326. Ed. by Burger, A. New-York: Dekker 1967

Haefely, W.: Electrophysiology of the adrenergic neuron. In: Handbook exp. Pharmacol., 33, 661–725. Berlin: Springer 1972

Kharkevich, D.A.: Ganglionic agents. Moskva: Medgiz 1962 (Russ.)

Kharkevich, D.A.: Ganglion-blocking substances in a series of bis-quaternary salts of the dialkylaminoalkyl esters of N-methyl-pyrrolidine carboxylic acid. Farmakol. i toxicol., 26, 172–179 (1963) (Russ.)

Kharkevich, D.A.: Ganglion-blocking and ganglion-stimulating agents. Oxford: Pergamon Press 1967 (translation from Russian edition, 1962)

Kharkevich, D.A. (ed.): New curariform and ganglion-blocking agents. Moskva: Meditsina 1970 (Russ.)

Klupp, H.: Pharmakologische Untersuchung eines neuen Ganglionblockers mit langer Wirkungsdauer, N-(γ-Trimethylammoniumpropyl)-N-methylcamphidinium-dimethylsulfat (Ha-106). Arzneimittel-Forsch., 7, 2, 123–128 (1957)

Langley, J.H.: On the reaction of cells and of nerve endigs to certain poisons chiefly as regards the reaction of striated muscle to nicotine and curare. J. Physiol., 33, 374–413 (1905)

Langley, J.H.: Croonian lecture. On nerve endings and on special exitable substances in cells. Proc. Roy. Soc., ser. B., 78170–194 (1906)

Langley, J.H.: The autonomic nervous system. London 1921

Langley, J.H., Dickinson, W.L.: On the local paralysis of the peripheral ganglia and on the connexion of different classes of nerve fibres with them. Proc. Roy. Soc. (London), 46, 423–431 (1889)

Larrabee, M.G.: Oxygen consumption of excised ganglia at rest and in activity. J. Neurochem., 2, 81–101 (1958)

Larrabee, M.G.: Glucose metabolism in ganglia and nerves. In: Biophysics of physiological and pharmacological actions, 199–213 (1961)

Larrabee, M.G.: Trans-synaptic stimulation of phosphatidylinositol metabolism in sympathetic neurons in situ. J. Neurochem., 15, 803–808 (1968)

Little, D.M.: Controlled hypotension in anesthesia and surgery. Springfield 1956
McBride, W.J., Klingman, J.D.: Effects of excitation on the metabolism of a simple neuronal
    system: The mammalian sympathetic ganglion. In: Progress in neurobiology, 3, 253–287. Ed.
    by G.A. Kerkut and J.W. Philips. Oxford: Pergamon 1974
McIntosh, F.C., Collier, B.: Neurochemistry of cholinergic terminals. In: Neuromuscular junc-
    tion. Ed. by E. Zaimis. Handbook of exp. Pharmacol., 42, 99–228. Berlin: Springer 1976
Mashkovsky, M.D., Rabkina, L.E.: Pharmacological properties of the alkaloid pachicarpine.
    Farmakol. i toxicol., 15, 23–31 (1952) (Russ.)
Nádor, R.: Ganglienblocker. In: Progress in drug research, 2, 298–416 (1960)
Osipov, V.P.: Artificial hypotension. Moskva: Medgiz 1967 (Russ.)
Paton, W.D.M., Zaimis, E.J.: Clinical potentialities of certain bis-quaternary salts causing neuro-
    muscular and ganglionic block. Nature (London), 162, 810 (1948)
Paton, W.D.M., Zaimis, E.J.: The methonium compounds. Pharmacol. Rev., 4, 3, 219–253 (1952)
Plummer, A.J., Trapold, I.H., Schneider, J.A., Maxwell, R.A., Earl, A.E.: Ganglionic blockade by
    a new bis-quaternary series including chlorisondamine dimethochloride. J. Pharmacol. exp.
    Ther., 115, 2, 173–184 (1955)
Randall, L.O., Peterson, W.G., Lehmann, G.: The ganglion blocking action of thiophanium
    derivatives. J. Pharmacol. exp. Ther., 97, 48–57 (1949)
Sharapov, I.M.: Pharmacology of ganglion-blocking agents, Dicolinum. Farmakol. i Toxicol.,
    21, 1, 19–24 (1958) (Russ.)
Sharapov, I.M.: Pharmacology of Dimecolinum, a new ganglion-blocking agents. Farmakol. i
    Toxicol., 25, 5, 533–538 (1962) (Russ.)
Skok, V.I.: Physiology of autonomic ganglia. Leningrad: Izdatelstvo "Nauka" 1970 (Russ.) and
    Tokyo: Igaku Shoin 1973 (translation from Russian edition, 1970)
Spinks, A., Young, E.H.P., Farrington, J.A., Dunlop, D.: The pharmacological actions of pempi-
    dine and its ethyl homologue. Brit. J. Pharmacol., 13, 501–520 (1958)
Syrneva, Yu.I.: Pharmacology of the alkaloids from the plant Nanophyton. Farmakol. i Toxicol.,
    13, 2, 26–28 (1950) (Russ.)
Stone, C.A., Torchiana, M.L., Navarro, A., Beyer, K.H.: Ganglionic blocking properties of 3-
    methyl-amino-isocamphane hydrochloride (mecamylamine): A secondary amine. J. Pharma-
    col. exp. Ther., 117, 2, 169–183 (1956)
Trčka, V., Vaněček, M.: Nektere nove typy ganglioplegic. Ceskoslov. Farmacie, 8, 6, 316–326
    (1959)
Trendelenburg, U.: Some aspects of the pharmacology of autonomic ganglion cells. Ergebn. der
    Physiol., 59, 1–85 (1967)
Vysotskaja, N.B.: Effect of gangliolytics on phosphoric fractions in the superior cervical gan-
    glion. Farmakol. i Toxicol., 20, 2, 12–15 (1957) (Russ.)
Vysotskaja, N.B.: Effects of ganglion-blocking substances on glycolytic processes in the superior
    cervical ganglion. Farmakol. i toxicol., 23, 2, 155–158 (1960) (Russ.)
Vysotskaja, N.B.: Effects of ganglion-blocking substances on metabolic processes connected with
    transmission in the superior cervical ganglion. Doct. thesis: Moskva 1963 (Russ.)
Volle, R.L.: Muscarinic and nicotinic stimulant actions at autonomic ganglia. Int. encyclop. of
    pharmacol. and therap., 1, Sect. 12, Oxford: Pergamon press 1966
Volle, R.L.: Ganglionic transmission. Ann. Rev. Pharmacol., 9, 135–146 (1969)

CHAPTER 1

Ganglionic Transmission: Morphology and Physiology

V. I. SKOK

A. Pathways in Autonomic Ganglia

I. Extramural Ganglia

Centrifugal pathways of the ganglia begin with preganglionic fibres. Their cell bodies are located in the lateral column of the spinal cord, particularly in the nucleus intermediolateralis (for sympathetic preganglionic fibres) or in the nuclei of the III, IV, IX, and X cranial nerves and in sacral segments of the spinal cord (for parasympathetic preganglionic fibres).

Figure 1 is a diagram of the main pathways found in the extramural ganglia: the preganglionic fibres make synaptic contacts with the neurones of the ganglion, which send their axons (postganglionic fibres) to peripheral organs. Some preganglionic fibres may pass through one or more ganglia, giving the collaterals that terminate in each ganglion crossed by the fibres. These pathways were first found by LANGLEY in a mammalian superior cervical ganglion and in lumbar and thoracic ganglia of the terminal sympathetic trunk. They are also present in the extramural parasympathetic ganglia, e.g., in the ciliary ganglion (for references see SKOK, 1973).

Some sympathetic ganglia contain peripheral reflex pathways in addition to centrifugal pathways. As shown in Fig. 1, these begin with the afferent fibres whose cell bodies are located peripherally to the ganglion (in the peripheral organs). The

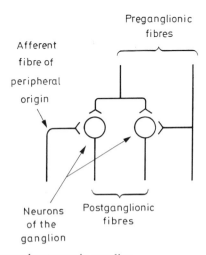

Fig. 1. Pathways of the extramural autonomic ganglion

afferent fibres enter the ganglion and terminate on its neurones. Such pathways have been found in the inferior mesenteric ganglion and in the solar plexus (Razenkov, 1926; Kuntz and Saccomanno, 1944; Bulygin, 1964; Skok, 1973). The afferent fibres of peripheral origins terminate on the same neurones of the ganglion as receive the preganglionic synaptic input (Oscarsson, 1955; Bulygin and Lemesh, 1971).

Through the pathways described above, the impulses are transmitted from pre-synaptic (preganglionic or afferent) to postsynaptic neurones; this finally results in the propagation of impulses in postganglionic fibres. In addition to this synaptic input, the neurones of the ganglion receive other influences that modulate the impulse transmission. These influences are not shown in Fig. 1. They will be described below (Sect. B). The organisation of the pathways transmitting the impulses through each particular ganglion has been discussed in a detailed review (Skok, 1973).

II. Intramural Ganglia

The pathways in the intramural ganglia have scarcely been studied, and it is impossible at present to give a complete diagram of them. Figures 2 and 3 illustrate the main centrifugal pathways and some intrinsic (particularly peripheral reflex) pathways, respectively. They have been found in the intramural ganglia of the mammalian intestine, which have been studied better than those in other organs.

As shown in Fig. 2, preganglionic parasympathetic cholinergic fibres form excitatory synaptic contacts with the cholinergic neurones of the ganglion. The function of this pathway is to evoke contraction of the longitudinal intestinal muscle (Paton and Zar, 1968; Wood, 1975). Besides this excitatory centrifugal pathway, there is also an inhibitory one. Preganglionic cholinergic fibres make excitatory synaptic contacts with the inhibitory neurones that inhibit intestinal muscle. The inhibitory neurones are thought to be purinergic, i.e., their inhibitory transmitter is ATP (Burnstock, 1972; Tomita and Watanabe, 1973; Vladimirova and Shuba, 1978).

According to the classic concept, sympathetic (adrenergic) fibres terminate in the gut muscle. However, it has been found that these fibres may form synaptic contacts with the neurones of the intramural ganglia (Norberg, 1964), and probably modu-

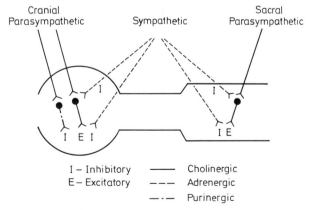

Fig. 2. Main centrifugal pathways of the intramural intestinal ganglia. (Modified from Burnstock, 1972)

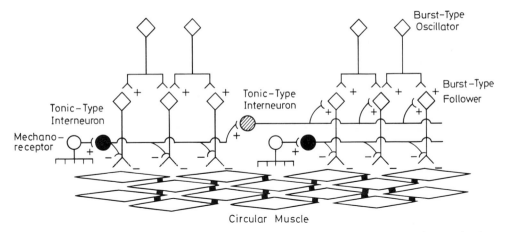

Fig. 3. Model of inhibitory nervous control of intestinal circular musculature, showing the intrinsic and peripheral reflex pathways of the intramural intestinal ganglia. −: inhibitory synapses; + : excitatory synapses. For details see text (WOOD, 1975)

late ganglionic transmission (HUKUHARA and FUKUDA, 1965; NORBERG and SJÖQVIST, 1966; BURNSTOCK, 1972). The adrenergic fibres terminate either on the internuncial neurones or on the presynaptic terminals (HIRST and MCKIRDY, 1974).

Important information on the pathways in the intestinal ganglia has been obtained from studying the patterns of spontaneous firing in single neurones (WOOD, 1975; WOOD and MAYER, 1978). Figure 3 is a diagram of interrelations between the neurones in the inhibitory pathways involved in the nervous control of intestinal circular musculature. The inhibitory (probably purinergic) neurones, the burst-type followers, are controlled by another group of neurones, the burst-type oscillators. These oscillators send several excitatory cholinergic fibres to each burst-type follower.

The burst-type followers are also controlled by enteric mechanoreceptors, which provide the synaptic input activating the tonic-type interneurones. These in turn provide a synaptic input, which in one type stimulates, and in another type inhibits the burst-type followers.

The model shown in Fig. 3 operates in the following way. Spontaneously active burst-type oscillators excite the inhibitory burst-type followers, which results in continuous suppression of the myogenic activity in the intestinal circular muscle. When enteric mechanoreceptors are activated, they inhibit some burst-type followers and excite others, causing contraction or relaxation of circular muscle, respectively. This model is thought to produce descending inhibition and thus to cause peristaltic propulsion from left to right on the diagram shown in Fig. 3 (WOOD, 1975).

III. Quantitative Relationship Between Preganglionic Fibres and Neurones of the Ganglion

There are a few ganglia in which the ratio of cells to preganglionic fibres does not exceed 2, e.g., the cat ciliary ganglion (WOLF, 1941). In most mammalian ganglia this ratio is much higher. It ranges from 11 to 17 in cat superior cervical ganglion (see Hillarp, 1960) and from 63 to 196 in human superior cervical ganglion (Ebbesson, 1963). This means that each preganglionic fibre has synaptic contacts with many neurones of the ganglion (divergence or muliplication).

The highest ratio of cells to preganglionic fibres has been found in intestinal ganglia: 6000 (see Kosterlitz, 1968). This is in keeping with the fact that, unlike extramural ganglia, the intestinal intramural ganglia contain not only efferent neurones but also afferent and internuncial neurones (Hirst et al., 1972; Holman et al., 1972; Burnstock, 1972; Nishi and North, 1973; Wood, 1975).

Each neurone of the ganglion is usually supplied with several preganglionic fibres (convergence). About 25–30 fibres converge on each neurone in cat superior cervical ganglion (Blackman, 1974), and up to ten fibres in guinea-pig pelvic ganglia (Crowcroft and Szurszewski, 1971). The impulse that arrives through one fibre evokes only subliminal excitation in the neurone of these ganglia, resulting in the appearance of an excitatory postsynaptic potential (EPSP). To evoke a discharge in the neurone, the impulses must arrive simultaneously through many preganglionic fibres converging on the neurone, e.g., through eight fibres in guinea-pig superior cervical ganglion (Sacchi and Perri, 1971).

Since each cell is innervated by several preganglionic fibres, the actual number of cells supplied by synaptic contacts from a single preganglionic fibre is higher than that obtained by dividing the number of cells by the number of preganglionic fibres that enter the ganglion. The actual number of cells innervated by a single preganglionic fibre in rabbit superior cervical ganglion is approaching 240 (Wallis and North, 1978).

There are ganglia in which no convergence of preganglionic fibres is observed. This is the case in ciliary neurones in chick ciliary ganglion (Martin and Pilar, 1963a; Landmesser and Pilar, 1974a) and in B neurones in amphibian sympathetic ganglia (Nishi et al., 1965b). In these ganglia, a depolarisation caused in a neurone by an impulse arriving through a single preganglionic fibre is large enough to evoke a discharge from the neurone.

What is the physiological role of the convergence of preganglionic fibres? There is a definite correlation between the degree of convergence and the degree of multiplication: an increasing number of preganglionic fibres converging upon a single neurone is accompanied by a rising ratio of cells to preganglionic fibres. On the basis of this, it has been suggested that the role of convergence is to ensure selective firing within a large neuronal population by a small number of preganglionic fibres. To fire a particular neurone, a preganglionic volley must arrive at the ganglion through a certain combination of preganglionic fibres, all of these fibres converging upon the necessary neurone. Other neurones of the ganglion, which receive some fibres of the combination but not a complete combination, would respond with an EPSP too slight to trigger a discharge (Skok, 1974). Such ineffective EPSPs have actually been observed in the natural activity of the ganglion neurones (see below).

IV. Morphology of Neurones in the Ganglia

There are myelinated and non-myelinated preganglionic fibres, their diameters and conduction velocities ranging from 0.5 μm and 0.55 m/s (Dunant, 1967) to 6.5 μm

(DE CASTRO, 1951) and 31 m/s (SKOK and HEEROOG, 1975). Each ganglion receives more than one group of preganglionic fibres, the groups differing in fibre diameters and in conduction velocities (ECCLES, J.C., 1935a; SHEVELEVA, 1961). Several groups of preganglionic fibres converge upon the same neurone of the ganglion (ECCLES, R.M., 1963; SKOK et al., 1966). The smallest of the presynaptic fibres are the afferent fibres of peripheral origin: their conduction velocities are 0.2–0.3 m/s (BROWN and PASCOE, 1952).

The neurones of the extramural ganglia are mostly of Dogiel I type, i.e., efferent neurones, with their dendrites wholly confined within a ganglion and their axons leaving the ganglion. Intramural ganglia also contain neurones of Dogiel II type, i.e., afferent neurones. Each neurone, together with its processes, is surrounded by glial cells located between the surface of the neurone and the connective tissue stroma.

The neurones in mammalian autonomic ganglia are multipolar. Each neurone has 2–10 dendrites (DE CASTRO, 1932). The diameter of soma ranges from 15 to 55 μm. A neurone of a mammalian sympathetic ganglion is shown in Fig.4A. In amphibian sympathetic ganglia the neurones are unipolar.

Postganglionic fibres are mostly non-myelinated; their conduction velocities range from 0.4 m/s (DUNANT, 1967) to 9 m/s (MELNICHENKO and SKOK, 1969).

Chronic section of preganglionic fibres is followed by the disappearance of all presynaptic terminals from the sympathetic ganglion unless there are peripheral reflex pathways. It has been concluded from this that the sympathetic ganglion does not contain internuncial neurones in centrifugal pathways (GIBSON, 1940; LAVRENTJEV, 1946; LAKOS, 1970). A similar conclusion was drawn from the analysis of intracellular responses of the ganglion neurones to single orthodromic stimuli (PERRI et al., 1970; SKOK and HEEROOG, 1975). In intramural ganglia synaptic contacts between the efferent cells have been found (ROPER, 1976).

However, there is a group of small, intensively fluorescent cells (SIF cells) in the superior cervical ganglion, with their axons not extending outside the ganglion. These cells receive a preganglionic input supply (HAMBERGER et al., 1963; NORBERG and SJÖQVIST, 1966; GRILLO, 1966; CSILLIK and KNYIHAR, 1967; MATTHEWS and RAISMAN, 1969; ERÄNKO and ERÄNKO, 1971). It has been suggested that SIF cells are inhibitory interneurones (LIBET and OWMAN, 1974).

Each preganglionic fibre entering the ganglion ramifies, giving many terminal branches or terminals 0.1–0.3 μm in diameter (ELFVIN, 1963b). The terminals spread over the surface of the dendrites and soma and make numerous synaptic contacts along their courses (Fig.4a). The synapses are much more often located at the dendrites than at the soma (DE CASTRO, 1951; ELFVIN, 1963a; BABMINDRA and DJACHKOVA, 1968).

Preganglionic terminals contain synaptic vesicles of two types: small and lucent, 500 Å in diameter; and large, with a dense core, 1000 Å in diameter (UCHIZONO, 1964). The lucent vesicles contain acetylcholine (UCHIZONO and OHSAWA, 1973). Recent studies show that acetylcholine may also be located in the intravesical space (BIRKS and FITCH, 1974).

At the synapses the protoplasm of a presynaptic neurone is separated from the protoplasm of a postsynaptic neurone by a distance of 150–300 Å (CAUSEY and BARTON, 1958; COUTEAUX, 1958), and there are areas of increased electron density on both pre- and postsynaptic sites (Fig.4b).

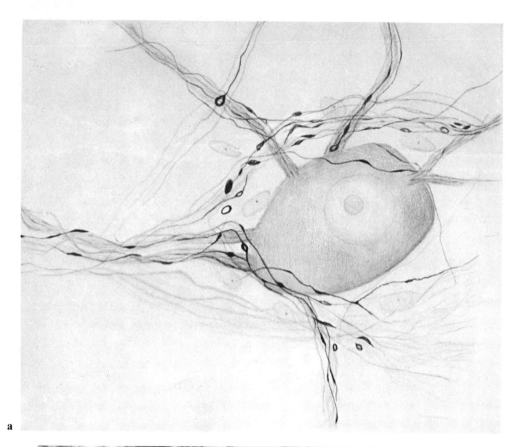

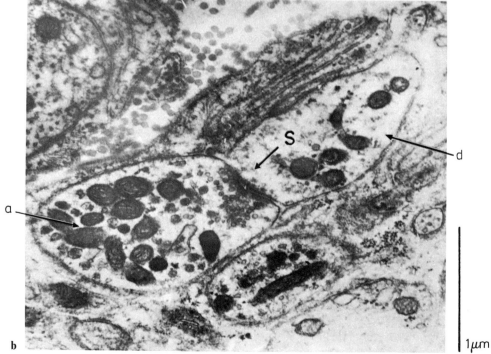

Regeneration of preganglionic fibres is followed by complete restoration of the structure and function of synapses in the ganglion, even if a sympathetic ganglion is reinnervated by parasympathetic preganglionic fibres (CECCARELLI et al., 1971).

There are receptors made up of afferent fibres of cerebrospinal origin in the autonomic ganglia (KOLOSOV, 1954, 1972). Their functions are not yet clear (see BULYGIN and KALYUNOV, 1974).

V. Embryogenesis and Development of Neurones in the Ganglia

The autonomic ganglia develop from the accumulations of cells (primordia) migrating from the embryoneural tube. The migration occurs along the nerves containing preganglionic fibres, e.g., the sympathetic cells migrate through the ventral roots of the spinal cord (KUNTZ, 1947).

It has been found recently that normal development of the neurones in the ganglia depends on their synaptic contacts with the target organs. There is a critical period in embryonic development during which axotomy causes atrophy and marked reduction in the total enzyme content of the ganglion (HENDRY, 1975). In avian ciliary ganglion, approximately half the total neuronal population suddenly dies, this half consisting of the neurones that have failed to form adequate peripheral connections with their target organs (LANDMESSER and PILAR, 1974a,b). In cell culture, the neurones of sympathetic ganglion establish synaptic contacts with each other that are inhibited by co-cultivation with the target tissue (KO et al., 1976). The selection of the transmitter to be employed by the autonomic neurone is influenced by interactions with the tissues it will innervate (BUNGE et al., 1978).

Salivary glands contain a special protein called nerve growth factor (NGF), which stimulates growth and differentiation of the neurones in sympathetic ganglia (LEVI-MONTALCINI, 1964; LEVI-MONTALCINI and ANGELETTI, 1968; BANKS et al., 1975). NGF has also been found in other organs that obtain sympathetic innervation (JOHNSON et al., 1972). It has been suggested that peripheral organs control the growth and differentiation of the neurones in the ganglion by NGF, which is taken up by adrenergic nerve terminals and moves in a retrograde direction towards their somata (HENDRY and IVERSEN, 1973; HENDRY et al., 1974; STOECKEL and THOENEN, 1975). In sympathetic neurones NGF causes selective induction of tyrosine hydroxylase and dopamine-β-hydroxylase (THOENEN et al., 1971; HENDRY and THOENEN, 1974).

The injection of antiNGF serum is followed by the degeneration of all sympathetic ganglia (immunosympathectomy): the number of neurones in sympathetic ganglia drops markedly and synaptic innervation disappears (KLINGMAN and KLINGMAN, 1969; YARYGIN et al., 1970; VARAGIĆ et al., 1970). The final effect is

◄ **Fig. 4. a** Neurone with synaptic contacts on its surface (Goldi-Deineke method; BABMINDRA and DYACHKOVA, 1968). **b** Electron micrograph of a synaptic contact from the cat superior cervical ganglion [s. synapse; *a*, acon; *d*, dendrite (BABMINDRA, unpublished)]. *Bar* represents 1 μm

similar to that observed in chemical sympathectomy produced in newborn animals by injection of 6-hydroxydopamine followed by reduction of peripheral noradrenergic terminals (GOLDMAN and JACOBOWITZ, 1971; PAPPAS, 1973).

The development of sympathetic ganglion neurones is also controlled by their preganglionic inputs. Trans-synaptic factors regulate the maturation of adrenergic nerve terminals and their innervation of target organs (BLACK and MYTILINEOU, 1976).

B. Synaptic Transmission in Autonomic Ganglia

I. Properties of Preganglionic Nerve Terminals

The range of conduction velocities in the terminals of preganglionic nerve fibres is 0.1–4 m/s, which is 0.02–1.0 of the conduction velocity in the preganglionic fibres to which these terminals belong (SKOK and HEEROOG, 1975). This reduction in conduction velocity is accounted for by a reduction in diameter.

Repetitive firing of preganglionic fibres is followed by long depolarisation in their terminals. This depolarisation is produced by acetylcholine liberated from the terminals during synaptic transmission. It is not large enough to cause in turn the liberation of acetylcholine from the terminal (KOKETSU and NISHI, 1968). Thus the membrane of preganglionic nerve terminals possesses cholinoceptive sites.

There are also adrenoceptive sites (NISHI, 1970; PUSHKAREV, 1970; CHRIST and NISHI, 1971) and sites sensitive to γ-aminobutyric acid (KATO et al., 1978) in sympathetic preganglionic nerve terminals. Adrenaline and dopamine, when applied to a sympathetic ganglion, depress transmission through the ganglion. This inhibitory effect occurs through α-adrenergic receptors (CHRIST and NISHI, 1971; DUN and NISHI, 1974). It is likely that adrenaline and dopamine decrease the release of acetylcholine from preganglionic nerve terminals (BIRKS and MACINTOSH, 1961). A similar inhibition has been observed in parasympathetic ganglia (DE GROAT and SAUM, 1972; WIKBERG, 1978).

II. Acetylcholine as Excitatory Transmitter in the Ganglia

Acetylcholine conforms to all requirements for a synaptic transmitter in the ganglia (see GRUNDFEST, 1964). It is released in the ganglia during synaptic transmission (FELDBERG and GADDUM, 1934). If applied to the ganglion with the perfusion solution (see EMMELIN and MACINTOSH, 1956) or if applied iontophoretically to a single neurone through a micropipette (see KOKETSU, 1969) acetylcholine causes a discharge in the ganglion neurones (Fig. 6A: 1 and 2).

The ionic mechanisms and the time course of the action of exogenous acetylcholine on the postsynaptic membrane are similar to those for the action of the excitatory transmitter in the ganglion (KOKETSU, 1969; DENNIS et al., 1971; SKOK and SELYANKO, 1978b; SELYANKO and SKOK, 1979). This similarity is illustrated in Fig. 6.

Preganglionic fibres contain acetylcholine (MURALT, 1946; MACINTOSH, 1959) and choline acetylase (BANNISTER and SCRASE, 1950; HEBB and WAITES, 1956). The postsynaptic membrane contains acetylcholinesterase (KOELLE et al., 1971). All substances that block synaptic transmission through the ganglion also block an excitatory action of exogenous acetylcholine on the ganglion neurones (VOLLE, 1966).

These facts constitute the main evidence that acetylcholine is a natural excitatory transmitter in the autonomic ganglia. It also acts as a transmitter in their peripheral reflex pathways (SYROMYATNIKOV and SKOK, 1968).

III. Release of Acetylcholine From Preganglionic Nerve Terminals

BIRKS and MACINTOSH (1961) have found that the rate of synthesis of acetylcholine in isolated superior cervical ganglion of the cat is about 4 ng/min. A small part of this amount (0.15–0.5 ng/min) is continuously released from the ganglion even in the absence of any stimulation of preganglionic fibres. This results in the appearance of spontaneous miniature potentials that have been recorded intracellularly from the ganglion neurones (NISHI and KOKETSU, 1960; BLACKMAN et al., 1963b,c; SACCHI and PERRI, 1976); this is a similar phenomenon to that observed in neuromuscular synapses (FATT and KATZ, 1952). Each miniature potential is a result of the sponta neous release of one or several quanta of acetylcholine. Miniature potentials appear at a frequency of 0.01/s, the frequency increasing with a rising calcium-to-magnesium ratio in the solution (DENNIS et al., 1971).

Repetitive stimulation of preganglionic fibres causes a marked increase in the rate of acetylcholine synthesis (BIRKS, 1978) and in the rate of acetylcholine release (BIRKS and MACINTOSH, 1961). When the frequency of stimulation is 20/s the rate of acetylcholine release is 30 ng/min. A single stimulus applied to preganglionic fibres is followed by the release of 1.6×10^{-16} g acetylcholine per single neurone in amphibian sympathetic ganglion (NISHI et al., 1967). This amount drops to 0.6×10^{-16} g when the frequency of stimulation is 10/s. Most neurones fail to fire when the frequency of preganglionic stimulation is higher than 10–15/s. Thus 0.6×10^{-16} g acetylcholine per neurone is probably close to a threshold amount for firing of the neurone.

It has been suggested that approximately 15–19% of the acetylcholine store in the ganglion is located in the intraganglionic part of the preganglionic fibres (stationary acetylcholine), while the rest of the store is located in their terminals (BIRKS and MACINTOSH, 1961; MACINTOSH, 1963).

When the synthesis of acetylcholine is not affected, the store of the transmitter in the ganglion does not decrease even after a long period of preganglionic stimulation at a frequency of 20/s, which is close to the maximal frequency of natural firing in preganglionic fibres. Thus there is no exhaustion of the acetylcholine store during the natural activity of the ganglion.

Most of the acetylcholine released from a continuously stimulated ganglion is newly synthesized (COLLIER, 1969; SACCHI et al., 1978). There is an alternative hypothesis, that it is pre-stored (BIRKS and MACINTOSH, 1961; BIRKS and FITCH, 1974).

As in other synapses, the release of the transmitter in the ganglion is enhanced by calcium and is depressed by magnesium ions (HUTTER and KOSTIAL, 1954). Sodium ions are important both for synthesis and for release of acetylcholine (BIRKS, 1963).

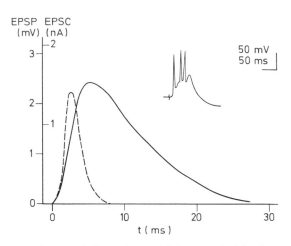

Fig.5. The EPSC *(broken line)* and the EPSP *(solid line)* evoked in the same neurone of the rabbit superior cervical ganglion by single preganglionic stimuli. The EPSC has been recorded by the voltage clamp technique (SKOK et al., in press). *Inset,* a response with three spikes to a supramaximal single preganglionic stimulus recorded from the neurone of the rabbit superior cervical ganglion (SKOK, 1973). *Horizontal line* represents 50 ms; *vertical line* represents 50 mV

IV. Nicotinic Cholinergic Transmission

The acetylcholine released by preganglionic fibres activates nicotinic receptors of the subsynaptic membrane, which results in the appearance of a fast EPSP (there is also a slow EPSP evoked by the activation of muscarinic receptors; it is described below). The time interval between the action potential of preganglionic nerve terminal and the onset of fast EPSP (the synaptic delay) is 1.5–2.5 ms in amphibian sympathetic ganglion (KOKETSU, 1969), and 1.6 ms (mean value) in mammalian sympathetic ganglion (SKOK and HEEROOG, 1975). Both these synaptic delays are much longer than in skeletal neuromuscular synapse (0.22 ms: HUBBARD and SCHMIDT, 1963) or in monosynaptic contact in spinal motoneurones (0.3–0.45 ms: BROOKS and ECCLES, 1947). The nature of the difference is not yet clear.

Figure 5 illustrates an EPSP evoked in the neurone of a mammalian sympathetic ganglion by a single preganglionic stimulus (solid line), and the excitatory postsynaptic current (EPSC) that produces this EPSP when passes through the postsynaptic membrane (broken line). The time course of decay in EPSP is exponential and corresponds to the membrane time constant (mean value 10 ms: SKOK, 1973).

An ESPC is generated by the increase in subsynaptic membrane ionic permeability caused by the activation of nicotinic receptors. Thus the time course of ESPC provides information on the time course of the·transmitter action on the subsynaptic membrane. The rising time of EPSC in rabbit superior cervical ganglion is 2.5–3.5 ms, and the half-decay time is 1.5–3.5 ms (SKOK, SELYANKO and DERKACH, to be published).

Comparison of the size of the EPSP evoked by a single preganglionic volley with the size of the postsynaptic potential evoked by one quantum of a transmitter (i.e., by an amount of a transmitter contained in single synaptic vesicle) has revealed that a single preganglionic volley releases 129 quanta in a B neurone and 79 quanta in a C neurone of amphibian sympathetic ganglion (NISHI et al., 1967) and 20 quanta in a neurone of chick ciliary ganglion (MARTIN and PILAR, 1964). Each of these neurones usually receives only one preganglionic fibre. In contrast to this, in a mammalian sympathetic ganglion a single preganglionic fibre releases only 1.5 quanta of a transmitter to a neurone. The small amount of the transmitter released can be explained by the few synaptic contacts formed by a single fibre with one neurone. To evoke a discharge of a neurone, eight or more preganglionic fibres converging on the neurone must fire simultaneously (SACCHI and PERRI, 1971).

A transmitter release to a neurone produced by single preganglionic volley can be imitated by a short application of acetylcholine through an iontophoretic micropipette. This results in the appearance of a depolarization, or acetylcholine potential, which resembles EPSP in its time course (Fig.6A: 1 and 3) and depends on the dose of acetylcholine for its size. Figure 7 illustrates the dose-response relationship of acetylcholine potential plotted on a double logarithmic scale. The slope is a Hill number indicating how many acetylcholine molecules combine with one receptor (see WERMAN, 1969; COLQUHOUN, 1975). The mean value of the Hill number in rabbit superior cervical ganglion is 2, suggesting that at least two molecules of a transmitter combine with one receptor (SELYANKO and SKOK, 1979).

The cholinomimetic drugs carbamylcholine and tetramethylammonium produce much longer depolarisation in the neurone of the ganglion than acetylcholine does, due to their stability to the action of acetylcholinesterase. In their depolarising effect, they are 7.8 and 4.6 times less effective than acetylcholine is, respectively (SELYANKO and SKOK, 1979).

The transmitter causes a marked drop in the membrane resistance of the neurone, from 456 $\Omega \cdot cm^2$ in the resting state (NISHI and KOKETSU, 1960) to 5 $\Omega \cdot cm^2$ (NISHI et al., 1967), as has been observed in amphibian sympathetic ganglion.

The transmitter increases membrane conductance for sodium and potassium ions (see KOKETSU, 1969; SKOK and SELYANKO, 1978b; SELYANKO and SKOK, 1979). Calcium ions determine the ratio of the sodium and potassium conductance changes (KOKETSU, 1969). The ionic mechanisms of nicotinic transmission in sympathetic ganglia are similar to those in skeletal neuromuscular synapses (cf. TAKEUCHI and TAKEUCHI, 1960; TAKEUCHI, 1963).

The mean reversal potential for EPSP is -14 mV both in amphibian (NISHI and KOKETSU, 1960; BLACKMAN et al., 1963a) and in mammalian (SKOK and SELYANKO, 1978b; SELYANKO and SKOK, 1979) sympathetic ganglion neurones. The reversal potential for nicotinic acetylcholine depolarisation is similar to that for fast EPSP (Fig.6B; see DENNIS et al., 1971).

In skeletal muscle, firm binding of α-bungarotoxin to a nicotinic acetylcholine receptor is always associated with an antagonism of nicotinic agonist action, but this is not necessarily so in mammalian sympathetic ganglion (MAGAZANIK et al., 1974; BROWN and FUMAGALLY, 1977) or, probably, in other ganglia (see BROWN and FUMAGALLY, 1977).

The disulphide bond-reducing agent ditiotreitol blocks the depolarising effect of nicotinic agonists, suggesting that this bond is important for the function of nicotinic acetylcholine receptors in mammalian sympathetic ganglion (BROWN and KWIATKOWSKI, 1976; TRINUS and SKOK, unpublished).

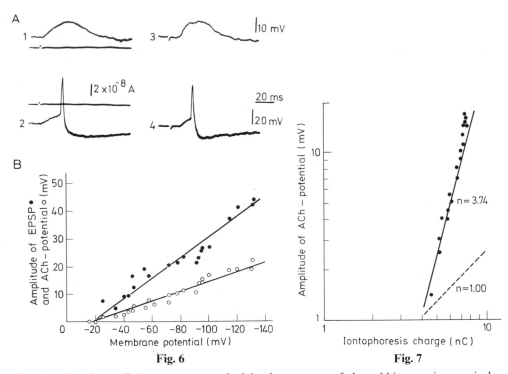

Fig. 6. **A** The intracellular responses evoked in the neurone of the rabbit superior cervical ganglion by iontophoretic application of a subthreshold (*1*) or threshold (*2*) dose of acetylcholine, compared with the responses evoked in the same neurone by a single subthreshold (*3*) or threshold (*4*) preganglionic stimulus. The iontophoretic current is monitored in the lower trace in (*1*) and in the upper trace in (*2*). *Vertical line* in (*2*) represents 2×10^{-8} A; *vertical line* in (*3*), 10 mV; *vertical line* in (*4*) represents 20 mV and *horizonal* line, 20 ms. **B** The reversal potentials for the EPSP and acetylcholine potential shown in **A**, as measured with the use of extrapolation method. Both EPSP (●) and acetylcholine potential (○) disappear at -15 mV. (Modified from SELYANKO and SKOK, 1979)

Fig. 7. Dose-response curve showing the relationship in a neurone of the rabbit superior cervical ganglion between the iontophoretic charge used to release acetylcholine and the amplitude of the acetylcholine potential, plotted in a double logarithmic scale. Hill number calculated as a slope (*solid line*) is about 3.7. A slope of 1.0 is indicated by the *broken line* (SELYANKO and SKOK, 1979)

When acetylcholine or nicotinic agonists are applied in the perfusion fluid they evoke an initial depolarisation followed by hyperpolarisation in mammalian sympathetic ganglion neurones (GEBBER and VOLLE, 1966; KOSTERLITZ et al., 1968; HAEFELY, 1974a,b). The hyperpolarisation is accounted for by the increased activity of the electrogenic sodium pump stimulated by sodium ions that enter the neurone during the initial depolarisation (BROWN and SCHOLFIELD, 1974a,b).

V. Electrical Transmission

The avian ciliary ganglion is the only one in which the impulse is transmitted from preganglionic fibres to the neurones of the ganglion by means of electrotonic spread.

A single stimulus applied to preganglionic fibres evokes two local potentials in the ganglion neurone. The first local potential (coupling potential) appears without a synaptic delay and does not decrease after treatment with d-tubocurarine. The coupling potential is produced in a postsynaptic cell by the action current of preganglionic fibre. The second local potential (EPSP) appears after a synaptic delay of 1.5–2.0 ms and is sensitive to d-tubocurarine. Thus there is both electrical and chemical transmission into the same neurone of the ganglion (MARTIN and PILAR, 1963a,b).

The electrical transmission occurs in ciliary neurones innervating ciliary muscle and pupil muscle, and does not occur in another group of neurones of ciliary ganglion, i.e., the choroid neurones innervating the smooth muscles of the blood vessels of the eye, which possess only chemical transmission. In ciliary neurones the electrical transmission develops later than the chemical transmission (LANDMESSER and PILAR, 1972).

The electrical transmission is bidirectional in chick ciliary ganglion (MARTIN and PILAR, 1963a,b) and unidirectional in pigeon ciliary ganglion (HESS et al., 1969). Both these types of electrical transmission have been found in other interneuronal contacts (FURSHPAN and POTTER, 1959; WATANABE and GRUNDFEST, 1961; BENNET, 1972).

It has been suggested that the electrical transmission occurs in avian ciliary ganglion because myelin sheath limits the spread of the current generated by preganglionic nerve terminal outside the postsynaptic neurone (HESS et al., 1969; MARWITT et al., 1971). No electrical transmission has been found in mammalian ciliary ganglion (WHITTERIDGE, 1937; MELNICHENKO and SKOK, 1969).

VI. Generation of Postsynaptic Spike. After-Hyperpolarization

When the amplitude of the depolarization produced in postsynaptic neurone by a chemical transmitter or by the action current of preganglionic fibre reaches a threshold level, a spike occurs (Fig. 6A: 2 and 4). The discharge from a soma is usually not preceded by the discharge from the initial segment, as has been observed in central neurones (ECCLES, R.M., 1955; cf. ECCLES, J.C., 1957).

A further increase in the strength of a stimulus applied to preganglionic fibres causes firing of high-threshold preganglionic fibres, evoking additional EPSPs with longer latencies and additional spikes (Fig. 5, inset). Long latencies of high-threshold EPSPs are due to slow conduction in the appropriate preganglionic fibres rather than to transmission through the internuncial neurones (PERRI et al., 1970; SKOK and HEEROOG, 1975; cf. ERULKAR and WOODWARD, 1968).

The spike is due to increased sodium conductance of the neuronal membrane. The ions of calcium and strontium can also serve as charge carriers in amphibian sympathetic ganglion (KOKETSU and NISHI, 1969). In mammalian intestinal ganglia, the neurones with increased sodium conductance indlude a group of neurones with increases in the conductance of both sodium and calcium during the action potential. This group does not have synaptic input, and is thought to be the group of afferent neurones (HIRST et al., 1972). Other afferent neurones also show calcium conductance during the action potential (NISHI et al., 1965a).

The spike is followed by after-hyperpolarisation, which in sympathetic ganglia continues for up to several hundred milliseconds and is due to increased potassium conductance of the membrane (NISHI and KOKETSU, 1960). A markedly long after-hyperpolarisation (up to 20 s) has been found in the presumed afferent neurones of mammalian intestinal ganglia mentioned above. The prolonged increase in potassium conductance in their membrane is triggered by the entry of calcium into the cell during spike generation (HIRST et al., 1972, 1974; NISHI and NORTH, 1973). The increase in membrane potassium conductance has also been observed during the effect of caffeine on amphibian (KUBA and NISHI, 1976) and mammalian (SKOK et al., 1978) sympathetic ganglion neurones, presumably as a result of intracellular calcium release.

VII. Muscarinic Cholinergic and Adrenergic Transmissions

When nicotinic transmission through the sympathetic ganglion is blocked by *d*-tubocurarine, a series of repetitive preganglionic stimuli makes the ganglion positive in relation to postganglionic fibres. This positive potential (P potential) was first observed in reptilian sympathetic ganglion (LAPORTE and LORENTE DE NÒ, 1950a,b).

In mammalian sympathetic ganglion, the P potential is followed by a late negative potential (LN potential), which is also resistant to *d*-tubocurarine, in contrast to depolarisation evoked by the activation of nicotinic receptors (N potential), as has been shown by ECCLES, R.M. (1952a,b). When recorded intracellularly, N, P, and LN potentials correspond to fast EPSP, slow IPSP, and slow EPSP, respectively.

As illustrated by Fig.8*1*, *d*-tubocurarine suppresses the spike transmission, leaving a small N potential. With the slower sweep, P and LN potentials are seen as

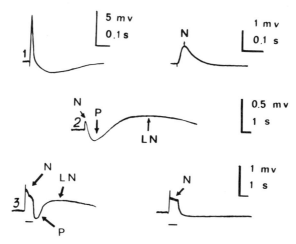

Fig.8. Effect of nicotinic and muscarinic blockers on the orthodromic responses recorded from the superior cervical ganglion of rabbit *(1, 2)* and of cat *(3)* with the sucrose-gap method. *1* Action potential *(left)* and N potential *(right)* evoked by single orthodromic stimuli before and after the application of *d*-tubocurarine (5×10^{-6} M), respectively; *2* response to single orthodromic stimulus recorded after the application of *d*-tubocurarine (5×10^{-6} M); note that the time scale is slower than in *(1)*; *3* response to repetitive stimulation (30/s during a period of 1 s, indicated by *horizontal line*) recorded after application of *d*-tubocurarine (5×10^{-6} M) before *(left)* and after *(right)* atropine (1×10^{-6} M) was added. Responses in *1–3* were obtained from three different ganglia (IVANOV and SKOK, unpublished). *Vertical lines* represent 5 mV (1, left), 1 mV (1, right, and 3) or 0.5 mV (2); *horizontal lines* 0.1 s (1) or 1 s (2 and 3)

evoked by single preganglionic stimulus (Fig. 8 2). All three potentials increase when a train of stimuli is used instead of single stimulus (Fig. 83, left).

Atropine selectively blocks P and LN potentials, not affecting the N potential (Fig. 83, right). The adrenergic blocking agents selectively block the P potential. On the basis of these findings, a hypothesis has been proposed that acetylcholine released by preganglionic fibres activates not only nicotinic but also muscarinic receptors of the ganglion neurone, evoking the slow EPSP. It also activates the muscarinic receptors of SIF cells, which respond by releasing adrenaline (ECCLES, R.M. and LIBET, 1961) or dopamine (LIBET and OWMAN, 1974), evoking slow IPSP in the neurones of the ganglion.

It is possible to observe slow IPSP even if nicotinic transmission is not blocked, when preganglionic stimuli that are subthreshold for fast EPSP are applied (TOSAKA et al., 1968; KOKETSU, 1969; LIBET and TOSAKA, 1969). In the C neurone of the amphibian sympathetic ganglion slow IPSP can be evoked by the same preganglionic C fibre that evokes fast EPSP (LIBET, 1970). There is no special group of preganglionic fibres responsible for slow IPSP.

There is morphological (SIEGRIST et al., 1968; WILLIAMS and PALAY, 1969; MATTHEWS, 1971) and physiological (LIBET and OWMAN, 1974) evidence that SIF cells are not chromaffin cells releasing the substances into the blood, but interneurones sending fibres to the neurones of the ganglion (see above). SIF cells are thought to be dopaminergic in mammals and adrenergic in amphibia (LIBET and KOBAYASHI, 1974).

An alternative hypothesis suggests that slow IPSP is the result of a direct action of acetylcholine released by preganglionic fibres on the muscarinic receptors of the ganglion neurone (WEIGHT and PADJEN, 1973a, b; see HARTZELL et al., 1977; cf. BUNGE et al., 1978).

A markedly long latency of the P potential (35–100 ms: LIBET, 1967; LIBET et al., 1968) is probably the result of slow activation of muscarinic receptors; other potentials evoked through the activation of muscarinic receptors, e.g., slow EPSP or slow acetylcholine potential, have latencies of the same order.

The electrogenesis of slow IPSP is somewhat different from that of fast IPSP observed in the neurones of the central nervous system, which is due to the increased potassium and chloride membrane conductances (see ECCLES, J.C., 1964). In amphibian sympathetic ganglion neurones slow IPSP consists of two components, namely, one component generated by an activation of the electrogenic sodium pump (NISHI and KOKETSU, 1968b; KOKETSU and AKASU, 1978), and one generated by an increase in membrane potassium permeability (KOKETSU and AKASU, 1978). Only the second component has been found in slow IPSP evoked in amphibian intracardial ganglion neurones by the activation of muscarinic receptors of the neuronal membrane. The increase in potassium conductance in intracardial ganglion neurones is voltage-sensitive (HARTZELL et al., 1977).

It seems likely that two similar mechanisms are involved in the generation of slow IPSP in mammalian sympathetic ganglion, although some authors deny the possibility of involvement of the electrogenic sodium pump (LIBET et al., 1977).

It has been suggested that the production of slow IPSP is mediated by cyclic AMP of the ganglion neurones (GREENGARD and KEBABIAN, 1974). But there is evidence against this hypothesis (GALLAGHER and SHINNICK-GALLAGHER, 1977; DUN et al., 1977).

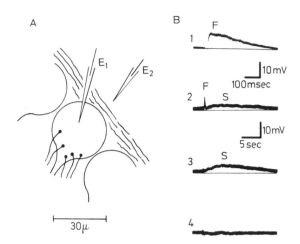

Fig. 9. A Schematic drawing of a superficially located ganglion cell and the position of recording and acetylcholine microelectrodes. Synaptic knobs are shown in the distal portion of the ganglion cell body. (*Bar* represents 30 μm.) **B** Fast (*F*) and slow (*S*) acetylcholine potentials evoked by iontophoretic application of acetylcholine to a bullfrog sympathetic ganglion cell. The strength of current pulses was 5×10^{-7} A with a duration of 15 ms (*records 1–4*); note the fast (*record 1*) and slow (*records 2–4*) time bases. *d*-Tubocurarine (0.015 mM) was given approximately 3 min before *record 3* was taken, and atropine (0.0014 mM) was added approximately 5 min before *record 4* was taken (KOKETSU, 1969). *Horizontal lines* represent 100 ms (**B** 2) or 5 s (**B** 3); *vertical lines*, 10 mV

The physiological role of the slow IPSP remains obscure. This slow process has no apparent inhibitory effect on transmission through the non-curarised amphibian sympathetic ganglion (KOKETSU and NISHI, 1967; LIBET et al., 1968). Slow IPSP has not been observed during the natural spontaneous activity of mammalian sympathetic ganglion neurones (MIRGORODSKI and SKOK, 1969; CROWCROFT and SZURSZEWSKI, 1971) or during the inhibition of efferent sympathetic activity caused by afferent stimulation (SKOK, 1973, 1976; SKOK et al., 1974). Thus it seems likely that slow IPSP does not have an inhibitory function similar to that of fast IPSP in the neurones of the central nervous system, but is rather related to some unknown metabolic processes.

Another potential evoked by activation of muscarinic receptors, slow EPSP, has been observed in all ganglia that show slow IPSP. The iontophoretic application of acetylcholine to the neurones of the amphibian sympathetic ganglion is followed by the appearance of two depolarising potentials (Fig. 9). The early one, fast acetylcholine potential, can be selectively blocked by *d*-tubocurarine, while the late one, slow acetylcholine potential, can be selectively blocked by atropine. It thus follows that fast and slow acetylcholine potentials are due to the activation of nicotinic and muscarinic receptors of the neuronal soma, respectively (KOKETSU, 1969). Some data indicate that the muscarinic receptors in the prinicipal neurone differ from those in the SIF cells described above (GARDIER et al., 1978). In contrast to this, no muscarinic receptors have been found in the soma of the mammalian sympathetic ganglion neurone (SELYANKO and SKOK, 1979). It thus seems likely that in neurones of mammalian sympathetic ganglion, muscarinic receptors are located only on the dendrites.

A similar location of muscarinic receptors has been found in the brain (KUHAR and YAMAMURA, 1976).

The synaptic delay in slow EPSP ranges from approximately 200 to 300 ms (LIBET, 1967). A comparable delay (120–500 ms) has been observed in depolarisation produced by iontophoretic application of acetylcholine to the muscarinic receptors of smooth muscle, and it has been shown that a long delay is not attributable to the diffusion time (PURVES, 1974). This implies that the activation of muscarinic receptors takes longer than the activation of nicotinic receptors.

Slow EPSP is produced by the same preganglionic fibres as fast EPSP. Occasionally it is possible to observe slow EPSP without fast EPSP in a non-curarised sympathetic ganglion when a preganglionic stimulus subthreshold for fast EPSP in this particular cell is used (LIBET and TOSAKA, 1969).

The electrogenesis of slow EPSP varies in different neurones of the ganglion. In some B neurones in amphibian sympathetic ganglion slow EPSP is due to decreased potassium conductance of the membrane (WEIGHT and VOTAVA, 1970; KUBA and KOKETSU, 1974). Other authors, however, consider that this mechanism is responsible for only an initial part of the slow EPSP (KOBAYASHI and LIBET, 1974). In other amphibian sympathetic B neurones the slow EPSP is due to increased sodium and calcium conductance of the membrane (KUBA and KOKETSU, 1974).

It has been suggested that cyclic GMP is the intracellular messenger of slow EPSP (GREENGARD, 1976; MCAFEE and GREENGARD, 1972), but recent results do not confirm this hypothesis (DUN et al., 1978).

Neither the slow EPSP evoked by a single preganglionic stimulus nor the slow acetylcholine potential can evoke a discharge from the ganglion neurone (KOKETSU, 1969), probably because of their small amplitude and slow rising phase. The neurones can be fired through their muscarinic receptors only if high-frequency (over 60/s) repetitive preganglionic stimulation is used (TAKESHIGE and VOLLE, 1962; VOLLE, 1966). This frequency is much higher than the natural firing frequency of preganglionic fibres (see below). Thus it seems unlikely that muscarinic receptors can transmit natural impulse activity through the ganglion.

There is evidence that the activation of muscarinic receptors may directly control the active sodium and potassium conductances of the cell membrane in amphibian sympathetic ganglion neurones, and in this way probably modulate synaptic transmission through the ganglion (KUBA and KOKETSU, 1975). On the other hand, the intra-arterial or intravenous injection of atropine in a dose high enough to block muscarinic transmission in the rabbit superior cervical ganglion has no effect on the frequency of spontaneous firing of the neurones in this ganglion evoked by spontaneous preganglionic impulses coming from the spinal cord (IVANOV and SKOK, unpublished). This confuses the issue as to whether activation of muscarinic receptors actually modulates natural transmission through the ganglion.

Slow synaptic processes mediated by muscarinic receptors have not yet been found in parasympathetic ganglia such as the ciliary ganglion (IVANOV and MELNICHENKO, 1971), pelvic ganglia (HOLMAN et al., 1971), and intestinal ganglia (NISHI and NORTH, 1973).

The late part of the slow EPSP recorded from the neurone of the amphibian sympathetic ganglion differs in some respects from the initial part of the slow EPSP. It has been suggested that the late part of the slow EPSP in amphibian sympathetic ganglion is due to non-cholinergic transmission (NISHI and KOKETSU, 1968a).

VIII. Role of Catecholamines in Transmission Through the Ganglia

The intravenous injection of adrenaline or the release of adrenaline from the adrenal medulla is followed by a depression of synaptic transmission through the mammalian sympathetic ganglion (MARRAZZI, 1939; POSTERNAK and LARRABEE, 1950; LUNDBERG, 1952; WEIR and McLENNAN, 1963). A similar effect has been observed in the parasympathetic ganglion (TUM SUDEN and MARRAZZI, 1951). The dose that depresses transmission does not exceed the normal level of catecholamines in the blood (SKOK, 1973, 1978).

Catecholamines may also be released within the sympathetic ganglion (BÜL-BRING, 1944; SHEVELEVA, 1961; REINERT, 1963). Some authors believe that these endogenous catecholamines can inhibit transmission through the ganglion (ECCLES, R.M. and LIBET, 1961; LIBET and OWMAN, 1974), while others deny that they can affect the transmission on the grounds that they are present in too-small amounts (REINERT, 1963; WEIR and McLENNAN, 1963).

The exogenous catecholamines can produce a small hyperpolarisation of the neuronal membrane (LUNDBERG, 1952) without any change in membrane resistance (KOBAYASHI and LIBET, 1970). But the inhibitory effect of exogenous catecholamines on synaptic transmission through the ganglion is probably due to their presynaptic rather than their postsynaptic effect, namely, to their depressant action on the preganglionic nerve terminals (see above). It should be noted that catecholamines and 5-hydroxytryptamine (5-HT) are considered possible inhibitory transmitters in the central sympathetic patways (DE GROAT and LALLEY, 1973; COOTE and MacLEOD, 1974).

IX. Other Chemoceptive Sites in the Ganglion Neurones

The neurones of mammalian sympathetic ganglion are sensitive to 5-HT and to γ-aminobutyric acid (GABA). The application of 5-HT to a soma membrane through an iontophoretic micropipette causes depolarisation and discharge in about half the neurones of rabbit superior cervical ganglion. The ionic mechanisms of 5-HT effect are probably similar to those of the nicotinic acetylcholine effect described above (SKOK and SELYANKO, 1978a; cf. WALLIS and WOODWARD, 1975). When 5-HT is applied in the perfusion fluid, a complicated effect consisting of depolarisation and hyperpolarisation is observed in sympathetic ganglion (MACHOVA and BOSKA, 1969; HAEFELY, 1974c). There are many cells containing 5-HT in the autonomic ganglia (ROBINSON and GERSHON, 1971), but their function is not clear.

The effect of GABA on sympathetic ganglion neurones is depolarisation, which is probably due to increased membrane chloride conductance (BOWERY and BROWN, 1974; ADAMS and BROWN, 1975). There is no evidence that GABA is involved in ganglionic transmission.

X. Inhibition in the Ganglia

A number of authors have suggested that there are inhibitory preganglionic fibres that produce the inhibitory effect in the neurones of the sympathetic ganglia (ECCLES, J.C., 1935b; SHEVELEVA, 1961; BECK et al., 1966; DUNANT, 1967; ERULKAR and WOODWARD, 1968). However, other experiments have not confirmed this suggestion.

The depression of transmission through the ganglion after orthodromic stimulation can be explained as an after-depression that occurs in the ganglion neurones after their firing but not as a direct inhibition (SKOK, 1967, 1973). No fast IPSP has been found in the sympathetic ganglion. There is no evidence for the inhibitory role of slow IPSP (see above; SKOK, 1976). Thus it seems likely that sympathetic ganglion does not receive purely inhibitory preganglionic fibres.

In the parasympathetic ganglion, the adrenergic fibres of sympathetic origin that enter the ganglion can inhibit transmission from parasympathetic preganglionic fibres into the neurones of the ganglion. Such a direct inhibitory effect has been observed in pelvic ganglia and in the ganglia of the urinary bladder (DE GROAT and SAUM, 1972), and also in the ganglia of the myenteric plexus (HIRST and McKIRDY, 1974; WOOD, 1975). The inhibition is mediated by α-adrenergic receptors thought to be located at a presynaptic site (HIRST and McKIRDY, 1974). It remains an open question whether this inhibition occurs in natural conditions.

No direct inhibiton has been found in mammalian ciliary ganglion, which does not receive adrenergic fibres (MELNICHENKO and SKOK, 1969, 1970).

In contrast to extramural ganglia, the intramural ganglia have IPSPs occurring separately from EPSP, both evoked and spontaneous; they are presumably due to increased membrane potassium conductance (HIRST and McKIRDY, 1975; HART-ZELL et al., 1977; WOOD and MAYER, 1978).

XI. Natural Activity of the Ganglia

The natural activity of the autonomic ganglia has been studied by recording the electrical activity from their nerves or their single neurones while the connections of the ganglia with the central nervous system are still intact.

Recording from nerves allows study of the activity of the pre- and postganglionic fibres in chronic experiments. However, with this method, only the activity of those fibres that fire synchronously can be revealed, for the action potential produced by a single fibre is too small to be recorded from the whole nerve. Two rhythms are present in the activity recorded from sympathetic nerves: the cardiac rhythm and the respiratory rhythm (PITTS et al., 1941; NOZDRACHEV, 1966). No cardiac or respiratory rhythm has been found in the parasympathetic nerves (MELNICHENKO and SKOK, 1970).

Recording from single preganglionic sympathetic neurones in acute experiments has revealed that most of them are not active spontaneously. In the resting condition, regular or irregular spontaneous firing has been observed with an average frequency of 1.4 impulses/s (POLOSA, 1968) and a range of 1–5 impulses/s (LEBEDEV, 1970). The highest frequencies recorded in the group are 20 impulses/s (LEBEDEV, 1970) and 30 impulses/s (IGGO and VOGT, 1960).

Intracellular recording from mammalian autonomic ganglia show spontaneous EPSPs of different amplitudes; large EPSPs generate spikes (MIRGORODSKI and SKOK, 1969; MELNICHENKO and SKOK, 1970). This activity is illustrated in Fig. 10. Section of preganglionic fibres abolishes all spontaneous activity of the ganglion neurones, indicating that all activity in the extramural autonomic ganglion is due to spontaneous preganglionic impulses.

The average frequency of spikes in natural spontaneous activity of cat superior cervical ganglion neurones is 3.4/s (Mirgorodski and Skok, 1969). A much lower frequency of spontaneous firing has been found in single postganglionic fibres of human skin nerve: 15/min. Emotional excitation increases it to 35/s (Hallin and Torebjörk, 1974). The highest frequency of firing in single parasympathetic neurones of cat intestinal ganglia is about 30/s (Wood, 1970).

Each spike in the natural activity of mammalian sympathetic ganglion neurones is the result of synchronous stimulation of a neurone by several preganglionic fibres. Preganglionic fibres of different conduction velocities participate in spontaneous stimulation of the same neurone (Mirgorodski and Skok, 1970).

Stimulation of afferent input to the central nervous system changes the spontaneous activity of the ganglion neurones. Figure 10A shows an example of the increase produced in the activity of the cat ciliary ganglion neurone by illumination of

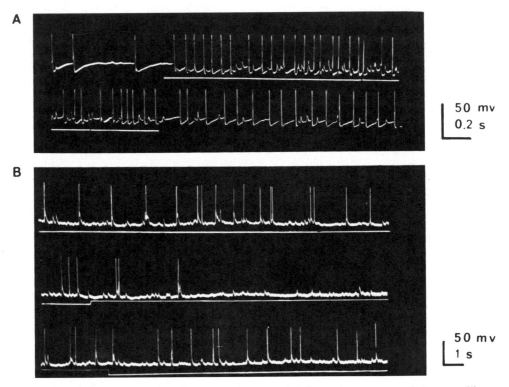

Fig. 10. A and B. Natural intracellular activity recorded from the neurone of the cat ciliary ganglion (**A**, Melnichenko and Skok, 1970) and from the neurone of rabbit superior cervical ganglion (**B**, Mirgorodski and Skok, unpublished). The activity was recorded in acute experiments under light urethane-chloralose anaesthesia; preganglionic fibres were left intact. Illumination of the eye causes an increase in spontaneous activity of the ciliary ganglion neurone **A**, and stimulation applied to the depressor nerve causes a decrease in spontaneous activity of the sympathetic ganglion neurone **B**. The time of stimulation is indicated by a *horizontal line* (**A**) or by rise in *horizontal line* (**B**). The parts of records between the top and bottom records shown in **A** (2.2 s) and between the middle and bottom records shown in **B** (9.0 s) are omitted. *Vertical lines* represent 50 mV (**A** and **B**); *horizontal lines*, 0.2 s **A** or 1 s **B**

the eye. Figure 10 B shows an example of the decreased activity of the rabbit superior cervical ganglion produced by stimulation of the depressor nerve. It follows from Fig. 10 that the increase in the frequency of firing in the neurone of the ganglion is due to an increase in the frequency of preganglionic firing. On the other hand, the decrease in the activity of the ganglion neurone is due to a decrease in the frequency of preganglionic firing. This agrees with reports of a decrease in the spontaneous activity of preganglionic fibres caused by stimulation of baroreceptor areas (RICHTER et al., 1970; SKOK and MIRGORODSKI, 1971). No IPSPs are observed during a decrease in the activity of the neurones of the ganglion caused by the afferent stimulation. Thus this decrease is due to an inhibition that has occurred in the central nervous system but not in the ganglion.

C. Summary

The main function of the extramural autonomic ganglion is distribution of the excitation that comes from the central nervous system through the relatively small number of preganglionic fibres among the much more numerous postganglionic fibres. In some groups of neurones of amphibian and avian ganglia this is attained by means of a simple schema by which a single preganglionic fibre fires many efferent neurones of the ganglion. But in mammalian autonomic ganglion there is a more complicated schema, with many preganglionic fibres converging on the same neurone, in which a synchronous firing of several preganglionic fibres is necessary to fire the neurone of the ganglion. This latter schema presumably has an advantage in ensuring selective firing within a large population of the ganglion neurones by a small number of preganglionic fibres. No internuncial neurones are involved in the transmission of centrifugal impulses through the extramural ganglion.

Besides the transmission of centrifugal impulses, some extramural and probably all intramural ganglia transmit the peripheral reflex impulses that come through the afferent fibres of peripheral origin entering the ganglion. In addition to the efferent neurones, the intramural ganglia contain afferent neurones, oscillators, and internuncial neurones.

The transmission of impulses from preganglionic fibres or from the afferent fibres of peripheral origin to the neurones of the ganglion is chemical in all ganglia except the group of ciliary neurones in the avian ciliary ganglion, where it is electrical.

Figure 11 summarizes all known synaptic inputs to the neurone of mammalian sympathetic ganglion. The impulse transmission through the ganglion occurs by means of acetylcholine released by preganglionic fibres and activating the nicotinic receptors of the neuronal membrane. Each nicotinic receptor combines with at least two acetylcholine molecules. This triggers an increase in sodium and potassium conductances of a subsynaptic membrane, resulting in the appearance of fast EPSP, which generates a spike.

The acetylcholine released by preganglionic fibres also activates the muscarinic receptors of the ganglion neurone and probably of the SIF cell. This results in the appearance of slow IPSP and slow EPSP in the neurone of the ganglion. Slow IPSP is thought to be mediated by the catecholamines released by the SIF cell. Slow IPSP is due to an increase in membrane potassium conductance, to increased activity of the

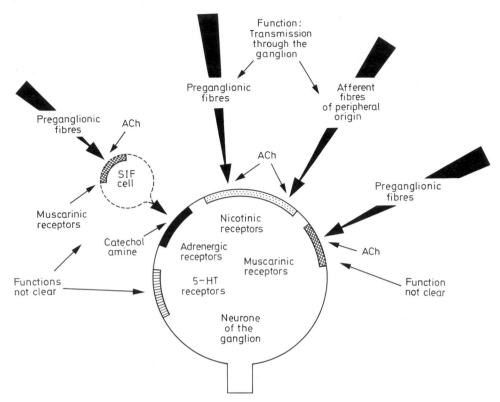

Fig. 11. Synaptic inputs to the neurone of a sympathetic ganglion. The types of transmitters and the types of synaptic receptors are indicated

electrogenic sodium pump, and, presumably, to a decrease in membrane sodium conductance. Slow EPSP is due to an increase in membrane sodium and calcium conductances and to a decrease in membrane potassium conductance. In some neurones of the ganglion somas possess 5-HT receptors. The functions of muscarinic, adrenergic, and 5-HT receptors are not yet clear. There is evidence that transmission through the sympathetic ganglion may be controlled by the level of catecholamines in the blood.

References

Adams, P.R., Brown, D.A.: Action of γ-aminobutyric acid on sympathetic ganglion cells. J. Physiol. (Lond.) *250*, 85–120 (1975)

Babmindra, V.P., Dyachkova, L.N.: On the structure of synapses in the extramural ganglia of autonomic nervous system (the data obtained by the light and electron microscopy). (Russian) Tsitologia *10*, 413–421 (1968)

Banks, B.E.C., Charlwood, K.A., Edwards, D.C., Vernon, C.A., Walter, S.J.: Effects of nerve growth factors from mouse salivary glands and snake venom on the sympathetic ganglia of neonatal and developing mice. J. Physiol. (Lond.) *247*, 289–298 (1975)

Bannister, J., Scrase, M.: Acetylcholine synthesis in normal and denervated sympathetic ganglia of the cat. J. Physiol. (Lond.) *3*, 437–444 (1950)

Beck, L., Du Charme, D.W., Gebberg, L., Levin, J.A., Pollard, A.A.: Inhibition of adrenergic activity at a locus peripheral to the brain and spinal cord. Circ. Res. [Suppl. 1] *18*, 55–59 (1966)

Bennet, M.V.L.: A comparison of electrically and chemically mediated transmission. In: Structure and function of synapses. Pappas, G., Purpura, D.P. (eds.). New York: Raven Press 1972

Birks, R.I.: The role of sodium ions in the metabolism of acetylcholine. Can. J. Biochem. Physiol. *41*, 2573–2597 (1963)

Birks, R.I.: Regulation by patterned preganglionic neural activity of transmitter stores in a sympathetic ganglion. J. Physiol. (Lond.) *280*, 559–572 (1978)

Birks, R.I., Fitch, S.J.G.: Storage and release of acetylcholine in a sympathetic ganglion. J. Physiol. (Lond.) *240*, 125–134 (1974)

Birks, R.I., MacIntosh, F.C.: Acetylcholine metabolism of a sympathetic ganglion. Can. J. Biochem. Physiol. *39*, 787–827 (1961)

Black, I.B., Mytilineou, C.: Trans-synaptic regulation of the development of end organ innervation by sympathetic neurons. Brain Res. *101*, 503–522 (1976)

Blackman, J.G.: Function of autonomic ganglia. In: The peripheral nervous system. Hubbard, J.I. (ed.). New York: Plenum Press 1974

Blackman, J.G., Ginsborg, B.L., Ray, C.: Synaptic transmission in the sympathetic ganglion of the frog. J. Physiol. (Lond.) *167*, 355–373 (1963a)

Blackman, J.G., Ginsborg, B.L., Ray, C.: Spontaneous synaptic activity in sympathetic ganglion cells of the frog. J. Physiol. (Lond.) *167*, 389–401 (1963b)

Blackman, J.G., Ginsborg, B.L., Ray, C.: On the quantal release of the transmitter at sympathetic synapse. J. Physiol. (Lond.) *167*, 402–415 (1963c)

Bowery, N.G., Brown, D.A.: Depolarising actions of γ-aminobutiric acid and related compounds on rat superior cervical ganglia in vitro. Br. J. Pharmacol. *50*, 205–218 (1974)

Brooks, C.M., Eccles, J.C.: Electrical investigation of the monosynaptic pathway through the spinal cord. J. Neurophysiol. *10*, 251–274 (1947)

Brown, C.L., Pascoe, J.E.: Conduction through the inferior mesenteric ganglion of the rabbit. J. Physiol. (Lond.) *118*, 113–123 (1952)

Brown, D.A., Fumagalli, L.: Dissociation of α-bungarotoxin binding and receptor block in the rat superior cervical ganglion. Brain Res. *129*, 165–168 (1977)

Brown, D.A., Kwiatkowski, D.: A note on the effect of ditiothreitol (DTT) on the depolarisation of isolated sympathetic ganglia by carbachol and bromo-acetylcholine. Br. J. Pharmacol. *56*, 128–130 (1976)

Brown, D.A., Scholfield, C.N.: Changes of intracellular sodium and potassium ion concentrations in isolated rat superior cervical ganglia induced by depolarizing agents. J. Physiol. (Lond.) *242*, 307–319 (1974a)

Brown, D.A., Scholfield, C.N.: Movements of labelled sodium ions in isolated rat superior cervical ganglia. J. Physiol. (Lond.) *242*, 321–351 (1974b)

Bülbring, E.: The action of adrenaline on transmission in the superior cervical ganglion. J. Physiol. (Lond.) *103*, 55–67 (1944)

Bulygin, I.A.: Closing function and receptory function of autonomic ganglia. (Russian) Minsk: Nauka i Teknika 1964

Bulygin, I.A., Kalyunov, V.N.: Receptor function of sympathetic ganglia. (Russian) Minsk: Nauka i Teknika 1974

Bulygin, I.A., Lemesh, R.G.: Microelectrode study of mechanisms involved in the closing of peripheral reflexes in cat caudal mesenteric ganglion. (Russian) Izv. Akad. Nauk. S.S.S.R. [Biol.] *3*, 102–106 (1971)

Bunge, R., Johnson, M., Ross, C.D.: Nature and nurture in development of the autonomic neuron. Science *199*, 1409–1416 (1978)

Burnstock, G.: Purinergic nerves. Pharmacol. Rev. *24*, 509–581 (1972)

Causey, G., Barton, A.A.: Synapses in the superior cervical ganglion and their changes under experimental conditions. Exp. Cell Res. [Suppl.] *5*, 338–346 (1958)

Ceccarelli, B., Clementi, F., Mantegazza, P.: Synaptic transmission in the superior cervical ganglion of the cat after reinnervation by vagus fibres. J. Physiol. (Lond.) *216*, 87–98 (1971)

Christ, D.D., Nishi, S.: Effect of adrenaline on nerve terminals in the superior cervical ganglion of the rabbit. Br. J. Pharmacol. *41*, 331–338 (1971)

Collier, B.: The preferential release of newly synthesized transmitter by sympathetic ganglion. J. Physiol. (Lond.) *205*, 341–353 (1969)

Colquhoun, D.: Mechanisms of drug action at the voluntary muscle endplate. Annu. Rev. Pharmacol. Toxicol. *15*, 307–325 (1975)

Coote, J.H., MacLeod, V.H.: The influence of bulbospinal monoaminergic pathways on sympathetic nerve activity. J. Physiol. (Lond.) *241*, 453–475 (1974)

Couteaux, R.: Morphological and cytochemical observations on the postsynaptic membrane at motor end-plates and ganglionic synapses. Exp. Cell Res. [Suppl.] *5*, 294–322 (1958)

Crowcroft, P.J., Szurszewski, J.H.: A study of the inferior mesenteric and pelvic ganglia of guinea-pigs with intracellular electrodes. J. Physiol. (Lond.) *219*, 421–441 (1971)

Csillik, B., Knyihar, E.: Cholinergic mechanism in the release of catecholamines from intra-ganglionic inhibitory terminals. Experientia *23*, 948 (1967)

De Castro, F.: Sympathetic ganglia normal and pathological. In.: Cytology and cellular pathology of nervous system. Penfield, W. (ed.), Vol. I, pp. 317–380. New York: Hoeber 1932

De Castro, F.: Aspects anatomiques de la transmission synaptique ganglionnaire chez les mammifères. Arch. Int. Physiol. Biochim. *59*, 479–511 (1951)

De Groat, W.C., Lalley, P.M.: Depression by *p*-methoxyphenylethylamine of sympathetic reflex firing elicited by electrical stimulation of the carotid sinus nerve or pelvic nerve. Brain Res. *64*, 460–465 (1973)

De Groat, W.C., Saum, W.R.: Sympathetic inhibition of the urinary bladder and of pelvic ganglionic transmission in the cat. J. Physiol. (Lond.) *220*, 279–314 (1972)

Dennis, M.J., Harris, A.J., Kuffler, S.W.: Synaptic transmission and its duplication by focally applied acetylcholine in parasympathetic neurons of the heart of the frog. Proc. R. Soc. Lond. [Biol.] *177*, 509–539 (1971)

Dun, N.J., Kaibara, K., Karczmar, A.G.: Dopamine and adenosine 3′,5′-monophosphate responses of single mammalian sympathetic neurons. Science *197*, 778–780 (1977)

Dun, N., Nishi, S.: Effects of dopamine on the rabbit's superior cervical ganglion. J. Physiol. (Lond.) *239*, 155–164 (1974)

Dun, N.J., Kaebara, K., Karczmar, A.G.: Muscarinic and cGMP induced membrane potential changes: differences in electrogenic mechanisms. Brain Res. *150*, 658–661 (1978)

Dunant, Y.: Organization tophographique et fonctionelle du ganglion cervical superieur chez le rat. J. Physiol. (Lond.) *59*, 17–38 (1967)

Ebbesson, S.O.: A quantitative study of human superior cervical sympathetic ganglia. Anat. Rec. *4*, 353–356 (1963)

Eccles, J.C.: The action potential of the superior cervical ganglion. J. Physiol. (Lond.) *85*, 179–206 (1935a)

Eccles, J.C.: Facilitation and inhibition in the superior cervical ganglion. J. Physiol. (Lond.) *85*, 207–238 (1935b)

Eccles, J.C.: The physiology of nerve cells. Baltimore: Johns Hopkins 1957

Eccles, J.C.: The physiology of synapses. Berlin, Göttingen, Heidelberg: Springer 1964

Eccles, R.M.: Action potentials of isolated mammalian sympathetic ganglia. J. Physiol. (Lond.) *117*, 181–195 (1952a)

Eccles, R.M.: Responses of isolated curarized sympathetic ganglia. J. Physiol. (Lond.) *117*, 196–217 (1952b)

Eccles, R.M.: Intracellular potentials recorded from a mammalian sympathetic ganglion. J. Physiol. (Lond.) *130*, 572–584 (1955)

Eccles, R.M.: Orthodromic activation of single cells. J. Physiol. (Lond.) *165*, 387–391 (1963)

Eccles, R.M., Libet, B.: Origin and blockade of the synaptic responses of curarized sympathetic ganglia. J. Physiol. (Lond.) *157*, 484–503 (1961)

Elfvin, L.-G.: The ultrastructure of the superior cervical sympathetic ganglion of the cat. I. The structure of the ganglion cell processes as studied by serial sections. J. Ultrastruct. Res. *8*, 403–440 (1963a)

Elfvin, L.-G.: The ultrastructure of the superior cervical sympathetic ganglion of the cat. II. The structure of the preganglionic end fibres and synapses as studied by serial sections. J. Ultrastruct. Res. *8*, 441–476 (1963b)

Emmelin, N., MacIntosh, F.C.: The release of acetylcholine from perfused sympathetic ganglia and skeletal muscles. J. Physiol. (Lond.) *131*, 477–496 (1956)

Eränko, O., Eränko, L.: Small, intensively fluorescent granule containing cells in the sympathetic ganglion of the rat. Prog. Brain Res. *34*, 39–52 (1971)

Erulkar, S.D., Woodward, J.K.: Intracellular recording from mammalian superior cervical ganglion in situ. J. Physiol. (Lond.) *199*, 189–204 (1968)

Fatt, P., Katz, B.: Spontaneous subthreshold activity at motor nerve endings. J. Physiol. (Lond.) *117*, 109–128 (1952)

Feldberg, W., Gaddum, J.H.: The chemical transmitter at synapses in a sympathetic ganglion. J. Physiol. (Lond.) *81*, 305–319 (1934)

Furshpan, E.J., Potter, D.D.: Transmission at the giant motor synapses of the crayfish. J. Physiol. (Lond.) *145*, 289–325 (1959)

Gallagher, J.P., Shinnick-Gallagher, P.: Cyclic nucleotides injected intracellularly into rat superior cervical ganglion cells. Science *198*, 851–852 (1977)

Gardier, R.W., Tsevdos, E.J., Jackson, D.B., Delaunois, A.L.: Distinct muscarinic mediation of suspected dopaminergic activity in sympathetic ganglions. Fed. Proc. *37*, 2422–2428 (1978)

Gebber, G.L., Volle, R.L.: Mechanisms involved in ganglionic blockade induced by tetramethylammonium. J. Pharmacol. Exp. Ther. *152*, 18–28 (1966)

Gibson, W.C.: Degeneration and regeneration of sympathetic synapses. J. Neurophysiol. *3*, 237–247 (1940)

Goldman, H., Jacobowitz, D.: Correlation of norepinephrine content with observations of adrenergic nerves after a single dose of 6-hydroxydopamine. J. Pharmacol. Exp. Ther. *176*, 119–123 (1971)

Greengard, P.: Possible role for cyclic nucleotides and phosphorylated membrane proteins in postsynaptic actions of neurotransmitters. Nature *260*, 101–108 (1976)

Greengard, P., Kebabian, J.W.: Role of cyclic AMP in synaptic transmission in the mammalian peripheral nervous system. Fed. Proc. *33*, 1059–1067 (1974)

Grillo, M.A.: Electron microscopy of sympathetic tissue. Pharmacol. Rev. *18*, 387–399 (1966)

Grundfest, H.: The chemical mediators. In: Unfinished tasks in the behavioral sciences. Abrams, A., Garner, H.H., and Torman, J.E.P. (eds.), pp. 61–110. Baltimore: Williams & Wilkin Company 1964

Haefely, W.: The effects of I,I-dimethyl-4-phenyl-piperazinium (DMPP) in the cat superior cervical ganglion in situ. Naunyn Schmiedebergs Arch. Pharmacol. *281*, 57–91 (1974a)

Haefely, W.: The effects of various "nicotine-like" agents in the cat superior cervical ganglion in situ. Naunyn Schmiedebergs Arch. Pharmacol. *281*, 93–117 (1974b)

Haefely, W.: The effects of 5-hydroxytryptamine and some related compounds of the cat superior cervical ganglion in situ. Naunyn Schmiedebergs Arch. Pharmacol. *281*, 145–165 (1974c)

Hallin, R.G., Torebjörk, H.E.: Single unit sympathetic activity in human skin nerves during rest and various manoeuvres. Acta Physiol. Scand. *92*, 303–317 (1974)

Hamberger, B., Norberg, K.-A., Sjöqvist, F.D.: Cellular localization of monoamines in sympathetic ganglia of the cat. A preliminary report. Life Sci. *9*, 659–661 (1963)

Hartzell, H.C., Kuffler, S.W., Stickgold, R., Yoshikami, D.: Synaptic excitation and inhibition resulting from direct action of acetylcholine on two types of chemoreceptors on individual amphibian parasympathetic neurons. J. Physiol. (Lond.) *271*, 817–846 (1977)

Hebb, C.O., Waites, G.M.H.: Choline acetylase in antero- and retro-grade degeneration of a cholinergic nerve. J. Physiol. (Lond.) *132*, 667–671 (1956)

Hendry, I.A.: The effects of axotomy on the development of the rat superior cervical ganglion. Brain Res. *90*, 235–244 (1975)

Hendry, I.A., Iversen, L.L.: Changes in tissue and plasma concentrations of nerve growth factor following removal of the submaxillary glands in adult mice and their effect on the sympathetic nervous system. Nature *243*, 500–504 (1973)

Hendry, I.A., Thoenen, H.: Changes of enzyme pattern in the sympathetic nervous system of adult mice after submaxillary gland removal, response to exogenous nerve growth factor. J. Neurochem. *22*, 999–1004 (1974)

Hendry, I.A., Stoeckel, K., Thoenen, H., Iversen, L.L.: Retrograde axonal transport of the nerve growth factor. Brain Res. *68*, 103–121 (1974)

Hess, A., Pilar, G., Weakly, J.N.: Correlation between transmission and structure in avian ciliary ganglion synapses. J. Physiol. (Lond.) *202*, 339–354 (1969)

Hillarp, N.A.: Pheripheral autonomic mechanisms. In: Handbook of physiology. Neurophysiology. Field, J., Magoun, H.W., Hall, V. (eds.), Vol. II, Sect. 1, pp. 919–1006. Baltimore: Williams & Wilkins 1960

Hirst, G.D.S., McKirdy, H.C.: Presynaptic inhibition at mammalian peripheral synapse? Nature 250, 430–431 (1974)

Hirst, G.D.S., McKirdy, H.C.: Synaptic potentials recorded from neurons of the submucous plexus of guinea-pig small intestine. J. Physiol. (Lond.) 249, 369–385 (1975)

Hirst, G.D.S., Holman, M.E., Prosser, C.L., Spence, I.: Some properties of the neurons of Auerbach's plexus. J. Physiol. (Lond.) 225, 60–61 (1972)

Hirst, G.D.S., Holman, M.E., Spence, I.: Two types of neurons in the myenteric plexus of duodenum in guinea-pig. J. Physiol. (Lond.) 236, 303–326 (1974)

Holman, M.E., Muir, T.C., Szurszewski, J.H., Yonemura, K.: Effect of iontophoretic application of cholinergic agonists and their antagonists to guinea-pig pelvic ganglia. Br. J. Pharmacol. 41, 26–40 (1971)

Holman, M.E., Hirst, G.D.S., Spence, I.: Preliminary studies of the neurons of Auerbach's plexus using intracellular microelectrodes. Aust. J. Exp. Biol. Med. Sci. 7, 795–801 (1972)

Hubbard, J.I., Schmidt, R.F.: An electrophysiological investigation of mammalian motor nerve terminals. J. Physiol. (Lond.) 166, 145–167 (1963)

Hukuhara, T., Fukuda, H.: The effects of thiamine tetrahydrofurfuril disulfide upon the movement of the isolated small intestine. J. Vitaminol. (Kyoto) 2, 253–260 (1965)

Hutter, O.F., Kostial, K.: Effect of magnesium and calcium ions on the release of acetylcholine. J. Physiol. (Lond.) 124, 234–241 (1954)

Iggo, A., Vogt, M.: Preganglionic sympathetic activity in normal and in reserpine-treated cats. J. Physiol. (Lond.) 150, 114–133 (1960)

Ivanov, A.Y., Melnichenko, L.V.: Effect of d-tubocurarine upon the synaptic transmission in cat ciliary ganglion. (Russian) Fiziol. Zh. 17, 94–95 (1971)

Johnson, D.G., Silberstein, S.D., Hanbauer, I., Kopin, I.J.: The role of nerve growth factor in the ramification of sympathetic nerve fibres into rat iris in organ culture. J. Neurochem. 19, 2025–2029 (1972)

Kato, E., Kuba, K., Koketsu, K.: Presynaptic inhibition by γ-aminobutiric acid in bullfrog sympathetic ganglion cells. Brain Res. 153, 398–402 (1978)

Klingman, G.I., Klingman, J.D.: Cholinesterases of rat sympathetic ganglia after immunosympathectomy, decentralisation, and axotomy. J. Neurochem. 16, 261–268 (1969)

Ko, C.P., Burton, M., Johnson, M.I., Bunge, R.P.: Synaptic transmission between rat superior cervical ganglion neurons in dissociated cell cultures. Brain Res. 117, 461–486 (1976)

Kobayashi, H., Libet, B.: Actions of noradrenaline and acetylcholine on sympathetic ganglion cells. J. Physiol. (Lond.) 208, 353–372 (1970)

Kobayashi, H., Libet, B.: Is inactivation of potassium conductance involved in slow postsynaptic excitation of sympathetic ganglion cells? Effects of nicotine. Life Sci. 14, 1871–1883 (1974)

Koelle, G.B., Davis, R., Smyrl, E.G.: New findings concerning the localization by electron microscopy of acetylcholinesterase in autonomic ganglia. Prog. Brain Res. 34, 371–375 (1971)

Koketsu, K.: Cholinergic synaptic potentials and the underlying ionic mechanisms. Fed. Proc. 28, 101–131 (1969)

Koketsu, K., Akasu, T.: Unique potential component of the slow IPSP of bullfrog sympathetic ganglion cells. International Brain Research Organization News 6, 4 (1978)

Koketsu, K., Nishi, S.: Characteristics of the slow inhibitory postsynaptic potential of bullfrog sympathetic ganglion cells. Life Sci. 6, 1827–1836 (1967)

Koketsu, K., Nishi, S.: Cholinergic receptors at sympathetic preganglionic nerve terminals. J. Physiol. (Lond.) 196, 293–310 (1968)

Koketsu, K., Nishi, S.: Calcium and action potentials of bullfrog sympathetic ganglion cells. J. Gen. Physiol. 53, 608–623 (1969)

Kolosov, N.G.: Innervation of visceral organs and of cardiovascular system. (Russian) Moscow, Leningrad: Izdatelstvo AN SSSR 1954

Kolosov, N.G.: Autonomic ganglion. (Russian) Leningrad: Nauka 1972

Kosterlitz, H.W.: Intrinsic and extrinsic nervous control of motility of the stomach and the intestines. In: Handbook of physiology, Sect. 6: Alimentary canal 4. Motility. Am. Physiol. Society (ed.), pp. 2147–2172. Baltimore: Williams & Wilkins 1968

Kosterlitz, H.W., Lees, G.M., Wallis, D.I.: Resting and action potentials recorded by the sucrose-gap method in the superior cervical ganglion of the rabbit. J. Physiol. (Lond.) *195*, 39–54 (1968)

Kuba, K., Koketsu, K.: Ionic mechanism of the slow excitatory postsynaptic potential in bullfrog sympathetic ganglion cell. Brain Res. *81*, 338–342 (1974)

Kuba, K., Koketsu, K.: Direct control of action potentials by acetylcholine in bullfrog sympathetic ganglion cells. Brain Res. *89*, 166–196 (1975)

Kuba, K., Nishi, S.: The rhythmic hyperpolarizations and the depolarization of sympathetic ganglion cells induced by caffeine. J. Neurophysiol. *39*, 547–563 (1976)

Kuhar, M.J., Yamamura, H.T.: Localization of cholinergic muscarinic receptors in rat brain by light microscopic radioautography. Brain Res. *110*, 229–244 (1976)

Kuntz, A.: The autonomic nervous system. Philadelphia: Lea & Febiger 1947

Kuntz, A., Saccomanno, G.: Inhibitory reflex of intestinal motility elicited through the decentralized prevertebral ganglion. J. Neurophysiol. *7*, 163–170 (1944)

Lakos, I.: Ultrastructure of chronically denervated superior cervical ganglion in the cat and rat. Acta Biol. Sci. Hung. *21*, 425–427 (1970)

Landmesser, L., Pilar, G.: The onset and development of transmission in the chick ciliary ganglion. J. Physiol. (Lond.) *222*, 691–713 (1972)

Landmesser, L., Pilar, G.: Synapse formation during embryogenesis of ganglion cells lacking a periphery. J. Physiol. (Lond.) *241*, 715–736 (1974a)

Landmesser, L., Pilar, P.: Synaptic transmission and cell death during normal ganglionic development. J. Physiol. (Lond.) *241*, 739–749 (1974b)

Laporte, Y., Lorente de No, R.: Properties of sympathetic B ganglion cells. J. Cell. Comp. Physiol. [Suppl.2] *35*, 41–60 (1950a)

Laporte, Y., Lorente de No, R.: Potential changes evoked in a curarized sympathetic ganglion by presynaptic volleys of impulses. J. Cell. Comp. Physiol. [Suppl2] *35*, 61–106 (1950b)

Lavrentjev, B.I.: Morphology of antagonist innervation in the nervous system. In: Morphology of autonomic nervous system. (Russian) Lavrentjev, B.I. (eds.), pp. 13–81. Moscow: Medgiz 1946

Lebedev, V.P.: Some patterns of lateral horn sympathetic neurons responses to anti- and orthodromic stimulation. In: Interneuronal transmission in autonomic nervous system. (Russian) Kostjuk, P.G. (ed.), pp. 76 90. Kiev: Naukova Dumka 1970)

Levi-Montalcini, R.: Growth control of nerve cells by a protein factor and its antiserum. Science *143*, 105 110 (1964)

Levi-Montalcini, R., Angeletti, P.U.: Nerve growth factor. Physiol. Rev. *48*, 534–569 (1968)

Libet, B.: Long latent periods and further analysis of slow synaptic responses in sympathetic ganglia. J. Neurophysiol. *30*, 494–514 (1967)

Libet, B.: Generation of slow inhibitory and excitatory postsynaptic potentials. Fed. Proc. *29*, 1945–1956 (1970)

Libet, B., Kobayashi, H.: Adrenergic mediation of slow inhibitory postsynaptic potential in sympathetic ganglia of the frog. J. Neurophysiol. *37*, 805–814 (1974)

Libet, B., Owman, C.: Concomitant changes in formaldehyde-induced fluorescence of dopamine interneurons and in slow inhibitory postsynaptic potentials of the rabbit superior cervical ganglion, induced by stimulation of the preganglionic nerve or by a muscarinic agent. J. Physiol. (Lond.) *237*, 635–662 (1974)

Libet, B., Chichibu, S., Tosaka, T.: Slow synaptic responses and excitability in sympathetic ganglia of the bullfrog. J. Neurophysiol. *31*, 383–395 (1968)

Libet, B., Tanaka, T., Tosaka, T.: Different sensitivities of acetylcholine-induced "after-hyperpolarization" compared to dopamine-induced hyperpolarization, to ouabain, or to lithiumreplacement of sodium, in rabbit sympathetic ganglia. Life Sci. *20*, 1863–1870 (1977)

Libet, T., Tosaka, T.: Slow inhibitory and excitatory postsynaptic responses in single cells of mammalian sympathetic ganglia. J. Neurophysiol. *32*, 43–50 (1969)

Lundberg, A.: Adrenaline and transmission in the sympathetic ganglion of the cat. Acta Physiol. Scand. *26*, 252–263 (1952)

Machova, J., Boska, D.: The effect of 5-hydroxytryptamine, dimethylpiperazinium and acetylcholine on transmission and surface potential in the cat sympathetic ganglion. Eur. J. Pharmacol. *7*, 152–158 (1969)

MacIntosh, F.C.: Formation, storage, and release of acetylcholine at nerve endings. Can. J. Biochem. Physiol. *37*, 343–356 (1959)

MacIntosh, F.C.: Synthesis and storage of acetylcholine in nervous tissue. Can. J. Biochem. Physiol. *41*, 2553–2571 (1963)

Magazanik, L.G., Ivanov, A.Y., Lucomskaya, N.Y.: Inability of snake venom polypeptides to block the cholinoreception in the isolated sympathetic ganglion of rabbit. (Russian) Neurophysiology *6*, 652–654 (1974)

Marrazzi, A.S.: Electrical studies on the pharmacology of autonomic synapses. II. The action of a sympathomimetic drug (epinephrine) on sympathetic ganglia. J. Pharmacol. Exp. Ther. *65*, 395–404 (1939)

Martin, A.R., Pilar, G.: Dual mode of synaptic transmission in the avian ciliary ganglion. J. Physiol. (Lond.) *168*, 443–463 (1963a)

Martin, A.R., Pilar, G.: Transmission through the ciliary ganglion of the chick. J. Physiol. (Lond.) *168*, 464–475 (1963b)

Martin, A.R., Pilar, G.: An analysis of electrical coupling and synapses in the ciliary ganglion. J. Physiol. (Lond.) *171*, 454–475 (1964)

Marwitt, R., Pilar, G., Weakly, J.N.: Characterization of two ganglion cells populations in avian ciliary ganglion. Brain Res. *25*, 317–334 (1971)

Matthews, M.R.: Evidence from degeneration experiment for the preganglionic origin of afferent fibres to the small granule-containing cell of the rat superior cervical ganglion. J. Physiol. (Lond.) *218*, 95 P–96 P (1971)

Matthews, M.R., Raisman, G.: The ultrastructure and somatic efferent synapses of small granule-containing cells in the superior cervical ganglion. J. Anat. *105*, 255–282 (1969)

McAfee, D.A., Greengard, P.: Adenosine 3′,5′-monophosphate: electrophysiological evidence for a role in synaptic transmission. Science *178*, 310–312 (1972)

Melnichenko, L.V., Skok, V.I.: Electrophysiological study of cat ciliary ganglion. (Russian) Neurofiziologiia *1*, 101–108 (1969)

Melichenko, L.V., Skok, V.I.: Natural electrical activity in mammalian parasympathetic ganglion neurons. Brain Res. *23*, 277–279 (1970)

Mirgorodsky, V.N., Skok, V.I.: Intracellular potentials recorded from a tonically active mammalian sympathetic ganglion. Brain Res. *15*, 570–572 (1969)

Mirgorodsky, V.N., Skok, V.I.: The role of different preganglionic fibres in tonic activity of mammalian sympathetic ganglion. Brain Res. *22*, 262–263 (1970)

Muralt, A.V.: Die Signalübermittlung in Nerven. Basel: Birkhäuser 1946

Nishi, S.: Cholinergic and adrenergic receptors at sympathetic preganglionic nerve terminals. Fed. Proc. *29*, 1956–1957 (1970)

Nishi, S., Koketsu, K.: Electrical properties and activities of single sympathetic neurons in frog. J. Cell. Comp. Physiol. *55*, 15–30 (1960)

Nishi, S., Koketsu, K.: Early and late after-discharges of amphibian sympathetic ganglion cells. J. Neurophysiol. *31*, 109–121 (1968a)

Nishi, S., Koketsu, K.: Analysis of slow inhibitory postsynaptic potential of bullfrog sympathetic ganglion. J. Neurophysiol. *31*, 717–728 (1968b)

Nishi, S., North, R.A.: Intracellular recordings from the myenteric plexus of the guinea-pig ileum. J. Physiol. (Lond.) *231*, 471–491 (1973)

Nishi, S., Soeda, H., Koketsu, K.: Effect of alkali-earth cations on frog spinal ganglion cell. J. Neurophysiol. *28*, 457–472 (1965a)

Nishi, S., Soeda, H., Koketsu, K.: Studies on sympathetic B and C neurons and patterns of preganglionic innervations. J. Cell. Comp. Physiol. *66*, 19–32 (1965b)

Nishi, S., Soeda, H., Koketsu, K.: Release of acetylcholine from sympathetic preganglionic nerve terminals. J. Neurophysiol. *30*, 114–134 (1967)

Norberg, K.A.: Adrenergic innervation of the intestinal wall studied by fluorescence microscopy. Int. J. Neuropharmacol. *3*, 379–382 (1964)

Norberg, K.A., Sjöqvist, F.D.: New possibilities for adrenergic modulation of ganglionic transmission. Pharmacol. Rev. *18*, 743–751 (1966)

Nozdrachev, A.D.: A study of electric activity in autonomic nerves by means of chronically implanted electrodes. Information material of the council "Human and Animal Physiology", Academy of Sciences of USSR, Vol. 9–10. (Russian) Leningrad: Nauka 1966

Oscarsson, O.: On the functional organisation of the two presynaptic systems to the colonic nerve neurons of the inferior mesenteric ganglion in the cat. Acta Physiol. Scand. *35*, 153–166 (1955)

Pappas, B.A.: Neonatal sympathectomy by 6-hydroxydopamine: cardiovascular responses in the paralyzed rat. Physiol. Behav. *10*, 549–554 (1973)

Paton, W.D.M., Zar, M.A.: The origin of acetylcholine released from guinea-pig intestine and longitudinal muscle strips. J. Physiol. (Lond.) *194*, 13–33 (1968)

Perri, V., Sacchi, O., Casella, C.: Electrical properties and synaptic connections of the sympathetic neurons in the rat and guinea-pig superior cervical ganglion. Pflügers Arch. *314*, 40–54 (1970)

Pitts, R.F., Larrabee, M.G., Bronk, D.W.: An analysis of hypothalamic cardiovascular control. Am. J. Physiol. *134*, 359–383 (1941)

Polosa, C.: Spontaneous activity of sympathetic preganglionic neurons. Can. J. Physiol. Pharmacol. *46*, 887–896 (1968)

Posternak, J.M., Larrabee, M.G.: Depression of synaptic transmission through sympathetic ganglia following temporary occlusion of the aorta: an effect of endogenous adrenalin. Johns Hopkins Hosp. Bull. *87*, 144–155 (1950)

Purves, R.D.: Muscarinic excitation: a microelectrophoretic study on cultured smooth muscle cells. Br. J. Pharmacol. *52*, 77–86 (1974)

Pushkarev, U.P.: Analysis of the effect of catecholamines and serotonine upon the autonomic ganglia. (Russian) Farmacol. Toksikol. *1*, 22–25 (1970)

Razenkov, I.P.: To the question on the independent reflexes in sympathetic nervous system. (Russian) Zh. Eksp. Biol. Med. *3*, 66–77 (1926)

Reinert, H.: Role and origin of noradrenaline in the superior cervical ganglion. J. Physiol. (Lond.) *167*, 18–29 (1963)

Richter, D.W., Keck, W., Seller, H.: The course of inhibition of sympathetic activity during various patterns of carotid sinus nerve stimulation. Pflügers Arch. *317*, 110–123 (1970)

Robinson, R.C., Gershon, M.D.: Synthesis and uptake of 5-hydroxytryptamine by the myenteric plexus of the guinea-pig ileum. A histochemical study. J. Pharmacol. Exp. Ther. *178*, 311–324 (1971)

Roper, S.: An electrophysiological study of chemical and electrical synapses on neurones in the parasympathetic cardial ganglion of the mudpuppy, Necturus maculosus: evidence for intrinsic ganglionic innervation. J. Physiol. (Lond.) *254*, 427–454 (1976)

Sacchi, O., Perri, V.: Quantal release of acetylcholine from the nerve endings of the guinea-pig superior cervical ganglion. Pflügers Arch. *329*, 207–219 (1971)

Sacchi, O., Perri, V.: Some properties of the transmitter release mechanism at the rat ganglionic synapse during potassium stimulation. Brain Res. *107*, 275–289 (1976)

Sacchi, O., Consolo, S., Peri, G., Prigioni, I., Ladinsky, H., Perri, V.: Storage and release of acetylcholine in the isolated superior cervical ganglion of the rat. Brain Res. *151*, 443–456 (1978)

Selyanko, A.A., Skok, V.I.: Activation of acetylcholine receptors in mammalian sympathetic ganglion neurons. In: Progress in brain research. Tuček, S. (ed.), Vol.49, The cholinergic synapse, pp. 241–252. Amsterdam: Elsevier/North-Holland: Biomedical Press 1979

Sheveleva, V.S.: Interneuronal transmission of excitation in sympathetic ganglia. (Russian) Leningrad: Medgiz 1961

Siegrist, G., Dolivo, M., Dunant, Y., Foroglon-Kerameus, C., Ribaupierre, F., Roniller, C.: Ultrastructure and function of the chromaffin cells in the superior cervical ganglion of the rat. Ultrastruct. Res. *25*, 381–407 (1968)

Skok, V.I.: Origin of the after-depression of the sympathetic ganglion. (Russian) Fiziol. Zh. *53*, 535–542 (1967), also in: Neurosci. Translations *1*, 40–46 (1967–1968)

Skok, V.I.: Physiology of autonomic ganglia. Tokyo: Igaku Shoin 1973

Skok, V.I.: Convergence of preganglionic fibres in autonomic ganglia. In: Mechanisms of neuronal integration in nervous center. (Russian) Kostjuk, P.G. (ed.). Leningrad: Nauka 1974

Skok, V.I.: On the physiological role of slow inhibitory postsynaptic potential in the neurons of sympathetic ganglia. In: Electrobiology of nerve, synapse, and muscle. Reuben, J.P., Purpura, D.P., Bennet, M.V.Z., Kandel, E.R. (eds.), pp. 123–128. New York: Raven Press 1976

Skok, V.I.: Synaptic transmission in the sympathetic ganglion. In: Modern problems of general physiology of excitable tissues, pp. 92–96. (Russian) Kiev: Naukova Dumka 1978

Skok, V.I., Heeroog, S.S.: Synaptic delay in superior cervical ganglion of the cat. Brain Res. *87*, 343–353 (1975)

Skok, V.I., Mirgorodski, V.N.: Activity of preganglionic sympathetic neurons recorded from cervical sympathetic nerve and superior cervical ganglion. In: Mechanisms of descending control of spinal cord activities. (Russian) Kostjuk, P.G. (ed.), pp. 181–185. Leningrad: Nauka 1971

Skok, V.I., Selyanko, A.A.: The effect of local iontophoretic application of acetylcholine and serotonine on the neurons of the rabbit superior cervical ganglion. (Russian) Neurophysiology *10*, 519–524 (1978 a)

Skok, V.I., Selyanko, A.A.: Ionic mechanisms of excitatory action of the transmitter, the exogenous acetylcholine and serotonine on the neurons of rabbit superior cervical ganglion. (Russian) Neurophysiology *10*, 637–644 (1978 b)

Skok, V.I., Ivanov, A.J., Bukolova, R.P.: Convergence in cat superior cervical ganglion. (Russian) Fiziol. Zh. *12*, 721–727 (1966)

Skok, V.I., Bogomoletz, V.I., Ivanov, A.J., Mirgorodski, V.N.: Electrical activity of sympathetic ganglia during depressor reflex. (Russian) Neirofiziologiia *6*, 519–524 (1974)

Skok, V.I., Storch, N.N., Nishi, S.: The effect of caffeine on the neurons of a mammalian sympathetic ganglion. Neuroscience *3*, 647–708 (1978)

Stoeckel, K., Thoenen, H.: Retrograde axonal transport of nerve growth factor: specificity and biological importance. Brain Res. *85*, 337–341 (1975)

Syromyatnikov, A.V., Skok, V.I.: Pathways in the sympathetic ganglia of cat solar plexus. (Russian) Fiziol. Zh. *54*, 1163–1170 (1968)

Takeshige, C., Volle, R.L.: Bimodal response of sympathetic ganglia to acetylcholine following eserine or repetitive preganglionic stimulation. J. Pharmacol. Exp. Ther. *138*, 66–73 (1962)

Takeuchi, A., Takeuchi, N.: Further analysis of relationship between end-plate potential and end-plate current. J. Neurophysiol. *23*, 397–402 (1960)

Takeuchi, N.: Some properties of conductance changes at the end-plate membrane during the action of acetylcholine. J. Physiol. (Lond.) *169*, 128–140 (1963)

Thoenen, H., Angeletti, P.U., Levi-Montalcini, R., Kettler, R.: Selective induction by nerve growth factor of tyrosine hydroxylase and dopamine β-hydroxylase in the rat superior cervical ganglia. Proc. Natl. Acad. Sci. USA *68*, 1598–1602 (1971)

Tomita, T., Watanabe, H.: A comparison of the effects of adenosinetriphosphate with noradrenaline and with the inhibitory potential of the guinea-pig taenia coli. J. Physiol. (Lond.) *231*, 167–177 (1973)

Tosaka, T., Chichibu, S., Libet, B.: Intracellular analysis of slow inhibitory and excitatory postsynaptic potentials in sympathetic ganglia of the frog. J. Neurophysiol. *31*, 396–409 (1968)

Tum Suden, C., Marrazzi, A.S.: Synaptic inhibitory action of adrenaline at parasympathetic synapses. Fed. Proc. *10*, 138 (1951)

Uchizono, K.: On different types of synaptic vesicles in the sympathetic ganglia of amphibia. Jpn. J. Physiol. *14*, 210–219 (1964)

Uchizono, K., Ohsawa, K.: Morpho-physiological considerations on synaptic transmission in the amphibian sympathetic ganglion. Acta Physiol. Pol. *24*, 205–214 (1973)

Varagic, V.M., Mrsulja, B.B., Stosic, N., Pasic, M., Terzic, M.: The glycogenolytic and hypertensive effect of physostigmine in the anti-nerve-growth-factor-serum-treated rats. Eur. J. Pharmacol. *12*, 194–202 (1970)

Vladimirova, I.N., Shuba, M.F.: Strichnine, hydrastine, and apamine effects on synaptic transmission in smooth muscle cells. (Russian) Neurophysiology *10*, 295–299 (1978)

Volle, R.L.: Muscarinic and nicotinic stimulating actions at autonomic ganglia. Oxford: Pergamon Press 1966

Wallis, D.I., North, R.A.: Synaptic input to cells of the rabbit superior cervical ganglion. Pflügers Arch. *374*, 145–152 (1978)

Wallis, D.I., Woodward, B.: Membrane potential changes induced by 5-hydroxytryptamine in the rabbit superior cervical ganglion. Br. J. Pharmacol. *55*, 149–212 (1975)

Watanabe, A., Grundfest, H.: Impulse propagation at the septal and comissural junctions of crayfish giant axons. J. Gen. Physiol. *45*, 167–308 (1961)

Weight, F.F., Padjen, A.: Slow synaptic inhibition: evidence for synaptic inactivation of sodium conductance in sympathetic ganglion cells. Brain Res. 55, 219–224 (1973a)

Weight, F.F., Padjen, A.: Acetylcholine and slow synaptic inhibition in frog sympathetic ganglion cells. Brain Res. 55, 225–228 (1973b)

Weight, F.F., Votava, J.: Slow synaptic excitation in sympathetic ganglion cells: evidence for synaptic inactivation of potassium conductance. Science 170, 755–757 (1970)

Weir, M.C.L., McLennan, H.: The action of catecholamines in sympathetic ganglia. Can. J. Biochem. Physiol. 41, 2627–2636 (1963)

Werman, R.: An electrophysiological approach to drug-receptor mechanisms. Comp. Biochem. Physiol. 30, 997–1017 (1969)

Whitteridge, D.: The transmission of impulses through the ciliary ganglion. J. Physiol. (Lond.) 89, 99–111 (1937)

Wikberg, J.: Localization of adrenergic receptors in guinea-pig ileum and rabbit jejunum to cholinergic neurons and to smooth muscle cells. Acta Physiol. Scand. 99, 190–207 (1978)

Williams, T.H., Palay, S.L.: Ultrastructure of the small neurons in the superior cervical ganglion. Brain Res. 15, 17–34 (1969)

Wolf, G.A.: The ratio of preganglionic neurons to postganglionic neurons in the visceral neurons system. J. Comp. Neurol. 75, 235–243 (1941)

Wood, J.D.: Electrical activity from single neurons in Auerbach's plexus. Am. J. Physiol. 219, 159–169 (1970)

Wood, J.D.: Neurophysiology of Auerbach's plexus and control of intestinal motility. Physiol. Rev. 55, 307–324 (1975)

Wood, J.D., Mayer, C.J.: Intracellular study of electrical activity of Auerbach's plexus in guinea-pig small intestine. Pflügers Arch. 374, 265–275 (1978)

Yarygin, V.N., Rodionov, I.M., Giber, L.M.: Changes in the number, in structure and in some cytochemical peculiarities of the sympathetic neurons in the stellate ganglia of the mouse and rat produced by inducing to the animals of antibodies specific to growth factor of nervous tissue. (Russian) Tsitologiia 12, 745–753 (1970)

CHAPTER 2

Ganglionic Metabolism

J.D. Klingman, D.T. Organisciak, and G.I. Klingman

Relatively few papers have been reported on ganglionic metabolism since our previous review (McBride and Klingman, 1975). Two short specific reviews are those of Marchisio (1974) on the metabolism of embryonic ganglia and Dolivo (1974) which discusses the physiologic parameters of the adult ganglion. For those interested in the effects of NGF on ganglionic biochemistry see Patterson et al. (1975, 1978) or Yu et al. (1978).

Of those autonomic ganglia investigated, their overall general respiratory response to excitation is not unlike that of the central nervous system (CNS). Since the superior cervical ganglion (SCG) is readily accessible for either in situ perfusion studies or can be surgically removed and remains active in vitro, it is a system of choice for studying metabolic events related to excitation (Larrabee, 1961).

One of the great advantages that an investigator has in using this tissue is the well-established morphological and physiologic parameters (see Chap. 1). The biochemical contents and those enzymes which have been measured for the rat SCG are given in Tables 1, 2, 4, and 7. Thus, the rat SCG, contains some 35,000–40,000 postganglionic neuronal cells (Klingman and Klingman, 1965a, b, 1967). The nerve cells and fibers are surrounded by smaller satellite cells which are separated from the extracellular space by a basement membrane of connective tissue cells. Interspersed, in clusters, are the small intensely fluorescent cells.

The preganglionic fibers have conduction velocoties of 2.6, 1.0 and 0.55 m/s (Dunant, 1967). The large postganglionic internal carotid fibers are mainly "C" type axons. The various types of synaptic connectives and the relationship of the small intensely fluorescent cells to the physiologic and biochemical responses are discussed in Chap. 1 (Table 1).

A. Carbohydrate Metabolism

Not unlike other neuronal systems, the SCG has a prerequisite requirement for a continuous supply of oxygen and glucose to maintain function (Larrabee and Bronk, 1952; Larrabee, 1970). The rat SCG, which weighs approximately 1 mg wet when stripped of its outer connective tissue sheath, can usually obtain enough oxygen and nutrients by diffusion from the bathing solution to maintain function. This is not so for those ganglia from larger species (e.g., cat, dog, or calf), which either have a larger amount of connective tissue slowing diffusion or their cross-sectional volume is too large. In these cases, the ganglia must be either perfused or sliced, similar to brain cortex.

The first documented evidence of the dynamics of oxygen utilization for rat, cat, and rabbit ganglia was reported by Larrabee (1958). The amount of oxygen utilized

Table 1. Activity of some enzymes in the superior cervical ganglion of the rat

Enzyme	Activity	
	nmol/mg protein/min	
Glucose 6-phosphate dehydrogenase	16.7 ± 0.2	Härkönen and Kauffman, 1974a, b
6-Phosphogluconate dehydrogenase	9.9 ± 0.4	Härkönen and Kauffman, 1974a, b
Ribose-5-phosphate isomerase	21.5 + 2.1	Härkönen and Kauffman, 1974a, b
Transketolase	4.9 ± 0.3	Härkönen and Kauffman, 1974a, b
Isocitrate dehydrogenase	25.1 ± 1.5	Härkönen and Kauffman, 1974a, b
Malic enzyme	4.8 ± 0.4	Härkönen and Kauffman, 1974a, b
Hexokinase	37.7 ± 3.3	Härkönen and Kauffman, 1974a, b
Phosphofructokinase	27.6 ± 2.4	Härkönen and Kauffman, 1974a, b
Pyruvate kinase	66.8 ± 6.0	Härkönen and Kauffman, 1974a, b
Prostaglandin E synthetase	0.154	Webb et al., 1978
	nmol/mg fresh tissue/min	
RNAase polymerase I	0.6 → 1.18×10^{-3}	Huf et al., 1978
RNAase polymerase II	0.57 → 1.16×10^{-3}	Huf et al., 1978
Lactate dehydrogenase	51.4 ± 8.0	Roch-Ramel and Dolivo, 1967
Succinic dehydrogenase	10.2 ± 2.51	Roch-Ramel and Dolivo, 1967
Glutamic-oxaloacetic transminase	20.5 ± 2.40	Roch-Ramel and Dolivo, 1967
	μmol substrate hydrolyzed/g wet tissue/min	
Choline esterase	28.8 ± 3.3	Klingman and Klingman, 1969
Acetylcholine esterase	18.5 ± 2.1	Klingman and Klingman, 1969
Pseudocholine esterase	9.6 ± 1.2	Klingman and Klingman, 1969
	μmol product formed/h/ganglion	
DOPA decarboxylase	0.175 ± 0.015	Klingman, 1965a
Monoamine oxidase	5.6 ± 1.9	Klingman, 1966
Catechol-O-methyl transferase	3.71 ± 0.63	Klingman, 1965b
Phenylethanolamine-N-Methyl transferase	2.8×10^{-3} newborn	Liuzzi et al., 1977
	0.29×10^{-3} adult	Liuzzi et al., 1977

was directly related to the frequency of preganglionic stimulation. This relationship in the rat was maximal at 15 Hz and the increased oxygen consumption was shown to be related to the mitochondrial cytochrome system. The delay between the rise of the action potential and the activation of the respiratory chain, after a single stimulus, is 280 ms (Dolivo and DeRibaupierre, 1973). This effect also was seen in myelinated nerve fibers (Larrabee and Bronk, 1952; Larrabee, 1958). After the maximum oxygen to frequency response had occurred, a further increase in frequency resulted in a diminished oxygen utilization. This also occurs in the rat SCG above 15 Hz, i.e., there is a fall-off in the rate at which oxygen is utilized. Whether this is a failure in the ionic or in the metabolic systems is not known.

The SCG glucose pool of 6 nmol/mg wet weight takes about 30 min to achieve a steady state with bathing solution glucose (Horowicz and Larrabee, 1962a). The utilization of this glucose carbon (Table 1) is predominantly as CO_2 and lactate

(LARRABEE and KLINGMAN, 1962; QUADFLIEG and BRAND, 1978). The rest of the glucose carbons are partitioned (in decreasing order of utilization) among the lipids, amino acids, other carbohydrates, nucleosides, and a minor component of volatile acids. When the resting SCG is switched from the normal unlabeled bathing solution to one containing ^{14}C-glucose, the time for the CO_2 to reach a constant ^{14}C output is about 45 min, while the CO_2 derived from the lipids is greater than 10 h. The lactate carbons are equilibrated with ^{14}C-carbons in 30 min (LARRABEE, 1967). In order to achieve a true picture of the partitioning of glucose carbons, one must account for the measurable amounts of carbohydrates, amino acids, and other materials which diffuse into the bathing medium (McBRIDE and KLINGMAN, 1972).

Since the functional use of glucose and oxygen is to maintain the tissue ATP and phosphocreatine levels, it is not surprising that they have been measured (Table 2). In freshly excised and quickly frozen SCG, the concentrations of ATP is about 1.5 nmol and of phosphocreatine 1.9 nmol per mg wet wt. (ORGANISCIAK and KLINGMAN, 1974b; HÄRKÖNEN et al., 1969; LARRABEE, 1961). Under in vitro conditions, the resting SCG still elicits a transsynaptic potential after 36 h of incubation in a glucose Krebs–Ringer, pH 7.4 medium. During this time, there is a gradual decline in the ATP levels, such that by 12 h only one third of the original concentration remains (LARRABEE, 1961). Glucose removal from the medium results in a depletion of the internal glucose in 30 min and by 2 h glucose is barely detectable. The glycogen pool falls at a slower rate. The decreased glucose concentration at 30 min is reflected in a failure of the

Table 2. Constituents of the rat superior cervical ganglia

H$_2$O water space	809.8	μg/mg wet	HÄRKÖNEN and KAUFMAN (1974a)
Protein	154.6	μg/mg wet	HÄRKÖNEN and KAUFFMAN (1974a)
TCA insoluble	91.7	μg/mg wet	McBRIDE and KLINGMAN (1972)
Glycogen	21.9	pg/mg wet	HÄRKÖNEN and KAUFFMAN (1974a)
Glucose	6.03	nmol/mg wet	ORGANISCIAK and KLINGMAN (1974a)
Glucose-6-P	1057	pmole/mg wet	HÄRKÖNEN and KAUFFMAN (1974a)
6-P-glucomate	36	pmole/mg wet	HÄRKÖNEN and KAUFFMAN (1974a)
Fructose	59	pmol/mg wet	HÄRKÖNEN and KAUFFMAN (1974a)
Lactate	2070	pmol/mg wet	HÄRKÖNEN and KAUFFMAN (1974a)
NAD	200	pmol/mg wet	HÄRKÖNEN and KAUFFMAN (1974a)
NADH	15	pmol/mg wet	HÄRKÖNEN and KAUFFMAN (1974a)
RNA	7.1	μg/mg wet	HÄRKÖNEN and KAUFFMAN (1974a)
DNA	0.6398	μg/mg wet	HÄRKÖNEN and KAUFFMAN (1974a)
ATP	1.48	nmol/mg wet	ORGANISCIAK and KLINGMAN (1974a)
Phosphocreatine	1.90	nmol/mg wet	ORGANISCIAK and KLINGMAN (1974a)
cAMP	1.6	pmol/mg wet	CRAMER et al. (1973)
cAMP neuronal	4	pmol/mg protein	WALLACE et al. (1978)
cAMP glial	14	pmol/mg protein	WALLACE et al. (1978)
Acetylcholine	0.0214	nmol/mg wet	HÄRKÖNEN and KAUFFMAN (1974a)
Norepinephrine	0.267	nmol/mg wet	LUTOLD et al. (1979)
Epinephrine	0.0016	pmol/mg wet	KLINGMAN, G. (1965)
GABA	47.77	mol/mg wet	BERTILSSON and COSTA (1976)
DOPAC	0.030678	nmol/mg wet	LUTOLD et al. (1979)
Dopamine	0.023	nmol/mg wet	LUTOLD et al. (1979)
Glucocorticoid receptor	1750	fmol/mg protein	TOWLE et al. (1979)
K$^+$	0.489	μmol/mg dry	GALVIN and TEN BRUGGENCOTTE (1979)

transynaptic action potential (DOLIVO and LARRABEE, 1958; HÄRKÖNEN et al., 1969; DERIBAUPIERE, 1968). The ATP and phosphocreatine levels do not follow this time course, being at 2 h 50% of their initial values. Anoxia dramatically lowers both ATP and phosphocreatine in 15 min to nonmeasurable levels (HÄRKÖNEN et al., 1969). Ganglia, to which the perfusion was stopped or which were perfused with deoxygenated media, showed reversible resting action potential failure in about 30 min; this failure was reversible when profusion was reinstituted or the medium was again oxygenated (LARRABEE and BRONK, 1952; LARRABEE et al., 1956). When rats are raised on lithium containing diets to achieve whole blood lithium levels of 0.5 mEq/liter (ORGANISCIAK and KLINGMAN, 1974b), the adult animal's SCG contained only approximately 42% of the normal ATP and about 75% of the normal phosphocreatine. Incubation of such chronic lithium SCG in normal medium initially elevates these values, regardless of whether the ganglia are rested or stimulated, but after 30 min both the ATP and phosphocreatine decline below normal values in rested and stimulated ganglia. In acute in vitro lithium experiments ganglia show lowered ATP and phosphocreatine levels by 20 min, being 10% and 30% of controls respectively, which do not recover to normal whether the ganglia are rested or stimulated. This lowered energy state in the acute and chronic lithium treated ganglion may partly explain the altered transynaptic action potentials seen in such ganglia (KLINGMAN, 1966).

B. Stimulation

As already stated, stimulation produces a rapid increase in the utilization of oxygen and glucose with an increased release of lactate and CO_2 (HOROWICZ and LARRABEE, 1958; LARRABEE, 1958; DOLIVO, 1974). The increased oxygen utilization abruptly ends as soon as the stimulation stops. The partitioning of glucose carbons into the various metabolic pools is similarly accelerated and changed from the normal resting state (MCBRIDE and KLINGMAN, 1972; HOROWICZ and LARRABEE, 1962a, b; ORGANISCIAK and KLINGMAN, 1976). Even though there are increased rates of incorporation of glucose carbons into the amino acids and lipids, the CO_2 that is being produced during excitation can still be accounted for as coming from the glucose carbons. It is this increased glucose uptake and use during stimulation which probably allows for the maintenance of the SCG in simple glucose buffered media for several hours (ROCH-RAMEL, 1962; LARRABEE, 1961).

If the apparent intracellular glucose concentration and the rate at which CO_2 is produced by the SCG, is used as a basis of calculation some 30% of the CO_2 can not be accounted for as coming directly from glucose carbons. Similarly, when the total lactate output is compared to the ^{14}C lactate carbon output it becomes apparent that about 40% of the lactate carbons do not come directly from glucose. From these types of data, it is apparent that other components besides glucose are being oxidized to CO_2 and lactate. The extent to which this labeled CO_2 comes directly from glucose via the oxidative Krebs cycle or from the pentose cycle is still being challenged. It seems that the sliced calf SCG (QUADFLIEG and BRAND, 1978) differs from the whole rat SCG since less than 1% of the CO_2 is derived from the HMP system. The extent to which the HMP system operates in neuronal tissue will undoubtedly become clearer when the experimental modeling experiments of LARRABEE (1978) are completed.

The effects of stimulation on SCG bathed in glucose-free bathing medium were first described by LARRABEE et al. (1956). The morphological alterations which occur during glucose lack was studied by NICOLASCU et al. (1966). Loss of the transynaptic action potentials occurs within 30 min of glucose withdrawal and complete, irreversible failure at 2.5–3 h. However, the pre- or postganglionic fibers retain their ability to conduct for 12 and 30 h, respectively, after glucose deprivation. Electron microscopic examination of the ganglionic cell bodies shows only minor alterations; ribosomes are dispersed, polysomes dissociated, mitochondria elongated, and enlarged Golgi areas. Within the presynaptic area more marked alteration in morphology were noted. Not only did this area appear swollen and lack fibrillar material, but there was a paucity of mitochondria and those mitochondria present had vesicated and were swollen. Throughout the presynaptic areas larger cytolysosomes, vesicles, and amorphous masses, as seen in myelin degeneration, were noted. DOLIVO and ROUILLER (1969) rarely saw synaptic vesicles or synapses in the most extensively damaged regions. That this structural deterioration was due to a lack of glucose was verified in two ways. If ganglia were incubated without glucose at 6 °C for 18 h and then returned to a glucose medium at 37 °C, normal action potentials were obtained. This would indicate that, presynaptically, glucose is involved in maintaining morphological intergrity. Furthermore, it seems that the presynaptic swelling and subsequent damage were not merely a derangement of osmotic equilibrium, since SCG bathed in electrolytes or polyvinylpyrrolidone media still showed the lesions (NICOLESCU et al., 1966). If ganglia were deprived of glucose, but given physostigimine, such that loss of function occurred, the subsequent addition of acetylcholine to the bathing medium produced postsynaptic axonal responses. Thus, even though the presynaptic area had been lesioned, the postsynaptic receptors for acetylcholine and the resultant action potentials were not damaged by lack of glucose. The only external chemical parameter which increased at the time of glucose lack failure was a slight increase in nitrogen although no decrease in the amount of oxygen consumed was noted. The failure can be delayed if the ganglia were first incubated in a medium containing high glucose concentrations. This obvious sparing action of high initial glucose concentrations was due to the increased amounts of glycogen found in such ganglia (DERIBAUPIERRE et al., 1966).

C. Nonglucose Metabolites Substrates

It is an accepted dictum that glucose is the required substrate for the CNS. Therefore, it is not surprising that the requirement for the SCG is similar. The reason that other compounds may not totally replace glucose in maintaining function and integrity can be due to numerous factors. The one factor that does not need to be considered with the in vitro SCG is a blood–brain barrier component, but this is replaced by a diffusion component. We do not know the effects of various metabolites, when substituted for glucose, on shifting the metabolic equilibria and producing thereby altered metabolism and structural defects. Some compounds can

Table 3. Substances restoring or maintaining the superior cervical ganglia in vitro[a]

Substrate	% of Glucose survival time	Substrate	% of Glucose survival time
Glucose	100	Aspartate + α-Ketoglutarate	72
Mannose	60–90	GABA + α-Ketoglutarate	59
Fructose	79	Alanine + α-Ketoglutarate	58
Lactate	82	Serine + α-Ketoglutarate	50
Pyruvate	80	Glutamate + α-Ketoglutarate	49
Oxaloacetate	70	Glutamate + Succinate	~48
Glutamine	55		

[a] Partial data from ROCH-RAMEL (1962).

maintain the oxygen utilization but not the action potentials (ROCH-RAMEL, 1962; LARRABEE et al., 1956). With perfused in situ cat SCG, KAHLSON and MACINTOSH (1939) noted a loss of the nictitating membrane response, when the ganglia were perfused with nonglucose containing medium. To reverse this loss of response, they tried numerous compounds but found that only mannose, lactate, and pyruvate would replace the glucose and allow for continued synthesis of acetylcholine while maintaining function. However, complete functional recovery was not attainable with these substrates (Table 3). LARRABEE et al. (1956) using in vitro rat SCG and following the postsynaptic responses of resting ganglia, showed that lactate and glutamine, but not glutamate or creatine phosphate, could replace glucose. An exhaustive substrate replacement study was carried out by ROCH-RAMEL (1962) on rat SCG trying to find a substrate or combination of substrates that would maintain the postsynaptic function. Mannose, lactate, pyruvate, and fructose were able to give 80% or greater of the survival time compared to ganglia incubated in the glucose-containing medium. A second category of substrates or combinations which produced shorter survival times were oxaloacetate, aspartate + α-ketoglutarate at the 70% range and, at the 50% range glutamine, GABA or alanine + α-ketoglutarate and then glutamate or serine + α-ketoglutarate.

Although the above studies have included a larger number of singular and combinations of substrates, they were by no means an exhaustive list of compounds. The critical question remains as to whether nonglucose substrates can really maintain ganglionic function during sustained maximal stimulation. For this latter purpose mannose, fructose, and lactate seemed to provide the best substitutes for glucose. Two observations from our laboratory would appear to be pertinent at this point. When the rat SCG was stimulated at 6 Hz, then pyruvate acted as a sufficient substrate for survival over a 2-h period. Yet, a different carbon distribution from pyruvate than from glucose occurred, suggesting that over prolonged time periods or at higher stimulation rates, physiologic lesion might well develop. The use of glucosamine as a sole carbon source, resulted in an immediate and irreversible loss of activity. One would suspect that this might be due to the irreversible phosphorylation of glucosamine.

The central theme in the glucose lack experiments, that must be kept in mind, is the loss of the structural integrity in the presynaptic area. The glucose must be metabolized to produce either the energy for the maintenance of these structures or it is providing a critical metabolite. A study was reported (PÁRDUCZ and FEHÉR, 1970) in which cat SCG were perfused with oxygenated Locke's solution until transynaptic action potential failure occurred. If, however, choline was added to such perfusion medium, failure did not occur. Remembering that HÄRKÖNEN et al. (1969) found both the ATP and phosphocreatine at 50% of their normal level at the time of failure, the above choline experiment might be merely a restudy of the NICOLESCU et al. (1966) experiment, indicating that the postganglionic receptors were still functional. The ATP value could be misleading in that it was primarily from the neuronal and satellite cells and not from the critical presynaptic region. This would lead one to surmise that the critical needs of the presynaptic areas for glucose lies in the production of ATP in maintenance of the ionic pumps. More precise critical studies need to be conducted in this area. These glucose lack studies are a prime example of how the SCG might be used to provide critical answers to general neuronal function.

D. Lipids

Ganglionic lipids exhibit marked alterations in their rates of uptake and patterns of incorporation of radioactive substrates following incubation in ionically modified media. These alterations can be explained, in part, by the multiplicity of cell types in the ganglia and differences in substrate pool size and cellular activity in response to stimulation or the addition of exogenous agents. Ionic influences, however, either directly at the enzyme–substrate level or mediated through effects on subcellular organelles should also be considered in the study of lipid metabolism. In ganglia, with a measurable and reproducible action potential, studies utilizing ^{32}P-inorganic phosphate, ^{14}C-glucose, pyruvate, glycerol or acetate or tritiated substrates have established that isotope incorporation generally increases in proportion to the length of the incubation period (LARRABEE et al., 1963; KLINGMAN, 1966; DEVINCENZO, 1968; BURT and LARRABEE, 1976; ORGANISCIAK and KLINGMAN, 1976; for review see McBRIDE and KLINGMAN, 1974). Depending upon the radioactive substrate utilized, however, and the relative turnover rates of the component parts of the lipid molecules, different lipid specific activities may be measured. For example, in double label experiments employing equal activities of ^{32}Pi and ^{14}C-glucose, KLINGMAN (1966) reported differential rates of incorporation of the two isotopes into phosphatidylcholine and ethanolamine following 2 to 4 h of incubation. BURT and LARRABEE (1976) measured different rates of phosphatidylinositol (PI) labeling with ^{3}H-inositol and ^{32}Pi in stimulated ganglia. They suggested that a fraction of the ganglionic PI turned over more rapidly than the remainder, supporting an earlier study in which they showed that upon stimulation, PI of mitochondrial and synaptosomal compartments was labeled preferentially with ^{32}Pi (BURT and LARRABEE,

Table 4. Rat superior cervical ganglionic lipids[a]

Lipid	nmol P/mg Dry w.
Phosphatidylethanolamine (PE)	30.1±4.7
Phosphatidic acid (PA)	7.2±1.7
Phosphatidylserine (PS)	9.4±1.0
Phosphatidylcholine (PC)	46.4±6.6
Phosphatidylinositol (PI)	8.4±1.0
Sphingomyelin	24.2±3.4
Cerebroside[b]	10.2
Sulfatide[b]	11.8
Cholesterol[c]	55.5±0.9
Cholesterol esters[c]	6.9±0.9

[a] Results are expressed as nanomoles P/mg tissue dry w. ±SD ($n=3$) for ganglia incubated 20 min in Krebs-Ringer buffer.
[b] Estimated as free sphingosine by the method of Siakotos.
[c] Determination by Liebermann–Burchard assay.

1973). The effects of ganglia excitation and its effect on PI metabolism have been reviewed (McBride and Klingman, 1974; Hawthorne and Pickard, 1979).

The ganglion phospholipid composition (Table 4) (Organisciak and Klingman, 1974a) is not unlike that of brain (Wells and Dittmer, 1967). Phosphatidylcholine and phosphatidylethanolamine constitute about 75% of the glycerophospholipids. Sphingomyelin is present in moderate amounts and cholesterol, about 10–15% of which is cholesterol esters, in substantial amounts. Under normal conditions the phospholipid pool does not change dramatically during incubations of ganglia, although stimulation for 4 h has been shown to result in an approximately 20% increase in phospholipid phosphorus (DeVincenzo, 1968). On a molar basis cerebrosides and sulfatides each represent about 5% of the total ganglionic lipids. Their combined incorporation of ^{14}C-pyruvate, however, represents no more than 3% of the sphingolipid class, which is otherwise extensively labeled (Table 5). The ganglioside concentration of SCG is only 0.3 nmol per ganglia; however, evidence has been obtained that ^{14}C-glucose, pyruvate, and glucosamine all label gangliosides to approximately the same extent (Harris and Klingman, 1972).

Since the overall size of the ganglionic lipid pool remains fairly constant during incubation but differential rates of lipid turnover exist, it can be seen that the choice of a radioactive substrate used in in vitro labeling studies can greatly affect the results (Table 5). Aside from the obvious labeling of glycerophospholipid phosphorus with ^{32}Pi (Larrabee et al., 1963; Larrabee and Leicht, 1965; Burt and Larrabee, 1973, 1976), ^{14}C-glucose is largely (70%) incorporated into the glycerol portion of the glycerophospholipids. On the other hand, ^{14}C-pyruvate incubation preferentially labels the fatty acids of the glycerophospholipids, while 94% of glucosamine carbons appear in the glycerol base. Glucose and pyruvate carbons are found in nearly identical proportions among the individual glycerophospholipids, with PC containing approximately 50% of the ^{14}C followed by PE > PI > PS > PA, while ^{14}C-glucosamine appears in most of the glycerophospholipids in nearly equal amounts.

Table 5. DPM/mg wet w

Substrate[a] 30 min Incubation	Phospholipid		Glycerophospholipid					Neutral lipids
	Glycerol Base	Fatty acid	PC	PE	PI	PS	PA	
Glucose	845	352	648	180	116	99	68	552
Pyruvate	718	2212	1529	570	435	227	166	—
Glucosamine	2578	167	576	471	455	515	304	951
^{32}Pi (2 h)	—	—	2600	200	—	—	500	—

[a] Substrate radioactivity 20 µCi each.

Sphingolipids are estimated to contain 10–20% of the total ganglia lipid radio-activity when ^{14}C-glucose is utilized, regardless of the duration of incubation or electric stimulation. With ^{14}C-pyruvate as the radioactive tracer, sphingomyelin labeling is much greater than the total incorporation of the entire glycero-phospholipid pool (Table 6). Only 4% of the ^{14}C-pyruvate carbons are localized in the sphingomyelin fatty acids with 90% in sphingosine itself (ORGANISCIAK and KLINGMAN, 1976). As expected from its relationship to the cholesterol precursor acetyl CoA, radioactive pyruvate labels the neutral lipid fraction of ganglionic lipids extensively while glucose and glucosamine labeling of the neutral lipids represents only about 25% of the total lipid radioactivity.

Table 6. Incorporation of ^{14}C-pyruvate into ganglionic lipids distintegrations/min/mg tissue dry w[a]

Lipid	Control				Acute lithium				Chronic lithium			
	Resting		Stimulated		Resting		Stimulated		Resting		Stimulated	
Phospholipids												
PE	236±	25	215±	24	416±	109	174±	27	287±	24	257±	24
PA	70±	2	114±	22	174±	48	132±	15	148±	16	186±	30
PS	92±	10	87±	17	146±	10	124±	30	87±	21	68±	20
PC	1,280±	130	1,265±	46	1,557±	390	1,545±	80	1,544±	38	846±	72
PI	212±	46	310±	27	249±	86	266±	32	279±	43	243±	30
Sphingolipids												
Sph	10,802±1,060		11,490±1,197		11,716±1,040		5,870±970		2,844±375		2,540±397	
Cer	284±	49	257±	57	377±	100	318±	80	221±	30	193±	72
Sulf	37±	4	20±	2	74±	27	47±	18	25±	6	34±	9
Neutral lipids												
Chol	1,531±	425	1.864±	590	1,247±	490	1,036±378		1,151±	50	919±266	
Chol E	117±	30	142±	69	212±	20	143±	17	318±	60	432±150	

[a] Values represent the mean ±SD of 3 or 4 determinations from individual ganglia incubated for 40 min. Abbreviations: PE, Phosphatidylethanolamine; PA, Phosphatidic Acid; PS, Phosphatidylserine; PC, Phosphatidylcholine, PI, Phosphatidylinositol; Sph, Sphingomyelin; Cer, Cerebrosides; Sulf, Sulfatides; Chol, Cholesterol; Chol E, Cholesterol Esters.

The fatty acid compositions of the individual ganglionic lipids have been measured (ORGANISCIAK and KLINGMAN, 1974a). In all lipids, the major saturated fatty acids of SCG include palmitic, stearic, and myristic acids while oleic and palmitoleic acids are the predominant unsaturated species. Together they account for about 90% of the ganglionic lipid fatty acids. In control media, marked compositional alterations of fatty acids have not been observed, but depending upon the radioactive substrate utilized and the incubation conditions, marked changes in fatty acid labeling have been determined (DeVINCENZO, 1968). The suggestion that separate pools of fatty acids may be utilized for the synthesis of ganglia glycerophospholipids and sphingolipids has also been advanced (ORGANISCIAK and KLINGMAN, 1976).

The effect of singularly lowering the incubation media cation concentration demonstrates they elicit differential rates on in vitro SCG lipid metabolism. When calcium is reduced in the bathing solution PC, PE, and PA ^{32}Pi incorporation declines 50% while PI labeling remains unchanged. Incorporation of ^{14}C-glucose carbons, on the other hand, increases in PI and remains unchanged in PC, PE, and PA (LARRABEE et al., 1963). In studies utilizing ^{45}Ca^{++}, ROBINSON and KABELA (1977) determined that calcium efflux occurred from separate compartments in the SCG. Assuming calcium efflux from SCG subcellular organelles also occurs at various rates, the differential rates of lipid metabolism may therefore be a result of different turnover rates in discrete cellular compartments.

In an extensive investigation of the effects of ions on phospholipid metabolism, KLINGMAN (1966) also measured a 50% reduction in ^{32}Pi incorporation with little change in ^{14}C-glucose labeling in PC from ganglia incubated in zero magnesium solution. In contrast to the effect of low calcium, however, PE labeling from both ^{32}Pi and ^{14}C-glucose increased in zero magnesium incubations. These studies suggest, therefore, that divalent cations may not only exhibit a compartmentalized effect on phospholipid metabolism, but that they may exert that effect at the substrate level on the metabolism of individual phospholipids. The effects of other divalent cations on the ganglionic electric activity have been determined (GUERRERO and RIKER, 1973), but their effects on lipid metabolism in ganglia have not yet been measured.

Removal of the monovalent cation potassium from the bathing solution reduces ^{32}Pi incorporation in PC, PE, and PA dramatically compared to control, while ^{14}C-glucose incorporation was little changed after 2 h of incubation (KLINGMAN, 1966). After 4 h of incubation in zero potassium solution, DeVINCENZO (1968) measured a 40% reduction in phospholipid label from ^{14}C-glucose. This decrease could be largely explained by a reduction in fatty acid label since radioactivity in the phospholipid glycerol bases was similar to controls. In these studies, the pattern of fatty acid labeling from ^{14}C-glucose also shifted upon incubation from 16 and 18 carbon fatty acids to those longer than 18 carbons, suggesting that a lack of potassium ion may lead to a decrease in de novo fatty acids synthesis. In contrast to the effects of lowered potassium ion, the addition of potassium (80 mM) to the incubation media of excised intact ganglia induced a rapid uptake of ^{32}Pi into all glycerophospholipids (NAGATA et al., 1973). Dramatic increases in oxygen consumption, glucose utilization and lactace production also accompanied the enhanced uptake of ^{32}Pi by ganglionic lipids. To a lesser extent, potassium ion stimulation of lipid metabolism, glucose utilization, and lactate production also occurred in previously axonimized ganglia, but oxygen consumption was not affected to the same extent as in intact tissues (NAGATA et al., 1973). It appears, therefore, that the concentration of K^+ ion directly stimulates the uptake of phosphate, yet decreases fatty acid metabolism in ganglionic glycerophospholipids.

When 50% of the bathing solution sodium is replaced with sucrose (to maintain osmolarity), a dramatic increase in ^{14}C-glucose labeling of the glycerophospholipid and neutral lipid pool occurs (KLINGMAN, 1966; DEVINCENZO, 1968). Among the glycerophospholipids, incorporation is increased 100% without a concomitant increase in the phospholipid phosphorus. The pattern of ^{14}C labeling from glucose also changes with respect to control, in that the ratio of fatty acid to glycerol base radioactivity approximates 1:1 instead of 70:30 (cf. Table 5). DEVINCENZO (1968) concludes that lowering the sodium concentration causes an increase in glucose utilization, presumably through a disinhibition of the enzymes hexokinase and pyruvate kinase (see RACKER and KRIMSKY, 1945; TAKAGAKI and TSUKADA, 1957).

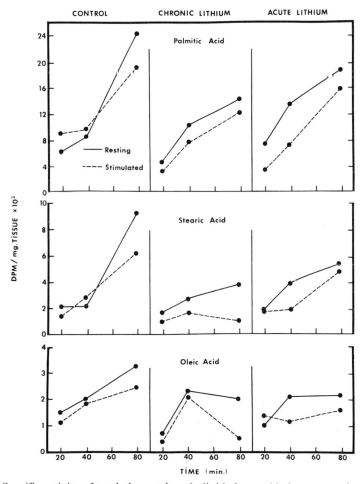

Fig. 1. Specific activity of total glycerophospholipids fatty acids from normal, acute and chronic lithium fed rat SCG incubated in vitro in Krebs–Ringers media, aerated with 95% O_2–5% CO_2, pH 7.4 and [U-^{14}C]-pyruvate (ORGANISCIAK and KLINGMAN, 1976)

When lithium ion is substituted for 50% sodium, instead of sucrose, the increase in phospholipid labeling from ^{14}C-glucose which occurs is not only greater than with sodium withdrawal alone, but the label is also distributed 70:30 between the fatty acid and glycerol base moieties of the glycerophospholipids (KLINGMAN, 1966; DEVINCENZO, 1968). In acute lithium ion exchange experiments, the same general effect from the fatty acid specific precursor ^{14}C-pyruvate was measured even though only 25% of the sodium was exchanged and the duration of the experiments was shorter (Table 6). In both the ^{14}C-glucose and pyruvate-containing incubations, lithium ion does not alter the ganglionic lipid fatty acid composition, although the distribution of radioactivity between fatty acids and glycerol base fragments among the phospholipids reportedly varies with glucose (DEVINCENZO, 1968). In contrast to acute lithium, incubation of ganglia from rats reared on a lithium-containing diet (ORGANISCIAK and KLINGMAN, 1974b), in 0.5 mM lithium (chronic lithium) for 80 min, depresses the uptake of ^{14}C-pyruvate in the major glycerophospholipid fatty acids (Fig. 1). Stimulation of ganglia further depresses the labeling of fatty acids in lithium media and particularly affects the processes of elongation (stearic acid) and desaturation (oleic acid) in chronic ganglia. It is unclear at this time, whether the lithium-induced inhibition of fatty acid metabolism is a site-specific phenomenon in endoplasmic reticulum and mitochondria or a result of the more general loss of ATP in lithium-treated ganglia (ORGANISCIAK and KLINGMAN, 1974b).

A dramatic reduction in sphingomyelin labeling from ^{14}C-pyruvate was also measurable in stimulated acute lithium-treated ganglia and in resting and stimulated chronic lithium ganglia (Table 6). Since the radioactivity from ^{14}C-pyruvate is largely contained in the sphingosine moiety of sphingomyelin, the loss of labeling in the presence of lithium may result from either a lithium-mediated effect on palmitate synthesis or serine metabolism. Acute lithium ion incubations are known to result in an increase in serine metabolism and its efflux from ganglia (McBRIDE and KLINGMAN, 1972) and in lower levels of high-energy phosphates (ORGANISCIAK and KLINGMAN, 1974b). It is possible, therefore, that the lithium effect on ganglion lipid metabolism may result from its effects on amino acid precursors of lipids as well as from a more generalized effect on energy metabolism in the ganglia.

E. Amino Acids

Aside from their role as supplementors of carbohydrate metabolism, the importance of amino acids in neuronal tissue is their involvement in the formation of transmitters and the extent to which amino acids are involved in the synthesis of general and unique proteins. Since the neurotransmitters are covered in other chapters, we shall restrict ourselves to other aspects of amino acids metabolism.

In freshly excised rat SCG, there exist a free amino acid pool composed mainly of glutamate, aspartate, glycine, serine, with lesser amounts of proline, ornithine, phenylalanine, and lysine followed by tracer amounts of leucine, isoleucine, and valine (McBRIDE and KLINGMAN, 1972; CANCALON and KLINGMAN, unpublished) (Table 7). After a 30 min incubation in glucose Krebs–Ringer, there was an increase in the amounts of free intraganglionic essential and other amino acids. This increase suggests the effects of either axotomy or of proteolysis due to the artificiality of the bathing medium. MCBRIDE and KLINGMAN (1972) tried to affect this increase by the addition of all amino acids, at the concentrations normally present in rat sera, to the bathing medium, but only achieved a significant increase in the intracellular concentrations of glutamate, aspartate, and lysine, whereas the others remained unaffected.

Table 7. Free intraganglionic amino acids in rat superior cervical ganglia[a]

Amino acid		nmole/mg wet w. of ganglia	
		0 h (CANCALON and KLINGMAN, unpublished)	0.5 h (MCBRIDE and KLINGMAN, 1972)
Alanine	(R)	1.69±0.004	1.9 ±0.1
	(S)		2.9 ±0.3δ
Serine	(R)	1.90±0.023	2.0 ±0.3
	(3)		1.2 ±0.3π
Glycine	(R)	2.30±0.018	3.1 ±0.3
	(S)		3.9 ±0.5
Aspartate (+asparagine)	(R)	2.06±0.046	2.3 ±0.2
	(S)		3.3 ±0.7
Glutamate (+glutamine)	(R)	4.09±0.044	4.2 ±0.4
	(S)		3.4 ±0.7
Proline	(R)	0.50±0.012	0.56±0.05
	(S)		0.60±0.09
Ornithine	(R)	0.28±0.048	0.20±0.08
	(S)		0.38±0.02
Threonine	(R)	0.52±0.011	0.81±0.07
	(S)		0.82±0.11
Valine	(R)	0.13±0.032	0.50±0.06
	(S)		0.41±0.07
Leucine	(R)	0.21±0.008	0.60±0.09
	(S)		0.44±0.06
Isoleucine	(R)	0.10±0.009	0.42±0.08
	(S)		0.43±0.23
Lysine	(R)	0.24±0.021	0.11±0.03
	(S)		0.29±0.10
Phenylalanine	(R)	0.08±0.004	0.23±0.02
	(S)		0.31±0.04π
Tyrosine	(R)	0.03±0.002	
Methionine	(R)	0.05±0.002	

[a] The data represents the mean ±SEM of four–six determinations for resting (R) and for stimulated (S) ganglia. Zero (0) h are freshly dissected desheathed ganglia which were then quick frozen. Those at 0.5 h are desheathed ganglia incubated in standard bathing media and in equilibrium with 95% O_2–5% CO_2 in the gas phase. The stimulated ganglia were stimulated for the entire period at a frequency of 5 Hz with rectangular pulses of 0.1–3 ms duration and 3–5 V. Significance of differences of levels in stimulated ganglia from those in resting ganglia are indicated as follows (Student's t-test): δ$P<0.002$; π $0.10>P>0.05$.

Several investigators (NAGATA et al., 1966; MASI et al., 1969; and MCBRIDE and KLINGMAN, 1972) were unable to detect GABA or its biosynthetic system in the rat SCG. Others (BERTILSSON et al., 1976; BOWERY et al., 1976) have recently reported the presence of GABA in ganglionic glial cells (Table 2).

When the initial glucose carbon balance studies on rat SCG were done (LARRABEE and KLINGMAN, 1962), analysis of the bathing media revealed the presence of amino acids. Subsequent quantitation of these amino acids (MCBRIDE and KLINGMAN, 1972; CANCALON and KLINGMAN, unpublished), under sterile conditions, showed that rested ganglia do leak amino acids into the media, such that by 1 h the mixture and concentration of amino acids are almost equivalent to the free intraganglia pool. Over a 4-h period the extraganglionic amino acid pool remains relatively constant both in total and individual concentrations.

F. Uptake and Efflux of Amino Acids

The uptake and efflux of amino acids from SCG has been studied mainly in vitro. Accumulation of L-glutamate is an energy dependent process, while that of L-aspartate appears not to be energy dependent (NAGATA et al., 1966). CANCALON and KLINGMAN (unpublished) agree with the L-aspartate uptake studies and they find that L-serine enters the ganglia more than either glutamate or aspartate.

Using [U-^{14}C]-L-glutamate, the initial 30 min uptake rate into resting ganglia was almost identical to that of stimulated ganglia (MCBRIDE and KLINGMAN, 1972). During the next 30-min period, stimulated ganglia acquired significantly more glutamate than rested ganglia. The presence of amino acids, equivalent in concentration to those in rat sera, increased the initial uptake rates and raised the resting ganglia concentrations by the end of 60 min, but not those of stimulated ganglia. It is interesting to note that when [U-^{14}C]-D-glucose was used, the rate of entry of glucose carbons into SCG free glutamate and aspartate took place at a rate greater than that from [U-^{14}C]-L-glutamate for both rested and stimulated ganglia. When [-^{14}C]-L-aspartate was studied (CANCALON and KLINGMAN, unpublished) and only the incorporation into the free intraganglionic amino acid pool was considered, rested ganglia had lower amounts of ^{14}C than did stimulated ganglia. There was no difference between the rested or stimulated ganglionic incorporation if the amount of ^{14}C in the intraganglionic and extraganglionic amino acid pools and the protein pools were considered. Considering only the incorporation into the intraganglionic free amino acids, the rested to stimulated ratio was 0.35, but when the total uptake was considered this ratio became 0.73. The nmol/g/h for ^{14}C-serine uptake was most interesting in that not only was more serine incorporated than aspartate or glutamate but stimulation produced a profound increase. The total ^{14}C incorporation for rested to stimulated ganglia was 0.36 and the free intraganglionic amino acids ratio was 0.27. Ganglia which had been stimulated for 30 min in normal bathing solution and then plunged into ^{14}C-serine bathing solution acquired almost five times the amount of serine as did ganglia similarily incubated but kept at rest.

Ganglia incubated in glucose Krebs–Ringer, as stated, slowly leaked amino acids into the bathing medium, the total concentration becoming similar to that of the free intraganglionic amino acid pool. Stimulation with time, over a 4-h period, does not increase this pool size but does change the composition of the pool. When examining only the 30-min period of incubation, the following intraganglionic amino acid labeling resulted: with [14]-C-glucose as the substrate glutamate, alanine and, glycine were labeled; with ^{14}C-aspartate as substrate glutamate, alanine, serine, and glycine received label; while with ^{14}C-glutamate as the substrate only aspartate, and alanine, while ^{14}C-serine gives glycine and lower but almost equivalent labeling of glutamate and aspartate.

Since unlabeled glucose is also present, to maintain ganglionic viability, during the metabolism of the added labeled amino acid, a dilution of the label by the unlabeled glucose carbons will occur. The amino acid labeling from ^{14}C-glucose represents the extent to which the transamination and the glutamate dehydrogenase reactions occur. The pattern of glucose carbon entry into rested ganglia amino acids is not surprising, nor is the fact that in stimulated ganglia the intraganglionic amino acids have lower specific activities. This latter effect may be due, in part, to their increased pool size. The observation that ^{14}C-glutamate labels only aspartate and alanine in the first 30 min, shows there is little flow of carbons to cytoplasmic oxalo-acetate and from the latter to serine. This lack of conversion is not because glutamate does not enter fast enough, since the internal glutamate and aspartate specific activities are, respectively, twofold higher or equivalent to those from ^{14}C-glucose. The flow of carbons from ^{14}C-aspartate measures both the cytosolic and mito-chondrial transaminases as well as the entry of aspartate carbons into the TCA cycle (glutamate). In this case, glycine and serine are labeled at about 66% of the aspartate specific activity while glutamate has about 50% of the aspartate activity. The only effects of stimulation on this distribution are a severe restriction of aspartate carbons entering glutamate and a slight but significant increase in glycine label. With ^{14}C-serine as the labeled substrate, a measure of not only the conversion to glycine but also the conversion to pyruvate and subsequent entry into the TCA or carboxylation to oxaloacetate can be made. As expected, among the various amino acids the highest specific activity is in glycine. However, the interesting observation is that in rested ganglia more serine carbons which enter glutamate (TCA cycle) are increased while fewer enter aspartate. Caution is indicated when interpreting single time point values as the rates through various metabolic pathways can not be ascertained. Comparison of the aspartate and serine data shows the following relationships: In rested ganglia, the glutamate specific activity from aspartate is only 50% or less of the aspartate specific activity which indicates a dilution by glucose carbons. This is borne out by stimulation which maintains the aspartate pool specific activity, but the glutamate pool is now only one-half the rested glutamate activity. Thus, more nonlabeled glucose carbons are flowing into the TCA cycle, diluting those derived from labeled aspartate. The labeled serine-glycine represents the amount of aspartate that is converted to pyruvate and then transaminated to serine which stays relatively constant and represents about 3% of the aspartate specific activity. The extent to which serine gives rise to pyruvate and which is then carboxylated and transaminated to aspartate, is seen in the ganglia rested in ^{14}C-serine medium. In this case, the aspartate specific activity is three times that of the glutamate. The carboxylation of the derived pyruvate from serine is decreased upon stimulation since the aspartate specific activity is now only 20% of the aspartate in rested ganglia. That this reduction is not merely due to dilution by glucose carbons

Table 8. The specific activity of some of the free intraganglionic amino acids found in rat superior ganglia from various labeled substrates

[U-^{14}C] Substrate added		dpm/nmol/mg wet w.				
		Alanine	Serine	Glycine	Glutamate (+gluta- mine)	Aspartate (+aspara- gine)
Glucose	(R)	250	22	3	849	435
(McBRIDE and KLINGMAN,	(S)	238	48	6	948	624
1972)						
Glutamate	(R)	19	—	—	1569	436
(McBRIDE and KLINGMAN,	(S)	10	—	—	1413	488
1972)						
Aspartate	(R)	317	111	139	1870	3670
(CANCALON and Klingman,	(S)	326	115	163	867	3860
unpublished)						
Serine	(R)	390	14,600	16,200	374	1380
(CANCALON and KLINGMAN,	(S)	173	16,400	14,300	1960	280
unpublished)						

Ganglia incubated in vitro in 1 ml of standard bathing media in equilibrium with 95% O$_2$–5% CO$_2$ at 37 °C for 30 min. The isotopic substrates were all [U-^{14}C] at: Glucose 307 mCi/mmol, 20 µCi; Glutamate, 195 mCi/mmol, 1 µCi; Aspartate, 156 mCi/mmol, 5 µCi; Serine, 125 mCi/mmol, 5 µCi, — = not detected.

is verified by the increased specific activity of the glutamate. By comparing other time periods one is led to speculate the possibility that in the SCG aspartate and serine may play a more important role in functional metabolism than we have previously assumed (Table 8).

G. RNA Protein

Most studies dealing with ganglionic RNA have been concerned with its measurements (GORELIKOV and EM, (1974); PEVZNER et al. (1973); or with the inductive effects of NGF on RNA and protein synthesis (KLINGMAN, 1966; LARRABEE, 1970; HENDRY, 1976; MIZEL and BAMBURG, 1976; OTTEN et al., 1978). The only substrate utilization studies on in vitro adult SCG using radioactive precursors are those of GISIGER and GAIGEN-HUGUENIN (1969), GISIGER (1971) and LEVEDEV (1977). According to these initial studies incorporation of ^{14}C-uridine into RNA was increased by both electric and acetylcholine stimulation. The addition of mecamine or tubocurarine blocked this incorporation. No attempts were made in these studies to discern the turnover of the RNA nor if the precursor pools were increased or decreased. An interesting complimentary study has been done on the nodose ganglion GUNNING et al. (1977a, b); KAYE et al. (1977).

More recently HUFF et al. (1978), have measured the RNA polymerases I and II of the rat neonate SCG when treated with NGF. They found that the Km for GTP for either polymerase was 10^{-5} M. Under the experimental conditions, the amount of poly(A)-containing RNA synthesized was about 4–5%. Treatment of the SCG with NGF caused an increase in the polymerases activities.

H. Protein

Assessments of ganglionic protein metabolism have been approached by either measuring the extent of amino acids incorporated into the general protein pool (MCBRIDE and KLINGMAN, 1972; BANKS, 1970), the effects stimulation may have on protein formation and catabolism (CANCALON and KLINGMAN, unpublished); or by assessing the particular effects of NGF (HENDRY, 1976) or more recently the effect of glucocorticoids (OTTEN and THOENEN, 1977; DIBNER and BLACK, 1978; COUGHLIN et al., 1978).

The use of labeled amino acids, regardless of whether they are essential or nonessential amino acids, have all shown an incorparation into ganglionic protein during rest. In chick embryonic ganglia (PARTLOW and LARRABEE, 1971), the incorporation of leucine into protein correspnds to the time course for incorporation of uridine into RNA for the first 10 days. At this time, both protein and RNA synthesis begin to decrease, but on day 12 when RNA synthesis only slowly increases, the formation of protein increases dramatically. THOENEN (OTTEN et al., 1978) and PATTERSON et al. (1975, 1978) have respectively shown the inductive synthesis of tyrosine hydroxylase and proteins due to NGF effects on SCG.

Taking into account that the water space does not increase in stimulated ganglia (NAGATA et al., 1966) and that the radioactivity in the amino acid pool of stimulated ganglia is greater than in rested ganglia, then protein synthesis in the stimulated ganglia is less than or equivalent to rested ganglia (MCBRIDE and KLINGMAN, 1972). Catabolism of SCG protein occurs, as indicated by the increase in both the amounts and types of amino acids found in the intra- and extraganglionic pools (MCBRIDE and KLINGMAN, 1972; CANCALON and KLINGMAN, unpublished). However, when stimulated ganglia are allowed to rest in ^{14}C-labeled amino acid containing bathing solution, there is a greater amino acid incorporation into the ganglionic protein after 5 or 30 min than in ganglia which are kept at rest or continuously stimulated. Thus, a period of rest following stimulation is a period of accelerated protein synthesis. What proteins are involved in this flux is inknown at this time. It is an interesting observation that RNA synthesis increases during stimulation (GISIGER, 1971). These data raise an interesting question: Is the neuron after stimulation then primed with mRNA to synthesize proteins, once the demand for ATP and the accompanying ionic fluxes have returned to normal, from the protein(s) which were catabolized during the biochemical processes associated with excitation?

References

Banks, P.: The effect of preganglionic stimulation on the incorporation of L-(U-^{14}C)-valine into the protein of the superior cervical ganglion of the guinea pig. Biochem. J. *118*, 813–818 (1970)

Bertilsson, L., Costa, E.: Mass fragmentographic quantitation of glutamic acid and gamma-aminobutyric acid in cerebellar nuclei and sympathetic ganglia of rats. J. Chromatog. *118*, 395–402 (1976)

Bowery, N.G., Brown, D.A., Collins, G.G., Galvin, M., Marsh, S., Yamini, G.: Indirect effects of amino acids on sympathetic ganglion cells mediated through the release of gamma-amino-butyric acid from glial cells. Br. J. Pharmacol. *57*, 73–91 (1976)

Burt, D.R., Larrabee, M.G.: Subcellular site of the phosphatidyl-inositol effect. Distribution on density gradients of labeled lipids from resting and active sympathetic ganglia of the rat. J. Neurochem. *21*, 255–272 (1973)

Burt, D.R., Larrabee, M.G.: Phosphatidylinositol and other lipids in a mammalian sympathetic ganglion: Effects of neuronal activity on incorporation of labeled inositol, phosphate, glycerol and acetate. J. Neurochem. *27*, 753–763 (1976)

Coughlin, M.D., Bibner, M.D., Boyer, D.M., and Black, I.B.: Factors regulating development of an embryonic mouse sympathetic ganglion. Dev. Biol. *88*, 513–528 (1978)

Cramer, H., Johnson, D.G., Hanbauer, I., Silberstein, S.D., Kopin, I.J.: Accumulation of adenosine, 3′,5′-monophosphate induced by catecholamines in the rat superior cervical ganglion in vitro. Brain Res. *53*, 97–104 (1973)

DeRibaupierre, F.: Localisation, synthese et utilisation du glycogene dans le ganglion sympatique cervical du rat. Brain Res. *11*, 42–64 (1968)

De Ribaupierre, F., Siegrist, G., Dolivo, M., Rouller, C.: Synthese et utilisation in vitro du glycogene dans le ganglion sympatique cervical du rat. Helv. Physiol. Pharmacol. Acta *24*, C 48–49 (1966)

DeVincenzo, G.D.: The effects of electrical stimulation and ionic alterations on phospholipid metabolism in rat superior cervical ganglion. Ph. D. Thesis, Department of Biochemistry, State University of New York at Buffalo, Buffalo, New York, 1968

Dibner, M.B., Black, I.B.: Biochemical and morphological effects of testosterone on developing sympathetic neurons. J. Neurochem. *30*, 1479–1484 (1978)

Dolivo, M.: Metabolism of mammalian sympathetic ganglia. Fed. Proc. *33*, 1042–1048 (1974)

Dolivo, M., DeRibaupierre, F.: Redox changes in sympathetic neurons after a single preganglionic shock. Experientia *29*, 5 (1973)

Dolivo, M., Larrabee, M.G.: Metabolism of glucose and oxygen in a mammalian sympathetic ganglion at reduced temperature and varied pH. J. Neurochem. *3*, 72–88 (1958)

Dolivo, M., Roullier, C.: Changes in ultrastructure and synaptic transmission in the sympathetic ganglion during various metabolic conditions. Brain Res. *31*, 111–123 (1969)

Dunant, Y.: Organisation topographique et functionelle du ganglion cervical superior chez le rat. J. Physiol. (Paris) *59*, 17–38 (1967)

Dunant, Y., Dolivo, M.: Relations entre les potentiels synaptiques lents et l'excitabilité du ganglion sympatique chez le rat. J. Physiol. (Paris) *59*, 281–284 (1967)

Galvin, M.G., Ten Bruggencote, Senekowitsch, R.: The effect of neuronal stimulation and GABA upon extracellular K^+ and Ca^{+2} levels in rat isolated superior cervical ganglia. Brain Res. *160*, 544–548 (1979)

Gisiger, V.: Triggering of RNA synthesis by acetylcholine stimulation of the postsynaptic membrane in a mammalian sympathetic ganglion. Brain Res. *33*, 139–146 (1971)

Gisiger, V., Gaide-Hugunin, A.C.: Effect of preganglionic stimulation upon RNA synthesis in the isolated sympathetic ganglion of the rat. In: Mechanisms of synaptic transmission, progress in brain research. Akert, K., Waser, P.G. (eds.), Vol. 31, pp. 125–129. Amsterdam: Elsevier 1969

Gorelikov, P.L., Em, V.S.: Dynamics of ribonucleic metabolism in the cat sympathetic ganglia during hypoxia and subsequent normalization studied by the method of optico-structural machine analysis. Arkhanat Anat Gistol Embriol. *66*, 91–97 (1974)

Guerrero, S., Riker, W.K.: Effects of some divalent cations on sympathetic ganglion function. J. Pharmacol. Exp. Ther. *186*, 152–159 (1973)

Gunning, P.W., Kaye, P.L., Austin, L.: In vivo RNA synthesis with the rat nodose ganglia. J. Neurochem. *28*, 1237–1240 (1977a)

Gunning, P.W., Kaye, P.L., Austin, L.: In vivo synthesis of rapidly-labeled RNA with the rat nodose ganglia following vagotomy. J. Neurochem. *28*, 1245–1248 (1977b)

Härkönen, M.H.A., Kauffman, F.C.: Metabolic alterations in the axotimized superior cervical ganglion of the rat: I Energy metabolism. Brain Res. 65, 127–139 (1974a)

Härkönen, M.H.A., Kauffman, F.C.: Metabolic alterations in the axotimized superior cervical ganglion of the rat: II Pentose phosphate pathway. Brain Res. 65, 141–157 (1974b)

Härkönen, M.H.A., Passonneau, J.V., Lowry, O.H.: Relationships between energy reserves and function in rat superior cervical ganglion. J. Neurochem. 16, 1439–1458 (1969)

Harris, J.U., Klingman, J.D.: Detection, determination and metabolism in vitro of gangliosides in mammalian sympathetic ganglia. J. Neurochem. 19, 1267–1278 (1972)

Hawthorne, J.N., Pickard, M.R.: Phospholipids in synaptic function. J. Neurochem. 32, 5–14 (1979)

Hendry, I.A.: Control mechanisms in the development of the vertebrate sympathetic nervous system. In: Reviews of neurosciences. Ehrenpreis, Kopin (eds.), Vol. 2, pp. 149–194. New York: Raven Press 1976

Hill, C.E., Hendry, I.A.: Development of neurons synthetizing noradrenaline and acetylcholine in the superior cervical ganglion of the rat in vivo and in vitro. Neurosciences 2, 741–750 (1977)

Horowicz, P., Larrabee, M.G.: Glucose consumption and lactate production in a mammalian sympathetic ganglion at rest and in activity. J. Neurochem. 2, 102–118 (1958)

Horowicz, P., Larrabee, M.G.: Metabolic partitioning of carbon from glucose by a mammalian ganglion. J. Neurochem. 9, 407–420 (1962a)

Horowicz, P., Larrabee, M.G.: Oxidation of glucose in a mammalian sympathetic ganglion at rest and in activity. J. Neurochem. 9, 1–22 (1962b)

Huf, K., Lakshmanan, J., Guroff, G.: RNA polymerase activity in the superior cervical ganglion of the neonatal rat: the effect of nerve growth factor. J. Neurochem. 31, 599–606 (1978)

Kaye, P.L., Gunning, P.W., Austin, L.: In vivo synthesis of stable RNA within the rat nodose ganglia following vagotomy. J. Neurochem. 28, 1241–1244 (1977)

Kahlson, G., MacIntosh, F.C.: Acetylcholine synthesis in a sympathetic ganglion. J. Physiol. 96, 277–292 (1939)

Klingman, G.I · Catecholamine levels and dopa decarboxylase activity in peripheral organs and adrenergic tissues in the rat after immunosympathectomy. J. Pharmacol. Exp. Ther. 148, 14–21 (1965a)

Klingman, G.I.: Monoamine oxidase and catechol-0-methyltransferase activities in peripheral organs and adrenergic tissues in immunosympathectomized rats. Pharmacologist 7, 157 (1965b)

Klingman, G.I.: Monoamine oxidase activity of peripheral organs and sympathetic ganglia of the rat after immunosympathectomy. Biochem. Pharmacol. 15, 1729–1736 (1966)

Klingman, G.I., Klingman, J.D.: The effect of immunosympathectomy on the superior cervical ganglion and other adrenergic tissues of the rat. Life Sci. 4, 2171–2179 (1965)

Klingman, G.I., Klingman, J.D.: Catecholamines in peripheral tissues of mice and cell counts of sympathetic ganglia after the prenatal and postnatal administration of the nerve growth factor antiserum. Int. J. Neuropharmacol. 6, 501–508 (1967)

Klingman, G.I., Klingman, J.D.: Cholinesterases of rat sympathetic ganglia after immunosympathectomy, decentralization and axotomy. J. Neurochem. 16, 261–268 (1969)

Klingman, G.I., Klingman, J.D.: Immunosympathectomy as an ontogenetic tool. In: Immunosympathectomy. Steiner, Schönbaum (eds.), pp. 91–95. London: Elsevier 1972

Klingman, J.D.: Ionic influences on rat superior cervical ganglion phospholipid metabolism. Life Sci. 5, 1397–1407 (1966)

Larrabee, M.G.: Oxygen consumption of excised sympathetic ganglion at rest and in activity. J. Neurochem. 2, 81–101 (1958)

Larrabee, M.G.: Conduction, transmission and metabolism in sympathetic ganglia excised from rat. In: Methods in medical research. Quastel, J.H. (ed.), Vol. 9, pp. 241–247. Chicago: Yearbook 1961

Larrabee, M.: The influence of neural activity on neural metabolism of glucose and phospholipid. In: Sleep and altered states of consciousness. Vol. 45, pp. 64–85. Baltimore: Williams & Wilkins 1967

Larrabee, M.G.: Metabolism of adult and embryonic sympathetic ganglia. Fed. Proc. 29, 1919–1928 (1970)

Larrabee, M.G.: A new mathematical approach to the metabolism of (^{14}C)-glucose with application to sensory ganglia of chick embryos. J. Neurochem. *31*, 461–492 (1978)

Larrabee, M.G., Bronk, D.W.: Metabolic requirements of sympathetic neurons. Cold Spring Harbor Symp. Quant. Biol. *17*, 245–266 (1952)

Larrabee, M.G., Horowicz, P.: Glucose and oxygen utilization in sympathetic ganglia. In: Molecular structure and functional activity of nerve cells. Grenell, R.G., Mullins, L.J. (eds.), pp. 84–102. Baltimore: Waverly 1956

Larrabee, M.G., Klingman, J.D.: Metabolism of glucose and oxygen in mammalian sympathetic ganglia at rest and in action. In: Neurochemistry. 2nd ed. Elliott, K.A.C., Page, I.H., Quastel, J.H. (eds.), pp. 150–176. Springfield, Ill.: Thomas 1962

Larrabee, M.G., Leicht, W.S.: Metabolism of phosphatidyl inositol and other lipids in active neurons of sympathetic ganglia and other peripheral nervous tissues. J. Neurochem. *12*, 1–13 (1965)

Larrabee, M.G., Horowicz, P., Stekiel, W., Dolivo, M.: Metabolism in relation to function in mammalian sympathetic ganglia. In: Metabolism of the nervous system. Richter, D. (ed.), pp. 208–220. Oxford: Pergamon 1856

Larrabee, M.G., Klingman, J.D., Leicht, W.S.: Effects of temperature, calcium and activity on phospholipid metabolism in sympathetic ganglion. J. Neurochem. *10*, 549–570 (1963)

Levedev, D.B.: Autoradiographic analysis of RNA synthesis by sympathetic neurocytes from a population depleted of nerve cells. Eksp. Biol. Med. *83*, 748–758 (1977)

Liuzzi, A., Poppen, P.H., Kopin, I.J.: Stimulation and maintenance by nerve growth factor of phenylethanolamine-N-methyltransferase in the superior cervical ganglia of adult rats. Brain Res. *138*, 309–315 (1977)

Lutold, B.E., Karoum, F., Neff, N.H.: Activation of rat sympathetic ganglia SIF cell dopamine metabolism by muscarinic agonists. Eur. J. Pharmacol. *54*, 21–26 (1979)

Mizel, S.B., Bamburg, J.R.: Studies on the action of nerve growth factor. III. Role of RNA and protein synthesis in the process of neurite outgrowth. Dev. Biol. *49*, 20–28 (1976)

Marchisio, P.C.: Embryological development of metabolic systems in sympathetic ganglia. Fed. Proc. *33*, 1039–1942 (1974)

Masi, I., Paggi, P., Pocchiari, F., Toschi, G.: Metabolism of labeled glucose in sympathetic ganglia in vitro, at rest and during sustained activity. Brain Res. *12*, 467–470 (1969)

McBride, W.J., Klingman, J.D.: The effects of electrical stimulation and ionic alterations on the metabolism of amino acids and proteins in excised superior cervical ganglia of the rat. J. Neurochem. *19*, 865–880 (1972)

McBride, W.J., Klingman, J.D.: Effects of excitation on the metabolism of a simple neuronal system: the mammalian sympathetic ganglion. In: Progress in neurobiology. Kerkut, Phillis (eds.), Vol. 3, pp. 251–278. New York: Pergamon Press 1975

Nagata, Y., Yokoi, Y., Tsukada, Y.: Studies on free amino acid metabolism in excised cervical sympathetic ganglia from the rat. J. Neurochem. *13*, 1421–1431 (1966)

Nagata, Y., Mikoshiba, K., Tsukada, Y.: Effect of potassium ions on glucose and phospholipoid metabolism in the rat's cervical sympathetic ganglia with and without axotomy. Brain Res. *56*, 259–269 (1973)

Nicolescu, P., Dolivo, M., Rouiller, C., Foroglou-Kerameus, C.: The effect of deprivation of glucose on the ultrastructure and function of the superior cervical ganglion of the rat in vitro. J. Cell. Biol. *29*, 267–285 (1966)

Organisciak, D.T., Klingman, J.D.: Lipid composition of rat superior cervical ganglion. Lipids *9*, 307–313 (1974a)

Organisciak, D.T., Klingman, J.D.: The effects of lithium on high energy phosphate and glucose levels in the rat superior cervical ganglion. J. Neurochem. *22*, 341–345 (1974b)

Organisciak, D.T., Klingman, J.D.: Lithium induced alterations in rat ganglionic lipids. Brain Res. *115*, 467–478 (1976)

Otten, U., Thoenen, H.: Effects of glucocorticoids on nerve growth factor-mediated enzyme induction in organ cultures of rat sympathetic ganglia: enhanced response and reduced time requirement to initiate enzyme induction. J. Neurochem. *29*, 69–76 (1977)

Otten, U., Katanaka, H., Thoenen, H.: Role of cyclic nucleotides in NGF-mediated induction of tyrosine hydroxylase in rat sympathetic ganglia and adrenal medulla. Brain Res. *140*, 385–389 (1978)

Parducz, A., Feher, O.: Fine structural alterations of presynaptic endings in the superior cervical ganglion of the cat after exhausting preganglionic stimulation. Experientia 26, 629–630 (1970)

Partlow, L.M., Larrabee, M.G.: Effects of a nerve growth factor, embryo age and metabolic inhibitors on growth of fibers and on ribonucleic acid and protein in embryonic sympathetic ganglia. J. Neurochem. 18, 2101–2118 (1971)

Patterson, P.H., Reichardt, L.F., Chun, L.L.: Biochemical studies on the development of primary sympathetic neurons in cell culture. Cold Spring Harbor Symp. Quant. Biol. 40, 389–397 (1975)

Patterson, P.H., Potter, D.D., Purshpan, E.J.: The chemical differentiation of nerve cells. Sci. Am. 239, 50–59 (1978)

Pevzner, L.Z., Nozdrachev, A.D., Glushchenko, T.S., Federova, L.D.: RNA content in the neuron-neurologia system of the sympathetic ganglion and characteristics of synaptic transmission. Dokl. Acad. Nauk. SSSR 213, 1458–1460 (1973)

Quadflieg, K.H., Brand, K.: Time-dependent partitioning of glucose carbons metabolized by the superior cervical ganglion from calves. J. Neurochem. 31, 211–216 (1978)

Racker, E., Krimsky, I.J.: Effect of nicotinic acid amide and sodium on glycolysis and oxygen uptake in brain homogenates. J. Biol. Chem. 161, 453–461 (1945)

Robinson, J.D., Kabela, E.: Distribution of ^{45}Ca in the superior cervical ganglion of the cat. J. Neurobiology 8, 511–522 (1977)

Roch-Ramel, F.: Metabolisme et "survival functionelle" du ganglion sympathique cervical isole du rat. Helv. Physiol. Acta. Suppl. 13, 1–64 (1962)

Roch-Ramel, F., Dolivo, M.: Activite de quelques enzymes et survie functionelle du ganglion sympathique isole du rat. Helv. Physiol. Pharmacol. Acta 25, 40–61 (1967)

Takagaki, G., Tsukada, Y.: Effect of some inorganic ions on brain slices metabolizing glucose or pyruvate. J. Neurochem. 2, 21–29 (1957)

Towle, A.C., Sze, P.Y., Lauder, J.M.: Cytosol glucocorticoid receptors in monoaminergic cell groups. Trans. Am. Soc. Neurochem. 10, 199 (1979)

Wallace, L.J., Partlow, L.M., Ferrendelli, J.A.: Comparisons of levels of adenosine 3',5'-monophosphate in highly purified and mixed primary cultures of neurons and non-neuronal cells from embryonic chick sympathetic ganglia. J. Neurochem. 31, 801–808 (1978)

Webb, J.G., Saelens, D.A., Halushka, P.V.: Biosynthesis of prostaglandin E by rat superior cervical ganglia. J. Neurochem. 31, 13–20 (1978)

Wells, M.A., Dittmer, J.C.: A comprehensive study of the postnatal changes in the concentration of the lipids of developing rat brain. Biochemistry 6, 3169–3174 (1967)

Yu, M.W., Lakshmann, J., Guroff, G.: Chemical control of neuronal growth – The nerve growth factor. Essays Neurochem. Neuro Pharmacol. 3, 33–48 (1978)

CHAPTER 3

Methods for the Examination of Ganglion-Blocking Activity

L. GYERMEK

A. Introduction

Ganglion-blocking agents are widely used by physiologists and pharmacologists as useful tools in the exploration of the basic mechanism of ganglionic transmission, which is a crucial field of the neurosciences. Methods utilizing ganglionic preparations therefore have been and still are of importance for two reasons: For the promotion of possible new drug development, and for assistance in basic research in the neurophysiology of synapses.

B. General Physiological and Pharmacological Aspects of the Evaluation of Ganglion-Blocking Agents

Functional characterization of autonomic ganglia can be achieved by many physiological and pharmcological methods. These include the study of: a) liberation of the specific neurotransmitter substance(s); b) formation and liberation of the other biologically active substances that may indirectly influence (e.g., modulate) ganglionic transmission; c) the electrophysiologic attributes of ganglionic transmission under normal, pathological or pharmacologically altered conditions; and, d) the pharmacological action of the transmitter substance per se on different autonomic ganglia, including the study of agents that are capable of mimicking, potentiating, or antagonising the action of the transmitter. In considering the many possibilities for use of the different, pharmacologically active classes of agents, one should realise that the application of blocking substances of autonomic ganglia as pharmacological tools, irrespective of their potential therapeutic use, presents a broad field of exploration.

The necessity for a wide array of pharmacological methods in the study of ganglionic transmission stems from the fact that it is now realised that the chemical transmission phenomena in these synapses are rather complex (ECCLES, 1964; TRENDELENBURG, 1967). Accordingly, in recent years, the scope of studies on ganglionic transmission has been expanded to include investigation of the following important aspects.

1) Electrophysiologic correlates of ganglionic transmission (ECCLES and LIBET, 1961; KOELLE, 1961; PAPPANO and VOLLE, 1962; TAKESHIGE and VOLLE, 1963; TRENDELENBURG, 1967; KOKETSU, 1969; COLLIER and KATZ, 1970; NISHI, 1970; LIBET, 1970; ALKADHI and McISAAC, 1973; HAEFELY, 1974b).

2) Blockade of ganglionic transmission by ganglionic stimulants of the nicotinic type (GINSBORG and GUERRERO, 1964; HANCOCK and VOLLE, 1969a and b; VOLLE and HANCOCK, 1970; HAEFELY, 1974a; see also Fig. 1).

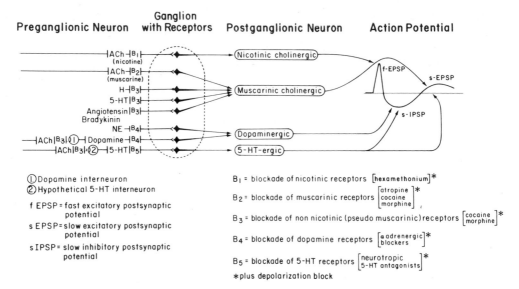

Fig. 1. Schematic diagram of pharmacological types of ganglionic stimulation and blockade

3) Agents modulating ganglionic transmission: a) The role of catecholamines in ganglionic transmission (MATTHEWS, 1956, cf. REINERT, 1963; MUSCHOLL and VOGT, 1958, cf. REINERT, 1963; ECCLES and LIBET, 1961; see also Fig. 1); b) The role of 5-HT, histamine and vasoactive peptides (angiotensin and bradykinin) in ganglionic transmission (TRENDELENBURG, 1967; GYERMEK, 1966; GYERMEK, 1967); c) The influence of potassium on ganglionic transmission (FELDBERG and VARTIAINEN, 1934; MINKER and KOLTAI, 1961 a; see also Fig. 1); d) The role of calcium ion in ganglionic transmission (SHAFER, 1939; KOMALAHIRANYA and VOLLE, 1962; JOHNSON, 1963; BLACKMAN and PURVES, 1968).

4) The role of various modalities of ganglionic stimulation in the assessment of ganglionic blockade: a) The critical frequency of electrical stimulation (SCHNEIDER and MOORE, 1955; RIKER and KOMALAHIRANYA, 1962; KHARKEVICH, 1962, 1967; ALKADHI and McISAAC, 1974): b) Comparison of the blockade of electrically stimulated ganglia and that of ganglia subjected to chemical stimuli (KEWITZ, 1954; KEWITZ and REINERT, 1954; DOUGLAS et al., 1960; MINKER and KOLTAI, 1961 b; VOLLE, 1962 a, b, c; FLACKE and GILLIS, 1968; HOLMAN et al., 1971, HAEFELY, 174 a, b); c) The role of different ganglionic receptors responding to various ganglionic stimulants (KHARKEVICH, 1962, 1967; TRENDELENBURG, 1967; HAEFELY, 1972; see also Tables 1 and 2, and Fig. 1).

5) The mechanism of ganglionic block (PATON and PERRY, 1953; GEBBER and VOLLE, 1966; HAEFELY, 1972). Various types of ganglionic blockade, e.g., depolarization block elicited by acetylcholine and TMA and blocked by atropine; hyperpolarisation block, (a) produced by acetylcholine and methacholine and blocked by atropine and (b) produced by large doses of acetylcholine and not blocked by atropine; post-depolarization block produced by large doses of TMA and not blocked by atropine (TAKESHIGE and VOLLE, 1964; JARAMILLO and VOLLE, 1967).

Table 1. Schematic representation of the effects of various drugs on the stimulation of the superior cervical ganglion of the cat by various ganglion-stimulating agents

	Nico-tine DMPP TMA	Musca-rinic agents	Hist-amine	5-HT	Angio-tensin	Brady-kinin	Potassium chloride
Non-depolarizing ganglion-blocking agents	−	0	0	0	0	0	0
Nicotine:							
depolarizing phase	−		−	−	−	−	−
non-polarizing phase	−	+	+	+	+	−[a]	0
Cocaine	0	−	−	−	−	−	0
Morphine, methadone	0	−	−	−	−	−	0
Atropine	0	−	0	0	0	0	0
Antihistaminic agents	0	0	−	0	−[a]	0	0
5-Hydroxy-3-indolacetamidine	0		−				
Facilitation after preganglionic stimulation	0	+	+	+	+	+	0

Adapted from TRENDELENBURG, 1967.
− : Inhibition of the effects of the ganglion-stimulating agent; +: potentiation of the effects of the ganglion-stimulating agent; 0: no change in the effects of the ganglion-stimulating agent.
[a] Partial inhibition.

6) Characterisation of the ganglionic sites involved in different types of ganglionic blockade by a) altering the blocking agents per se (GYERMEK and BINDLER, 1962); b) changing the timing of administration, (TRENDELENBURG, 1957b); and c) modifying the dosage (PELIKAN, 1960; PAPPANO and VOLLE, 1962; PATON and THOMPSON, 1964).

7) Selectivity of ganglionic block (RIKER and SZRENIAWSZKI, 1959; PATON and ZAIMIS, 1951; HERTTING et al., 1962; ELLIOTT and QUILLIAM, 1964; KELKAR et al., 1964; GYERMEK, 1967; BOWMAN and WEBB, 1972).

8) Tolerance to ganglion-blocking agents (MOHANTY, 1955; ZAIMIS, 1956; VOLLE, 1962b).

9) Reversal of ganglionic block (KOPPANYI et al., 1936; CHOU and DE ELIO, 1947; KAMIJO and KOELLE, 1952; GRIMSON et al., 1955; MINKER and KOLTAI, 1961a).

C. Pharmacological Methods

I. In vivo and in situ Preparations

1. Preparation of Superior Cervical Ganglia of Cat

These preparations originated from the early studies of LANGLEY and DICKINSON (1889; cf. KHARKEVICH, 1967), who established that local application of nicotine to the ganglionic surface on cat blocked transmission across the ganglion. Through a large number of successive studies, this preparation underwent several modifications, and has so far proved to be the most useful and widely used preparation for the study

Table 2. The type and mode of action of different ganglionic stimulant agents on various automatic ganglia

Agents	Type	Method	Notes	References
ACh, choline nicotine arecoline, hordenine methoidie	N receptors	Perfused cat superior cervical ganglion	All block transmission in larger doses	FELDBERG and VARTIAINEN, 1934
ACh, methacholine	M and N^a	Superior cervical ganglion	Besides stimulation, blockade by various mechanisms	TAKESHIGE et al., 1963
ACh	Presynaptic	Superior cervical ganglion	May enhance ganglionic transmission by liberating more ACh at the presynaptic terminals– produces antidromic firing	KOELLE, 1961
ACh	M and N	Superior cervical ganglion	Biphasic action, first hexamethonium-sensitive phase, followed by second, atropine-sensitive phase	TAKESHIGE and VOLLE, 1963
ACh, carbaminoylcholine, and TMA	M and N	Superior cervical ganglion	Postganglionic responses are enhanced by repetitive electrical stimulation	VOLLE, 1962c
Arecoline	M	Superior cervical ganglion	Stimulant action is atropine-sensitive	KRSTIĆ, 1971
ACh, carbaminoylcholine, nicotine TMA	M and N	Sympathetic ganglia of frog	All depress ganglionic transmission by depolarising block	GINSBORG and GUERRERO, 1964
ACh, carbaminoylcholine, muscarone, pilocarpine, arecoline, and furthretonium	M and N	Pelvic ganglia of dog	Atropine is only partially effective or ineffective to block stimulant response	GYERMEK, 1961
Muscarine	M	Perfused superior cervical ganglion	Stimulant effect blocked with atropine	KONZETT and ROTHLIN, 1949
Muscarinic agents	M	Superior cervical ganglion	Ganglionic stimulant action is enhanced by denervation	AMBACHE, 1955
Muscarine, ACh, carbaminoylcholine, muscarone, nicotine, DMPP	M	Inferior mensenteric ganglion of cat	Muscarine is ineffective on atropinised preparation. Others are effective, blocked by hexamethonium	HERR and GYERMEK, 1960

Compound	Receptor	Preparation	Effect	Reference
Muscarine	M	Perfused superior cervical ganglion	Muscarine potentiates the action of ACh	KONZETT and WASER, 1956
Muscarine and isomers	M	Inferior mensenteric and superior cervical ganglia	Postganglionic discharges blocked by atropine. Isomers of muscarine are inactive	GYERMEK et al., 1963
Muscarine	M	Superior cervical ganglion	Muscarinic ganglionic stimulation and potentiation of preganglionic electrical stimulation	SANGHVI et al., 1963
Muscarine and muscarinic stimulants	M	Superior cervical ganglion	Facilitate submaximal preganglionic electrical stimulation. Depolarising block by nicotine and TMA is inhibitory	JONES, 1963
Muscarinic ganglionic stimulants (McN-A-343 and AHR-602)	M receptors		Not blocked by non-depolarising block. Cocaine, morphine and depolarising block inhibit	JONES et al. 1963
Muscarinic stimulants	M	Superior cervical ganglion	Tetanic conditioning, anticholinesterases and moderate degree of depolarisation intensify action. Postsynaptic LN wave is associated to M-type transmission	HAEFELY, 1974c
McN-A-343	M	Superior cervical ganglion pressor response	Ganglionic stimulation resistant to hexamethonium blocked by atropine	ROSZKOWSKI, 1961
McN-A-343	M	Superior cervical ganglion, inferior mesenteric ganglion, cat	Similar to pilocarpine mexamethonium ineffective. Atropine blocks.	MURAYAMA and UNNA, 1963
Muscarone and derivatives	N	Superior cervical ganglion and pelvic ganglia of dog	Nicotinic type of stimulation	GYERMEK and UNNA, 1960
Nicotine, DMPP and TMA	N receptors	Guinea-pig ileum	Actions other than ganglionic	DAY and VANE, 1963
Nicotine and DMPP	N receptors	Heart ganglia of dog	Different susceptibility to ganglionic block	CHIBA et al., 1972

Table 2 (contnued)

Agents	Type	Method	Notes	References
DMPP	N	Isolated guinea-pig ileum	Blocking depolarising action follows stimulation	Ling, 1959
DMPP	N	Cardiac functions	Non-ganglionic actions	Maxwell et al., 1963
DMPP, pilocarpine neostigmine and McN-A-343	M and N	Blood pressure	Two pharmacologically different ganglionic stimulant types: 1) hexamethonium-sensitive (DMPP), 2) atropine-sensitive (others listed)	Levy and Ahlquist, 1962
Nicotinic stimulants	M receptor	Hypogastric ganglion of guinea-pig	Action on M receptors is suggested for the development of tachyphylaxis	Bentley, 1972
m-Hydroxyphenyl-propyl-trimethyl-ammonium and 3–4 dihydroxy-phenyl-ethyl-trimethyl ammonium	N receptors	Isolated guinea-pig ileum	More selective ganglionic stimulants than nicotine and DMPP, but affect the myoneural junctions	Barlow et al., 1974
Nicotine, histamine, 5-HT	N and non-chilinergic	Guinea-pig ileum	Each has stimulant action at different intramural ganglionic sites	Harry, 1963
Neostigmine	M	Superior cervical ganglion	Its ganglionic activating effect is enhanced by d-tubocurarine and blocked by atropine	Takeshige and Volle, 1963
Neostigmine	?	Superior cervical ganglion	Neostigmine enhances the depolarising type of block produced by ACh but suspends the block produced by acetylthiocholine	Wurzel et al., 1964
DFP	?	Superior cervical ganglion	Postganglionic discharges are blocked by CaCl$_2$	Komalahiranya and Volle, 1962
Veratrine	?	Superior cervical ganglion	Stimulates only DFP-treated ganglion	Komalahiranya and Volle, 1962
EDTA	?	Superior cervical ganglion	Atropine and hexamethonium-resistant stimulation	Komalahiranya and Volle, 1962

Stimulant	Receptor type	Preparation	Comments	Reference
KCl	?	Superior cervical ganglion	Stimulant action is blocked by $CaCl_2$	KOMALAHIRANYA and VOLLE, 1962
Anticholinesterases	N and M	Rat sympathetic ganglion		DREW and LEACH, 1972
5-HT	5-HT	Guinea-pig ileum	Ganglionic, nerve plexus M receptors are sensitive to morphine and atropine. Muscular (D receptors) are sensitive to LSD and dibenzyline	GADDUM and PICARELLI, 1957
5-HT	5-HT	Inferior mesenteric ganglion of cat; pelvic ganglion of dog	Non-depolarizing blocking agents ineffective; morphine cocaine and particularly neurotropic 5-HT antagonists are effective	GYERMEK and BINDLER, 1962; GYERMEK, 1962; GYERMEK, 1966
5-HT	5-HT	Superior cervical ganglion	Different electrophysiological features than with N and M stimulants (desensitisation and tachyphylaxis)	HAEFELY, 1974c
5-HT, H, KCl, pilocarpine	Non-nicotinic receptors	Superior cervical ganglion	Depolarising nicotine block is effective against these stimulants	TRENDELENBURG, 1957a
Angiotensin	Non-cholinergic	Caudal cervical ganglion	Effects on heart are resistant to atropine and hexamethonium	FARR and GRUPP, 1971
Adrenergic neurone-blocking agents	M receptors	Superior cervical ganglion	Inhibition of the block by NA	FARMER et al., 1966
Various agents	Direct and latent	Miscellaneous	Different classes are reviewed	KONZETT and ROTHLIN, 1953
Various agents	Variable	Miscellaneous	Different classes are reviewed	HAEFELY, 1972
Various agents	N	Miscellaneous	Different chemical classes are reviewed	KHARKHEVICH, 1967
Various agents	N, M and non-cholinergic	Miscellaneous	Different chemical classes are reviewed	GYERMEK, 1966
Various non-nicotinic stimulants, muscarinic agents H, 5-HT, angiotensin	M and possibly other types	Miscellaneous	Potentiate the effect of preganglionic stimulation. Stimulant effects are blocked by depolarising nicotine block, cocaine, and morphine	TRENDELENBURG, 1967

[a] N: Nicotinic; M: Muscarinic.

of autonomic ganglionic transmission and of ganglion-stimulating and -blocking agents. An early version of the preparation was that of Bykov (1912; cf. Kharkevich, 1967), who used preganglionic electrical stimulation and recorded the resulting contraction of the nictitating membrane. No systematic studies using the superior cervical ganglion–nictitating membrane preparation were undertaken prior to the detailed pharmacological evaluation of TEA by Acheson and Moe (1946), however. Besides the cat, the superior cervical ganglia were extensively studied in rabbit and rat. Guinea-pig (Perri et al., 1970) and dog (Chandrasekhar et al., 1959; Marlier, 1960; Kharkevich, 1967) were only rarely used.

a) Cat Superior Cervical Ganglion–Nictitating Membrane Preparation

The cat is selected for this purpose primarily because in this species the number of nonsynapsing (through) nerve fibres is negligible [although collateral fibres to the neighbouring nodose ganglion may occur (Kharkevich, 1967)]. Anatomically, isolation of the postganglionic nerve is not as easy in cat as in rabbit, where the postganglionic portion is considerably longer, but this is usually not necessary when the response of the nictitating membrane is utilized as an end point. The cat is anaesthetised, preferably with an anaesthetic that does not noticeably influence ganglionic transmission. Both chloralose and urethane are suitable for this purpose. Spinal cats can also be used; however, it should be kept in mind that aether and chloroform have been shown to influence ganglionic transmission in anaesthetic concentrations (Larrabee and Posternak, 1952) and therefore some considerable time should be allowed to elapse after trans-section of the cord under aether or chloroform anaesthesia. Through a midline incision in the neck the trachea is exposed and cannulated for artificial respiration. Usually the common carotid artery on the opposite side of the ganglionic set-up or a femoral artery and a femoral vein are cannulated for the purposes of recording the systemic blood pressure and intravenous drug administration, respectively. The head of the animal is placed in a suitable head holder, preferably clamped on the upper jaw, which allows no mobility of the head. A suture is placed in the middle of the rim of one nictitating membrane, which is connected through a pulley to an isotonic recording lever or force displacement transducer. The vagosympathetic trunk running along the common carotid artery is bluntly separated from the artery and the surrounding tissues. The sympathetic nerve is separated from the vagus and both of them are cut caudally. The preganglionic portion of the sympathetic nerve is placed on bipolar platinum electrodes and the nerve is immersed in mineral oil, either within a pool formed by the edges of the neck incision or surrounded with gauze soaked in mineral oil. There are various options for ganglionic stimulation. The majority of investigators use electrical stimulation to the preganglionic nerve with supramaximal square-wave stimuli at a frequency of 5–10 s, which activates the entire pool of fibres and results in sustained maximal contraction of the nictitating membrane. The ganglion-blocking agent to be studied is injected, usually intravenously, during the sustained contraction. The stimulation is shut off at the moment when the membrane starts to contract, following the drug-induced relaxation. After several minutes of resting period the sensitivity of the membrane to preganglionic stimulation is retested, and when its sensitivity has returned to normal a second, increased or decreased, dose of the blocking agent

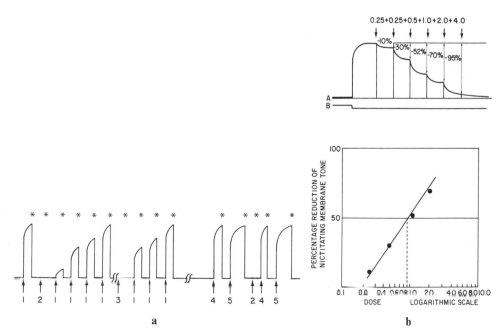

Fig. 2a and b. Different methods of analysing the qualitative and quantitative aspects of ganglionic blockade. Superior cervical ganglion-nictitating membrane preparation. **a** Intermittent electrical stimulation: *1*, Preganglionic electrical stimulation 50 c/s, 0.1 ms. *2*, Ganglion-blocking agent, e.g. hexamethonium, 1 mg/kg injected; *3*, Ganglion-blocking agent, e.g. hexamethonium, 0.5 mg/kg injected; *4*, Postganglionic electrical stimulation 50 c/s, 1 ms; *5*, Noradrenaline injected intra-arterially close to the ganglion.
* Stop recording for 2 min; SS: time interval for recovery
b Continuous stimulation at supramaximal strength, 5 c/s, 0.2 ms, single shock duration. At *arrows*, IV injection of blocking agent, e.g. hexamethonium (doses in mg/kg) (KHARKEVICH, 1967)

is administered (Fig. 2a). The relative potency of the new agent is determined by direct comparison with a known, standard drug, e.g., TEA, hexamethonium. This experimental arrangement does not provide for the estimation of duration of action. For this purpose, intermittent preganglionic stimulation with a high (usually 20–50 cps) rate and shorter trains of stimuli, e.g., 3–5 s in every 2–3 min, is a suitable procedure. This technique allows assessment of agents with intermediate or long duration of action. The duration of action of more evanescent agents can be determined fairly accurately with continuous, low-frequency preganglionic stimulation during which the entire response pattern of the nictitating membrane is depicted (Fig. 2b). With the conventional cat superior cervical ganglion–nictitating membrane preparation, proof of a ganglionic site of action of the agent in question can be obtained in two different ways: a) by electrical stimulation of the postganglionic nerve; and b) by stimulation of the postganglionic α-adrenergic site of the nictitating membrane with adrenaline or noradrenaline. The first method, although technically more involved, seems to be the more appropriate (unfortunately, the postganglionic nerves of cat are relatively short and lie fairly deep before entering the cranium). A useful modification of the superior cervical ganglion–nictitating membrane preparation is the arrangement for localized intra-arterial injections, as described by Tren-DELENBURG (1956). With this method, separate injections into the external and inter-nal carotid artery can be made, whereby the drug is delivered as required either to the nictitating membrane or to the ganglion. This modification is particularly useful for the study of stimulant agents or of blocking agents when only minute quantities are available for use. For the intra-arterial injections, the lingual artery is tied and the cannula is inserted pointing towards the centre. Injections are made when the external or internal carotid arteries are occluded or left open. Experiments have indicated that during occlusion of the external carotid artery the flow goes primarily to the superior cervical ganglion, and when the internal carotid artery is obstructed, the agent injected reaches primarily the nictitating membrane.

b) Isolated Perfused Superior Cervical Ganglion Preparation of Cat

KIBJAKOW described this preparation in 1933, and it has since become one of the most useful and often-used techniques in the study of ganglionic transmission. The original method, which was soon modified by FELDBERG and VARTIAINEN (1934) and FELDBERG and GADDUM (1934), was not used for testing ganglion-blocking agents by the early investigators, who were mainly concerned with the exploration of humo-ral transmission in the ganglia. The isolation of the superior cervical ganglion is essentially a circulatory one. All branches of the carotid artery except a few small twigs leading to the ganglion are tied and cut, along with the main trunk cephalad. The caudal end is cannulated and perfused with oxygenated Ringer-Locke solution at 38 °F. The branches of the internal jugular vein leaving the superior cervical ganglion are similarly isolated, and the cannula is inserted at the caudal end to collect the perfusate of the ganglion (Fig. 3). The preganglionic portion of the cervical sympathetic nerve is cut and stimulated with bi-polar electrodes. (In the original work, a slide inductorium was used for the stimulation, which was later replaced by stimulators delivering square-wave pulses through capacitor discharges.) The post-ganglionic portion of the cervical sympathetic nerve is left intact and connected to the nictitating membrane. (The arrangement of the cannulation and the anatomy of the vessels involved is illustrated in Fig. 3.) The majority of investigators who used the isolated superior cervical ganglion preparation recorded the end organ response, i.e., contraction or relaxation of the nictitating membrane evoked by pre- or postgan-glionic electrical stimuli or by drugs.

There are several methodological aspects to consider with this perfusion tech-nique. The first is the surgical preparation per se, with an aim to a) produce the least possible trauma to the vessels and the ganglion; and, b) make the isolation as complete as possible. To achieve this goal, familiarity with the anatomical, particu-larly vascular, topography of the region around the ganglion is necessary. The im-portant branches of the common carotid artery and their relationships to the sur-rounding structures are presented in Fig. 4. The branches of the common carotid from caudad to cephalad are: A comparatively large muscular branch (18 in Fig. 4) (subsequent numbers also refer to this figure), which supplies the cervical muscles and enters the spinal canal; the superior thyroid artery (26) branches off at the same level in the medial direction. Approximately 0.5 in. higher a branch leads medially to the laryngeal muscles (2). The occipital artery (19) and the small internal carotid (11)

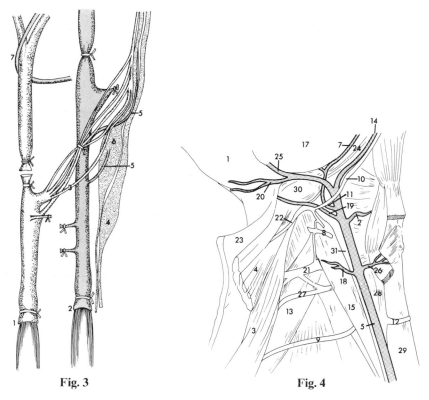

Fig. 3   Fig. 4

Fig. 3. Diagram of the relationships of blood vessels to the superior cervical ganglion and ganglion nodosum of cat. *1*, Common carotid artery (cannulated); *2*, Internal jugular vein (cannulated); *4*, Nodose ganglion; *5*, Veins draining the superior cervical ganglion; *6*, Superior cervical ganglion; *7*, Hypoglossal nerve (KIBJAKOW, 1933)

Fig. 4. The anatomical relationship of the common carotid artery in cat to the surrounding structures. Adapted from GILBERT, S.G.: Pictorial Anatomy of the Cat, 1968. University of Washington Press, Seattle.

1, Auricular cartilage	*17*, Masseter
2, Branch to laryngeal muscles	*18*, Muscular branch
3, Clavotrapezius	*19*, Occipital artery
4, Cleidomastoid	*20*, Posterior auricular artery
5, Common carotid artery	*21*, Second cervical nerve
6, External carotid artery	*22*, Spinal accessory nerve
7, External maxillary artery	*23*, Sternomastoid
8, First cervical nerve	*24*, Styloglossus
9, Fourth cervical nerve	*25*, Superficial temporal artery
10, Hypoglossal nerve	*26*, Superior thyroid artery
11, Internal carotid artery	*27*, Third cervical nerve
12, Isthmus of thyroid gland	*28*, Thyroid gland
13, Levator scapulae ventralis	*29*, Trachea
14, Lingual artery	*30*, Tympanic bulla
15, Longus capitis	*31*, Vagus nerve and sympathetic trunk
16, Mandible	

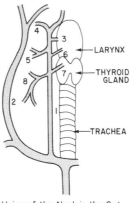

Veins of the Neck in the Cat

Fig. 5. Veins of the neck in cat. *1*, Internal jugular vein; *2*, External jugular vein; *3*, Vein from the spinal column; *4*, Vein from the bulla auditiva; *5*, Vein from lymph node; *6*, Vein from the thyroid cartilage; *7*, Vein from thyroid gland; *8*, Veins from neck muscles and spinal canal

leave either close together or from a common trunk at about the same level. The lingual artery (14) is the most substantial branch besides the external carotid (6), which runs laterally between the masseter m. (17) and the tympanic bulla (30). Its branches in the upper neck are the posterior auricular artery (20) and the superficial temporal artery (25). The external maxillary artery (7) may branch off from either the internal or the external carotid artery.

The blood supply of the superior cervical ganglion is shared by the ganglion nodosum of the vagus nerve. In most cases, the arteries originate from the common trunk of the internal carotid and occipital arteries. Less frequently, they arise from branches running to the base of the skull. There are some arteries that ascend along the vagus nerve and the sympathetic trunk and also contribute to the blood supply of the ganglia.

The veins consist of superficial and deep branches (Fig. 5). The main superficial veins are the large external jugular (2), uniting with the internal jugular (1) and subclavian veins. The internal jugular vein is frequently very small as it emerges from the skull through the jugular foramen. It is joined by a fairly large vein from the spinal column (3) and a similarly large vein running anteriorly from the medial aspect of the *bulla auditiva* (4). Veins from the lymph node lying lateral to the internal jugular vein (5) and from the region of the thyroid cartilage (6), the thyroid gland (7), and the veins from the neck muscles and spinal canal (8) all empty into the internal jugular vein.

The other important technical problems encountered with this preparation concern the composition, perfusion pressure, and temperature of the perfusing solution. It was soon recognised that in order to keep the perfused ganglion in good working condition, the above criteria have to be satisfied. Thus, FELDBERG and GADDUM (1934) adjusted the potassium chloride content of the Locke solution from 0.042% to 0.02%, employed 100 mg Hg perfusion pressure, filtered the perfusing fluid through a glass-wool filter, and warmed it by means of an electrically heated warming coil placed around the arterial cannula. This was described in detail by FELDBERG and

VARTIAINEN (1934). The temperature was maintained at 38–39 °C. The same authors called attention to adjustments of perfusing pressure and the size of the injections given into the perfusing tube, because prolonged perfusion and extreme pressures produce oedema of the ganglion and, as a consequence, wide variations occur in the rate at which drugs reach and leave the ganglia. The detailed study by BIRKS and MACINTOSH (1961) on the acetylcholine metabolism in the superior cervical ganglion required further refinement of the perfusion technique. They took particular care to leave the postganglionic trunk and its arterial twigs intact. Perfusion pressure was maintained at below 100 mg Hg so that a flow of 0.2–0.4 ml/min through the ganglion was maintained. The perfusion fluid consisted of modified Locke solution containing (g/liter) sodium chloride 9.0; $KHCO_3$ 0.56; calcium chloride 0.24; and eserine sulphate 0.005. The fluid was saturated with O_2 at room temperature and had a pH of approximately 8.5. When perfusion with plasma is indicated, pooled heparinised cat plasma is preferred, although human plasma or plasma dialysates can be used. The study of BIRKS and MACINTOSH (1961) indicated that for optimal synthesis of acetylcholine at the ganglion, perfusion with Locke solution and choline is required, while adequate release of acetylcholine is assured only in the presence of additional factors, e.g., CO_2 and plasma. Performance of the ganglion also depended heavily on the extent and volume of electrical stimulation. Although the perfused superior cervical ganglion preparation is not ideally suitable for the measurement of ganglion-blocking activity, because of the difficulty of obtaining reliable dose-response relationships, the preparation has often been used in basic studies in relation to the mechanism of ganglionic stimulation and blockade. In addition to the early studies of FELDBERG and GADDUM (1934), in which acetylcholine was identified as the neurotransmitter substance at the ganglion, and of FELDBERG and VARTIAINEN (1934), confirming the ganglionic site of action of acetylcholine, nicotine, and other stimulants, more recent studies on this preparation have contributed to the exploration of muscarinic ganglionic receptors (KONZETT and ROTHLIN, 1949; KEWITZ, 1954), to the analysis of inhibitory action of catecholamines on the ganglionic transmission (KEWITZ and REINERT, 1954), and to clarification of the mechanism of action of nicotine (PELIKAN, 1960). COLLIER and KATZ (1970) used isotope-labelled acetylcholine on this preparation in the exploration of the possible presynaptic site of action of acetylcholine.

c) Superior Cervical Ganglion Preparations With Electrical Recording
of Postganglionic Nerve Activity

Several investigations of ganglion-blocking agents have been performed on preparations belonging to this category. The most frequently used species are cat, rabbit, and rat. Ganglionic activity and its blockade, as with some other ganglionic preparations, can be assessed in situ when the ganglion is supplied by the animal's own circulation or in a completely isolated form when the excised ganglion is placed in a wet chamber and drug delivery to the ganglion is maintained by diffusion. The in vivo method is more suitable for testing the potency and duration of action of ganglion-blocking agents, while the in vitro method is satisfactory and even sometimes preferred when the aim is to analyse the neurophysiological correlates of ganglionic transmission as influenced by changes in chemical (e.g., ionic and drug) and other (e.g., temperature, stimulus parameters) conditions.

Preparation of the animals for in situ experiments is basically as described for the cat superior cervical ganglion–nictitating membrane preparation, except that the postganglionic nerve is also isolated and cut cephalad as far as possible; even so the postganglionic portion is relatively short in cat. Recordings for routine purposes can be made through bi-polar platinum electrodes or by a "unipolar" moving electrode placed on the ganglionic surface or on the postganglionic nerve. (For other special electrophysiologic recordings techniques, see the comprehensive review on the electrophysiology of the adrenergic neurone by Haefely, 1972.) The stimulation of the ganglion in its simplest form can be performed with single supramaximal volleys, resulting in a compound postganglionic action potential (orthodromic spike), the components of which are depressed (or altered) by ganglion-blocking agents. Dose-response relationships can be established by using several doses, measuring the height of the compound action potential, and plotting the heights against the dose (Fig.6a). Although these postganglionic action potentials are easy to obtain, the relevance of their pharmacological blockade is limited. The reasons are twofold: (1) this potential consists of several components, which are complex in nature as far as their origin and pharmacological sensitivity is concerned; (2) the physiological

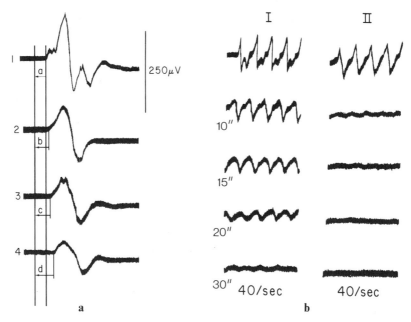

Fig. 6a and b. Superior cervical ganglion in situ; evoked post-ganglionic action potentials (oscilloscopic recording). (Modified from Kharkevich, 1967).
a Stimulation: Single preganglionic volleys (supramaximal strength, 0.1 ms duration) at arrows. *1*, Post-ganglionic compound action potential, prior blocking agent; *2*, Same, 2 min. after hexamethonium 2 mg/kg; *3*, Same, 2 min. after hexamethonium 4 mg/kg; *4*, Same, 2 min. after hexamethonium 7 mg/kg. a–d latency periods. **b** Stimulation: *repetitive* pre-ganglionic volleys (40/s, 0.1 ms duration, supramaximal stimuli). *I*, Postganglionic potentials before blocking agent; *II*, Postanglionic potentials two minutes after pentamethonium 2 mg/kg IV. Numbers in each frame show duration of stimulation to illustrate fatigue of ganglionic transmission at the chosen 40/s stimulus frequency. There is no noticeable fatigue at lower (e.g., 5–20/s) stimulation frequency

activation in autonomic ganglia normally takes place differently through trains of low-voltage physiologic stimuli travelling through the preganglionic nerve.

More appropriate parameters of electrical stimulation of the preganglionic nerve, for the purposes of testing ganglion-blocking agents, are those recommended for the superior cervical ganglion–nictitating membrane preparation. KHARKEVICH (1962, 1967) emphasised the importance of optimal frequency, duration, and intensity of stimulation at the level of ganglionic "lability" (utilizing those parameters of stimulation at which the ganglion is most sensitive ·to blockade). Frequencies varying between 5 and 50 c/s were recommended. The preganglionic fibres are stimulated at these frequencies in periods of up to one minute intermittently before and after administration of the ganglion-blocking agent. With the selected frequencies of stimulation, for example, the blocking effect of TEA is manifest even with doses as low as 0.05–0.1 mg/kg, and marked blockade can be obtained at the 1 mg/kg dose level. Measurements are made by comparing the heights of the series of action potentials produced (Fig. 6 b). The third method of stimulation is by injection of ganglion-stimulating drugs, preferably close to the ganglion, intra-arterially. These, e.g., ACh, nicotine or DMPP, produce bursts of ganglionic discharge. Recordings can be made on the entire, preferably desheathed postganglionic nerve or on isolated filaments or single fibres. In the former case, the increase in height of the train of postganglionic potentials and their duration of action can be measured with slow sweep speed on a storage oscilloscope and integrated, preferably planimetrically (Fig. 7a), while in the case of single fibres, the frequency response of firing is measured (Fig. 7b). The

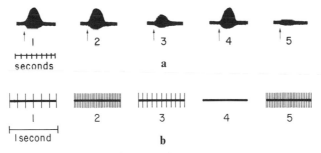

Fig. 7a and b. Superior cervical ganglion in situ, spontaneous postganglionic activity **a** Stimulation by ganglion-stimulating drugs, recording from the entire postganglionic trunk. *1*, Firing pattern of the postganglionic nerve following intra-arterial injection of a nicotonic ganglionic stimulant DMPP (↑); *2*, Firing pattern of the postganglionic nerve following injection of a non-cholinergic ganglionic stimulant (e.g., 5-HT); *3*, Same as *1*, 2 min after small dose of hexamethonium (50% blockade by planimetry); *4*, Same as *2*, 2 min after small dose of hexamethonium (no noticeable block); *5*, Same as *1*, 2 min after large dose of hexamethonium (90% bockade by planimetry).
Figure illustrates selectivity of hexamethonium as blocking agent. **b** Stimulation by ganglion-stimulating drugs, recording from isolated single postganglionic fibre. *1*, Single-fibre firing before ganglionic stimulant; *2*, Same as *1*, following ganglionic stimulant, e.g., nicotine; *3*, Partial blockade of single-fibre firing following small dose of ganglion-blocking agent (e.g., hexamethonium) + nicotine as stimulant; *4*, Complete blockade of single-fibre firing following large dose of hexamethonium + nicotine; *5*, Single-fibre firing following a non-cholinergic ganglion-blocking agent, e.g., 5-hydroxyindoleacetamidine (effective against 5-HT stimulation but ineffective against nicotine) + nicotine.
Figure illustrates selectivity of nicotine as a stimulant agent

responses before and after administration of the ganglion-blocking drug are compared. Selection of the proper stimulant agent is important, since not only different classes of stimulant agents, e.g., nicotinic and muscarinic, cholinergic, and noncholinergic, exist, but because even within a class, individual agents, e.g., nicotine or ACh, may differ in their spectrum and mechanism of stimulant action.

2. Other Sympathetic Ganglion Preparations

a) Stellate Ganglion

Like the superior cervical ganglion, this ganglion has frequently been used, not so much in routine pharmacological investigations as in neurophysiological experiments studying the basic mechanisms of ganglionic transmission. Research involving this ganglion (mostly in dog and cat) was stimulated following the observations of LIDDEL and SHERRINGTON (1929), who studied the changes in heart rate following stimulation of the stellate ganglion through the thoracic sympathetic chain. The anatomic relationships around the stellate ganglion of cat were described by HOLMES and TORRANCE (1959), who noted that in addition to the fibres connecting this ganglion to the cervical and thoracic sympathetic chain, some afferents came from the muscle spindles of the neck muscles (e.g., *longus colli*), and some from receptors in the lungs and the mediastinum. The anatomy of the cardiac nerves that leave the stellate ganglion and middle cervical ganglion is not constant, and up to three cardiac nerves may be present. The preparation of the cat's stellate ganglion for neurophysiological and neuropharmacological studies was described by BRONK et al. (1938), who analysed the conduction characteristics of the pre- and postganglionic fibres, and by LARRABEE and POSTERNAK (1952) and LARRABEE and HOLADAY (1952), who described the depressant action of general anaesthetics on this ganglion preparation. These investigators, and also TOLLACK et al. (1971), noted that, in addition to axons that terminate in synaptic contact with the ganglion itself, other axons that enter the ganglion traverse it without synapsing with it. This allows differentiation between drug effects influencing ganglionic as opposed to axonal conduction. This ganglion, as interpreted by HOLMES and TORRACE (1959), is shown in Fig. 8. The preparation of the isolated ganglion is as follows: The left stellate ganglion of cat is prepared by anaesthetising the animals with pentobarbital and keeping them under artificial respiration. The thoracic sympathetic trunk, the presynaptic fibres, the inferior cardiac nerve, the postsynaptic fibres, and the cervical sympathetic trunk (direct fibres) are sectioned at a distance from the ganglion, freed from the surrounding tissue, and placed on suitable electrodes. The thoracic trunk is stimulated by brief electric shocks. Stimuli of supramaximal strength are preferable, in order to ensure excitation of a constant number of preganglionic fibres throughout an experiment. [Action potentials were recorded alternately from the inferior cardiac nerve and the cervical sympathetic nerve by LARRABEE and POSTERNAK (1952).] The stellate ganglion can be perfused through a cannula directed towards the heart inserted in the axillary artery. The left subclavian artery is clamped near to its origin from the aorta and its vertebral, mammary and thyrocervical branches are ligated. To maintain a suitable temperature, the entire enclosure in which the experiments were conducted was heated to approximately 36 °C and was controlled thermostatically. More recently, KHARKEVICH (1960) analysed the actions of different ganglion-blocking

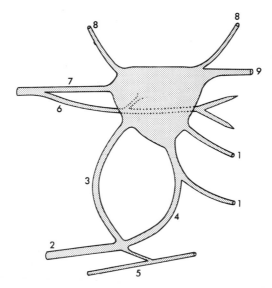

Fig. 8. Diagram of the stellate ganglion (left) of cat. *1*, Cardiac nerves; *2*, Cervical sympathetic trunk; *3*, Dorsal limb of ansa subclavia; *4*, Ventral limb of ansa subclavia; *5*, Depressor nerve with connection to sympathetic trunk; *6*, Nerve to longus colli from C_7 and C_8 with connection to stellate ganglion; *7*, Vertebral nerve; *8*, Sympathetic rami of first and second thoracic nerves; *9*, Thoracic sympathetic trunk. (HOLMES and TORRANCE, 1959)

agents in comparison with amobarbital and procaine on this preparation with different modalities of stimulation. BELMONTE et al. (1972) found that the action of ganglion-blocking agents was dependent on the frequencies of preganglionic stimulation, while conduction velocity was not influenced in this ganglion. They used different sites of preganglionic stimulation. The majority of studies involving the stellate ganglion used cardiac or vascular mechanical responses, as influenced by preganglionic electrical stimulation to one of the afferent nerves. The slightly different methods used by various authors were modifications of the early experiments described by LIDDEL and SHERRINGTON (1929). Among these, FLACKE and GILLIS (1968) used anaesthetised dogs, and utilized the heart rate changes as the end point. They found only incomplete block of the preganglionic electrical stimulation by nicotinic ganglion-blocking agents. The residual effect was blocked by atropine or scopolamine. Observations with anticholinesterase agents also indicated the existence of muscarinic receptors at the stellate ganglion. GRACA et al. (1970) used DMPP and nicotine as stimulants of the stellate ganglion. Their results indicated that hexamethonium was effective only in combination with atropine. They suggested that there is a population of ganglionic receptors with varying sensitivity to hexamethonium and atropine, the majority being sensitive only to the combination of the two agents. A recent study on the stellate ganglion of cat (GILLIS et al., 1975) emphasizes the functional importance of both nicotinic and muscarinic receptor sites in this ganglion. The study of AIKEN and REIT (1969) utilised cardiac acceleration and changes in sweat secretion, which followed the stimulation of adrenergic or cholinergic neurones of the stellate ganglion of cat. They demonstrated that the cholinergic neurones were more readily blocked by chorisondamine than the adrenergic ones, indicating functional heterogeneity of the nerve cell population of the stellate ganglion.

A simple in vivo preparation that indicates vascular change (vasodilation) in the guinea-pig ear was described by GIONO and CHEVILLARD (1962). Guinea-pig ears were denervated on one side by removing the stellate ganglion. After the animals recovered, the ganglion-blocking agents were given parenterally to the awake animal. The resulting vasodilation was measured by the change in the temperature of the innervated ear. In contrast to ganglion-blocking agents, spasmolytic agents produce bilateral vasodilation. The inhibitory effect of the jugular ganglia of frog was studied with ganglionic stimulation and blockade by KIBIAKOW et al. (1974), and the existence of postganglionic intracardial parasympathetic neurones was suggested. Similarly, the negative (and also positive) inotropic responses to ganglionic stimulants were blocked by hexamethonium and tetrodotoxin on the SA node of dog. Atropine blocked only the negative and propranalol only the positive response (CHIBA et al., 1972). The authors called attention to the differences in the stimulating pattern on the SA node by DMPP and nicotine.

b) Inferior Mesenteric Ganglion Preparations

The anatomy and physiology of the inferior mesenteric ganglion of the cat has been described by LLOYD (1937).

Method of Preparation. On decerebrated cats, the inferior mesenteric ganglia were exposed through a left lateral abdominal incision without entering the peritoneal cavity. The preparation was enclosed in a box and kept warm and moist. Stimulation was through different routes, e.g., orthodromically and antidromically. Different pathways through the inferior mesenteric ganglia of cat were recognised when different routes of electrical stimulation of the pre- and postganglionic nerves were used and oscilloscopic recordings of the evoked potentials made, and also when nicotine was used as a blocking agent of ganglionic transmission. Temporal but not spatial facilitation was observed, and occlusion was demonstrable between the ganglion cell pools of the ipsilateral preganglionic nerves. The suggested forms of synaptic relationships between preganglionic fibres and ganglion cells were presented in a simplified scheme by LLOYD (1937) (Fig. 9). In contrast to the original preparation, most subsequent investigations utilized a wide midline incision for better exposure of the ganglia. ACHESON and REMOLINA (1955) and HERR and GYERMEK (1960) used cats anaesthetised with pentobarbital, or urethane. The animals were eviscerated prior to the recording of nerve activity. Pre- and postganglionic nerves were exposed, usually on the left side, and isolated. If electrical stimulation is employed through the preganglionic nerves, these should be cut. ACHESON and REMOLINA (1955) studied the effect of postganglionic axotomy and found that the sensitivity of axotomised ganglia had changed, in that they became more sensitive to ganglionic blockade. Recovery of function of the ganglia begins 3 weeks after axotomy and seems to be complete between 72 and 100 days after trans-section, of the nerve. For chemical stimulation of the mesenteric ganglia, an injection of ganglionic stimulants, e.g., nicotine, ACh, or DMPP is made intra-arterially into the coeliac or inferior mesenteric artery via an in-dwelling polyethylene catheter. Study of chemically produced ganglionic stimula-

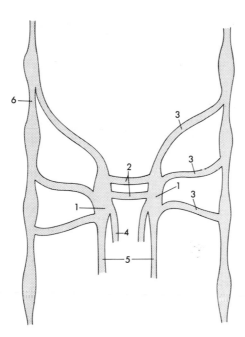

Fig. 9. Diagram of the inferior mesenteric ganglia of the cat with their neural connections. *1*, Inferior mesenteric ganglia; *2*, Interganglionic commissures; *3*, First, second and third inferior splanchnic nerves; *4*, Colonic nerve; *5*, Hypogastric nerve; *6*, Lumbar sympathetic chain. (LLOYD, 1937)

tion does not always necessitate severance, of the preganglionic nerves. The acquisition of quantitative data on the degree of ganglionic stimulation and blockade when chemical stimulants are used is dependent on the spontaneous firing of a few postganglionic nerve filaments. The postganglionic nerves are dissected under a microscope to filaments containing one to ten fibres. During dissection and recording the nerves are kept in a warm mineral oil pool made within the abdominal cavity. Bipolar platinium electrodes are used for recording. The frequency of impulses is counted before and after the administration of ganglionic stimulants. Evaluation of the ganglion-blocking agents can be made, as in other preparations in which electrophysiological recording techniques are used, by determining: (a) the degree of supression of the number of spikes on spontaneous firing; (b) the degree of block of the number of spikes following chemical ganglionic stimulation; and (c) the degree of supression of the height of the electrically evoked compound post-ganglionic action potential. Besides the nicotinic receptors, receptor sites sensitive to muscarine (GYERMEK et al., 1963) and to 5-HT (GYERMEK and BINDLER, 1962) were also detected in this ganglion preparation.

Several other preparations are available that utilise the postganglionic nerve activity of neurones connected to the lumbar sympathetic chain. OBRADOR and ODORIZ (1936) conducted experiments on decerebrate cats for the study of transmission through the lumbar sympathetic ganglia, and were among the first to call attention to the possible technical problems deriving from the existence of collateral and through fibres in the lumbar sympathetic chain, which can complicate the evaluation of ganglion-blocking agents on a routine basis, recording mainly changes in the height of compound evoked action potentials. The more recent study of 'Nishi et al. (1965) demonstrated the presence of fast- (B) and slow- (C)-conducting neurones, which connect with two types of ganglion cells in the isolated lumbar sympathetic ganglion of toad, which also has to be taken into consideration when such a preparation is used for the assay of ganglion-blocking agents.

c) Coeliac Ganglion

MALMEJAC (1955) described perfusion of the adrenal-renal region of an anaesthetised dog, including the coeliac plexus, from a donor dog. In the original experiments the donor dog's splanchnic nerve was electrically stimulated or the dog received epinephrine, which, in small doses, produced an increase in synaptic transmission and in adrenal glandular transmission. The effect on the coeliac ganglion was measured by recording vasomotor reactions in the neurally connected, but vascularly separated, kidney of the recipient by measuring kidney volume. The output of the adrenal gland was measured by blood pressure and spleen volume changes in a third adrenalectomised dog, which was perfused from the adrenal vein of the recipient. The method, although technically involved, lends itself to studies of ganglion-blocking drugs, particularly if electrophysiological recordings would be applied to measure postganglionic nerve activity. SAITO (1961) studied the effects of a series of ganglion-blocking agents on the coeliac ganglion by measuring the changes in splenic volume as indicator. Pre- and postganglionic electrical stimulation was employed to ascertain the ganglionic site of action of the agents.

d) Hypogastric Nerve–Vas Deferens and Seminal Vesicle Preparation (in situ)

This preparation (SAXENA, 1970) offers the possibility of comparison between the reactivity of two end organs at the same time. Fairly large, male guinea-pigs were used. The animals were anaesthetised with urethane or pentobarbital. After insertion of a cannula in the external jugular vein for intravenous injections, a midline incision on the abdomen was made, and the right seminal vesicle and the left vas deferens identified. The intraseminal-vesicle pressure was recorded with a pressure transducer connected to a small, saline-filled latex balloon, while contractions of the vas were registered by means of a force-displacement transducer connected with threads through the middle of the duct via a small hook. Hypogastric nerves on both sides were tied centrally, and placed on a pair of electrodes about 2 cm away from the innervated organs. The nerves were stimulated for 5 s every 1 or 2 min. In this preparation, hexamethonium produced complete blockade of the responses of both organs. Further pharmacological analysis showed that the postganglionic innervation through these organs is mainly adrenergic; however, a cholinergic portion is also suggested. A similar preparation, in which the hypogastric nerve and vas deferens were used without the seminal vesicle, was described by MANTEGAZZA and NAIMZADA (1967).

3. Parasympathetic Ganglion Preparations (in vivo and in situ)

a) Ciliary Ganglion Preparation

Parasympathetic ganglia usually form a network of many small ganglia and nerve fibres. Exceptions are the ciliary, otic, and sphenopalatine ganglia. Usually they are supplied with very short, postganglionic nerves, and therefore pharmacological examination of these ganglia is often restricted to preparations in which the end organ response is recorded following preganglionic stimulation. Because of the acetylcholinergic nature of the parasympathetic end organ receptors, agents with a postganglionic parasympathetic (atropine-like) action are usually not suitable for analysis on the parasympathetic ganglia. Recording of postganglionic potentials is possible with the ciliary ganglion, where the postganglionic portion is relatively accessible. WHITTERIDGE (1937) described the anatomic arrangement around the ciliary ganglion of cat and monkey and the isolation of the pre- and postganglionic aspects of the ganglion, and he analysed the synaptic threshold and conduction velocity of the postganglionic nerves, while PERRY and TALESNIK (1953) adopted the following method for the analysis of ganglion-blocking agents: Cats were anaesthetised with aether or chloralose, decerebrated and the ciliary ganglion (whose anatomic layout is shown in Fig. 10) was exposed between the lateral and superior aspects of the rectus

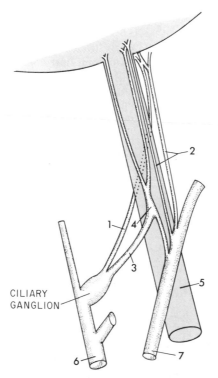

Fig. 10. Diagram of the ciliary ganglion of the cat with its neural connections. *1,* Medial short ciliary nerve; *2,* Lateral short ciliary nerve; *3,* Long ciliary nerves; *4,* Accessory ciliary ganglion; *5,* Optic nerve; *6,* Oculomotor nerve; *7,* Nasociliary branch of the Vth nerve. (WHITTERIDGE, 1937)

muscles by removal of the orbital plate. WHITTERIDGE (1937) removed the eyeball after cutting the optic nerve, while PERRY and TALESNIK (1953) left the globus and optic nerve intact and applied only adequate forward traction on the eyeball by means of sutures placed on its anterior surface. The short ciliary nerve was isolated from the optic nerve, cut, and cleaned. The oculomotor nerve was divided at its origin from the brainstem. All the other nerve trunks of the ciliary ganglion were cut. Recordings were made with silver-silver chloride electrodes from the short ciliary nerve or the body of the ganglion, while stimulation was produced by bi-polar platinum electrodes placed on the oculomotor nerve. Recording was by the conventional cathode-follower, D.C. amplifier-oscilloscope set-up. In experiments where, instead of postganglionic nerve activity, the responses of the end organ (pupil) are recorded, the influences of sympathetic innervation to the pupil have to be eliminated. For this purpose, PERRY and TALESNIK (1953) aseptically removed the superior cervical ganglion ten days before setting up the ciliary ganglion preparation. (On the cat ciliary ganglion preparation, acetylcholine was found to potentiate the electrically evoked potentials following submaximal stimuli. Nicotine produced initial stimulation, followed by depolarising block, while hexamethonium blocked the ganglia without depolarisation.) Several subsequent studies utilised the cat ciliary ganglia preparation, mainly for the purpose of comparative pharmacological evaluation of ganglion-blocking drugs on parasympathetic versus sympathetic ganglia. LUCO and MARCONI (1949) used the pupillary response following preganglionic electrical stimulation. SCHNEIDER and MOORE (1955) compared the efficacy of hexamethonium, pentapyrrolidinium, and chlorisondamine and found the blockade produced by the last two more stimulus rate-dependent than that obtained with hexamethonium. PERRY and WILSON (1956) utilized several ganglionic preparations in the comparison of a few well-known ganglion-blocking agents, and found that pentamethonium had more potent effects on the parasympathetic than on sympathetic ganglia. (In addition, they gave a critical appraisal of the ganglionic preparations available.) The studies of ALONSO DE FLORIDA, et al. (1960) on the cat ciliary ganglion were also done with the primary purpose of comparing the ganglion-blocking drugs on sympathetic versus parasympathetic ganglia. (Only minor differences in sensitivity between different compounds were found with respect to their blocking potency for the two sets of ganglia.) Using the same techniques, PARDO et al. (1963) analysed the mechanism of ganglionic action of sympathomimetics amines and found essentially no difference in reactivity between the two ganglia. (Epinephrine was the most potent depressor of ganglionic transmission among the agents studied.)

b) Urinary Bladder Preparation

The mechanism of autonomic innervation of the bladder is unusual and has been the subject of numerous investigations, among which one of the earliest and also most comprehensive was that of ELLIOTT (1907). He described in detail the differences among species in the motor innervation of the bladder (Fig. 11), which offers at least a partial explanation for the divergent pharmacological results reported by some later authors. The effect of pelvic nerve stimulation on the tone of the bladder wall has been known since the early experiments of LANGLEY and ANDERSON (1895, cf. VANOV, 1965), and the pelvic nerve bladder preparation of several species has since

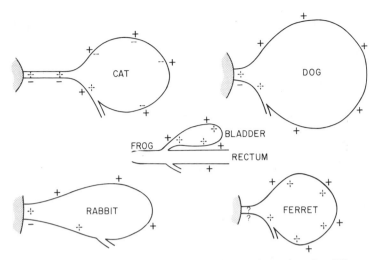

Fig. 11. Diagram of the innervation of the bladder and urethra in different mammals. Distribution of the pelvic (sacral) nerves is shown outside the organ, and distribution of the hypogastric nerves is indicated inside the organ. *Shaded area, prostate overlying* the urethrea. + indicates a stimulatory response, — an inhibitory response. Adapted from ELLIOTT, 1907

been utilised by many investigators studying ganglionic transmission and agents affecting autonomic ganglia. A characteristic feature of this organ is the prevalence of atropine-resistant receptors. Both the effects of ganglionic stimulant agents and those of electrical stimulation of the pelvic nerves are more sensitive to ganglion-blocking agents than to atropine-like drugs (URSILLO and CLARK, 1955; STILLE and HILFIKER, 1961; GYERMEK, 1961). The presence of muscarinic parasympathetic receptors in the bladder in addition to the nicotinic type of receptors was demonstrated by GYERMEK (1961), TAIRA et al. (1971), and SAXENA (1972). The relationship of these atropine-sensitive muscarinic receptors, which, under certain conditions, behave like ganglionic receptors, and the resistance of the neurally stimulated bladder to atropine has not yet been explained. The possibility of non-cholinergic transmission between the pelvic nerves and the bladder wall has been entertained by several investigators [for review, see TAIRA (1972)], and DE GROAT and SAUM, 1976, but has not been firmly established. The dog bladder was used by COOK et al. (1950), CHEN et al. (1951), URSILLO and CLARK (1955), and GYERMEK (1961, 1962). Similar preparations were used in cat (EDGE, 1955; GYERMEK, 1961; SAXENA, 1972; DESY, 1972), rabbit (STILLE and HILFIKER, 1961), ringtail possum (BURNSTOCK and CAMPBELL, 1963), and pithed rat (VANOV, 1965).

Most methods for preparation of the animal are similar. Usually anaesthetised female animals are used. The urethra is cannulated and connected to a recording system with a water- or saline-filled tube. A lower midline abdominal incision is made to expose the bladder, which is kept free from contact with the abdominal wall. The muscle margins are covered by warm, moist gauze and attached to a frame. The ureters may or may not be ligated, and the intestines may be removed. The nerves of the pelvic plexus are freed and cut on one side, and either bi-polar platinium or silver-silver chloride electrodes are placed on the cut peripheral end of the nerve. Stimulation is by rectangular pulses lasting 1–2 ms, 10–50 c/s for 3–10 s in each period of 1–3 min. Injections are administered preferably into the abdominal aorta via the inferior mesenteric or the femoral artery, to minimise any systemic effects of the drug. Stimulation of the bladder can also be achieved by intra-arterial adminis-tration of acetylcholine, nicotine, DMPP, or other ganglion-stimulating agents. Di-rect recording of postganglionic nerve activity, its neurophysiologic patterns and the effect of different blocking agents on the pelvic parasympathetic ganglia of the cat has been recently described by DE GROAT and SAUM (1976).

c) Parasympathetic Ganglia of Salivary Glands

The parasympathetic ganglia that supply the secretory postganglionic fibres to sali-vary glands are the otic ganglion, the end organ of which is the parotid gland, the sublingual ganglion connected to the sublingual gland, and the submaxillary gan-glion, which is related to the submaxillary gland. The otic ganglion is not easily amenable to pharmacological analysis by means of a technique of electrical stimula-tion of the preganglionic nerve. This nerve, the lesser superficial petrosal branch of the glossopharyngeal, branches off soon after it leaves the medulla, so that its isola-tion is rather difficult. According to KHARKEVICH (1967), use of the submaxillary gland, where the influence on the secretory function is measured in response to the electrical stimulation of the *chorda tympani*, is simpler. The quantity of salivary secretion is measured before and after the administration of a ganglion-blocking agent. Since agents with postganglionic, parasympathetic blocking (atropine-like properties) very effectively block the postganglionic portion of this autonomic neural pathway, control measurements, including stimulation by muscarinic stimulants, is required and the blocking agent in question should prove to have no effect against this chemical stimulation. For the measurement of salivary flow and its blockade, the method of BÜLBRING and DAWES (1945) can be recommended. They anaesthetised cats with pentobarbital or chloralose, after which the Wharton's duct was cannu-lated and connected through a water-filled bottle to a drop recorder. An IV infusion of pilocarpine, or preferably carbaminolycholine 0.004%, was given to increase the salivary flow. Intermittend small doses of atropine and atropine-like agents sup-pressed salivary flow. Atropine was highly effective in small (2–5 µg) doses. Although the preparation as described was originally designed for the testing of atropine-like drugs, it could be modified by infusing a suitable ganglionic stimulant, e.g., DMPP, to elicit salivation and to depress it with the ganglion-blocking agent in question.

4. Comparative Sensitivity of Sympathetic and Parasympathetic Ganglia to Ganglionic Blockade

Although there are recognized differences in the ratio of pre- to postganglionic neurones connected to each preganglionic neurone in the two divisions of the auto-nomic nerves, the basic transmission phenomena in sympathetic and parasympa-thetic ganglia are considered to be identical. Numerous pharmacological studies have been aimed at comparative evaluation of ganglion-blocking agents at the two divisions of autonomic ganglia. The possible therapeutic significance of blocking agents that would block the sympathetic or parasympathetic divisions selectively is obvious, and provoked several studies along these lines. Certain reports published in the 1940s indicated selectivity of a few agents, mainly at certain parasympathetic ganglia. Thus, SHÄFER (1939) reported that sodium citrate blocked parasympathetic ganglia preferentially. LUCO and MARCONI (1949) found that TEA blocked the ciliary ganglion more than the cervical sympathetic ganglion, as judged by changes in the pupil size in cat. PARDO et al. (1956) described ethyl-methyl-iso-octenylamine as a selective parasympathetic ganglion-blocking agent against vagal stimulation in the cat. KADATZ and KLUPP (1956) found that Q-160, a quaternary ammonium dioxolane derivative, acted more potently on the parasympathetic than on the sympathetic ganglia. SHIMAMOTO et al. (1958) noted that the submaxillary ganglia were much more vulnerable to ganglionic blockade than other ganglia, particularly the response of the adrenal gland. GINZEL et al. (1954) also reported relative selectivity to vagal ganglia by a series of polymethylene bis-phosphonium derivatives. Although in the study of PERRY and WILSON (1956) the differences between the two divisions of ganglia were not marked with most of the agents studied, they found pentamethonium to act considerably more potently on the parasympathetic ganglia in the heart preparation of cat. Although PERRY and WILSON (1956) and SHIMAMOTO et al. (1958) claimed that the salivary secretion as an indicator for parasympathetic activity is extremely vulnerable to depression of the corresponding ganglia, MASON and WIEN (1955) reported lack of selectivity with hexamethonium and pentapyrrolidinium when they used the *chorda tympani* stimulation-salivary flow response as compared to the mydriatic response and to blockade of the superior cervical ganglion of cat. When comparisons of sympathetic and parasympathetic ganglia are made in different species of animals, and in vivo and in vitro, differences in sensitivity are more likely to occur (PATON and ZAIMIS, 1949; WIEN and MASON, 1953b). In disagreement with the above data, many investigators concluded that there was no significant difference between the potency of many structurally different ganglion-blocking agents in the parasympathetic as against the sympathetic ganglia. This has been shown in cat (PARDO et al. 1963; MASON and WIEN, 1955; CUMMINGS et al., 1963) and dog (CHANDRASEKHAR et al., 1959; GARRETT, 1963). Some investigations explored the role of the rate of stimulation (SCHNEIDER and MOORE, 1955), and it was noted that certain agents, e.g., chlorisondamine and pentapyrrolidinium, did not produce blockade at low rates of stimulation, while others, such as hexamethonium, acted even at the low-frequency range of stimulation. The clinical studies of MAXWELL and CAMPBELL (1953) tested a series of bis-quaternary ammonium compounds in man and concluded that there were moderate but still well-defined differences among these agents with respect to vagal (achlorhydria) and sympathetic (hypotension) effects. Some of the agents were considerably more potent in producing mydriasis than in producing achlorhydria. In the clinical set-up, these differences are even more dependent on factors not directly related to ganglionic blockade per se than in animal experiments. The absorption following oral administration and the habituation that follows repeated administration are only two of the many causes for the discrepancies observed. Even in animal experiments that can be better controlled, the reasons for possible differences in sensitivity of the two divisions of autonomic ganglia or among ganglia of the same division can often be extraganglionic. Among the many possibilities are an unrecognised action in the end organ (provided a ganglion-end organ preparation is used), difference in access to the ganglion receptors, particularly in the whole animal, different parameters of electrical stimulation in the different ganglia studied, various dose-response curves of the agents, as related to the previous and possibly other factors, e.g., different temperatures of the differently exposed ganglia, reflex-modulating influences acting upon one set of ganglia as compared with others, different degrees of interference with ganglionic perfusion, depending upon the nature of the preparation. Clearly these factors are so numerous that the question of substantial and basic differences in sensitivity of ganglia to blocking agents cannot be answered with certainty. The vast majority of experimental and clinical observations have indicated that no agent has yet been discovered that, by blocking autonomic ganglionic transmission, exerts its effect following systemic administration selectively enough to be practically useful for the pharmacological blockade either of one division of the autonomic nervous system or of any organ selected for such a blockade.

II. Isolated Organ and Isolated Ganglion Preparations

Of the many preparations used in the past for assessing the potency and mode of action of ganglion-blocking agents, the isolated intestinal stips of rabbit, guinea-pig, and rat account for a sizeable proportion. Some of these, and also the vagus nerve-atrium preparation, the pelvic nerve-bladder preparation, and the intestinal peristaltic reflex preparation are of significant practical importance, since they allow the investigation of parasympathetic ganglionic function, which usually meets with technical difficulties because of the limited length of the postganglionic neuron. In addition to these, several other isolated preparations are available for testing sympathetic ganglionic function, e.g., the superior cervical ganglion, the stellate ganglion of various species, and the hypogastric nerve-vas deferens preparation, which has often been used in the pharmacological analysis of adrenergic neuron-depressant agents. A few other isolated organ methods are available, but are not widely accepted.

1. Isolated Smooth-Muscle Preparations of Gastrointestinal Tract

The isolated rabbit jejunum and ileum, the guinea-pig ileum, and the rat duodenum can all be used. The intestinal strips are suspended in an isolated organ bath according to the original method of Magnus (1904), or to one of its modifications, e.g., the superfusion technique of Gaddum (1953). Rather than the isolated intestine of cat, which was used by Magnus (1904), the guinea-pig ileum is now used most often, because of the relative lack of peristaltic movements, which allows the production of well-defined and quantifiable contractions of the longitudinal muscles. Most of these preparations are primarily suited to the analysis of postganglionic, parasympathetic (muscarinic) drugs and their antagonists, and only to a limited extent to the assessment of ganglion-blocking activity, unless the agents to be analysed affect exclusively the nicotinic ganglionic receptors and lack any activity at the sites of the muscarinic postganglionic, parasympathetic receptors. (Theoretically, agents with potential blocking action at the muscarinic ganglionic receptors could also be tested against a specific muscarinic ganglionic stimulant, e.g., McN-A-343. In practice, however, all agents so far proved to be effective against the ganglion-stimulant action of such an agent are also highly potent in surpressing the muscarinic postganglionic, parasympathetic receptors, thus masking the potential interaction at the ganglionic sites by blocking the end organ response to be measured.) The above-mentioned preparations were used in the past for testing ganglion-blocking activity against nicotinic ganglionic stimulants, e.g., nicotine- and DMPP-induced intestinal contractions. In this respect, rabbit jejunum or ileum may be superior to guinea-pig ileum, since in this species and in the dog *muscularis mucosae* preparation the nicotine-induced contractions are relatively insensitive to atropine blockade (ELLIS and RASMUSSEN, 1951). Nevertheless, caution should be exercised in interpreting the data from blockade obtained in this and other similar intestinal preparations stimulated chemically by DMPP or nicotine, as the possibility of a postganglionic blocking effect must be excluded. Details of the techniques, including data on the efficacy of several ganglion-blocking agents, are found in several studies, e.g., those by GADDUM (1953), LECHAT et al. (1961), LEE et al. (1958), LEVY et al. (1958), URSILLO (1961), DAY and VANE (1963), SETHI and GULATI (1973). For selection of the ganglionic stimulation in guinea-pig ileum, para-amino-phenylethyl-trimethylammonium is recommended by BARLOW and FRANKS (1971). Routine application of this stimulant may improve the above-mentioned technique. The isolated inferior mesenteric ganglion-colon preparation in the guinea-pig has been recently described by WEEMS and SZURSZEWSKI (1978). Blocking agents have not yet been investigated on this preparation.

a) Peristaltic Reflex Preparations

MAGNUS (1904) was the first to observe that the peristaltic movements of isolated intestines are largely under the control of the intraneural ganglionic network. TRENDELENBURG in 1971 conducted a thorough study on the physiology and pharmacology of intestinal peristalsis, utilizing strips of small intestines of guinea-pig, dog, cat, and rabbit. The peristaltic movements were elicited by changing the intraluminal pressure of the intestinal pieces by closing one end and connecting the other to a tube attached to a reservoir filled with the nutrient Tyrode solution, the height of which was adjustable above the level of the organ bath. The tissue was suspended in the organ bath under aeration and at a constant temperature. The reactivity of guinea-pig intestine to drugs was found to resemble that of man more closely than that of any other species, and guinea-pig intestine became frequently used. PATON and ZAIMIS (1949) were among the first to use the peristaltic reflex preparation of rabbit in the pharmacological analysis of ganglion-blocking drugs. Several other investigators, e.g., FELDBERG and LIN (1949) and WIEN and MASON (1953b) used the corresponding guinea-pig preparation for the analysis of *d*-tubocurarine and other ganglion-blocking agents. More recent studies embarked on the physiological analysis of the peristaltic reflex per se, which is primarily attributed to the function of the circular musculature of the intestine; thus HARRY (1963) pointed out that stimulant agents, including nicotine, 5-HT, and probably also histamine, act at different receptors of the postsynaptic membranes of the intestinal nerve plexus. Later GONELLA and VIENOT (1972), in an electromygraphic study of rabbit intestine, pointed out the different action of DMPP and hexamethonium on the longitudinal as against the circular musculature, and emphasised that in the development of peristalsis two mechanisms operate, both involving the circular muscles. Several details of the experimental set-up of the isolated guinea-pig peristaltic reflex preparation were out-

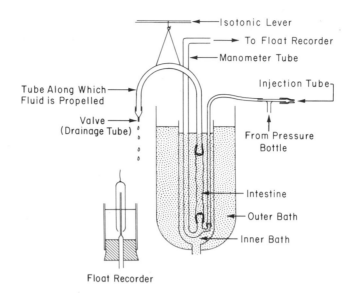

Float Recorder

Fig. 12. The apparatus for recording the peristaltic reflex in isolated guinea-pig ileum. BÜLBRING et al., 1953

A loop of guinea-pig ileum is suspended in an isolated organ bath of 50-ml capacity. The oral end is tied to the short end of a J-shaped tube with an internal diameter of 4 mm. The caudal end is tied to an inverted U-shaped tube fitted with a valve, The inverted U-tube is then suspended from a suitably counter-weighted lever connected with a frontal writing system. The long limb of the J-tube is used as a manometer, transferring the pressure changes of the intestinal segments by air transmission connected to a float recorder. The float is made from a thin-walled glass tube with the mouth turned in. This, and the use of a 1-mm capillary inlet tube prevents the two surfaces approaching each other, so the float cannot touch the inlet tube. Tyrode solution from a Marriott bottle is used, entering the lumen of the intestine trough a thin Portex tube into which a fine polyethylene tube, about 0.5 mm in diameter, has been inserted to allow intraluminal injections. An electromagnetic vibrator is fixed to the vertical rod from which the levers are suspended to minimise artifacts due to friction. Volume changes are recorded with a specifically designed volume recorder

lined by BÜLBRING et al. (1958) and BELESLIN and RAKIC (1969). For a description of this preparation, see Fig. 12 and its legend. The transmurally stimulated isolated guinea-pig ileum offers additional options for pharmacological analysis, beyond those offered by chemically or reflexly stimulated isolated guinea-pig ileum (PATON, 1955, cf. LEACH, 1966). With this preparation, it is possible to differentiate between the effects of postganglionically acting, atropine-like blocking agents and ganglionically acting inhibitors such as hexamethonium. The specifically arranged ileum preparation is electrically stimulated through transmurally placed platinum electrodes at low and elevated (1,5–3 cm water) intraluminal pressures. [The tissue is suspended in neostigmine (0.025 µg/ml)-sensitised Krebs solution at 34 °C.] While at resting tension the electrical stimulation only elicits a twitch-like longitudinal muscle response, in the distended stage the stimulation evokes a coordinated emptying response in which both the longitudinal and the circular fibres participate. The non-stimulated ileum responds to increased intraluminal pressure with the typical peristaltic reflex response. While atropine preferentially blocks the twitch response, hexamethonium

selectively inhibits the emptying response. Further details of the technique and evaluation of the data are given by LEACH (1966). The isolated longitudinal muscle of the
guinea pig ileum with its attached myenteric plexus can also be activated by electrical field stimulation (BURSZTAJN and GERSHON, 1977), and may lend itself to the
study of blocking agents of ganglionic transmission.

b) Isolated Guinea-Pig Oesophagus (THOMAS and TROUNCE, 1960)

A cholinergic ganglionic site of action was found in the lower smooth muscle portion
of the oesophagus. This is stimulated by acetylcholine and nicotine and was sensitive
to hexamethonium. Since atropine also produces blockade, the usefulness of this
preparation for the purpose of testing ganglion-blocking agents is limited.

c) Isolated Vagus Nerve-Stomach Preparation

Both rats and guinea-pig can be used. The responses of guinea-pig, kitten, rat and
mouse isolated stomach preparations in vitro were studied in detail by PATON and
VANE (1963) They investigated the responses to transmural stimulation, to excitation of the vagus nerves or of the peri-arterial nervous network, and also to stimulant
drugs and different blocking agents. The experimental set-up for this preparation
was as follows: The animals were killed, and the stomach rapidly removed and
washed out with cold Krebs solution, after which the pylorus and oesophagus were
tied. The stomach was placed on a wide-necked glass t-cannula through a hole
approximately 2 cm long cut in the side of the organ near to the greater curvature. A
small polyethylene tube was passed through the centre of the cannula for the removal of fluid. An internal electrode was coiled around this polyethylene tube. The
stomach was suspended from the cannula in a bath of warmed Krebs solution, which
was gassed with 95% O_2 and 5% CO_2. The bath was usually filled to capacity, which
was 140 ml. The volume of fluid within the stomach varied between 5 and 50 ml. The
bath was rinsed with fresh Krebs solution approximately every 10 min. Injections
were administered by syringe into the external fluid. The movements of the stomach
were measured by means of a float recorder or a water manometer. In the experiments, when the vagus nerve was stimulated, the oesophagus with the vagus trunk
was dissected out. After the oesophagus had been tied at its junction with the
stomach, the vagus nerve trunk was excluded from the ligature and the oesophagus
was pulled up into an electrode holder made of polyethylene tubing, which contained
two rings of platinum wire electrodes spaced approximately 0.5 cm apart. The electrodes were connected to the stimulator by a shielded wire. The resistance of the
preparation was usually about 1000 Ω. Square-wave pulses were used for stimulation
lasting 0.125 ms. The frequency of stimulation ranged from less than one shock/min
to 100 shocks/s. In the detailed study of PATON and VANE (1963), a large number of
stimulant agents were used. One of the blocking agents, hexamethonium, reduced
the transmural stimulation response and inhibited the response to vagal stimulation.
DELLA BELLA et al. (1962) investigated the effects of curare-like drugs in a similar rat
preparation, but no systematic study of ganglion-blocking agents has been performed by them. GREEF et al. (1962) also used the isolated vagus-stomach preparation of guinea-pig, with particular emphasis on analysis of the inhibitory vagal
effects. They found that ganglion-blocking agents were effective against the inhibi-

tory effects that develop in the atropinised preparation and postulated the existence of sympathetic neurones in the vagus in this species. In guinea-pig, the assay of ganglion-blocking drugs may be complicated by the fact that besides the vagal stimulatory pathway, inhibitory fibres to the stomach synpase at both cholinergic and serotoninergic ganglia (Bülbring and Gershon, 1967; Campbell, 1966). On a similar vagus-stomach preparation of frog (R. Tigrina), Singh (1964) reported that neural stimulation in addition to ACh, produces the release of 5-HT, H, and substance P. Further, there were marked changes in the relative amounts of these substances released, dependent upon seasonal variations as reflected in varying sensitivity to the corresponding blocking agents, e.g., atropine, bromolysergic acid diethylamide, tryptamine, and mepyramine.

d) Isolated Nerve-Bladder Preparations

α) Guinea-Pig Hypogastric Nerve-Bladder Preparation
(Mantegazza and Naimzada, 1967)

After sacrifine of the guinea-pig, the abdomen was opened and the intestines moved to one side to expose the bladder and hypogastric nerves. The nerves are easily identified in the mesentery of the colon. The urinary bladder and the hypogastric nerves were dissected free and placed in a 50 ml organ bath containing Krebs solution. The solution was aerated at 32 °C with a mixture of 95% oxygen and 5% carbon dioxide. A short (approximately 0.5 cm) strip of the interior wall of the bladder was dissected and the open organ was placed in a bath with threads on each edge of the dissected wall. One of the threads was connected to an isotonic lever, and the other end was connected to the bottom of the bath. This allowed recording of contractions of the circular muscles of the bladder. These muscle fibres are stronger than the longitudinal ones, and survive longer in vitro. The nerves were passed through platinum electrodes and were stimulated at 5–50 cs with pulses lasting 1 ms, with a supramaximal voltage for 5 s in every 2 min. The resulting contractions were blocked by ganglion-blocking agents such as hexamethonium and tetraethyl-ammonium.

β) Guinea-Pig Pelvic Nerve-Bladder Preparation (Weetman and Turner, 1973)

In the isolated pelvice nerve–bladder preparation of the guinea-pig, which is set up at 33 °C in a 100 ml organ bath gassed with 5% CO_2 and 95% oxygen, the nerves are stimulated by rectangular pulses through platinum electrodes with a frequency of 8/s. The duration of each shock is 0.5 ms, with a maximum voltage administered in trains for 5 s at 2 min intervals. In this preparation, typical ganglion-blocking agents such as hexamethonium, pentolinium and mecamylamine produced only incomplete blockade, indicating that as in in vivo bladder experiments, details of the neurohumoral transmission between pelvic nerves and the bladder still remain to be elucidated.

γ) Rabbit Pelvic Nerve–Bladder Preparation (Ursillo and Clark, 1955)

The course of the nerve fibres to the detrusor muscle in the rabbit follows that of the vascular supply to that muscle. These fibres are too fine to be isolated from the adjoining tissue, and they may be dissected out together with the artery and vein and stimulated without further dissection. The rabbits are killed and bled, and the urinary bladder well exposed. Ligatures are passed into the bladder. One ligature is placed at the vertex, and one at the middle of the fundus just below the dissected tissue. As the ligatures are retracted in opposite directions, a rectangular strip, whose corners are described by the ligatures, is dissected out. If the ligatures are not used, or are tied before the dissection, or not retracted during the dissection, the desired anatomic relationships are lost. The preparation is mounted on an L-shaped plastic holder in a bath containing 50 ml Krebs solution at 37 °C. The solution is aerated with a mixture of oxygen and CO_2. The nerves are stimulated with platinum wire-loop electrodes completely immersed in the bath. A light recording lever with a gravity writing point was used by the authors and the optimum tension was found to be around 1 g. The thickness of the strip in this arrangement was approximately 2 mm. Stimulation with slightly supramaximal stimuli of 12 V, of 1 ms duration at the frequency of 30 cs, was applied for 5 s every 2 min. Technical difficulties of interpreting the data obtained with ganglion-blocking agents in in vivo bladder preparations are shared with the isolated nerve bladder preparations. The parasympathetic ganglia of certain species, e.g., dog, contained both muscarinic and nicotinic receptor sites. The response to nicotinic stimulants is inhibited in most species by typical ganglion-blocking agents, but the effect of pelvic nerve stimulation is resistant, to varying extents, to postganglionic parasympathetic (atropine) blockade (URSILLO, 1961; URSILLO and CLARK, 1956; GYERMEK, 1961). Although specific 5-HT-sensitive receptors are present in the bladder (GYERMEK, 1962), there is no direct proof that 5-HT serves as a neurotransmitter substance, either in the nervous supply or in the muscle tissues of the bladder. Even according to recent studies and reviews (AMBACHE and ZAR, 1970; WEETMAN and TURNER, 1973; TAIRA, 1972), the exact nature of neural transmission between the pelvic nerves and the bladder remains undetermined.

2. Other Isolated Organ Preparations

a) Isolated Hypogastric Nerve-Vas Deferens Preparations

This preparation of guinea-pig and sometimes of rat has frequently been used for the study of both ganglion-blocking and adrenergic neurone-blocking agents. Since ganglion-blocking drugs inhibit the motor response of the vas deferens to hypogastric nerve stimulation, it was proposed that peripheral cholinergic synaptic mechanisms are involved in the sympathetic hypogastric innervation of this organ. The results of experiments with denervation and reserpine treatment supported this hypothesis (SJÖSTRAND, 1962). The method of preparation of the test organ is given below, as described by HUKOVIC (1961). Guinea-pigs were sacrificed by a blow on the head and bled. The animal was placed on an operating table supine, the abdomen opened, the gut displaced to the right. The testes were pushed out by pressure on the scrotum and while one testis was held the ductus deferens was freed from the surrounding tissues and cut from the epididymis. The testes were removed. The cut and of the ductus deferens was held with a forceps, and it was separated from the adjacent tissues. Then the hypogastric nerves were identified. The right and left nerves can easily be seen in the middle of the mesentery of the colon. One nerve was tied and cut 5 cm from the

ductus deferens. This was cleaned to within 0.5 cm of the organ. The remainder of the
nerve was preserved by isolating the piece of peritoneum that contained it. The
ductus deferens was then cut from the urethra, removed together with the nerve and
the small piece of peritoneum, and placed in an isolated tissue bath. Two preparations can be made from the same animal if necessary. The ductus deferens was tied by
its proximal end to a hollow glass rod. The isolated organ bath contained 12 ml of
Krebs solution at 30 °C. This war aerated with a mixture of oxygen (95%) and CO_2
(5%). The distal end of the ductus was attached to a lever that wrote on a smoked
paper. The hypogastric nerve was passed through the channel of a pair of electrodes
situated below the meniscus of the bath fluid. Usually a vibrator needs to be attached
to the frame of the organ bath to improve recordings. The electrical stimulation
consists in submaximal rectangular pulses of 2–3 V, lasting 2 ms at a frequency of 80/s.
The preparation is stimulated for 2 or 3 s in every minute. The author states that
similar preparations can be made from rabbits, rats, and mice. WATANABE (1969) and
BENTLEY (1972) modified this hypogastric nerve–vas deferens preparation by isolating the neural portion from the end organ. WATANABE used a specifically constructed
plastic capsule, which can be fitted with an electrode assembly for pre- and postganglionic stimulation. The little capsule containing the ganglion of the neural part is
shown in Fig. 13. This modification makes it possible to perfuse the ganglion. WA-
TANABE tested the typical ganglion-stimulating and -blocking agents in this preparation, and suggested that the method could be routinely used for the study of ganglionically active agents. BENTLEY's modification of the method involves separating
part of the vas deferens with a thin rubber membrane from the part on which the
hypogastric nerve is attached and the stimulation given. (The specially designed
isolated hypogastric nerve–vas deferens preparation bath in shown in Fig. 13.) Drugs
are added to the outer bath and contractions are recorded only from the part of the
vas deferens that lies within the inner bath. Thy hypogastric nerve was stimulated
through platinum electrodes in these experiments for periods of 5 s every 2 min, with

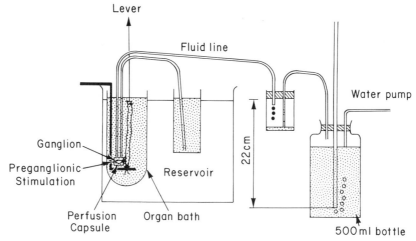

Fig. 13. The apparatus for the isolated hypogastric nerve–vas deferens preparation. WATANABE,
1969

supramaximal voltage, at a frequency of 15–20 cs for the guinea-pig, and 15–10 cs for the rat. [BENTLEY, 1972, also described a perfused preparation of a similar nature. YAMASHITA compared the effects of various drugs on the contraction of the excised vas deferens by using both hypogastric nerve and transmural stimulation (1967). As a critique of the above method, is should be noted that BENTLEY and SABINE (1963) called attention to the adrenergic neurone-blocking action of DMPP in this preparation. (Similar observations were made by WILSON 1962, about the guinea-pig ileum preparation.)

b) Isolated Vagus Nerve-Atrium Preparations

HUKOVIĆ (1960) described a rabbit atrium preparation in which the influences of both sympathetic and parasympathetic nerve stimulations can be studies. The rabbit is sacrificed, the vagus nerve and the sympathetic chain on the right side are identified and tied, and the trachea and the oesophagus are divided where they enter the thorax. The interior wall of the chest is removed without disturbing the thymus and adjacent tissues. The cervical sympathetic nerve is tied and freed of connective tissue as far as the stellate ganglion by blunt dissection, freeing the ganglion as well as possible. The vagus nerve is placed on a pair of electrodes approximately in the middle of the plate, and the second pair of electrodes is placed around the stellate ganglion itself. The other end of the atria is tied to a spring lever. The stimulus applied was 0.5 mA at a frequency of 20 pulses/s. Each stimulus lasted 5 s, and stimulation was maintained for between 15 and 30 s. The preparation is fixed on an L-shaped rod and then immersed in the nutrient solution at 30 °C. No ganglion-blocking agents were tested in this preparation in its original from, but WHITACRE et al. (1966) reported on the effect of hexamethonium, using a similar isolated preparation in which chronotrophic and inotropic effects of vagus nerve stimulation and those of transmural stimulation were compared. While atropine was effective against both types of stimulation, hexamethonium inhibited only the slowing produced by vagal stimuli and was ineffective against transmural stimulation. GREEFF et al. (1962) used the isolated vagus nerve-auricle preparation of guinea-pig for the evaluation of different ganglionic drugs. They have found blockade with hexamethonium and chlorisondamine against the paradoxical stimulant action that follows vagus stimulation. Nicotine produced a bi-phasic action, while guanethidine was ineffective against vagal stimulation. More recently BHAGAT (1966) used the same test organ for the analysis of nicotinic and muscarinic ganglionic stimulants, and concluded that their action on the atria is not ganglionic, but originates in the catecholamine stores at the nerve endings. Consequently, ganglion-blocking agents were ineffective against the externally applied chemical stimuli. On the isolated rat vagus nerve-atrium preparation, CHIANG and LEADERS (1965) noted that nicotinic ganglion stimulants produced a bi-phasic response consisting of an inhibitory phase followed by stimulation. The stimulant phase of nicotine but not that of DMPP was blocked by hexamethonium and hemicholinium. It was suggested that part of the effect of DMPP was related to catacholamine release, and part took place through a direct stimulant effect on the atrial musculature. This observation presents another example for the questionable selectivity of DMPP as a ganglionic stimulant, and calls for caution in interpreting data obtained with this agent under certain circumstances.

3. Isolated (Excised) Ganglion Preparations

It has been known for some time that completely isolated, excised ganglia, particularly those of cold-blooded animals, can be kept in a good functional condition for several hours. In a suitable experimental set-up, even mammalian ganglia can be well maintained and made suitable for the analysis of ganglion-blocking agents. According to ECCLES (1952) complete isolation of the ganglion offers certain advantages, namely freedom to position the stimulating and recording electrodes without electrical interference from surrounding tissues and the opportunity of exposing the ganglion to a given drug concentration. Against these advantages, one has to consider the problem of a gradually deteriorating preparation that equilibrates only slowly with the surrounding fluids and its drug medium. The slow diffusion can be partially overcome by desheathing the ganglia. The advantage of using rabbit superior cervical ganglion is that it contains a relatively long postganglionic trunk. Something of a disadvantage is the fact that occasionally two connecting superior cervical ganglia exist, one of which is connected to the vagus (ECCLES, 1952). The presence of some preganglionic fibres running through this ganglion presents another technical problem (DOUGLAS and RITCHIE, 1956). Nevertheless, the rabbit preparation has been successfully used by several investigators.

a) Isolated Rabbit Superior Cervical Ganglion Preparation (ECCLES, 1952)

The ganglia were removed from rabbits anaesthetised with paraldehyde. The preganglionic trunk was freed, and the postganglionic trunk was separated from the internal carotid artery, freed from the surrounding connective tissue, and cut at its point of entry into the base of the skull. During this surgical procedure, the blood supply of the ganglion was preserved. Finally, the ganglion was quickly immersed in Krebs solution at room temperature. The sheath was removed carefully to allow free diffusion of substances into and out of the ganglion. A perspex recording chamber was constructed, which incorporated an air-tight seal with tubes for gas entry and outflow to allow maintenance of a constant, predetermined atmosphere for long periods. The chamber provides for fixation of the preparation on the electrodes with the facility to adjust the position of the electrode without opening the chamber; the preparation can be immersed in the solution or lifted up as required; the nutrient Krebs solution was bubbled through with 95% oxygen and 5% CO_2. The pH of the solution was 8.3–8.4 before the addition of CO_2 and fell to 7.7 after the gas mixture was bubbled through. Attention was called to reducing the bicarbonate concentration to 13.6 mM because the original concentration of bicarbonate in the Krebs solution produced deterioration of ganglionic transmission.

A properly prepared isolated ganglion can respond adequately for up to 24 h. ECCLES (1952) found that d-tubocuranine selectively blocked synaptic transmission without depressing the preganglionic spike potential and that it produced posttetanic facilitation in the ganglion. KOSTERLITZ and WALLIS (1966), in their study of the ganglionic actions of hexamethonium and morphine, used essentially the same preparation, with the exception that the animals were anesthetized with urethane. These authors analysed mainly changes in the slow negative N potentials. Hexamethonium in concentrations of 275–550 µM produced an almost complete or complete block of ganglionic transmission. ELLIOTT (1965) and ELLIOTT and QUILLIAM (1964)

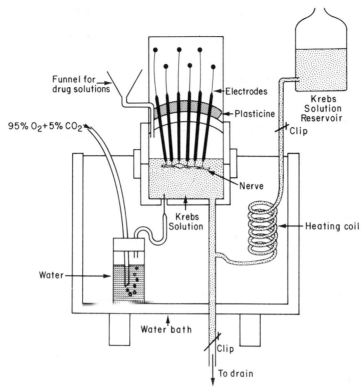

Fig. 14. Diagram of the apparatus used to record potentials from the rabbit isolated superior cervical ganglion preparation. ELLIOTT and QUILLIAM, 1964

investigated a large series of centrally active drugs in this preparation (the nerve chamber used by these authors is shown in Fig. 14), and found among them three characteristic types of blocking action. With the same preparation, ALKADI and McISAAC (1974) recently investigated the action of the venom of the black widow spider and found selective suppression of only certain spike population of the post-ganglionic potentials evoked. Thus, in the analysis of different ganglion-blocking agents by means of this technique, one has to consider the different components of the compound action potentials evoked.

b) Isolated Rat Superior Cervical Ganglion Preparation

The rat ganglion is set up much like the rabbit ganglion in an organ chamber filled with oxygenated Locke solution. During exposure to the drugs, the nerve lying on the electrode assembly is bathed in the fluid and during recording it is lifted out from the bath. Technical modifications of this and of similar isolated preparations include those of HERTZLER (1961), who used an electronically regulated switch that provided for periodic immersing and removal of the nerve into and out of the bath, and NILWISES and SCHMIDT (1965) who added small amounts (0.66%) of bovine hemoglobin to the oxygenated Tyrode solution nutrient during the procedure to improve oxygenation. Besides being used to measure the ganglion-blocking action of various substances (QUILLIAM and SHAND, 1964; NILWISES and SCHMIDT, 1965; HARADA et al., 1974) this ganglion has also frequently been used by investigators studying the basic mechanisms of ganglionic transmission (HANCOCK and VOLLE, 1969a; VOLLE and HANCOCK, 1970; HAEFELY, 1972; ECCLES and LIBET, 1961; LIBET, 1970; NISHI, 1970). ROCH-RAMEL (1962) conducted a very thorough study of the metabolism of the isolated rat ganglion.

c) Isolated Stellate Ganglion–Pulmonary Artery Preparation (BEVAN, 1963)

This preparation allows the measurement of changes in the vascular reaction to nerve stimulation across the ganglion. Rabbits are killed and exsanguinated. The chest is opened, the right lung is removed, and the abdominal inferior *vena cava* is cut out to prevent subsequent bleeding. The right thoracic sympathetic chain is separated from the posterior thoracic wall. The recurrent cardiac nerve is traced from its origin at the recurrent laryngeal nerve to its disappearance behind the pericardium. The right vagus nerve is sectioned 1 cm above and below the right subclavian artery and the recurrent laryngeal nerve is cut distal to its junction with the recurrent cardiac nerve. Finally, the right subclavian artery is cut both at its origin and at the level of the first rib. The whole complex tissue, containing the right thoracic chain, the stellate ganglion, the *ansa subclavia*, the inferior cervical ganglion, and part of the right vagus and the recurrent laryngeal nerve is freed from the prevertebral muscles. The recurrent cardiac nerve is dissected to within 2–3 mm of the pulmonary artery bifurcation and the whole of the main and the proximal few millimeters of the right and left pulmonary arteries linked by the recurrent cardiac nerve to the complex of tissue described above is removed to a dissection bath of cold oxygenated Krebs-bicarbonate solution. The pulmonary artery is dissected in such a way that a ring approximately 5 mm wide is left, containing the main vessel with the attachment of the recurrent cardiac nerve. The tissue is suspended on an L-shaped tissue holder, the recurrent cardiac nerve is placed on platinum electrodes, and the right thoracic sympathetic chain pulled through a pair of ring electrodes to within 5 mm of the stellate ganglion. The whole preparation is immersed in Krebs-bicarbonate solution. Direct and postganglionic stimulating electrodes are placed in one half of a divided tissue bath, and the ganglion and preganglionic electrodes in the other (see Fig. 15). Stimulation was performed with 80–120 V with a frequency of 25/s and a duration of 2 ms.

d) Other Isolated Ganglionic Preparations

Ganglionic preparations that have been set up on ganglia related to the heart and other than the stellate ganglion are the median nerve trunk-cardiac muscle preparation of the crustacea limulus. In this preparation, FUKUHARA et al. (1960) studied the effects of acetylcholine and atropine, using the cardiac pacemaker ganglion cells, but no specific ganglion-blocking agent was used in this study. In the pleural ganglion preparation of the mollusc aplysia, KEHOE (1972) described three different types of acetylcholine receptors. The majority of them were found to be of the nicotinic type,

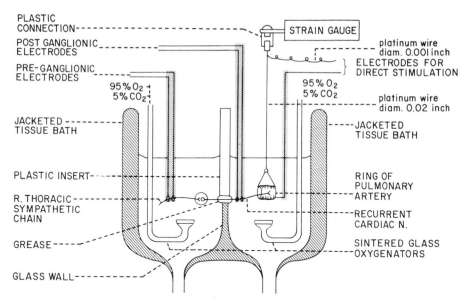

Fig. 15. Organ bath and recording set-up for the sympathetic ganglion–pulmonary artery preparation. The contractile response of the arterial ring to pre- and postganglionic and direct muscle stimulation is measured isometrically. BEVAN, 1963

showing sensitivity to both tetraethylammonium and hexamethonium. The visceral ganglia of the garden snail (helix aspersa) have been studied by several investigators using intracellular recording techniques (PIGGOTT et al., 1975; JUDGE et al., 1977). In this species glutamate plays a significant role as excitatory neurotransmitter therefore the significance of these ganglia in the study of ganglionic blocking agents, affecting cholinergic neurotransmission, is limited. The cholinergic visceral ganglionic system regulating ciliary activity in the gill of the mussel, Mytilus edulis has been studied by HAMBURG and PAPARO (1975). Recording of ganglionic unit activity or of the end organ response (e.g., ciliary activity) can be made. The excitatory responses following direct application of ACh can be blocked by hexamethonium. Measuring end organ response is complicated in this preparation by the endogenous release of and response to dopamine and 5-HT.

The lumbar sympathetic ganglia of the bullfrog have ben frequently used in neurophysiologic studies. The pharmacological behavior of isolated cell types can be assessed by using intracellular microelectrodes; for example the inhibitory action of atropine on muscarinic cell receptors of the B type ganglion cells (NISHI et al., 1965) has been analyzed recently by KUBA and KOKETSU (1976). The isolated, excised ciliary ganglion preparation of few-day-old chicks has been described by MARTIN and PILAR (1963), but no systematic study of ganglion-blocking agents in this preparation has been published. Intracellular recording of the synaptic potentials in the isolated inferior mesenteric ganglion of the guinea pig has been recently described by WEEMS and SZURSZEWSKI (1978). Their neurophysiological study did not include a pharmacological analysis of the neuronal activity but a suggestion for the existence of noradrenergic neurons in this ganglion has been made.

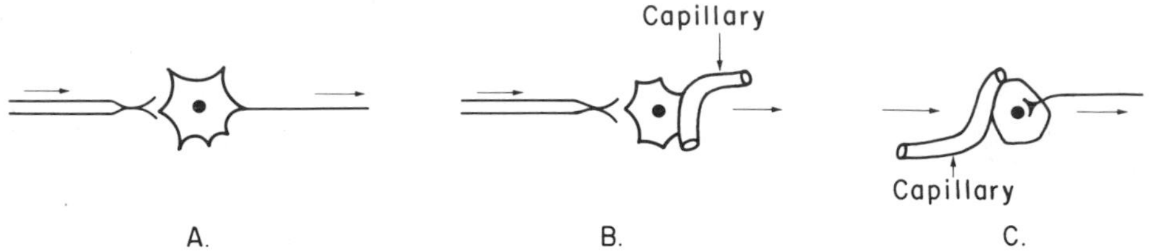

Fig. 16. Schematic illustration of the anatomical differences between autonomic ganglia (*A*), the adrenal gland (*B*) and the carotid body (*C*). Adopted from KONZETT and ROTHLIN, 1953

D. Preparations Other Than Autonomic Ganglia Used for Evaluation of Ganglion-Blocking Agents

The effects of ganglion-blocking drugs have been tested in the past in several preparations other than autonomic ganglionic preparations in which the organ in question contained cholinergic, mostly nicotinic-type receptor sites. Stimulation of these receptors usually evoked activation of a neural pathway or liberation of other chemical transmitter substances, such as catacholamines. Ganglion-stimulating and -blocking agents are effective in all these structures, and therefore it can be assumed that the receptors in question bear considerable similarity to one or more of the recognised "typical" ganglionic receptor sites. For these reasons, enumeration of certain preparations involving the adrenal and the glomus cells seems appropriate. There are two particularly significant specific structural elements of the autonomic nervous system, i.e., the cells of the adrenal medulla and the epitheloid cells of the carotid glomus. While, in the typical autonomic ganglion, a neural impulse is transmitted to another neurone (neuro-neural connection) in the adrenal medulla, the preganglionic nerve activates secretory cells (neuro-humoral connection) and in the glomus cell a humorally delivered chemical stimulus activates the afferent nerve fibers (humoral-neural connection). Figure 16 depicts the general features of the three prototype synapses.

I. Preparations of Adrenal Gland and Adrenal Medulla

Activation of the adrenal medulla in anaesthetised animals (cat and dog) can be achieved by stimulating the afferent (splanchnic) nerve electrically or chemically. Acetylcholine, nicotine, and other nicotine-like ganglionic stimulants can be used for chemical stimulation (for review, see KONZETT and ROTHLIN, 1953). A convenient and reproducible end point is the rise of systemic blood pressure. This reaction can be blocked by ganglion-blocking agents, as demonstrated for TEA by BURN and DALE as early as 1914. Since then, a large number of investigators have used this simple method to demonstrate a blocking action on the adrenal gland. The electrical and chemical stimuli, provided they are not intensive, can be repeated at fairly short intervals, indicating that the adrenals have a large capacity for rapid replenishment of the depleted catacholamine stores.

The adrenal medulla also responds to several non-nicotinic ganglionic stimulants, e.g., the muscarinic stimulant agents; McN-A-343 and pilocarpine; histamine, 5-HT, and angiotensin, particularly when these are given intra-arterially via the superior mesenteric or coeliac artery. The ensuing pressor responses are abolished by adrenalectomy, but are not usually blocked by the conventional, non-depolarising ganglion-blocking agents. Depolarisation block by nicotine is effective against all these stimulants. Cocaine, morphine, and methadone, which are effective in blocking ganglionic stimulation by non-nicotinic stimulants, are ineffective. This seems to be an important pharmacological difference between the behaviour of adrenal medullary cells and that of the sympathetic ganglia (TRENDELENBURG, 1967). Atropine is a specific blocking agent against pilocarpine on the adrenal gland, as is pyrilamine against histamine-induced stimulation (TRENDELENBURG, 1957a). No information is available on the adrenal action of the neurotrophic blocking agents that have been shown to be potent against 5-HT stimulation of autonomic ganglia (GYERMEK and BINDLER, 1962; GYERMEK, 1966).

An interesting method that measures the amount of catecholamines released from the adrenals following electrical stimulation of the left splanchnic nerve of cat was described by MARLEY and PATON (1961). Anaesthetised cats are eviscerated and artificially ventilated. The adrenal lumbar vein is cannulated and samples are taken from the adrenal venous blood before and after splanchnic nerve stimulation. The samples have to be heparinised, certifuged, and frozen until the bioassay for catacholamines is performed, either in isolated rat stomach or in spinal rat blood pressure preparation. The catecholamine output is in proportion to the frequency of electrical stimulation and ganglion-blocking drugs proved to be blocking the catecholamine output. This preparation allows the pharmacological differentiation of various catecholamine-releasing stimuli at the adrenal gland by the use of specific blocking agents. This aspect seems to be of importance, since in the mechanism of catecholamine release in the adrenal glands there may be more than one neural receptor mechanism. Thus, FELDBERG et al. (1934) found that the stimulating effect of ACh on the adrenal medulla is sensitive to atropine block, indicating the possible significance of muscarinic receptors at this synapse.

II. Preparations Using the Response of Chemoreceptors of Carotid and Aortic Bodies

These receptors are sensitive to oxygen lack and are also activated by stimulants of autonomic ganglia, e.g., acetylcholine, nicotine, nicotine-like ganglionic stimulants, lobeline, and KCL (KONZETT and ROTHLIN, 1953) but not by muscarinic ganglion-stimulants, e.g., McN-343 (PENNA and AVIADO, 1962). The chemoreceptors can be utilised in the study of ganglion-blocking substances by measuring reflex changes in blood pressure and respiration in anaesthetised animals (MOE et al., 1948; GINZEL et al., 1954; SUWANDI and BEVAN, 1966). The relationship of chemoreceptors to autonomic ganglia and their blockade was more fully outlined by KONZETT and ROTHLIN (1953).

Effects on the carotid body can be measured by recording the electrical activity of the sinus nerve (KAINDL and WERNER, 1948) or by the end organ response, e.g., respiratory stimulation. In order to avoid systemic effects of the stimulants or blocking agents, intra-arterial administration close to the sinus node or perfusion of the carotid sinus and carotid body following surgical isolation is recommended. DOUGLAS (1952), who studied the action of hexamethonium on cat carotid body, used a modification of the traditional technique of carotid sinus isolation, whereby venous drainage from the perfused area was permitted in order to avoid venous stagnation, which proved to be detrimental to continuing responsiveness of the chemoreceptors. Essentially, the technique consists in surgical exposure of the sinus region and ligation of all arterial branches around, except the common carotid, through which a donor cat's heparinised blood is perfused from its femoral artery. Further details of the method are found in the original article. For the purpose of testing the ganglion-blocking agents, the carotid body has to be stimulated by intra-arterially injected ganglionic stimulants, e.g., acetylcholine, nicotine, lobeline, or DMPP, because the responses to oxygen lack (and also to KCl and cyanide) are refractory to ganglion blockade (DOUGLAS, 1952). Utilizing changes in reflex vascular resistance of dog HENDERSON and UNGAR (1978) in a recent, elegant study of carotid perfusion technique were able to point at the primarily muscarinic receptor mechanisms in chemoreceptor stimulation (by sodium dithionite) and at the nicotinic nature of baroreceptor activation.

III. Other Preparations

Certain cutaneous sensory pathways are stimulated by acetylcholine, nicotine, and lobeline (and also by other substances such as histamine and 5-HT); this effect can be detected along the afferent nerve by conventional electrophysiologic recording. Using a cat preparation in which intra-arterial injections of the above-mentioned stimulants were administered into the superficial femoral artery and oscilloscopic recording of the nerve activity was taken from the saphenous nerve, DOUGLAS and GRAY (1953) reported that both hexamethonium and tubocurarine block the activation of the cutaneous sensory pathways. Pain and inflammation produced by locally administered nicotine to the eyes or rat and guinea-pig can also be selectively inhibited by ganglion-blocking agents (JANCSO et al., 1961). BURN et al. (1959) described several methods by which the effect of acetylcholine or nicotine on chromaffin cells releasing catacholamines, usually norepinephrine, can be studied. The effects of nicotine on the isolated nerve-nictitating membrane preparation of cat, on isolated perfused rabbit ear, and on the localized pilomotor response of cat's tail has been studied by these investigators. Although no ganglion-blocking agents were employed in this study, these methods, with suitable modifications, may lend themselves to the analysis of ganglion-blocking agents (DOMER, 1971). Pentolinium was found to be effective in dilating the tracheobronchial tree on newborn lambs, as determined by cineradiography. This effect seems to be relatively specific for the ganglion-blocking agent, since other bronchodilators, e.g., atropine and epinephrine were less potent. This method (ISABEL et al., 1972) may also be adopted as an auxiliary procedure in the analysis of ganglion-blocking agents.

IV. Antagonism Against the CNS Effects of Nicotine

Nicotine, being a tertiary-amine base, elicits considerable CNS toxicity on parenteral administration, by stimulating central cholinergic receptors of the nicotinic type. Ganglion-blocking agents can be tested against several central effects of nicotine.

1. Nicotine Convulsions and Toxicity

LAWRENCE and STACEY (1952) observed protective effects of members of the methonium-type ganglion-blocking agents against nicotine-induced convulsions in mice and rats. Hexamethonium was found to be fairly selective against nicotine convulsions; lobeline-, metrazol-, cocaine-, and strychnine-induced convulsions were not affected by it. The nicotine convulsion test has been used routinely as part of the screening profile of a large series of new ganglion-blocking agents (SPINKS et al., 1958). The tertiary and secondary amine-type ganglion-blocking agents are sometimes highly potent in this test, but hexamethonium, even though it is a quaternary ammonium salt, consistently proved to be effective (STONE et al., 1958; SPINKS et al., 1958). The antinicotinic potency of ganglion-blocking agents is not usually parallel with their peripheral ganglion-blocking activity. Chlorisondamine is only partially effective, and TEA has no effect (STONE et al., 1958). The test is usually performed on groups of mice, which are pretreated with various IP or IM doses of the blocking agents to be tested. IV doses of nicotine are then given, and the animals are observed for signs of running, jumping, and convulsing. The antinicotinic potency may run parallel with the peripheral ganglion-blocking potency within a certain series of compounds, as was the case within the group of mecamylamine analogs (STONE et al., 1962), but usually the central and peripheral effects are quantitatively different. The protection of nicotine convulsion, however, parallels the potency for preventing nicotine lethality (YAMAMOTO et al., 1966 ACETO et al., 1969). In order to improve the penetrability of the quaternary ammonium compounds into the brain, KRATSKIN (1973) used the intraventricular route of administration in mice and rabbits.

2. Behavioural Effects of Nicotine

Nicotine-induced changes in the bar-pressing performace of rats can be blocked by previous administration of mecamylamine. Quaternary ammonium-type ganglion-blocking agents are much less potent (MORRISON et al., 1969). The efficacy of even mecamylamine depends on the type of behavioural methods used. Thus, AVIS and PERT (1974) observed that mecamylamine and scopolamine both interfere with the conditioned fear reaction, while only scopolamine is effective in habituation experiments. Ganglion-blocking agents were used in this and in similar behavioural experiments as tools to clarify whether the behavioural responses could have been attributed to specific "nicotinic" CNS receptors or not. Present evidence indicates that both muscarinic and nicotinic ACh receptors have a functional role in the central nervous system.

E. Screening for Ganglion-Blocking Activity

In the search for new ganglion-blocking agents, as in the case of any other drug, establishment of the pharmacological efficacy, at least in a semiquantitative manner, is of paramount importance. Screening methods usually consist of procedures that are simple to perform and are reasonably economical. In the case of ganglion-blocking agents, methods that meet these criteria are rare, and usually either inaccurate or non-specific. For initial exploration of the agents, observational methods can be used: for example the degree of *relaxation of the nictitating membrane in the unanaesthetised animal* (e.g., cat and dog) can give an approximate estimate of the sympathetic ganglion-blocking potency of an agent. Trained dogs with indwelling intravenous catheters can be used and can be injected repeatedly.

I. Blood Pressure Responses in Anaesthetised Animals

Experiments in which blood pressure responses are measured have frequently been used in the pharmacological screening of ganglion-blocking agents. A pressor response as a result of stimulation of sympathetic ganglia (and of the adrenal medulla) can be elicited by appropriate doses of nicotine, TMA, DMPP, or other suitable ganglion-stimulating agents. In order to minimise the compensatory cardiovascular reflex changes, spinal cats or dogs are preferred. As early as 1914, Burn and Dale observed that the pressor effects of TMA is blocked by TEA, but this observation was not explored further until the systematic pharmacological evaluation of TEA 30 years later. Since several barbiturates depress ganglionic transmission, in the preparation of the animals for testing the pressor responses and their antagonism, this type of anaesthetic should preferably be avoided (Garrett, 1963). Chloralose and urethane are the preferred anaesthetics. Repeated small doses of DMPP (in the range of 3–10 μg/kg) produce reproducible pressor responses, which can be blocked or reduced by ganglion-blocking agents. The pressor response is due partly to the catecholamine released from the adrenals, because removal of the adrenals reduces the pressor responses to ganglionic stimulants significantly (Chen et al., 1951). Instead of chemical stimulation of sympathetic ganglia, the splanchnic sympathetic nerves can be electrically stimulated, preferably with tetanic frequencies, for 5–10 s to elicit pressor responses. To exclude any action on the adrenals, these have to be ligated. The degree of ganglionic blockade can be estimated by comparing the degrees of inhibition of a serially-evoked pressor response following different doses of the blocking agents. There are several limitations of the methods for measuring pressor responses. The well-recognized complexity of vasomotor regulation, even in anaesthetized or spinal animals and the necessity of using generally larger doses of blocking agents than in other preparations (e.g., superior cervical ganglion) to obtain a measurable degree of blockade are only two of the problems encountered with these methods.

Screening methods also include the observation or measurement of mydriasis in intact, unanaesthetised animals (mouse, rat, cat, or dog). The method used in mouse yields quantitative data that can be statistically analysed (Edge, 1953; Gyermek, 1959).

II. Mouse Pupil Mydriasis Test

The degree of parasympathetic ganglionic blockade (on the ciliary ganglion) can be measured in mice by means of the pupil dilation reaction following the injection of ganglion-blocking agents (Edge, 1953). Since parasympathetic blocking (atropine-like) drugs are highly potent in this respect, differentiation between the ganglionically and postganglionically induced mydriasis is necessary. This can be achieved by pretreating the animals with carbaminoylcholine. This method, described by Gyer-

MEK (1959), is as follows. Albino mice of both sexes and weighing 20–30 g can be used. Carbaminoylcholine in a dose of 2 ml/kg is given subcutaneously, 15 min before the blocking agents are given. This dose of carbaminoylcholine alone produces intense salivation, lacrimation, and defaecation, and is lethal to about 5% of the animals. Within 30 min of administration, this dose decreases the pupil size by 44%. The cholinergic blocking compounds are administered intraperitoneally. Each of the blocking agents is given in three or four logarithmically spaced doses to groups of five to ten mice each. The measurements are made under a microscope lamp illumination with a binocular microscope of 20 fold magnification before, and 15 and 30 min after administration of the blocking agents. The maximal changes (in pupillary diameter) after 15 and 30 min are determined. As the mice may differ in weight and pupillary size, expression of the maximal pupillary change as a percentage of the normal pupillary size is recommended. Each ganglion-blocking agent to be evaluated is subjected to two tests: one without carbaminoylcholine, and one with carbaminoylcholine. The pretreatment with carbaminylcholine does not alter the mydriasis produced by atropine or atropine-like drugs such as scopolamine and benactizine. On the other hand, typical ganglion-blocking agents such as hexamethonium and mecamylamine do not produce mydriasis following carbaminoylcholine administration. The interaction between carbaminoylcholine and cholinergic blocking drugs acting on the mouse pupil thus appears to be useful in determining the site of cholinergic blocking action. The method is not suitable for measuring the absolute quantity of the ganglion-blocking action of drugs that can effect both ganglionic and postganglionic blockade, but may give an approximate estimate of the predominance of one action over the other. Compounds that belong to this intermediary category are methylatropinium bromide, homatropinemethyl bromide, butylscopolaminium bromide, paraphenylbenzylatropinium bromide, and methantheline bromide.

F. Evaluation of Non-Nicotinic Ganglion-Blocking Agents

The effect of non-nicotinic ganglion-blocking agents often cannot be adequately analysed by the use of preganglionic electrical stimulation unless special arrangements are made, e.g., blockade of the nicotinic ganglionic receptors to unmask the response on the non-nicotinic receptors. With single, preganglionic volleys, the behaviour of the slow excitatory postsynaptic potentials (SEPSP) can be investigated under the influence of the appropriate blocking agent, e.g., atropine. No quantitative studies comparing various agents by means of this recording method have been developed, however. Quantitation of the blocking effect of agents that interfere with non-nicotinic receptor functions in the ganglia can be made more conveniently by using the appropriate stimulant agents with close, intra-arterial injections to the ganglia and by measuring either the end organ responses, for example in the modified superior cervical ganglion-nictitating membrane preparation (TRENDELENBURG, 1957) or pelvic nerve-bladder preparation (GYERMEK, 1962), or by measuring pressor responses in the whole animal (TRENDELENBURG, 1967) or ganglionic discharges in the superior cervical ganglion preparation (MURAYAMA and UNNA, 1963; HAEFELY, 1974c) and in the inferior mesenteric ganglion preparation (GYERMEK and BINDLER,

1962; MURAYAMA et al., 1963). The pressor effects of non-nicotinic stimulants have been explored particularly thoroughly, and a fair amount of data are available on the characteristics of blockade to these stimulants on autonomic ganglionic sites. Thus, the pressor effects of muscarinic stimulants such as McN-A-343, AHR-602, and pilocarpine can be abolished by nicotine-induced depolarizing block. In contrast, non-depolarizing ganglion-blocking agents and the non-depolarizing-phase nicotinic block enhance the responses of these agents. Cocaine, morphine, and methadone are also depressant, but their specificity, because of a possible axonal depressant action and a depressant action on acetylcholine release, is questionable (TRENDELENBURG, 1967). The end organ response (pressor response) is mediated through the liberation of catacholamines at the sympathetic nerve endings, so that an adrenal medullary depression of their release with adrenergic neurone-blocking agents (e.g., xylocholine) or by blockade of sympathetic α-receptors can also cause blockade that is obviously unrelated to the ganglionic sites (TRENDELENBURG, 1967). As discussed earlier, there are some additional, more or less specific blocking agents that can be utilized, e.g., antihistamines against histamine-induced ganglionic or adrenal activation and neurotrophic 5-HT antagonists against 5-HT-induced ganglionic stimulation. The only type of blockade that was effective against the ganglionic response to angiotensin was the depolarizing phase of nicotinic block (LEWIS and REIT, 1965; TRENDELENBURG, 1967).

G. Methods for the Determination of Absorption, Distribution, and Excretion of Ganglion-Blocking Agents

Determination of ganglion-blocking agents in tissues or in excreta, as with other drugs, depends heavily on the chemical nature of the compounds and on their pharmacological potency. The majority of ganglion-blocking agents are fully ionized quaternary ammonium compounds. Consequently, their oral absorption is generally limited and their penetration through the blood-brain barrier is negligible and/or slow. The intestinal absorption of quaternary ammonium-type compounds can be studied by the method of LEVINE et al. (1955), which utilises intestinal loops of rats into which the agent to be tested is injected. After a certain time interval, the animal is reanaesthetised, the loop is removed and the nonabsorbed amount of the quaternary ammonium salt is measured colorimetrically. If greater specificity and sensitivity is required, radioactive labelling of the compound and radioassay are recommended. Hexamethonium has been successfully analysed in biological fluids, (e.g., urine) by bioassay in the cat nictitating membrane preparation following intra-arterial injection (MORRISON and PATON, 1953). Chemical and biological assays showed the rate of absorption of quaternary ammonium-type blocking agents, mostly polymethylene bis-ammonium salts, to be limited and variable. In the case of hexamethonium, oral absorption in man varied between 0.2% and 34% (PATON and ZAIMIS, 1951). A few quaternary ammonium salts were reported to show better oral efficacy ratios than the methonium salts, indicating a higher degree of oral absorption (PLUMMER et al., 1955; FROMMEL et al., 1955; McKENDRICK and JONES, 1958). The distribution of ganglion-blocking agents can be studied most conveniently by radioassay. McISAAC (1962) reported on the fate of ^{14}C-labelled hexamethonium in cats. The highest concentrations occur in the kidney soon after IV administration. The plasma concentrations necessary for blockade at a certain type of ganglion varied considerably between 2.2 and 23 µg/ml. Similar data on other ganglion-blocking agents are lacking, and it is difficult to generalise on the relationship of tissue uptake and distribution related to the degree of ganglionic block. Quaternary ammonium-type agents are excreted almost exclusively through the kidneys by filtration. Again, those that have been most actively investigated are the methonium class (PATON and ZAIMIS, 1951; WIEN and MASON, 1951). More than half the injected methonium compounds appear in the urine in the first few hours, and excretion through the kidney accounts for about 90% or more in the first 24 h. Thus, chemical and biological assay of the urine can adequately analyse the degree of excretion. The absorption, distribution, and excretion patterns of tertiary and secondary amine-type ganglion-blocking agents are quite different from those of quaternary ammonium compounds. They are absorbed better and distributed between extra- and intracellular spaces more readily following oral administration, and thus they enter the brain and pass to the foetus more easily (PLUMMER et al., 1954; SPINKS et al., 1958; LEE et al., 1958; STONE et al., 1956a,b; CUMMINGS et al., 1963). Although excreted largely through the kidney, they are liable to metabolic changes (e.g., de-alkylation, N-oxidation) and in studies of their distribution and excretion it seems important to identify metabolic intermediates and end products. Radioactive tracer methods coupled with different methods of separation, e.g., thin-layer or gas chromatography, therefore seem to be more useful in this class of agents. In the case of highly potent agents, the chemically unchanged excreted portion can be measured by bioassay, but bioassay is of obviously limited value if performed alone. In the study of excretion of this class of agents, it is necessary to consult the appropriate research articles, which describe the general pharmacology of a given agent and also the corresponding analytical chemical references.

H. Clinical Testing of Ganglion-Blocking Agents

Methods for analysis of these agents are limited and lack the accuracy of animal tests. The use of invasive techniques, e.g., direct measurements of blood pressure through arterial cannulation, placing stimulating or recording electrodes to corresponding nerves, inserting balloons into visceral hollow organs, is usually not readily available to the investigator. Furthermore, the application of electrical or chemical ganglionic stimulation is not feasible. For the above reasons, testing of ganglion-blocking agents in the past, particularly in the 1950s, when therapeutic exploration of this class of agents was pursued with more enthusiasm, was restricted to measuring changes in systemic, resting blood pressure, observing the incidence of orthostatic changes in normotensive (MORRISON and PATON, 1953) and hypertensive patients (SMIRK, 1952; MORRISON, 1953; SMIRK, 1953, 1960, 1964; LOCKET, 1956), determining the degree of vagolytic action by measuring gastric achlorhydria (MAXWELL and CAMPBELL, 1953; MASEVICH, 1960), and measuring changes in pupil size and reaction to light (MORRISON and PATON, 1953; RUBINSTEIN et al., 1958). Most other clinical signs that follow the administration of ganglion-blocking agents, after either single or repeated doses, are even less quantifiable, and include changes in cardiac size, development of dry mouth, blurring vision, constipation, and reduction in the occurrence and intensity of hypertensive headaches, in shortness of breath, in arrhythmias, and in fundus changes. In the clinical evaluation of ganglion-blocking drugs, the routes of administration played important roles. Oral versus parenteral dosage and efficacy were studied often (Smirk, 1952, 1953; McKendrick and Jones, 1958; Maxwell and Campbell, 1953). With the development of newer, tertiary and secondary amine-type agents (mecamylamine and pempidine) oral efficacy has been improved, but CNS side effects appeared (Smirk, 1964). Chronic administration presents the common problem of tolerance. Even without this, either the efficacy of the ganglion-blocking agents was inadequate or the side effects required the addition of supplementing agents. Combinations with rauwolfia alkaloids and diuretics were most often used (Moyer and Brest, 1961; Smirk, 1964). Other potent drugs often used concurrently in the management of hypertensive cardiovascular disease, such as cardiac glycosides, adrenergic blocking agents, and anti-arrhythmic drugs, make the clinical evaluation of ganglion-blocking drugs even more cumbersome and unreliable. For the above reasons and because of their questionable long-term therapeutic value, ganglion-blocking drugs are very rarely used nowadays. Present therapeutic applications include treatment of acute hypertensive crises and the induction of controlled hypotension during anaesthesia. Even in this field, however, other agents, e.g., sodium nitroprusside, are gaining favour over the ganglion-blocking drugs (e.g., trimethaphan and trophenium) used so far.

J. Critical Appraisal of the Experimental Methods Used in the Evaluation of Ganglion-Blocking Agents

No ideal method exists for the assessment of ganglionic-blocking activity. This is related only partly to the limitations of the existing preparations. More importantly, the investigator still lacks methods that could measure ganglionic blockade in a pathological state capable of imitating a certain disease condition with underlying autonomic ganglionic disturbance. The pathophysiology in the motor innervation of the smooth muscles of the vascular system or gastrointestinal or genitourinary tract, and of gland secretions in various diseases, e.g., neurogenic hypertension, or in peptic ulcer disease are not clearly confined to autonomic ganglionic sites. Thus, the animal models used so far have not been appropriate even to the partial solution of the therapeutic problems presented. (Other failures of the research approach, e.g., false avenues of new chemical drug design or of clinical diagnosis are not treated in this discussion.) Even if we confine ourselves to the basic requirements of pharmacological research, i.e., the definition of potency and site or type of action of a given agent, the limitations of our existing methods are obvious. These limitations reside partly in the characteristics of the biological system, and partly in the drugs to be analysed or used as tools of the analysis. Thus, for example, the affinities of blocking agents to ACh receptors may vary in dependence on the test organ and/or on the agent (Barlow et al., 1972). Furthermore, the mode of action, even within the group of non-depolarising ganglion-blocking agents, e.g., hexamethonium vs mecamylamine, may be different (Trendelenburg, 1961a,b). In some preparations, particularly when end organ responses are measured, an abnormal degree of sensitivity or resistance is observed. Thus, it has been noted that the salivary secretion is a far more sensitive indicator of blockade of the submaxillary or submandibular ganglionic function than of blockade of other ganglia (PERRY and WILSON, 1956; SHIMAMOTO et al., 1958), while other parasympathetic ganglia do not show more than average sensitivity to ganglionic blockade. This phenomenon of abnormal responsiveness of one organ is contrasted by the resistance of some motor pathways of the urinary bladder to ganglionic and even postganglionic pharmacological blockade (for review see TAIRA, 1972). Resistance may not only lie in the organ system per se, but may develop to one particular drug on repeated administration, but not to another of the same type or class. Such tachyphylaxis has been noted with the effect of hexamethonium on the blood pressure of rat (BLACKMAN and LAVERTY, 1961). Sensitisation to catecholamines may be the explanation for this, and the phenomenon may have nothing to do with the ganglionic action of the agent per se (MANTEGAZZA et al., 1958; MAWJI and LOCKETT, 1963). Correspondingly, parasympathetic ganglia do not develop tolerance to agents like hexamethonium (ZAIMIS, 1956). Similar misleading information may arise from the use of other in vivo preparations, such as changes in systemic blood pressure, whose regulation depends on many factors, one of which may be a central inhibitory mechanism sensitive to TEA but not to other types of ganglion-blocking agents (LAPE and HOPPE, 1956). Chemically atypical agents with ganglion-blocking activity may produce unusual results: for example trimethaphan, a sulphonium compound, was shown to have excessive hypotensive potency, partly due to direct peripheral vasodilation McCUBBIN and PAGE, 1952). γ-Amino butyric acid (GABA) depresses ganglion transmission only in relatively large doses and only at some ganglia (MATTHEWS and ROBERTS, 1961). Thus, the true ganglionic action of such an agent remains questionable. Most testing methods for ganglionic blockade have been applied to anaesthetised animals. These were often given anaesthetics that were shown to profoundly influence (depress) ganglionic transmission, sometimes even in subanaesthetic concentrations. Among the better known ones, chloroform aether (LARRABEE and POSTERNAK, 1952) fluothane (RAVENTOS, 1956), amobarbital

Table 3. Concentrations of anaesthetics required for surgical anaesthesia and depression of sympathetic ganglia. Adapted from LARRABEE and POSTERNAK, 1952.

Anaesthetic Substance	Surgical Anaesthesia[a] mM/liter (in blood)	Depression of sympathetic ganglia[a] (mM/liter)[b]	
		Perfusion of cat stellate ganglion	Isolated superior cervical ganglion of rabbit
Chloroform	2.7	3.5	0.25
Aether	18	20	9.6
Nembutal	0.2	< 0.2	0.35
Ethyl alcohol	76	400	550
Urethane	10[c]	10	112

[a] Blood concentrations given mainly for man; doses by weight for animals.
[b] Concentrations reducing amplitude of postganglionic potentials by 20%.
[c] mM/kg.

(ELLIOTT and QUILLIAM, 1964), butabarbital (EXLEY, 1954), and pentobarbital (GAR-RETT, 1963) are known to be highly effective, and thus they could adversely influence evaluation of a blocking agent, particularly if their level is not kept constant during the experiment (Table 3). Temperature and ionic composition are well known to influence virtually all mammalian organ functions. Therefore, particularly in isolated organ preparations, the necessity of maintaining these at constant levels is obvious. Reduction of the calcium ion and increase of the magnesium ion concentration reduce neural output of ACh (JOHNSON, 1963), and correspondingly sodium citrate, binding calcium, was shown to interfere with ganglionic transmission (SHAFER, 1939). The role of potassium in ganglionic transmission has been emphasised since 1934 (BROWN and FELDBERG, 1934). Potassium interferes with the action of many gan-glion-blocking agents (MINKER and KOLTAI, 1961 b). Conversely, these agents may clinically alter serum potassium levels (LUEBECK, 1962), thereby altering the sensitiv-ity of ganglia to subsequently administered doses. Observations concerning the par-ticipation of catecholamines (e.g., noradrenaline and dopamine) in ganglionic trans-mission processes indicate that drugs that deplete catecholamines may indirectly influence synaptic transmission (SJÖSTRAND, 1962).

     Some of the limitations, particularly with in vivo preparations, are due to the relatively intensive anatomical complexity of the neuronal network that surrounds many autonomic ganglia. For example, several interconnected afferent nerves supply the stellate ganglia, and furthermore, the anatomy of its efferent outflow (the cardiac nerves) also lacks constancy (HOLMES and TORRANCE, 1959). There is a similar lack of a direct one-to-one connection at ganglia of the abdominal sympathetic chain with the presence of several collateral and also preganglionic fibres passing through the ganglia, which presents an obvious source of major error in recording (OBRADOR and ODORIZ, 1936). LLOYD (1937) also called attention to a similar complexity of fibres around the mesenteric ganglia, while more recently DOUGLAS and RITCHIE (1956) pointed out the existence of direct preganglionic fibres in the postganglionic trunk of the superior cervical ganglion of the rabbit, a ganglionic system conceived earlier as a prototype of simple, straight-forward "one-relay" ganglionic transmission. In addi-tion, an interesting, and not much explored, subject is the variation of the ganglionic transmission with seasonal changes. Although no such data on mammals have ap-peared, the observations of SINGH (1964) on frog merit attention. He noted that there are significant seasonal changes in the relative proportion of neurotransmitter sub-stances (e.g., 5-HT, substances P and H) released as a result of vagal stimulation. The sensitivity of such preparations to specific blocking agents accordingly underwent seasonal variation.

K. Conclusions

A substantial number of techniques are available for the study of ganglion-blocking agents. Most of them utilise mammalian ganglia, either in vivo or in vitro. Several methods rely on the response of an end organ innervated by the postganglionic nerve appropriate to the ganglion to be studied, while others measure postganglionic nerve activity in the forms of a) trains of impulses (usually elicited by chemical stimula-tion), or b) compound action potentials (evoked by preganglionic electrical stimuli).

The technical requirements, accuracy, specificity, and limitations of the methods vary widely. The object of this chapter was to outline these aspects, in addition to enumerating and evaluating the methods available. Hopefully, it will offer some useful guide to those who are interested in the pharmacological analysis and practical application of ganglion-blocking agents.

References

Aceto, M.D., Bentley, H.C., Dembinski, J.R.: Effects of ganglion-blocking agents on nicotine extensor convulsions and lethality in mice. Br. J. Pharmacol. 37, 104–111 (1969)

Acheson, G.H., Moe, G.K.: The action of TEA ion on the mammalian circulation. J. Pharmacol. Exp. Ther. 87, 220–236 (1946)

Acheson, G.H., Remolina, J.: The temporal course of the effects of postganglionic axotomy on the inferior mesenteric ganglion of the cat. J. Physiol. (Lond.) 127, 603–616 (1955)

Aiken, J.W., Reit, E.: A comparison of the sensitivity to chemical stimuli of adrenergic and cholinergic neurons in the cat stellate ganglion. J. Pharmacol. Exp. Ther. 169, 211–217 (1969)

Alkadhi, K.A., McIsaac, R.J.: Non-nicotinic transmission during ganglionic block with chlorisondamine and nicotine. Eur. J. Pharmacol. 24, 78–85 (1973)

Alkadhi, K.A., McIsaac, R.J.: Effect of preganglionic nerve stimulation on sensitivity of the superior cervical ganglion to nicotinic blocking agents. Br. J. Pharmacol. 51, 533–539 (1974)

Alonso-de Florida, F., Cato, J., Ramirez, L., Pardo, E.G.: Effects of several blocking agents on the sympathetic and parasympathetic postganglionic action potentials. J. Pharmacol. Exp. Ther. 129, 433–437 (1960)

Ambache, N.: The use and limitations of atropine for pharmacological studies on autonomic effectors. Pharmacol. Rev. 7, 467–494 (1955)

Ambache, N., Zar, M.A · Non-cholinergic transmission by postganglionic motor neurons in the mammalian bladder. J. Physiol. (Lond.) 210, 761 783 (1970)

Avis, H.H., Pert, A.: A comparison of the effects of muscarinic and nicotinic anticholinergic drugs on habituation and fear conditioning in rats. Psychopharmacologia 34, 209–222 (1974)

Barlow, R.B.: Introduction to chemical pharmacology, Vol. VI. New York: Wiley and Sons 1964

Barlow, R.B., Franks, F.: Specificity of some ganglion stimulants. Br. J. Pharmacol. 42, 137–142 (1971)

Barlow, R.B., Franks, F.M., Pearson, J.D.: A comparison of the affinities of antagonists for acetylcholine receptors in the ileum, bronchial muscle and iris of the guinea-pig. Br. J. Pharmacol. 46, 300–312 (1972)

Barlow, R.B., Bowman, F., Ison, R.R., McQueen, D.S.: The specificity of some agonists and antagonists for nicotine-sensitive receptors in ganglia. Br. J. Pharmacol. 51, 585–597 (1974)

Beleslin, D.B., Rakic, M.M.: Stimulant action of tetraethylammonium on the peristaltic reflex. Br. J. Pharmacol. 37, 245–250 (1969)

Belmonte, C., Simon, J., Gallego, R., Baron, M.: Sympathetic fibres in the aortic nerve of the cat. Brain Res. 43, 25–35 (1972)

Bentley, G.A.: Pharmacological studies on the hypogastric ganglion of the rat and guinea-pig. Br. J. Pharmacol. 44, 492–509 (1972)

Bentley, G.A., Sabine, J.R.: The effects of ganglion-blocking and postganglionic sympatholytic drugs on preparations of the guinea-pig vas deferens. Br. J. Pharmacol. 21, 190–201 (1963)

Bevan, J.A.: Action of tetraethylammonium chloride on the sympathetic ganglia-pulmonary artery preparation. J. Pharmacol. Exp. Ther. 140, 193–198 (1963)

Bevan, J.A.: Ganglionic blocking agents in selected pharmacological testing methods, Vol. III, pp. 136–254. New York: M. Dekker 1968

Bhagat, B.: Response of isolated guinea-pig atria to various ganglionstimulating agents. J. Pharmacol. Exp. Ther. 154, 264–270 (1966)

Birks, R., MacIntosh, F.C.: Acetylcholine metabolism of a sympathetic ganglion. Can. J. Biochem. Physiol. 39, 787–827 (1961)

Blackman, J.G., Laverty, R.: Peripheral actions of hexamethonium in relation to the decreasing effects of repeated doses on the blood pressure of anesthetized rats. Br. J. Pharmacol. 17, 124–130 (1961)

Blackman, J.G., Purves, R.D.: Ganglionic transmission in the autonomic nervous system. N.Z. Med. J. 67, 376–384 (1968)

Bowman, W.C., Webb, S.N.: Neuromuscular blocking and ganglion blocking activites of some acetylcholine antagonists in the cat. J. Pharm. Pharmacol. 24, 762–772 (1972)

Bronk, D.W., Tower, S.S., Solandt, D.Y., Larrabee, M.G.: The transmission of trains of impulse through a sympathetic ganglion and in its postganglionic nerves. Am. J. Physiol. 122, 1–15 (1938)

Brown, G.L., Trendelenburg, W.: Action of potassium on ganglion. J. Physiol. (Lond.) 86, 290–305 (1936)

Bülbring, E., Dawes, G.S.: A method for the assay of atropine substitutes on the salivary secretion. J. Pharmacol. Exp. Ther. 84, 177–183 (1945)

Bülbring, E., Gershon, M.D.: 5-hydroxytryptamine participation in the vagal inhibitory innervation of the stomach. J. Physiol. (Lond.) 192, 823–846 (1967)

Bülbring, E., Crema, A., Saxby, O.B.: A method for recording peristalsis in isolated intestine. Br. J. Pharmacol. 13, 440–443 (1958)

Burn, J.H., Dale, H.H.: The action of certain quaternary ammonium bases. J. Pharmacol. Exp. Ther. 6, 417–438 (1914)

Burn, J.H., Leach, E.H., Rand, M.J., Thompson, J.W.: Peripheral effects of nicotine and acetylcholine resembling those of sympathetic stimulation. J. Physiol. (Lond.) 148, 332–352 (1959)

Burnstock, G., Campbell, G.: Comparative physiology of the vertebrate autonomic nervous system and innervation of the urinary bladder of the ringtail possum (pseudocheirus peregrinus). J. Exp. Biol. 40, 421–436 (1963)

Bursztajn, S., Gershon, M.D.: Discrimination between nicotinic receptors in vertebrate ganglia and skeletal muscle by alpha-bungarotoxin and cobra venoms. J. Physiol. 269, 17–31 (1977)

Bykov, K.M.: Application of a graphic method in the study of the cells of the sympathetic nervous system. Neurol. vestnik. (Russ.) 19/4, 735–764 (1912)

Campbell, G.: The inhibitory nerve fibres in the vagal supply to the guinea-pig stomach. J. Physiol. (Lond.) 185, 600–612 (1966)

Chandrasekhar, G.R., Soyka, L.F., Gyermek, L.: Sensitivity of different ganglia to ganglionic blockade. Physiologist 2, 23 (1959)

Chen, G., Portman, R., Wickel, A.: Pharmacology of 1,1-Dimethyl-4-Phenylpiperazinium iodide, a ganglion-stimulating agent. J. Pharmacol. Exp. Ther. 103, 330–336 (1951)

Chiang, T.S., Leaders, F.E.: Mechanism for nicotine and DMPP on the isolated rat atria-vagus nerve preparation. J. Pharmacol. Exp. Ther. 149, 225–232 (1965)

Chiba, S., Tamura, L., Kubota, K., Hashimoto, K.: Pharmacologic analysis of nicotine and dimethylphenylipiperazinium on pacemaker activity of SA node in the dog. Jpn. J. Pharmacol. 22, 645–651 (1972)

Chou, T.C., De Elio, F.J.: The blocking effect of bis-triethylammonium salts in transmission in the perfused superior cervical ganglion of the cat. Br. J. Pharmacol. 2, 268–270 (1947)

Collier, B., Katz, H.S.: The release of acetylcholine by acetylcholine in the cat's superior cervical ganglion. Br. J. Pharmacol. 39, 428–438 (1970)

Cook, D.L., Hambourger, W.E., Bianchi, R.G.: Pharmacology of a new autonomic ganglion-blocking agent, 2,6-dimethyl-1-diethyl peperidinium bromide. (SC-1950). J. Pharmacol. Exp. Ther. 99, 435–444 (1950)

Cummings, J.R., Grace, J.L., Latimer, C.N.: Ganglioplegic activity of Di-Tert.-Butylnitroxide, a stable free radical, and analogues. J. Pharmacol. Exp. Ther. 141, 349–355 (1963)

Day, M., Vane, J.R.: An analysis of the direct and indirect actions of drugs on the isolated guinea-pig ileum. Br. J. Pharmacol. 20, 140–170 (1963)

Della Bella, D., Rognoni, F., Teotino, U.N.: Curare-like drugs and vagal synapses: Comparative study in vitro on the isolated vagus-stomach preparation of the rat. J. Pharmacol. 14, 701–706 (1962)

De Groat, W.C., Saum, W.R.: Synaptic transmission in parasympathetic ganglia in the urinary bladder of the cat. J. Physiol. 256, 137–158 (1976)

De Sy, W.A.: Pharmacological interference with the autonomic innervation of the urinary bladder of the cat. Arch. Int. Pharmacodyn. Ther. *196*, 99–101 (1972)

Domer, F.R.: Animal experiments in pharmacological analysis. Springfield, Illinois: Thomas 1971

Douglas, W.W.: The effect of a ganglion-blocking drug, hexamethonium, on the response of the cat's carotid body to various stimuli. J. Physiol. (Lond.) *118*, 373–383 (1952)

Douglas, W.W., Gray, J.A.B.: The excitant action of acetylcholine and other substances on cutaneous sensory pathways and its prevention by hexamethonium and d-tubocurarine. J. Physiol. (Lond.) *119*, 118–128 (1953)

Douglas, W.W., Ritchie, M.: The conduction of impulses through the superior cervical and accessory cervical ganglia of the rabbit. J. Physiol. *113*, 220–231 (1956)

Douglas, W.W., Lywood, D.W., Straub, R.W.: On excitant effect of acetylcholine on structures in the preganglionic trunk of the cervical sympathetic: with a note on the anatomical complexities of the region. J. Physiol. (Lond.) *153*, 250–264 (1960)

Drew, G.M., Leach, G.D.: The effects of anticholinesterases on synaptic transmission through nicotinic and muscarinic receptors in rat sympathetic ganglia in vivo. Br. J. Pharmacol. *52*, 51–59 (1972)

Eccles, J.C.: The physiology of synapses. New York: Academic Press 1964

Eccles, R.M.: Action potentials of isolated mammalian sympathetic ganglia. J. Physiol. (Lond.) *117*, 181–195 (1952)

Eccles, R.M., Libet, B.: Origin and blockage of the synaptic responses of curarized sympathetic ganglia. J. Physiol. (Lond.) *157*, 484–503 (1961)

Edge, N.D.: Mydriasis in the mouse: a quantitative method of estimating parasympathetic ganglion block. Br. J. Pharmacol. *8*, 10–14 (1953)

Edge, N.D.: A constribution to the innervation of the urinary bladder of the cat. J. Physiol. (Lond.) *127*, 54–68 (1955)

Elliott, R.C.: Centrally active drugs and transmission through the isolated superior cervical ganglion preparation of the rabbit when stimulated repetitively. Br. J. Pharmacol. *24*, 76–88 (1965)

Elliott, R.C., Quilliam, J.P.: Some actions of centrally active and other drugs on the transmission of single nerve impulses through the isolated superior cervical ganglion preparation of the rabbit. Br. J. Pharmacol. *23*, 222–240 (1964)

Elliott, T.R.: The innervation of the bladder and urethra. J. Physiol. (Lond.) *35*, 368–445 (1907)

Ellis, S., Rasmussen, H.: The atropine fast nicotine stimulation on the rabbit's intestine and of the muscularis mucosae of the dog's intestine. J. Pharmacol. Exp. Ther. *103*, 259–268 (1951)

Exley, K.A.: Depression of autonomic ganglia by barbituates. Br. J. Pharmacol. *9*, 170–181 (1954)

Farmer, J.D., Rand, M.J., Wilson, J.: Facilitation of ganglionic transmission by some adrenergic neurone blocking drugs. Int. J. Neuropharmacol. *5*, 241–246 (1966)

Farr, W.C., Grupp, G.: Ganglionic stimulation: mechanism of the positive inotropic and chronotropic effects of angiotensin. J. Pharmacol. Exp. Ther. *177*, 48–55 (1971)

Feldberg, W., Gaddum, J.H.: The chemical transmitter at synapses in a sympathetic ganglion. J. Physiol. (Lond.) *81*, 305–319 (1934)

Feldberg, W., Lin, R.C.Y.: The action of local anesthetic and d-tubocurarine on the isolated intestine of the rabbit and guinea-pig. Br. J. Pharmacol. *4*, 33–44 (1949)

Feldberg, W., Minz, B., Tsudzimura, H.: The mechanism of the nervous discharge of adrenaline. J. Physiol. (Lond.) *81*, 286–304 (1934)

Feldberg, W., Vartiainen, A.: Further observations on the physiology and pharmacology of a sympathetic ganglion. J. Physiol. (Lond.) *83*, 103–128 (1934)

Flacke, W., Gillis, R.A.: Dual transmission in the stellate ganglion of the dog. Naunyn Schmiedebergs Arch. Pharmacol. *259*, 165–166 (1968)

Frommel, E., Vincent, D., Gold, P., Melkonian, D., Radouco-Thomas, C., Meyer, M., De Quay, M.B., Vallette, F.: Le diiodure de β-(N-diéthyl-méthylamino) éthoxy-éthyl-N-(méthyl-pyrrolidine): nouveau ganglioplégique. Helv. Physiol. Pharmacol. Acta *13*, 217–244 (1955)

Fukuhara, T., Okada, H., Yamagami, M.: The action of atropine and acetylcholine on the pacemaker ganglion cells of Limulus heart. Jpn. Acta Med. Okayama *14*, 265–270 (1970) (JAP)

Gaddum, J.H.: The technique of superfusion. Br. J. Pharmacol. *8*, 321–326 (1953)

Gaddum, J.H., Picarelli, Z.P.: Two kinds of tryptamine receptor. Br. J. Pharmacol. *12*, 323–328 (1957)

Garrett, J.: Selective blockade of sympathetic or parasympathetic ganglia. Arch. Int. Pharmacodyn. *144*, 381–391 (1963)

Gebber, G.L., Volle, R.L.: Mechanisms involved in ganglionic blockade induced by tetramethylammonium. J. Pharmacol. Exp. Ther. *152*, 18–28 (1966)

Gillis, R.A., Jolson, H., Thibodeaux, H., Levitt, B.: Antagonism of deslanatoside-induced cardiotoxicity by combined nicotinic and muscarinic blockade of autonomic ganglia. J. Pharmacol. Exp. Ther. *195*, 126–132 (1975)

Ginsborg, B.L., Guerrero, S.: On the action of depolarizing drugs on sympathetic ganglion cells of the frog. J. Physiol. (Lond.) *172*, 189–206 (1964)

Ginzel, K.H., Klupp, H., Kraupp, O., Werner, G.: Ganglionär blockierende Wirkungen von polymethylen-bis-phosphonium-verbindungen. Arch. Exp. Pathol. Pharmakol. *221*, 336–350 (1954)

Giono, H., Chevillard, H.: Method for study of ganglion-blocking substances. C. R. Soc. Biol. (Paris) *156*, 1048–1050 (1962)

Gonella, J., Vienot, J.: Action of ganglioplegics on duodenal peristalsis propagation. J. Physiol. (Paris) *64*, 623–630 (1972)

Gráca, A.S., Hilton, J.G., Silva, A.J.: Effects of muscarinic ganglionic stimulation and blockade upon ganglion responses to DMPP and nicotine. Arch. Int. Pharmacodyn. Ther. *186*, 379–387 (1970)

Greeff, K., Kasperat, H., Osswald, W.: Paradoxical effects of electrical stimulation of the vagus nerve on the isolated stomach and atrial preparation of the guinea-pig and its alteration by ganglionic-blocking agents, sympatholytics, reserpine and cocaine. Naunyn Schmiedebergs Arch. Pharmacol. *243*, 528–545 (1962) (GER)

Grimson, K.S., Tarazi, A.K., Frazer, J.W.: Ganglion blocking actions of new quaternary ammonium compound Su 3088 in dog and man. Angiology *6*, 507–512 (1955)

Guyonneau, M.: Relation between chemical constitution and some pharmacological actions. Reciprocal influence of some structural factors encumbrance, polar groups, distances between the active centers on the spasmolytic, synaptotropic and curariform properties. J. Physiol. (Paris) *54*, 1–88 (1962) (FRE)

Gyermek, L.: Differences between atopine-like and ganglionic blocking agents in their action on the mouse pupil. J. Pharmacol. Exp. Ther. *127*, 313–316 (1959)

Gyermek, L.: Cholinergic stimulation and blockade on the urinary bladder. Am. J. Physiol. *201*, 325–328 (1961)

Gyermek, L.: Action of 5-Hydroxytryptamine on the urinary bladder of the dog. Arch. Int. Pharmacodyn. *137*, 137–144 (1962)

Gyermek, L.: Drugs which antagonize 5-Hydroxytryptamine and related indolealkylamines. In: Handbuch der Exp. Pharmakol. Ergänswk. XIX. Erspamer, V. (Ed.) Heidelberg: Springer 1966

Gyermek, L.: Ganglionic stimulant and depressant agents. In: Drugs affecting the peripheral nervous system. Burger, A. (Ed.), Vol. I, pp. 149–326. New York: Dekker 1967

Gyermek, L., Bindler, E.: Blockade of the ganglionic stimulant action of 5-Hydroxytryptamine. J. Pharmacol. Exp. Ther. *135*, 344–348 (1962)

Gyermek, L., Unna, K.R.: Pharmacological comparison of muscarine and muscarone with their dehydro derivatives. J. Pharmacol. Exp. Ther. *128*, 37–40 (1960)

Gyermek, L., Sigg, E.B., Bindler, E.: Ganglionic stimulant action of muscarine. Am. J. Physiol. *204*, 68–70 (1963)

Haefely, W.: Electrophysiology of the adrenergic neurone, pp. 662–725. In: Handb. Exp. Pharmakol., Blaschko, H., Muscholl, E. (Eds.), Vol. XXXIII. Heidelberg: Springer 1972

Haefely, W.: The effects of 1, 1-dimethyl 4 phenyl piperazinium (DMPP) in the cat superior cervical ganglion in situ. Naunyn Schmiedebergs Arch. Pharmacol. *281*, 57–91 (1974a)

Haefely, W.: Muscarinic postsynaptic events in the cat superior cervical ganglion in situ. Naunyn Schmiedebergs Arch. Pharmacol. *281*, 199–143 (1974b)

Haefely, W.: The effects of 5-Hydroxytryptamine and some related compounds on the cat superior cervical ganglion in situ. Naunyn Schmiedebergs Arch. Pharmacol. *281*, 145–165 (1974c)

Hamburg, M.D., Paparo, A.: Cholinergic influence on unit activity of the visceral ganglion of the mussel, mytilus edulis, and the control of ciliary movement -II. Comp. Biochem Physiol. *51 C*, 41–47 (1975)

Hancock, J.C., Volle, R.L.: Blockade of conduction in vagal fibres by nicotinic drugs. Arch. Int. Pharmacodyn. *178*, 85–98 (1969a)

Hancock, J., Volle, R.L.: Enhancement by cesium of ganglionic hyperpolarization induced by dimethylphenylpiperazinium (DMPP) and repetitive preganglionic simulation. J. Pharmacol. Exp. Ther. *169*, 201–210 (1969b)

Harada, M., Ozaki, Y., Sato, M.: Ganglion blocking effect of indole alkaloids contained in uncaria genus and amsonia genus and related synthetic compounds on the rat superior cervical ganglion in situ. Chem. Pharm. Bull. (Tokyo) *22*, 1372–1377 (1974)

Harry, J.: The action of drugs on the circular muscle-strip from the guinea-pig isolated ileum. Br. J. Pharmacol. *20*, 399–417 (1963)

Henderson, C.G., Ungar, A.: Effect of cholinergic antagonists on sympathetic ganglionic transmission of vasomotor reflexes from the carotid baroreceptors of the dog. J. Physiol. *277*, 379–385 (1978)

Herr, F., Gyermek, L.: Action of cholinergic stimulants on the inferior mesenteric ganglion of the cat. J. Pharmacol. Exp. Ther. *129*, 338–342 (1960)

Hertting, G., Potter, L.T., Axelrod, J.: Effect of decentralization and ganglionic blocking agents on the spontaneous release of H^3-norepinephrine. J. Pharmacol. Exp. Ther. *136*, 289–292 (1962)

Hertzler, E.: 5-HT and transmission in sympathetic ganglia. Br. J. Pharmacol. *17*, 406–413 (1961)

Holman, M.E., Muir, T.C., Szurszewszki, J.H., Yonemura, K.: Effects of iontophoretic application of cholinergic agonists and their antagonists to guinea-pig pelvic ganglia. Br. J. Pharmacol. *41*, 26–40 (1971)

Holmes, R., Torrance, R.W.: Afferant fibres of the stellate ganglion. Q. J. Exp. Physiol. *44*, 271–281 (1959)

Huković, S.: The action of sympathetic blocking agents on isolated and innervated atria and vessels. Br. J. Pharmacol. *15*, 117–121 (1960)

Huković, S.: Responses of the isolated sympathetic nerv ductus deferens preparation of the guinea pig. Br. J. Pharmacol. *16*, 188–194 (1961)

Isabel, J.B., Towers, B., Adams, F.H., Gyepes, M.T.: The effects of ganglionic blockade on tracheobronchial muscle in fetal and newborn lambs. Respir. Physiol. *15*, 255–267 (1972)

Jancso, N., Jancso-Gabor, A., Takats, I.: Pain and inflammation induced by nicotine, acetylcholine, and structurally related compounds and their prevention by desensitizing agents. Acta. Physiol. Acad. Sci. Hung. *19*, 113–132 (1961)

Jaramillo, J., Volle, R.L.: Ganglion blockade by muscarine, oxotremorine, and AHR-692. J. Pharmacol. Exp. Ther. *158*, 80–88 (1967)

Johnson, E.S.: The origin of the acetylcholine released spontaneously from the guinea-pig isolated ileum. Br. J. Pharmacol. *21*, 555–568 (1963)

Jones, A.: Ganglionic actions of muscarinic substances. J. Pharmacol. Exp. Ther. *141*, 195–205 (1963)

Jones, B., Gomez Alonso, B., Trendelenburg, U.: The pressor response of the spinal cat to different groups of ganglion-stimulation agents. J. Pharmacol. Exp. Ther. *139*, 312–320 (1963)

Judge, S.E., Kerkut, G.A., Walker, R.J.: Properties of an identified synaptic pathway in the visceral ganglion of helix aspersa. Comp. Biochem. Physiol. *57 C*, 101–106 (1977)

Kadatz, R., Klupp, H.: Die pharmakologischen Wirkungen des 2-(p-Butoxyphenyl)-2-(Tetrahydro-1, 4-Oxazino-methyl)-Dioxolan-(1,3)-Methylbromids, (Q 160). Arch. Exp. Pathol. Pharmakol. *227*, 383–392 (1956)

Kaindl, F., Werner, G.: Über die Wirkung von Eserin auf die Aktionsströme der Carotistinusnerven. Arch. Int. Pharmacodyn. *76*, 205–212 (1948)

Kamijo, K., Koelle, G.B.: The relationship between cholinesterase inhibition and ganglionic transmission. J. Pharmacol. Exp. Ther. *105*, 349–357 (1952)

Kehoe, J.: Three acetylcholine receptors in aplysia neurones. J. Physiol. (Lond.) *225*, 115–146 (1972)

Kelkar, V.V., Gulati, O.D., Gokhale, S.D.: Effects of ganglion-blocking drugs on the responses of the rabbit aortic strip to adrenaline, noradrenaline and other vasoactive substances. Arch. Int. Pharmacodyn. *149*, 209–222 (1964)

Kewitz, H.: Zur Bedeutung des Acetylcholins als Übertragersubstanz sympatischer Ganglien. Arch. Exp. Pathol. Pharmakol. *222*, 323–329 (1954)

Kewitz, H., Reinert, H.: Wirkung verschiedener Sympathicomimetica auf die chemisch und elektrisch ausgelöste Erregung des oberen Halsganglions. Arch. Exp. Pathol. Pharmakol. *222*, 311–314 (1954)

Kharkevich, D.A.: Effects of ganglioplegics on after-discharges. Byull. Eksp. Biol. I. Med. *49*, 62–66 (1960) (RUSS.)

Kharkevich, D.A.: Ganglionic agents. Moskva: "Medgiz" 1962 (RUSS.)

Kharkevich, D.A.: Ganglion-blocking and ganglion-stimulating agents. Oxford: Pergamon Press 1967 (translated from Russian edition, 1962)

Kibiakov, A.V., Eremeev, V.S., Mel'Man, IaI.: Efferent inhibitory effect of sensory nerves on the heart. Fiziol. Zh. S.S.S.R. *60*, 1434–1438 (1974) (RUSS.)

Kibjakow, A.W.: Über humorale Übertragung der Erregung von einem Neuron auf das andere. Pflügers Arch. *232*, 432–443 (1933)

Koelle, G.B.: A proposed dual neurohumoral role of acetylcholine: its functions at the pre- and postsynaptic sites. Nature *190*, 208–211 (1961)

Koketsu, K.: Cholinergic synaptic potentials and the underlying ionic mechanisms. Fed. Proc. *28*, 101–112 (1969)

Komalahiranya, A., Volle, R.L.: Actions of inorganic ions and veratrine on asynchronous post-ganglionic discharge in sympathetic ganglia treated with diisopropyl, phosphorofluoridate (DFP). J. Pharmacol. Exp. Ther. *138*, 57–65 (1962)

Komalahiranya, A., Volle, R.L.: Alterations of transmission in sympathetic ganglia treated with a sulfhydryl-group inhibitor, N-Ethylmaleimide (NEM). J. Pharmacol. Exp. Ther. *139*, 304–311 (1963)

Konzett, H., Rothlin, E.: Beeinflussung der nikotinartigen Wirkung von Acetylkolin durch Atropin. Helv. Physiol. Pharmacol. Acta 7, 46–47 C (1949)

Konzett, H., Rothlin, E.: Die Wirkung synaptotroper Substanzen auf gewisse efferente und afferente Strukturen des autonomen Nervensystems. Experientia 9, 405–412 (1953)

Konzett, H., Waser, P.G.: The ganglionic action of muscarine. Helv. Physiol. Pharmakol. Acta *14*, 202–206 (1956)

Koppanyi, T., Dille, J.M., Linegat, C.R.: Studies on synergism and antagonism of drugs; action of physostigmine on autonomic ganglion. J. Pharmacol. Exp. Ther. *58*, 105–110 (1936)

Kosterlitz, H.W., Wallis, D.I.: The effects of hexamethonium and morphine on transmission in the superior cervical ganglion of the rabbit. Br. J. Pharmacol. *26*, 334–344 (1966)

Kratskin, I.L.: A study of central nicotine-sensitive cholinoreceptors by introducing bis-quaternary ammonium compounds into the lateral cerebral ventricles. Farmakol. Toksikol. *36*, 261–266 (1973) (RUSS.)

Krstic, M.K.: The action of arecoline on the superior cervical ganglion of the cat. Arch. Int. Pharmacodyn. *194*, 238–252 (1971)

Kuba, K., Koketsu, K.: The muscarinic effects of acetylcholine on the action potential of bullfrog sympathetic ganglion cells. Jap. J. Physiol. *26*, 703–716 (1976)

Langley, J.N., Dickinson, W.L.: On the local paralysis of the peripheral ganglia and on the connexion of different classes of nerve fibres with them. Proc. Roy. Soc. (Lond.) *46*, 423–431 (1889)

Lape, H.E., Hoppe, J.O.: The use of serial carotid occlusion, nictitating membrane and cross-circulation technics in the investigation of the central hypotensive activity of ganglionic blocking agents. J. Pharmacol. Exp. Ther. *116*, 453–461 (1956)

Larrabee, H.G., Holaday, D.A.: Depression of transmission through sympathetic ganglia during general anesthesia. J. Pharmacol. Exp. Ther. *105*, 400–408 (1952)

Larrabee, H.G., Posternak, J.M.: Selective action of anesthetics on synapses and axons in mammalian sympathetic ganglia. J. Neurophysiol. *15*, 91–114 (1952)

Lawrence, D.R., Stacey, R.S.: Effect of methonium compounds on nicotine convulsions. Br. J. Pharmacol. 7, 80–84 (1952)

Leach, G.D.H.: The electrically stimulated ileum of the guinea-pig for measuring acetylcholine antagonism at different sites. J. Pharm. Pharmacol. *18*, 265–270 (1966)

Lechat, P., Lamarche, M., Renier-Cornec, A.: Contribution à l'étude pharmacodynamique de la mécamylamine. Therapie *16*, 252–264 (1961)

Lee, G.E., Wragg, W.R., Corne, S.J., Edge, N.E., Reading, H.W.: Pentamethylpiperidine: a new hypotensive drug. Nature *181*, 1717–1719 (1958)

Levine, R.M., Blair, M.R., Clark, B.B.: Factors influencing the intestinal absorption of certain monoquaternary anticholinergic compounds with special reference to benzomethamine [n-diethylaminoethyl-n'-methyl-benzilamide methobromide (MC-3199)]. J. Pharmacol. Exp. Ther. *114*, 78–86 (1955)

Levy, B., Ahlquist, R.P.: Sympathetic ganglion stimulants. J. Pharmacol. Exp. Ther. *137*, 219–228 (1962)

Levy, J., Mathieu, N., Michel-Ber, E.: Relations entre la constitution chimique et les actions parasympathomimétiques, nicotiniques et curarisantes de quelques ammoniums quáternaires de formide générale. J. Physiol. (Paris) *50*, 1043–1065 (1958)

Lewis, G.P., Reit, E.: The action of angiotensin and bradykinin on the superior cervical ganglion of the cat. J. Physiol. (Lond.) *179*, 538–553 (1965)

Libet, B.: Generation of slow inhibitory and excitatory postsynaptic potentials. Fed. Proc. *29*, 1945–1956 (1970)

Liddel, E.G.T., Sherrington, C.: Mammalian physiology. New York: Oxford Press 1929

Ling, H.W.: Actions of dimethylphenylpiperazinium. Br. J. Pharmacol. *14*, 505–511 (1959)

Lloyd, D.P.C.: The transmission of impulses throug the inferior mesenteric ganglion. J. Physiol. (Lond.) *91*, 296–313 (1937)

Locket, S.: Two new ganglion-blocking agents in treatment of hypertension. Br. Med. J. *1956 II*, 116–122

Luco, J.V., Marconi, J.: Effects of tetraethylammonium bromide on parasympathetic neuroeffector system. J. Pharmacol. Exp. Ther. *95*, 171–176 (1949)

Luebeck, I.: The serum potassium level under ganglion block as a problem of the intravasal volume output. Z. Gesamte Inn. Med. *17*, 908–910 (1962) (GER)

Magnus, R.: Versuche am überlebenden Dünndarm von Säugethieren. Pflügers Arch. *102*, 123 (1904)

Malmejac, J.: Action of adrenaline on synaptic transmission and on adrenal medullary secretion. J. Physiol. (Lond.) *130*, 497–512 (1955)

Mantegazza, P., Naimzada, K.M.M.: Observations on an isolated preparation of guinea-pig urinary bladder stimulated through the hypogastric nerves. Eur. J. Pharmacol. *1*, 396–401 (1967)

Mantegazza, P., Tyler, C., Zaimis, E.: The peripheral action of hexamethonium and of pentolinium. Br. J. Pharmacol. *13*, 480–484 (1958)

Marley, E., Paton, W.D.M.: The output of sympathetic amines from the cat's adrenal gland in response to splanchnic nerve activity. J. Physiol. (Lond.) *155*, 1–27 (1961)

Marlier, R.: Action ganglioplégiques sur le ganglion cervical supérieur chez le chien. Arch. Int. Pharmacodyn. *129*, 371–380 (1960)

Martin, A.R., Pilar, G.: Transmission through the ciliary ganglion of the chick. J. Physiol. (Lond.) *168*, 464–475 (1963)

Masevich, S.G.: Effect of ganglion-blocking substances (tetamon-I hexonium) on basic stomach functions in clinic and laboratory. Tr. Leningr. Sanit-Gigien. Med. Inst. *59*, 285–289 (1960) (RUSS.)

Mason, D.F.J., Wien, R.: The actions of heterocyclic bisquaternary compounds, especially of a pyrrolidinium series. Br. J. Pharmacol. *109*, 124–132 (1955)

Matthews, R.J.: The effect of epinephrine, levarterenol and dl-isoproterenol on transmission in the superior cervical ganglion of the cat. J. Pharmacol. exp. Ther. *116*, 433–443 (1956)

Metthews, R.J., Roberts, B.J.: The effect of γ-aminobutyric acid on synaptic transmission in autonomic ganglia. J. Pharmacol. Exp. Ther. *132*, 19–22 (1961)

Mawji, S., Lockett, M.F.: Pressor effect of adrenaline, noradrenaline and reflex vasoconstriction sensitised by low concentrations of ganglion blocking drugs. J. Pharm. Pharmacol. *15*, 45–55 (1963)

Maxwell, G.M., Kneebone, G.M., Elliott, R.B.: Pharmacology of 1,1-dimethyl-4-phenylpiperazinium iodide in the intact dog. Arch. Int. Pharmacodyn. Ther. *143*, 431–437 (1963)

Maxwell, R.D.G., Campbell, A.J.M.: New sympathicolytic agents. Lancet 1953 *CCLXIV*, 455–457

McCubbin, J.W., Page, I.H.: Nature of the hypotensive action of a thiophanium derivative (RO 2-2222) in dogs. J. Pharmacol. *105*, 437–444 (1952)

McIsaac, R.J.: Relation between distribution and pharmacological activity of hexamethonium-N-methyl-C^{14}. J. Pharmacol. Exp. Ther. *135*, 335–343 (1962)

McKendrick, C.S., Jones, P.O.: Pentacynium bis-methylsulphate (presidal) in the management of hypertension. Lancet 1958 *I*, 340–343

Minker, E., Koltai, M.: Effect of ganglion excidation after treatment with-ganglion-blocking agents. Acta Physiol. Acad. Sci. Hung. *20*, 411–420 (1961a) (GER.)

Minker, E., Koltai, M.: Reciprocal effects of ganglionic blocking agents and potassium salts. Acta Physiol. Acad. Sci. Hung. *20*, 187–195 (1961b) (GER.)

Moe, G.K., Capo, L.R., Peralta, R.B.: Action of TEA on chemoreceptor and stretchreceptor mechanisms. Am. J. Physiol. *153*, 601–605 (1948)

Moe, G.K., Freyburger, W.A.: Ganglionic blocking agents. Pharmacol. Rev. *2*, 61–95 (1950)

Mohanty, J.K.: The development of tolerance and cross-tolerance to methonium compounds in laboratory animals. Br. J. Pharmacol. *10*, 279–287 (1955)

Morrison, B.: Parenteral hexamethonium in hypertension. Br. Med. J. 1953 *VII*, 1289–1299

Morrison, B., Paton, W.D.M.: Effects of hexamethonium on normal individuals in relation to its concentration in the plasma. Br. Med. J. 1953 *VII*, 1299–1305

Morrison, C.F., Goodyear, J.M., Sellers, C.M.: Antagonism by antimuscarinic and ganglion-blocking drugs of some of the behavioural effects of nicotine. Psychopharmacologia *15*, 341–350 (1969)

Moyer, J.H., Brest, A.N.: Drug therapy of hypertension. V. Observations on the results with ganglion-blocking agents given in combination with rauwolfia and chlorothiazide. Arch. Intern. Med. *108*, 231–247 (1961)

Murayama, S., Unna, K.R.: Stimulant action of 4-(m-chlorophenylcarbamoyloxy)-2-butynyltri-methylammonium chloride (McN-A-343) on sympathetic ganglia. J. Pharmacol. Exp. Ther. *140*, 183–192 (1963)

Muscholl, E., Vogt, M.: The action of reserpine on the peripheral sympathetic system. J. Physiol. *141*, 132–155 (1958)

Nádor, K.: Ganglienblocker. Prog. Drug Res. *2*, 303–411 (1960)

Nilwises, N., Schmidt, G.: Effects of atropine compounds on the synaptic transmission in the isolated rat cervical ganglion. Naunyn Schmiedebergs Arch. Pharmacol. *251*, 335–343 (1965)

Nishi, S.: Cholinergic and adrenergic receptors at sympathetic preganglionic nerve terminals. Fed. Proc. *29*, 1957–1971 (1970)

Nishi, S., Soeda, H., Koketsu, K.: Studies on sympathetic B and C neurons and patterns of preganglionic innervation. J. Cell. Comp. Physiol. *66*, 19–32 (1965)

Obrador, S., Odoriz, I.B.: Transmission through a lumbar sympathetic ganglion. J. Physiol. (Lond.) *86*, 269–276 (1936)

Pappano, A.J., Volle, R.L.: The reversal by atropine of ganglionic blockade produced by acetyl-choline or methacholine. Life Sci. *1*, 677–682 (1962)

Pardo, E.G., Mendez, J., Vargas, R., Laguna, C., Laguna, J.: Pharmacologic actions of ethyl-methyl-isooctenyl amine (EMOA), new parasympathetic ganglionic blocking agent. J. Pharmacol. Exp. Ther. *116*, 377–386 (1956)

Pardo, E.G., Cato, J., Gijon, E., Alonso-de Florida, F.: Influence of several adrenergic drugs on synaptic transmission through the superior cervical and the ciliary ganglia of the cat. J. Pharmacol. Exp. Ther. *139*, 296–303 (1963)

Paton, W.D.M., Perry, W.L.M.: Relationship between depolarization and block in cat's superior cervical ganglion. J. Physiol. (Lond.) *119*, 43–57 (1953)

Paton, W.D.M., Thompson, J.W.: The ganglion blocking action of procainamide. Br. J. Pharmacol. *22*, 143–153 (1964)

Paton, W.D.M., Vane, J.R.: An analysis of the responses of the isolated stomach to electrical stimulation and to drug. J. Physiol. (Lond.) *165*, 10–46 (1963)

Paton, W.D.M., Zaimis, E.J.: Pharmacological actions of polymethylene bistrimethylammonium salts. Br. J. Pharmacol. *4*, 381–400 (1949)

Paton, W.D.M., Zaimis, E.J.: Paralysis of autonomic ganglia by methonium salts. Br. J. Pharmacol. *6*, 155–158 (1951)

Paton, W.D.M., Zaims, E.J.: The methonium compounds. Pharmacol. Rev. 4, 219–253 (1952)

Pelikan, E.W.: The mechanism of ganglionic blockade produced by nicotine. Ann. N.Y. Acad. Sci. 90, 52–69 (1960)

Penna, M., Aviado, D.M.: Stimulation of aortic body chemoreceptors by ganglion stimulants. Arch. Int. Pharmacodyn. Ther. 140, 269–280 (1962)

Perri, V., Sacchi, O., Cosella, C.: Synaptically mediated potentials elicited by the stimulation of post-ganglionic trunks in the guinea-pig superior cervical ganglion. Pflügers Arch. 314, 55–67 (1970)

Perry, W.L.M.: Central and synaptic transmission. Annu. Rev. Physiol. 18, 279–308 (1956)

Perry, W.L.M.: Transmission in autonomic ganglia. Br. Med. Bull. 13, 220–226 (1957)

Perry, W.L.M., Talesnik, J.: The role of acetylcholine in synaptic transmission at parasympathetic ganglia. J. Physiol. (Lond.) 119, 445–469 (1953)

Perry, W.L.M., Wilson, C.W.M.: The relative effects of ganglion-blocking compounds on the sympathetic and parasympathetic ganglia supplying the cat heart. Br. J. Pharmacol. 11, 81–88 (1956)

Piggott, S.M., Kerkut, G.A., Walker, R.J.: Structure-activity studies on glutamate receptor sites of three identifiable neurones in the suboesophageal ganglia of helix aspersa. Comp. Biochem. Physiol. 51 C, 91–100 (1975)

Plummer, A.M., Schneider, J.A., Barrett, W.E.: A series of tris(dialkylaminoalkyl) amines with ganglionic blocking activity. Arch. Int. Pharmacodyn. 97, 1–13 (1954)

Plummer, A.J., Trapold, J.H., Schneider, J.A., Maxwell, R.A., Earl, A.E.: Ganglionic blockade by new bisquaternary series, including chlorisondamine dimethochloride. J. Pharmacol. Exp. Ther. 115, 172–184 (1955)

Quilliam, J.P., Shand, D.G.: The selectivity of drugs blocking ganglionic transmission in the rat. Br. J. Pharmacol. 23, 273–284 (1964)

Raventos, J.: The action of fluothane – a new volatile anesthetic. Br. J. Pharmacol. 11, 394–409 (1956)

Reinert, H.: Role and origin of noradrenaline in the superior cervical ganglion. J. Physiol. (Lond.) 167, 18–29 (1963)

Riker, W.K., Komalahiranya, A.: Observations on the frequency dependence of sympathetic ganglion blockade. J. Pharmacol. Exp. Ther. 137, 267–274 (1962)

Riker, W.K., Szreniawski, Z.: The pharmacological reactivity of presynaptic nerve terminals in a sympathetic ganglion. J. Pharmacol. Exp. Ther. 126, 233–238 (1959)

Roch-Ramel, F.: Metabolisme et "survie functionelle", du ganglion sympathique cervical isolé du rat. Helv. Physiol. Pharmacol. Acta 13, 1–64 (1962)

Roszkowski, A.P.: An unusual type of sympathetic ganglionic stimulant. J. Pharmacol. Exp. Ther. 132, 156–170 (1961)

Rubinstein, K., Pederson, J.G.A., Fakstorp, J.: Hypotensive and ganglion blocking action of methyl substituted 3-amino-norcamphanes. Experientia 14, 222–223 (1958)

Saito, H.: The blocking effect of autonomic ganglionic blocking agents upon the celiac ganglion. II. Comparative observations on the celiac ganglion blocking effects of autonomic ganglionic blocking agents with the splenic volume change as an indicator. Nippon Yakurigaku Zasshi 57, 32–51 (1961) (JAP)

Sanghvi, I., Murayama, S., Smith, C.M., Unna, K.R.: Action of muscarine on the superior cervical ganglion of the cat. J. Pharmacol. Exp. Ther. 142, 192–199 (1963)

Saxena, P.R.: Effect of some drugs on the responses of the vas deferens and seminal vesicle to hypogastric nerve stimulation in guinea pig in vivo. Pharmacology 3, 220–228 (1970)

Saxena, P.R.: Contraction of the urinary bladder by muscarinic ganglionic stimulants: possible existence of muscarinic receptor sites on its parasympathetic ganglia. Arch. Int. Pharmacodyn. Ther. 199, 16–28 (1972)

Schneider, J.A., Moore, Jr., R.F.: Electrophysiological investigation of chlorisondamine dimethochloride (ecolid). New ganglionic blocking agent. Proc. Soc. Exp. Biol. 89, 450–453 (1955)

Sethi, O.P., Gulati, O.D.: Analysis of mode of action of some nicotinic blocking drugs. Jpn. J. Pharmacol. 23, 437–451 (1973)

Shafer, G.D.: Calcium ions necessary to synaptic transmission in parasymphatetic, not in sympathetic, ganglia. J. Pharmacol. Exp. Ther. 67, 341–352 (1939)

Shimamoto, K., Inoue, K., Ogiu, K.: Relative pharmacological effects of a series of quaternary alkaloids isolated from magnolia and cocculus plants. Jpn. J. Pharmacol. 7, 135–156 (1958)

Singh, I.: Seasonal variations in the nature of neurotransmitters in a frog vagus-stomach muscle preparation. Arch. Int. Physiol. Biochem. *72*, 843–851 (1964)

Sjöstrand, N.O.: Effect of reserpine and hypogastric denervation on the noradrenaline content of the vas deferens and the seminal vesicle of the guinea-pid. Acta Physiol. Scand. *56*, 376–380 (1962)

Smirk, F.H.: Hypotensive actions of hexamethonium bromide and some of its homologues; their use in high blood pressure. Lancet *1952 II*, 1002–1005

Smirk, F.H.: Action of a new methonium compound in arterial hypertension; pentamethylene 1:5 bis-n-(n-methyl-pyrrolidinium) bitartrate (M. & B. 2050A). Lancet *1953 I*, 457–464

Smirk, F.H.: Hypertension therapy. In: Current therapy. Conn, H.F. (Ed.). Philadelphia: Saunders 1964

Smirk, F.H., Hodge, J.V.: Six new hypotensive chemical relatives of pempidine. Clin. Pharmacol. Ther. *1*, 610–616 (1960)

Spinks, A., Young, E.H.P., Farrington, J.A., Dunlop, D.: The pharmacological actions of pempidine and its ethyl homologue. Br. J. Pharmacol. *13*, 501–521 (1958)

Stille, G., Hilfiker, H.: The testing of parasympathetic-ganglioplegic substances on the urinary bladder of the rabbit in situ. Arch. Int. Pharmacodyn. *130*, 211–219 (1961) (GER.)

Stone, C.A., Torchiana, M.L., Navarro, A., Beyer, K.H.: Ganglionic blocking properties of 3-methylaminoisocamphane hydrochloride (mecamylamine): a secondary amine. J. Pharmacol. Exp. Ther. *117*, 169–183 (1956a)

Stone, C.A., Torchiana, M.L., O'Neill, G.Q., Beyer, K.H.: Ganglionic blocking properties of 3-methylaminoisocamphane hydrochloride (mecamylamine): a secondary amine. J. Pharmacol. Exp. Ther. *116*, 54–55 (1956b)

Stone, C.A., Meckelnburg, K.L., Torchiana, M.L.: Antagonism of nicotine-induced convulsions by ganglionic blocking agents. Arch. Int. Pharmacodyn. *117*, 419–434 (1958)

Stone, C.A., Torchiana, M.L., Meckelnberg, K.L., Stavorski, J., Sletzinger, M., Stein, G.A., Ruyle, W.V., Reinhold, D.F., Gaines, W.A., Arnold, H., Pfister, K., III: Chemistry structure-activity relationships of mecamylamine and derivatives. J. Med. Pharm. Chem. *5*, 665–690 (1962)

Suwandi, I.S., Bevan, J.A.: Antagonism of lobeline by ganglion-blocking agents at afferent nerve endings. J. Pharmacol. Exp. Ther. *153*, 1–7 (1966)

Taira, N.: The autonomic pharmacology of the bladder. Annu. Rev. Pharmacol. *12*, 197–208 (1972)

Taira, N., Matsumura, S., Hashimoto, L: Excitation of the parasympathetic ganglia of the canine urinary bladder through a muscarinic mechanism. J. Pharmacol. Exp. Ther. *176*, 93–100 (1971)

Takeshige, C., Volle, R.L.: Asynchronous postganglionic firing from the cat superior cervical sympathetic ganglion treated with neostigmine. Br. J. Pharmacol. *20*, 214–220 (1963)

Takeshige, C., Volle, R.L.: A comparison of the ganglion potentials and block produced by acetylcholine and tetramethylammonium. Br. J. Pharmacol. *23*, 80–89 (1964)

Takeshige, C., Pappano, A.J., De Groot, W.C., Volle, R.L.: Ganglionic blockade produced in sympathetic ganglia by cholinomimetic drugs. J. Pharmacol. Exp. Ther. *141*, 333–342 (1963)

Thomas, G.A., Trounce, J.R.: The effect of neuromuscular and ganglion blockade on the function of the guinea-pig esophagus. Guy's Hosp. Repts. *109*, 21–28 (1960)

Tollack, J.L., Grupp, G., Farr, W.C.: Functional studies of right cardiac sympathetic nerves and ganglia in the dog. Proc. Soc. Exp. Biol. Med. *137*, 772–775 (1971)

Trendelenburg, P.: Physiologische und pharmakologische Versuche über die Dünndarmperistaltik. Arch. Exp. Pathol. Pharmakol. *81*, 55–119 (1917)

Trendelenburg, U.: The action of 5-dydroxytryptamine on the nictitating membrane and on the superior cervical ganglion of the cat. Br. J. Pharmacol. *11*, 74–80 (1956)

Trendelenburg, U.: The action of histamine, pilocarpine, and 5-hydroxypytamine on transmission through the superior cervical ganglion. J. Physiol. (Lond.) *135*, 66–72 (1957a)

Trendelenburg, U.: Reaktion sympathischer Ganglien während der Ganglienblockade durch Nicotin. Arch. Exp. Pathol. Pharmakol. *230*, 448–456 (1957b)

Trendelenburg, U.: Mode of action of some nondepolarizing ganglion-blocking substances. Arch. Exp. Pathol. Pharmakol. *241*, 452–466 (1961a)

Trendelenburg, U.: Pharmacology of autonomic ganglia. Annu. Rev. Pharmacol. *1*, 219–238 (1961b)

Trendelenburg, U.: Some aspects of the pharmacology of autonomic ganglion cells. Ergeb. Physiol. *59*, 1–85 (1967)

Ursillo, R.C.: Investigation of certain aspects of atropine-resistant nerve effects. J. Pharmacol. Exp. Ther. *131*, 231–236 (1961)

Ursillo, R.C., Clark, B.B.: Pharmacology of anticholinergic quaternary ammonium compound benzomethamine [N-diethylaminoethyl-N′methylbenzilamide methobromide (MC 3199) with note on tertiary amine analogue (MC 3137)]. J. Pharmacol. Exp. Ther. *114*, 54–62 (1955)

Vanov, S.: Responses of the urinary bladder in situ to drugs and to nerve stimulation. Br. J. Pharmacol. *24*, 591–600 (1965)

Volle, R.L.: The actions of several ganglion blocking agents on the postganglionic discharge induced by diisopropyl phosphorofluoridate (DFP) in sympathetic ganglia. J. Pharmacol. Exp. Ther. *135*, 45–53 (1962a)

Volle, R.L.: The responses to ganglionic stimulating and blocking drugs of cell groups within a sympathetic ganglion. J. Pharmacol. Exp. Ther. *135*, 54–61 (1962b)

Volle, R.L.: Enhancement of postganglionic responses to stimulating agents following repetitive preganglionic stimulation. J. Pharmacol. Exp. Ther. *136*, 68–74 (1962c)

Volle, R.L., Hancock, J.C.: Transmission in sympathetic ganglia. Fed. Proc. *29*, 1913–1918 (1970)

Watanabe, M.: A modification of the isolated hypogastric nerve-vas deferens preparations from the guinea-pig for assay of ganglionic actions. Naunyn Schmiedebergs Arch. Pharmacol. *262*, 221–227 (1969)

Weems, W.A., Szurszewski, J.H.: An intracellular analysis of some intrinsic factors controlling neural output from inferior mesenteric ganglion of guinea-pigs. J. Neurophysiol. *41*, 305 (1978)

Weetman, D.F., Turner, N.: The effects of ganglion blocking agents on the isolated, innervated bladder of the guinea pig. Arch. Int. Pharmacodyn. *201*, 100–105 (1973)

Whitacre, T.S., Long, J.R., Whalen, W.J.: Transmural and vagal nerve stimulation of the right atrium of the cat. Am. J. Physiol. *210*, 557–562 (1966)

Whitteridge, D.: The transmission of impulses through the ciliary ganglion. J. Physiol. (Lond.) *89*, 99–111 (1937)

Wien, R., Mason, D.F.J.: Some actions of hexamethonium and certain homologues. Br. J. Pharmacol. *6*, 611–630 (1951)

Wien, R., Mason, D.F.J.: Pharmacology of M. and B. 2050. Lancet *1953a CCLXIV*, 454–455

Wien, R., Mason, D.F.J.: The pharmacological actions of a series of phenyl alkane p-a-bis (trialkylammonium) compounds. Br. J. Pharmacol. *8*, 306–315 (1953b)

Wien, R., Mason, D.F.J., Edge, N.D., Langston, G.T.: Relation of chemical structure of compounds to their action on autonomic ganglia. Arch. Int. Pharmacodyn. *97*, 395–406 (1954)

Wilson, A.B.: Adrenergic neurone blocking action of dimethylphenylpiperazinium. J. Pharm. Pharmacol. *14*, 700 (1962)

Würzel, M., Efird, A.G., Goldberg, L.I.: Blocking effects of thiocholine-, choline-, and β-methyl-choline esters on transmission through the superior cervical ganglion of the cat. Arch. Int. Pharmacodyn. *148*, 53–60 (1964)

Yamamoto, I., Otori, K., Inoki, R.: Pharmacological studies on antagonists against nicotine-induced convulsions and death. Jpn. J. Pharmacol. *16*, 402–415 (1966)

Yamashita, T.: Effects of various drugs on the contraction of the excised vas deferens by hypogastric nerve and transmural stimulations in guinea pig. Folia Pharmacol. Jpn. *63*, 360–373 (1967)

Zaimis, E.: A possible explanation for the development of "tolerance" to ganglion-blocking substances. In: Hypotensive drugs. Harington, M. (Ed.). London: Pergamon Press 1956

CHAPTER 4a

Relationship Between Chemical Structure and Ganglion-Blocking Activity a) Quarternary Ammonium Compounds

V. TRČKA

A. Introduction

The discovery of drugs bringing about blockade of sympathetic ganglia has been an important step in the development of modern antihypertensive therapy. Partially successful clinical use of tetraethylammonium had initiated the synthesis and pharmacological studies on more than one thousand new substances with one or two quaternary nitrogen atoms in the molecule. It has been intended to find a drug with higher ganglion-blocking activity and long lasting hypotensive effect with less side-effects. These studies have led to the development of several drugs which were used for some years in therapeutic practice. Tetraethylammonium (1), hexamethonium (2), pentolinium (3), chlorisondamin (4), azamethonium (5), trimethydinium (6) and pentacynium (7) were the most important of them (see Fig. 1).

All these drugs brought about decrease of blood pressure in hypertensive patients. This benefitial action was accompanied by the drawback of an unpredictable effect stemming from poor and variable absorption from the gastro-intestinal tract. Unpleasant side-effects, orthostatic hypotension, obstipation, mydriasis etc., were caused by concomittant blockade of parasympathetic ganglia.

The development of better absorbed and parasympathetic ganglia less affecting non-quaternary ganglion-blocking drugs (mecamylamine, pempidine etc.) has put hexamethonium, pentolinium etc. into the background. However, parallel study of hypotensive drugs with a different mechanism of action has led to better tolerated, more reliable drugs with long lasting effect (reserpine, guanethidine, alpha-methyldopa etc.). Clinical experience has proved the superiority and advantages of these new therapeutics. Thus the ganglion-blocking drugs almost disappeared from clinical practice approximately 15 years ago; chemical and pharmacological studies of ganglionic blocking drugs during the past 15 years have been very rare.

Quaternary ammonium compounds do not act only on the sympathetic ganglia. They also affect, in part, other structures in which acetylcholine mediates neural stimuli. Therefore in many papers describing pharmacology of newly synthesized ganglion-blocking substances hypotensive, parasympatholytic, muscle-relaxant (curare-like) and other effects are presented.

This review refers only to the blocking activity in sympathetic ganglia. Because the nature of the effect of many compounds discussed in this review has not been studied by their authors, no attempt was made to classify the ganglion-blocking agents according to their mechanism of blocking effect at ganglionic cholinergic receptors, i.e. depolarizing, competitively or noncompetitively blocking drugs (VAN ROSSUM, 1962). Analysis of structural relationships in respect to activities in

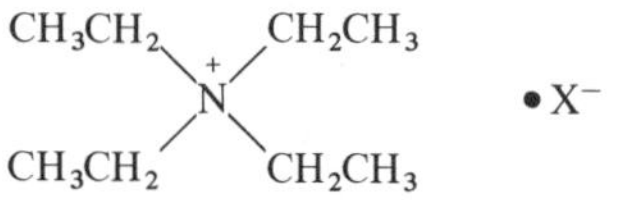

CH_3CH_2, CH_2CH_3
$\overset{+}{N}$
CH_3CH_2 CH_2CH_3 • X^- 1

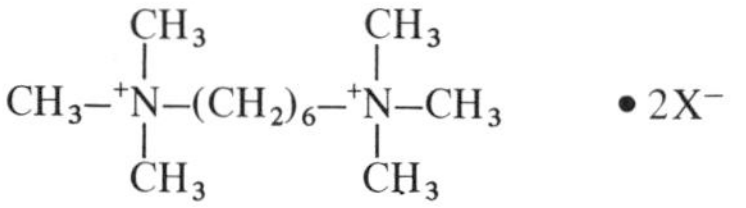

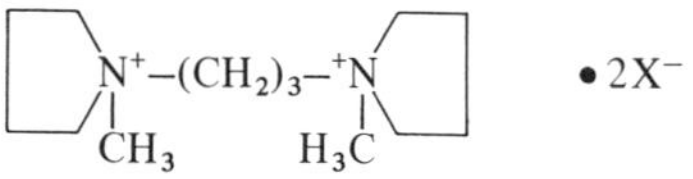

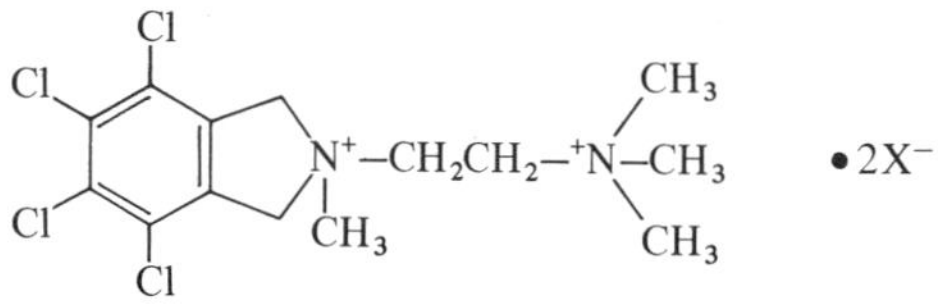

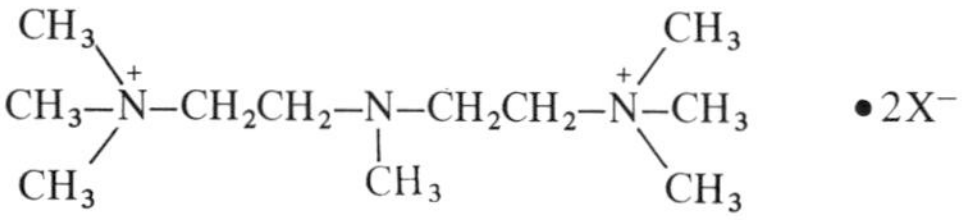

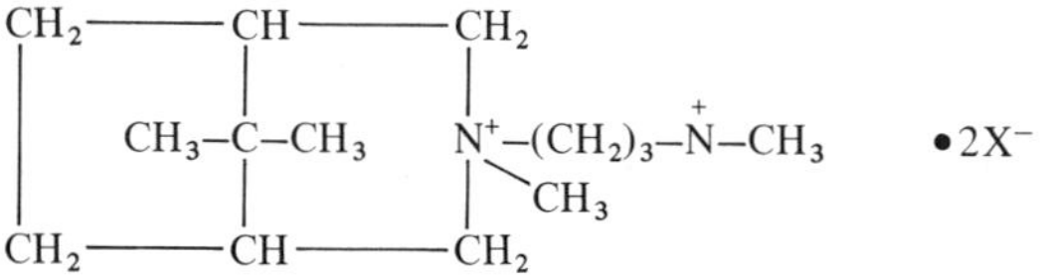

$CH_3-\overset{CH_3}{\underset{CH_3}{\overset{|}{\underset{|}{N}}}}{}^+-(CH_2)_6-{}^+\overset{CH_3}{\underset{CH_3}{\overset{|}{\underset{|}{N}}}}-CH_3$ • $2X^-$ 2

$N^+-(CH_2)_3-{}^+N$
$\underset{CH_3}{}$ $\underset{H_3C}{}$ • $2X^-$ 3

$N^+-CH_2CH_2-{}^+N(CH_3)_2$ with tetrachloro isoindole, CH_3 • $2X^-$ 4

$CH_3-\overset{CH_3}{\underset{CH_3}{\overset{|}{\underset{|}{N}}}}{}^+-CH_2CH_2-\overset{CH_3}{\underset{|}{N}}-CH_2CH_2-{}^+\overset{CH_3}{\underset{CH_3}{\overset{|}{\underset{|}{N}}}}-CH_3$ • $2X^-$ 5

$N^+-(CH_2)_3-\overset{+}{N}-CH_3$, CH_3 (with bicyclic structure CH_3-C-CH_3)   • $2X^-$ 6

$C-(CH_2)_4-\overset{+}{N}-(CH_2)_2-{}^+N$ (morpholine, O), CN, CH_3 CH_3, CH_3 • $2X^-$ 7

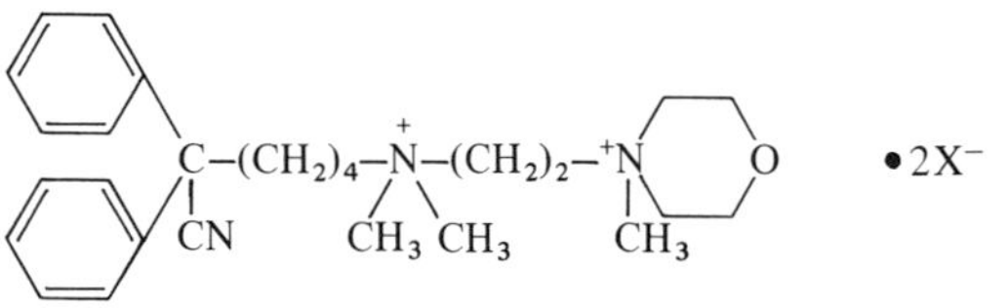

Fig. 1. The structure of the relevant compounds, the number identifies the substance, see text

other vegetative functions would need a more complex analysis, which is beyond the scope of this chapter. The ratio of sympathetic to parasympathetic blockade is not considered because of different methodological approaches in most papers, giving noncomparable data. The bulk of synthetic and pharmacological studies in the ganglion-blocking compounds has been between 1950–1965. In this period several extensive reviews have appeared which reflect the course of the research in this field (MOE and FREYBURGER, 1950; PATON and ZAIMIS, 1952; PATON, 1953; ZAIMIS, 1955; ING, 1957; CAVALLITO and GRAY, 1960; NÁDOR, 1960; VEJDĚLEK, 1960;

TRENDELENBURG, 1961; D'ARCY and TAYLOR, 1962; KHARKEVICH, 1962; TRIGGLE, 1965, 1971; JANNASCH, 1967).

Most of the compounds synthesized up to 1960 are mentioned in the reviews of NÁDOR (1960) and KHARKEVICH (1962). The present review introduces, therefore, only the most representative structural variations described. Drugs which have had information published about them more recently are mentioned only when they contribute to the question of the structure-activity relationship of quaternary ganglion-blocking agents.

The data on the activity of individual substances in the following tables are based on estimated values for ED_{50} in cat nictitating membrane (blockade of contractions elicited by preganglionic stimulation).

To provide a uniform view on structure-activity relationships, the activity of all mono-quaternary compounds was expressed in terms of the activity of tetraethyl-ammonium, and of those of bis-quaternary derivatives in terms of the activity of hexamethonium. Data collected in studies of mono-quaternary compounds in which the activity was related to hexamethonium, were converted to relative activity of tetraethylammonium.

The relative activity of tetraethylammonium (TEA) regarding to hexametho-nium was derived from the study of PATON and ZAIMIS (1949, 1951) on cats despite that different data on relative activities were found by other authors by similar methods (Table 1). The values of relative activity in the tables have to be considered as approximate. Several sources of inaccuracies are involved in compilation of data from papers by different authors:

1. Different modifications of the estimation of ganglion-blocking potency in electrically stimulated cat nictitating membrane give different relative activities (sustained or intermittend preganglionar stimulation, variable frequencies of stimu-lation, perfusion of the superior cervical ganglion, etc.).

2. The dose-response curves of structurally different compounds may be not parallel. Some of the compared agents are competitive, others non-competitive, ganglion-blocking drugs (VAN ROSSUM, 1962).

Table 1. Relative activities of standard quaternary ganglion-blocking agents

Drug	Percentage activity (activity of hexamethonium = 100%)	References
Cat nictitating membrane		
Tetraethylammonium	5.0	PATON and ZAIMIS (1949)
		PATON and ZAIMIS (1951)
	30	DI GREGORIO and DIPALMA (1967)
	20	LAPE and HOPPE (1956)
Azamethonium	40	LAPE and HOPPE (1956)
Pentapyrrolidinium	300	PLUMMER et al. (1955)
	500	MASON and WIEN (1955)
Chlorisondamin	600	PLUMMER et al. (1955)
Dog nictitating membrane		
Tetraethylammonium	3.0	LAPE and HOPPE (1956)
Azamethonium	54	LAPE and HOPPE (1956)

3. Individual reactivity of cats varies considerably, e.g. Cook et al. (1950), have found individual ED_{50} of TEA in the range of 0.22–1.40 mg/kg.

4. The ED_{50} is given in mg/kg without mentioning the anion in many papers.

In spite of all these inconsistencies, the transformed data reflect significant changes in relative activity induced by submission of one chemical group by another substituent and allow comparison of the effects on ganglion-blocking activity of similar structural changes in different types of compounds.

Several series of compounds related to quaternary ammonium compounds were evaluated by their hypotensive effect or by other criteria. These substances are not included in this reviews as the hypotensive activity is not parallel to the degree of blockade of sympathetic ganglia. The ratio of sympathetic to parasympathetic ganglion-blockade is not considered because of different methodological approaches in most papers, which gives noncomparable data.

The anions of quaternary compounds described here are not mentioned as they do not play any important role in the pharmacological activity.

B. Structure-Activity Relationships in Different Structural Types of Quaternary Ganglion-Blocking Agents

I. Mono-Quaternary Ammonium Derivatives

1. Aliphatic Quaternary Ammonium Derivatives

Cook et al. (1950), Robinson (1951), Winbury (1952) and Winbury et al. (1954), have described a series of aliphatic quaternary ammonium compounds related to tetraethylammonium enabling one to follow the influence of the length and branching and of different substituents of the alkyl chains on the sympathetic ganglion-blocking activity. Here only the most important derivatives are mentioned to show the main structure-activity relationships. Nádor (1960) and Kharkevich (1962) have given a full account of these compounds in their reviews. The replacement of two ethyl groups of the tetraethylammonium molecule (Table 2, No. 1) by propyl groups to the diethyl-di-n-propylammonium (No. 2) does not bring about significant change in the activity. In contrast to this, the diethyldiisopropylammonium (No. 4) is twelve times more active than tetraethylammonium. This is the most active substance of this series. Larger branched substituents are less active (No. 7 and 8).

Total number of carbon atoms does not play any systemic role in structure-activity relationships in tetraalkylammonium derivatives but the length and branching of N-alkyl substituents affects the ganglion-blocking activity. The introduction of an hydroxyl group on the terminal carbon of an N-ethyl group reduced the activity (No. 9 and 10). Substitution of one or two of the ethyl groups of tetraethylammonium molecule by one or two benzyl groups decreased partially the potency (Table 3).

Introduction of larger heterocycle in the molecule of tetraalkylammonium (9-xanthene or phenothiazine, Tables 4 and 5) did not change the activity very much. In contrast to this, substitution by 3-azabicyclononane increased the activity considerably (Table 6). Branching of the ethylene chain in the phenothiazine derivatives doubled the activity (Table 5, Nos. 5 and 6) while prolongation was

Table 2. Tetraalkylammonium derivatives[a]

$$R^4 \diagdown \overset{R^1}{\underset{+}{N}} \diagup \qquad \bullet X^-$$
$$R^3 \diagup \diagdown R^2$$

Compound no.	R^1	R^2	R^3	R^4	Percentage activity (activity of TEA = 100%)
1 (TEA)	CH_2CH_3	CH_2CH_3	CH_2CH_3	CH_2CH_3	100
2	CH_2CH_3	CH_2CH_3	$CH_2CH_2CH_3$	$CH_2CH_2CH_3$	90
3	CH_2CH_3	CH_2CH_3	CH_2CH_3	$CH(CH_3)_2$	260
4	CH_2CH_3	CH_2CH_3	$CH(CH_3)_2$	$CH(CH_3)_2$	1210
5	CH_3	CH_2CH_3	$CH(CH_3)_2$	$CH(CH_3)_2$	590 670
6	CH_3	CH_3	$CH(CH_3)_2$	$CH(CH_3)_2$	190
7	CH_3	CH_2CH_3	$CH_2CH(CH_3)_2$	$CH_2CH(CH_3)_2$	140 110
8	CH_3	CH_2CH_3	$CH_2CH_2CH(CH_3)_2$	$CH_2CH_2CH(CH_3)_2$	40
9	CH_2CH_3	CH_2CH_2OH	CH_2CH_3	CH_2CH_3	20
10	CH_2CH_3	CH_2CH_2OH	$CH(CH_3)_2$	$CH(CH_3)_2$	280

[a] Robinson, 1951, Winbury, 1952; Winbury et al., 1954

Table 3. Benzene substituted tetraalkylammonium derivatives.

$$R^4 \diagdown \overset{R^1}{\underset{+}{N}} \diagup \qquad \bullet X^-$$
$$R^3 \diagup \diagdown R^2$$

Compound no.	R^1	R^2	R^3	R^4	Percentage activity (activity of TEA = 100%)	References
1	CH_2CH_3	CH_2CH_3	CH_2CH_3	CH_2	80 42	Gyermek and Nador, 1952; Winbury et al., 1954
2	CH_2CH_3	CH_2CH_3	CH_2	CH_2	40	Gyermek and Nador, 1952
3	CH_3	CH_3	CH_2	CH_2	20	Gyermek and Nador, 1952

Table 4. 9—Xanthene substituted tetraalkylammonium derivatives Winbury et al., 1954.

Compound no.	R^1	R^2	R^3	Percentage activity (activity of TEA = 100%)
1	CH_3	CH_2CH_3	CH_2CH_3	80
2	CH_3	$CH(CH_3)CH_3$	$CH(CH_3)CH_3$	120

Table 5. Phenothiazine substituted tetraalkylammonium derivatives[a].

Compound no.	R^1	R^2	R^3	Z	Percentage activity (activity of TEA = 100%)
1	CH_3	CH_3	CH_3	CH_2CH_2	100
2	CH_3	CH_3	CH_2CH_3	CH_2CH_2	110
3	CH_3	CH_2CH_3	CH_2CH_3	CH_2CH_2	120
4	CH_2CH_3	CH_2CH_3	CH_2CH_3	CH_2CH_2	100
5	CH_3	CH_3	CH_3	CH_2CH-CH_2	250
6	CH_3	CH_3	CH_3	$CH_2CH-CH_2CH_3$	200
7	CH_3	CH_3	CH_3	$(CH_2)_3$	140
8	CH_3	CH_3	CH_3	$(CH_2)_4$	110

[a] Winbury, 1952; Winbury et al., 1954.

Table 6. 3—Azabicyclo—(3.3.1)—nonane substituted tetraalkylammonium derivatives TOMMASINI and PASSERINI, 1959.

$$CH_2 \text{—} CH \text{—} CH_2$$

	n	Percentage activity (activity of TEA = 100%)
	1	30
	2	1700
	3	1900

without effect (Nos. 7 and 8). Prolongation of the ethylene chain by one or two carbon atoms in 3-azabicyclo-nonane derivatives brought about a very high increase of the potency (Table 6, compare Nos. 1 vs 2, and 3).

When one of the methyl-groups in the tetramethylammonium molecule was substituted by the *cis-* or *trans-*2-hydroxycyclopentyl or 2-hydroxycyclohexyl group, the ganglion-stimulant activity of tetramethylammonium was replaced by a ganglion-blocking one, not differing very much by its intensity from that of tetraethyl-ammonium (STANDAERT et al., 1959).

In order to increase the absorption of ganglion-blocking agents from the intestinal tract, esters or ether derivatives of tetraethylammonium were studied.

Trialkylammoniumethyl esters of tropic acid (Table 7) and of diphenylacetic acid (Table 8) are less active than the corresponding aliphatic congeners.

In another series of ester derivatives, trialkylammoniumethyl esters of N-benzyl-N-phenylcarbonic acid (Table 9), several substances with high activity were found. Most interesting were compounds with two isopropyl groups (Nos. 5 and 6). 9-xanthenecarbonyloxy (Table 10), 9-fluorenecarbonyloxy (Table 11) substituents did not improve the activity. Only a different derivative, a metho salt of the beta-diisopropylaminoethyl N-(2-furfuryl)-N-phenylcarbamate (Table 12, No. 1) equalled the parent substance, the diethyldiisopropylammonium, both having 12-fold of the

Table 7. Trialkylammoniumethyl esters of tropic acid[a].

Compound no.	R^1	R^2	R^3	Percentage activity (activity of TEA = 100%)
1	CH_3	CH_3	CH_3	40
2	CH_3	CH_2CH_3	$CH_2(CH_3)_2$	50
3	CH_3	$CH(CH_3)_2$	$CH(CH_3)_2$	350

[a] Cusic and Robinson, 1951; Winbury et al., 1954.

Table 8. Trialkylammoniumethyl esters of diphenylacetic acid[a].

Compound no.	R^1	R^2	R^3	Percentage activity (activity of TEA = 100%)
1	CH_3	CH_3	CH_3	90
2	CH_3	CH_3	CH_2CH_3	40
3	CH_3	$CH(CH_3)_2$	$CH(CH_3)_2$	180

[a] Cusic and Robinson, 1951; Winbury et al., 1954.

Table 9. Trialkylammoniummethyl esters of N—pentyl—N—benzylcarbamic acid[a].

Compound no.	R[1]	R[2]	R[3]	R[4]	Percentage activity (activity of TEA = 100%)
1	CH_2CH_3	CH_2CH_3	CH_2CH_3	H	260
2	CH_3	CH_2CH_3	$CH(CH_3)_2$	H	290
3	CH_3	$CH_2CH_2CH_3$	$CH_2CH_2CH_3$	H	170
4	CH_3	$CH_2CH_2CH_3$	$CH_2CH_2CH_3$	Cl	440
5	CH_3	$CH(CH_3)_2$	$CH(CH_3)_2$	H	730
6	CH_3	$CH(CH_3)_2$	$CH(CH_3)_2$	Cl	710

Cusic and Robinson, 1951; Winbury et al., 1954.

Table 10. Trialkylammoniumalkyl esters of 9—xanthenecarboxylic acid[a].

Compound no.	R[1]	R[2]	R[3]	n	Percentage activity (activity of TEA = 100%)
1	CH_2CH_3	CH_2CH_3	CH_2CH_3	2	170
2	CH_2CH_3	CH_2CH_3	CH_2CH_3	3	240
3	CH_2CH_3	CH_2CH_3	$CH_2CH_2CH_3$	2	150
4	CH_2CH_3	CH_2CH_3	$CH(CH_3)_2$	2	140
5	CH_3	$CH(CH_3)_2$	$CH(CH_3)_2$	2	200
6	CH_3	CH_3	$CH(CH_3)_2$	2	200
7	CH_3	CH_3	CH_3	2	53

[a] Cusic and Robinson, 1951; Winbury et al., 1954.

Table 11. Trialkylammonium ethyl esters of
9–fluorenecarboxylic acid[a].

Compound no.	R^1	R^2	R^3	Percentage activity (activity of TEA = 100%)
1	CH_3	CH_3	CH_3	80
2	CH_3	CH_3	CH_2CH_3	80
3	CH_3	$CH(CH_3)_2$	$CH(CH_3)_2$	10

[a] Cusic and Robinson, 1951; Winbury et al., 1954.

Table 12. Trialkylammoniumalkyl esters of miscellaneous acids
Winbury et al., 1954.

Compound no.		Percentage activity (activity of TEA = 100%)
1		1 200
2		210
3		120

Table 13. Substituted cholinephenyl ethers
FAKSTORP and PEDERSEN, 1958.

Compound no.	R^1	R^2	R^3	Percentage activity (activity of TEA = 100%)
1	CH_3	CH_3	CH_3	250
2	CH_2CH_3	CH_3	CH_3	200
3	CH_2CH_3	CH_2CH_3	CH_2CH_3	300
4	H	CH_3	CH_3	30

Table 14. Biphenylyl ethers of tetraalkylammonium
CAVALLINI et al., 1953,

Compound no.	R^1	R^2	R^3	Percentage activity (activity of TEA = 100%)
1	CH_2CH_3	CH_2CH_3	CH_3	130
2	CH_2CH_3	CH_2CH_3	CH_2CH_3	250

activity of tetraethylammonium (Table 2, No. 4). This compound is closely related to the very active compound No. 5 of Table 9. However the introduction of the mentioned cyclic components into the molecule of tetraethylammonium influenced the quality of effects, mostly increasing the blocking activity in parasympathetic ganglia. The introduction of an arylether substituent into one of the ethyl groups of tetraethylammonium did not bring any substantial increase of activity (Tables 13, 14, 15).

Table 15. Stilbene derivatives of tetraalkylammonium
Cavallini et al., 1953.

Compound no.	R^1	R^2	R^3	Percentage activity (activity of TEA = 100%)
1	CH_3	CH_2CH_3	CH_2CH_3	250
2	CH_2CH_3	CH_2CH_3	CH_2CH_3	250
3	CH_2CH_3	CH_2CH_3	CH_2	0

Table 16. Piperidinium derivatives[a].

Compound no.	R^1	R^2	Percentage activity (activity of TEA = 100%)
1	CH_3	CH_3	200 250
2	CH_3	CH_2CH_3	320
3	CH_2CH_3	CH_2CH_3	950 1010
4	CH_2CH_3	CH_2CH_3OH	90
5	CH_3	$CH_2CH_2CH_3$	330
6	CH_3	$CH_2-\bigcirc$	240
7	CH_3	$CH_2CH_2OOC-N\underset{S}{}$	220

[a] Robinson, 1951; Winbury, 1952.

2. Heterocyclic Mono-Quaternary Derivatives

Very high activity of diisopropyldiethylammonium led ROBINSON (1951) to the
synthesis of cyclic analogues, namely piperidinium, pyrrolidinium or isoquinolinium
derivatives. In a series of piperidinium derivatives (Table 16), the compound No. 3,
closely related to diisopropyldiethylammonium, was the most active, being ten
times more potent than tetraethylammonium. The corresponding pyrrolidinium
derivative (Table 17, No. 1) was less active. Compounds containing the 9-xanthe-
carbonyloxy and phenothiazinecarbonyloxy group did not differ very much from
the standard drug (Table 16, No. 7, Table 17, Nos. 4 and 5).

Among quaternary tetrahydroisoquinoline derivatives (Table 18), several highly
active compounds were found, especially in derivatives with hydroxyl groups in the
position 7 and 8 of the isoquinoline nucleus. In contrast to the compound No. 3
of Table 18, the 2-phenylquinolinium methiodide was less active (DI GREGORIO and
DIPALMA, 1967).

NÁDOR (1960) has summarized the results of his studies of ganglion-blocking
and other pharmacological effects of more than 80 quaternary derivatives of

Table 17. Pyrrolidinium derivatives[a].

Compound no.	R¹	R²	Percentage activity (activity of TEA = 100%)
1	CH_2CH_3	CH_2CH_3	640
2	CH_2CH_3	CH_2CH_3OH	78
3	CH_3	CH_2CH_3OH	36
4	CH_3	CH_2CH_2OOC-	100
5	CH_3	CH_2CH_2OOC-N	350

[a] ROBINSON, 1951; WINBURY, 1952.

Table 18. Tetrahydroisoquinolinium derivatives Robinson, 1951.

Compound no.	R^1	R^2	R^3	R^4	R^5	Percentage activity (activity of TEA = 100%)
1	CH_2CH_3	CH_2CH_3	CH_3	H	H	65
2	CH_3	CH_3	$CH(CH_3)_2$	H	H	190
3	CH_3	CH_3	(ring)	H	H	160
4	CH_3	CH_3	$(CH_2)_6CH_3$	OH	OH	380
5	CH_3	CH_3	CH_2-(phenyl)	OH	OH	960
6	CH_3	CH_2CH_3	CH_2-(phenyl)	OH	OH	780
7	CH_2CH_3	CH_2CH_3	CH_2-(phenyl)	OH	OH	460
8	CH_3	CH_3	CH_2-(phenyl)	OCH_3	OCH_3	400

tropane, homatropine, tropeine and tropine. Table 19, which represents only a fraction of derivatives under study, illustrates main structure-activity relationships in these derivatives (e.g. Nos. 1, 2, 5). The introduction of the benzyl substituent on the quaternary nitrogen atom increases the blocking activity (e.g. Nos. 7, 8, 9). Further increase of activity could be reached by introducing a halogen or a phenyl group into the p-position of the benzyl substituent (Nos. 11, 12). The most active substance of this series of quaternary derivatives is compound No. 12.

II. Bis-Quaternary Derivatives

1. Symmetrical Polymethylene Bis-Trialkylammonium Derivatives

Barlow and Ing (1948) and Paton and Zaimis (1948) studying the curare-like activity of the quaternary bis-ammonium salts in which the ammonium groups were separated by polymethylene chain of different length, have discovered a new

Table 19. Quaternary tropane derivatives[a].

$$CH_2—CH—CH_3$$
$$\overset{+}{N}\underset{R^1}{\overset{CH_3}{\diagdown}}\qquad CHOR^2 \quad \bullet X^-$$
$$CH_2—CH—CH_2$$

Compound no.	R^1	R^2	Percentage activity (activity of TEA = 100%)
1	CH_3	$COCH_3$	30
2	CH_3	$CONH_3$ with two CH_3	20
3	H	OC—⬡	10
4	H	$OCCH_2$—⬡	35
5	CH	OC—⬡	200
6	CH	$OCCH_2$—⬡	450
7	CH_2	$COCH_3$	200
8	CH_2—⬡	CON with two CH_3	300
9	CH_2—⬡	CO ⬡	300
10	CH_2—⬡	CO—⬡—NH_2	800
11	⬡—Cl	CO—⬡—NH_2	2200
12	⬡—CH_2	CO—CH(OH)—⬡	4000

[a] NADOR, 1960; GYERMEK and NADOR, 1953; 1957

Table 20. Symmetrical polymethylene—bis(trialkylammonium) derivatives.

$$R^2\text{—}\overset{\overset{\displaystyle R^1}{|}}{\underset{\underset{\displaystyle R^3}{|}}{N^+}}\text{—}(CH_2)_n\text{—}\overset{\overset{\displaystyle R^1}{|}}{\underset{\underset{\displaystyle R^3}{|}}{N^+}}\text{—}R^2 \quad \bullet\, 2X^-$$

Compound no.	R^1	R^2	R^3	n	Percentage activity (activity of hexamethonium = 100%)	References
1	CH_3	CH_3	CH_3	4	2 1	Paton and Zaimis, 1949 Wien et al., 1952
2	CH_2CH_3	CH_3	CH_3	4	10	Wien et al., 1952
3	CH_2CH_3	CH_2CH_3	CH_3	4	100	Wien et al., 1952
4	CH_2CH_3	CH_2CH_3	CH_2CH_3	4	5	Wien et al., 1952
5	CH_3	CH_3	CH_3	5	65 80	Wien et al., 1952 Paton and Zaimis, 1949
6	CH_2CH_3	CH_3	CH_3	5	150	Wien et al., 1952
7	CH_2CH_3	CH_2CH_3	CH_3	5	125	Wien et al., 1952
8	CH_2CH_3	CH_2CH_3	CH_2CH_3	5	7 1	Wien et al., 1952 Chou and de Elio, 1948
9 (hexa-methonium)	CH_3	CH_3	CH_3	6	100	Paton and Zaimis, 1949
10	CH_2CH_3	CH_3	CH_3	6	150	Wien et al., 1952
11	CH_2CH_3	CH_2CH_3	CH_3	6	75	Wien et al., 1952
12	CH_2CH_3	CH_2CH_3	CH_2CH_3	6	5	Wien et al., 1952
13	CH_3	CH_3	CH_3	7	10	Paton and Zaimis, 1949
14	CH_3	CH_3	CH_3	12	25	Barlow and Zoller, 1964
15	CH_3	CH_3	CH_3	14	80	Barlow and Zoller, 1964
16	CH_3	CH_3	CH_3	16	400	Barlow and Zoller, 1964
17	CH_3	CH_3	CH_3	18	400	Barlow and Zoller, 1964
18	CH_3	CH_3	CH_3	20	80	Barlow and Zoller, 1964

class of ganglion-blocking compounds. While the curare-like activity reaches its maximum when the polymethylene chain is formed by 10 methylene groups, maximum of ganglion-blocking activity have compounds with 5 or 6 carbon atoms (Table 20). The hexamethylene-bis-trimethylammonium, hexamethonium (Table 20, No. 9), had found clinical use for some years. Activity of later synthesized bis-quaternary compounds was mostly compared to hexamethonium as a standard. Also in this review hexamethonium is used as the reference substance for the bis-quaternary ammonium derivatives.

The activities of different combinations of length of the connection chain and length of the alkyl groups attached to the quaternary nitrogen atom (Table 20) show, that in compounds with the 4 carbon chain, two ethyl groups attached to the quaternary nitrogen atom are necessary to reach the activity of the standard, hexamethonium. One ethyl group in both ammonium groups enhances the activity in compounds with the five- or six-membered polymethylene chain (WIEN, 1954). Substitution of one alkyl of the trialkylammonium group by ethoxyethyl group increased the activity (PALAZZO and VIRNO, 1959).

2. Symmetrical Polymethylene-Bis-Quaternary Cyclic Compounds

Substitution of the trialkylammonium groups by pyrrolidinium group brings about increase of activity up to five-fold in the pentamethylene-bis-(1-methylpyrrolidi-nium), (pentapyrrolidinium, pentolinium, Table 21, No. 3). This substance was used clinically with success. Corresponding piperidinium and morpholinium derivatives are less active (Tables 22 and 23).

Table 21. Polymethylene—bis(pyrrolidinium) derivatives
MASON and WIEN, 1955.

$$\left[\begin{array}{c} N-(CH_2)_n-N \\ | \\ R \end{array}\right] \cdot 2X^-$$

Compound no.	R	n	Percentage activity (activity of hexamethonium = 100%)
1	CH_3	3	5
2	CH_3	4	50
3 (Pentapyrro-lidinium)	CH_3	5	500
4	CH_3	6	300
5	CH_2CH_3	6	60
6	CH_3	10	75

Table 22. Polymethylene—bis(piperidinium) derivatives
MASON and WIEN, 1955.

$$\langle \rangle \overset{+}{N}-(CH_2)_n-\overset{+}{N} \langle \rangle \quad \bullet\, 2X^-$$
$$\qquad | \qquad\quad |$$
$$\qquad R \qquad\quad R$$

Compound no.	R	n	Percentage activity (activity of hexamethonium = 100%)
1	CH_3	3	7
2	CH_3	4	80
3	CH_3	5	90
4	CH_3	6	90
5	CH_2CH_3	6	<10
6	CH_3	7	30
7	CH_3	10	5

Table 23. Polymethylene—bis(morpholinium) derivatives
MASON and WIEN, 1955.

$$O\langle \rangle \overset{+}{N}-(CH_2)_n-\overset{+}{N} \langle \rangle O \quad \bullet\, 2X^-$$
$$\qquad\quad | \qquad\quad |$$
$$\qquad\quad R \qquad\quad R$$

Compound no.	R	n	Percentage activity (activity of hexamethonium = 100%)
1	CH_3	4	20
2	CH_3	5	100
3	CH_3	6	100
4	CH_3	7	80
5	CH_3	10	60
6	CH_2CH_3	6	6

3. Modifications of the Polymethylene Chain

Different substitutions of one or more methylene groups of the polymethylene chain in symmetrical bis-quaternary ammonium compounds by nitrogen, oxygen or sulphur has produced several interesting aspects on the structure-activity relationships.

Replacement of the central methylene group in the five carbon chain by the tertiary nitrogen atom has led to a clinically used compound – azamethonium (pendiomide) (Table 24, No. 2) – in spite of lower activity than that of hexamethonium. The activity of compounds in which one methylene group was substituted by oxygen atom (Table 25) depends largely from the character of alkyl groups attached to the quaternary nitrogen atoms. The derivative in which nitrogen atom is substituted by three ethyl or by two ethyl and one methyl group are the most active (Table 25, No. 6). Compounds with an asymmetrical number of methylene groups in corresponding oxapentane derivatives did not surpass the range of activity of compounds in Table 26 (FAKSTORP and PEDERSEN, 1957). Corresponding substitution by sulphur atom gave slightly more active substance (Table 26). Substitution of two methylene groups by the —S—S— or S—O bridge was less effective (FAKSTORP and PEDERSEN, 1957).

A part of the polymethylene chain can be replaced by phenyl group without lost of activity as can be seen in a series of phenylalkane p-ω-bis-trialkylammonium derivatives (Table 27). Related bis-quaternary dialkylaminoethyl-aryl ethers did not reach the activity of hexamethonium (Table 28). Compounds with two phenyl substituents in polymethylene chain are also active as can be shown in diphenyl-tetramethylene-bis-trimethylammonium, which is as active as hexamethonium (TRČKA and VANĚČEK, 1959).

$$CH_3-\overset{+}{\underset{CH_3}{\overset{CH_3}{N}}}-CHCH_2CH_2CH-\overset{+}{\underset{CH_3}{\overset{CH_3}{N}}}-CH_3 \cdot 2X^-$$

4. Asymmetrical Bis-Quaternary Compounds

Asymmetrical bis-quaternary derivatives with one ammonium and with one pyridinium group substituted on the pyridine nucleus by a bicyclo-ethyl group have proved to block sympathetic ganglia in significantly lower doses than hexamethonium (Table 29). One cationic head of the asymmetrical bis-quaternary derivatives can be represented by different quaternary nitrogen containing polycyclic systems (isoindolinium Table 30, isoquinoline Table 31, azabicyclooctane Table 32, tropane Table 33, harman Table 34). Compounds presented in Table 35 indicate that the ester bond between both cationic heads does not interfere with ganglion-blocking activity.

The length of the methylene chain and of the alkyl substituents on the second quaternary ammonium atom seems to play an important role in the activity of all these types of compounds. Lack of systematic studies in this respect gives no possibility of more exact conclusions.

Table 24. Aza–polymethylene–bis(trialkylammonium) derivatives BEIN and MEIER, 1950.

$$R^2-\overset{\overset{\displaystyle R^1}{|}}{\underset{\underset{\displaystyle R^3}{|}}{N^+}}-(CH_2)_n-\overset{\overset{\displaystyle }{|}}{\underset{\underset{\displaystyle CH_3}{|}}{N}}-(CH_2)_n-\overset{\overset{\displaystyle R^1}{|}}{\underset{\underset{\displaystyle R^3}{|}}{N^+}}-R^2 \quad \bullet 2X^-$$

Compound no.	R^1	R^2	R^3	n	Percentage activity (activity of hexamethonium = 100%)
1	CH_3	CH_3	CH_3	2	8
2 (Azamethonium)	CH_2CH_3	CH_3	CH_3	2	40
3	CH_2CH_3	CH_2CH_3	CH_2CH_3	2	10
4	CH_3	CH_3	CH_3	3	0

Table 25. Bis–quaternary 3–oxapentane derivatives FAKSTORP et al., 1957.

$$R^2-\overset{\overset{\displaystyle R^1}{|}}{\underset{\underset{\displaystyle R^3}{|}}{N^+}}-CH_2CH_2-O-CH_2CH_2-\overset{\overset{\displaystyle R^4}{|}}{\underset{\underset{\displaystyle R^6}{|}}{N^+}}-R^5 \quad \bullet 2X^-$$

Compound no.	R^1	R^2	R^3	R^4	R^5	R^6	Percentage activity (activity of hexamethonium = 100%)
1	CH_3	CH_3	CH_3	CH_3	CH_3	CH_3	10
2	CH_3	CH_3	CH_2CH_3	CH_3	CH_3	CH_2CH_3	32
3	CH_3	CH_3	CH_3	CH_3	CH_2CH_3	CH_2CH_3	53
4	CH_3	CH_3	CH_2CH_3	CH_3	CH_2CH_3	CH_2CH_3	58
5	CH_3	CH_3	CH_2CH_3	CH_2CH_3	CH_2CH_3	CH_2CH_3	140
6	CH_3	CH_2CH_3	CH_2CH_3	CH_2CH_3	CH_2CH_3	CH_2CH_3	170
7	CH_2CH_3	CH_2CH_3	CH_2CH_3	CH_2CH_3	CH_2CH_3	CH_2CH_3	6

Table 26. Bis–quaternary 3–thiopentane derivatives.

$$R^2-\overset{\overset{\displaystyle R^1}{|}}{\underset{\underset{\displaystyle R^3}{|}}{N}}{}^{+}-CH_2CH_2-S-CH_2CH_2-\overset{\overset{\displaystyle R^4}{|}}{\underset{\underset{\displaystyle R^6}{|}}{N}}{}^{+}-R^5 \quad \bullet\, 2X^-$$

Compound no.	R^1	R^2	R^3	R^4	R^5	R^6	Percentage activity (activity of hexamethonium = 100%)	References
1	CH_3	CH_3	CH_3	CH_3	CH_3	CH_3	70	Fakstorp and Pedersen, 1957
							30	Trčka and Lorencova, 1957; Trčka and Vaněček, 1957
2	CH_3	CH_3	CH_2CH_3	CH_3	CH_3	CH_2CH_3	250	Trčka and Lorencova, 1957; Trčka and Vaněček, 1957
3	CH_3	CH_3	CH_2CH_3	CH_2CH_3	CH_2CH_3	CH_2CH_3	140	Fakstorp and Pedersen, 1957
4	CH_3	CH_2CH_3	CH_2CH_3	CH_3	CH_2CH_3	CH_2CH_3	300	Trčka and Lorencova, 1957; Trčka and Vaněček, 1957
5	CH_2CH_3	CH_2CH_3	CH_2CH_3	CH_2CH_3	CH_2CH_3	CH_2CH_3	30	Trčka and Lorencova, 1957; Trčka and Vaněček, 1957

Table 27. Phenylalkane—p, ω—bis(trialkylammonium) derivatives.

$$R^2-\underset{\underset{R^3}{|}}{\overset{\overset{R^1}{|}}{N}}\!\!\!\!\!\!\!\!\!\!\!\!\!\!\!\!\!\!\!-\!\!\!\langle\text{phenyl}\rangle\!-(CH_2)_n-\underset{\underset{R^3}{|}}{\overset{\overset{R^1}{|}}{N}}-R^2 \quad \bullet\, 2X^-$$

Compound no.	R^1	R^2	R^3	n	Percentage activity (activity of hexamethonium = 100%)	References
1	CH_3	CH_3	CH_3	1	5	Wien and Mason, 1953
2	CH_3	CH_3	CH_3	2	300 200	Wien and Mason, 1953
3	CH_3	CH_3	CH_2CH_3	2	330	Trčka and Vaněček, 1959
4	CH_3	CH_2CH_3	CH_2CH_3	2	180	Wien and Mason, 1953
5	CH_3	CH_3	CH_3	3	25	Wien and Mason, 1953
6	CH_3	CH_3	CH_3	4	<5	Wien and Mason, 1953

Table 28. Bis—quaternary substituted choline phenylethers Fakstorp and Pedersen, 1958.

$$\text{phenyl}(R^3-N^+(R^3)(R^4))-O-CHCH-\underset{\underset{R^2}{|}}{\overset{\overset{R^1}{|}}{N}}-R^1 \quad \bullet\, 2X^-$$

Compound no.	R^1	R^2	R^3	R^4	Percentage activity (activity of hexamethonium = 100%)
1	CH_3	CH_3	CH_3	CH_3	35
2	CH_3	CH_2CH_3	CH_3	CH_2CH_3	45
3	CH_2CH_3	CH_3	CH_2CH_3	CH_3	5
4	CH_3	CH_3	CH_2CH_3	CH_3	51

Table 29. Bis—quaternary piperidine derivatives o'DELL and NAPOLI, 1957.

Compound no.	R	Position	Percentage activity (activity of hexamethonium = 100%)
1	$CH_2CH_2—$	2	400—600
2	$—CH_2CH_2—$	2	200
3		4	100
4	$—CH_2CH_2—$	2	400
5		4	400—600
6	$—CH_2CH_2—$	2	200—400

5. Phosphonium and Sulphonium Derivatives

The ganglion-blocking activity is not limited only to the quaternary ammonium derivatives. GINZEL et al. (1954) have shown that also polymethylene-bis-trialkyl or -triarylphosphonium derivatives block the contractions of electrically stimulated cat nictitating membrane.

$$R_3 \overset{+}{P}—(CH_2)_n—\overset{+}{P}R_3 \cdot 2X^-$$

More attention was paid to the sulphonium derivatives (PROTIVA et al., 1953; DELLA BELLA, 1955; BARLOW and VANE, 1956; TRČKA and VANĚČEK, 1959). Several examples of relative activity of polymethylene-bis-(dialkyl sulphonium)

Table 30. Isoindoline derivatives Plummer et al., 1955.

Compound no.	R^1	n	Percentage activity (activity of hexamethonium = 100%)
1 (Chlorisond- amine)	CH_3	2	650
2	CH_2CH_3	2	110
3	CH_2CH_3	4	80
4	CH_2CH_3	5	40

Table 31. Isoquinoline derivatives o'Dell et al., 1955[b].

Compound no.	R	n	Percentage activity (activity of hexamethonium = 100%)
1	$-\overset{+}{N}(CH_3)_3$	3	50
2	(pyrrolidinium, CH₃)	3	70
3	(morpholinium, CH₃)	3	70
4	(pyridinium)	3	0

Table 32. Azabicyclooctane bis—quaternary derivatives
TOMMASINI and PASSERINI, 1959

$$
\begin{array}{l}
CH_2\text{——}CH\text{——}CH_2 \\
\quad\quad\quad CH_2 \\
\quad\quad\quad CH_2 \\
CH_2\text{——}CH_2\text{——}CH_2
\end{array}
\quad
\overset{+}{N}-CH_2-(CH_2)_n-\overset{+}{N}\underset{CH_3}{\overset{CH_3}{<}}CH_3 \quad \bullet 2X^-
$$

Compound no.	n	Percentage activity (activity of hexamethonium = 100%)
1	1	5
2	2	350
3	3	380

Table 33. Bisquaternary tropane derivatives LAPE et al., 1956.

$$
\begin{array}{l}
CH_2\text{——}CH\text{——}CH_2 \\
\quad CH_3-\overset{+}{N}-R^1 \quad\quad CH-N-(CH_2)_n-\overset{+}{N}\underset{R^2}{\overset{R^1}{<}}R^1 \quad \bullet 2X^- \\
\quad\quad\quad\quad\quad\quad\quad\quad R^3 \\
CH_2\text{——}CH\text{——}CH_2
\end{array}
$$

Compound no.	R^1	R^2	R^3	n	Percentage activity (activity of hexamethonium = 100%)
1	CH_2CH_3	CH_3	CH_3	2	10
2	CH_2CH_3	CH_2CH_3	CH_3	2	< 3
3	CH_2CH_3	CH_3	CH_3	3	30
4	CH_2CH_3	CH_2CH_3	H	2	110
5	Piperidyl		H	2	170

Table 34. Harman derivatives.

Compound no.	R^1	R^2	R^3	R^4	n	Percentage activity (activity of hexamethonium = 100%)	References
1	CH$_3$	CH$_3$	CH$_3$	H	3	200	Cavallito et al., 1955
2	CH$_2$CH$_3$	CH$_3$	CH$_2$CH$_3$	H	3	100	Cavallito et al., 1955
3	CH$_2$CH$_3$	CH$_2$CH$_3$	CH$_2$CH$_3$	H	3	<50	Cavallito et al., 1955
4	CH$_3$	CH$_3$	CH$_3$	CH$_3$	3	50	o'Dell et al., 1955a
5	CH$_3$	CH$_3$	CH$_3$	H	6	200	o'Dell et al., 1955a
6				H	3	50	o'Dell et al., 1955a
7				CH$_3$	3	400	o'Dell et al., 1955a

derivatives in Table 36 show that replacement of nitrogen by sulphur reduced the activity. Derivatives with only one sulphonium group were without any blocking effect (Protiva et al., 1953; Trčka and Vaněček, 1959). In contrary to these findings, replacement of only one ammonium group in tetramethylene-bis-trialkyl ammonium derivatives by one sulphonium group gave compounds with activity higher than that of hexamethonium. The diethylsulphonium-tetramethylene-triethylammonium was three times more active than hexamethonium (Brown and Turner, 1959).

Table 35. Bisquaternary esters.

Compound no.		Percentage activity (activity of hexamethonium = 100%)	References
1	[piperidinium: H₃C–N⁺–CH₃ ring]–COO(CH₂)₃–N⁺(CH₃)(CH₃)–CH₃ • 2X⁻	active	BUCKLEY et al., 1960; BICKERTON et al., 1960
2	[H₃C–piperidinium: H₃C–N⁺–CH₃ ring]–COOCH₂CH₂N⁺(CH₃)(CH₂CH₃)–CH₂CH₃ • 2X⁻	8000	SHARAPOV, 1958
3	[quinuclidine-type: CH₂CH₂ bridge, H₃C–N⁺–CH₃]–CHCOOCH₂CH₂N⁺(CH₃)(CH₂CH₃)–CH₂CH₃ • 2X⁻	4000	SHARAPOV, 1957, 1958

Table 36. Bis—sulphonium derivatives.

$$\underset{R^2}{\overset{R^1}{\diagdown}}\!\!\overset{+}{S}\!-\!(CH_2)_n\!-\!\overset{+}{S}\!\underset{R^2}{\overset{R^1}{\diagup}} \quad \bullet 2X^-$$

Compound no.	R^1	R^2	n	Percentage activity (activity of hexamethonium = 100%)	References
1	CH_3	CH_3	3	<1	BARLOW and VANE, 1956
2	CH_3	CH_3	4	<1	BARLOW and VANE, 1956
3	CH_3	CH_3	5	<1	BARLOW and VANE, 1956
4	CH_3	CH_3	6	5	TRČKA and VANĚČEK, 1959
5	CH_3	CH_2CH_3	6	30	TRČKA and VANĚČEK, 1959
6	CH_2CH_3	CH_2CH_3	6	50	TRČKA and VANĚČEK, 1959

C. Conclusions

1. Mono-Quaternary Compounds

The most active mono-quaternary compounds include a common structural fragment

which fits well to the diethylisopropyl ammonium (Table 2, No. 2) to the 2,6-dimethyl-1,1-diethylpiperidinium (Table 16, No. 3), both these compounds being ten times more active than tetraethylammonium. This structural feature can be partially found also in quaternary tetrahydroisoquinoline and tropane derivatives (Tables 18 and 19).

Compared to the activity of tetraethylammonium, the branching on alpha carbon of two ethyl groups has a positive effect on the ganglionic blocking potency. Prolongation of the alkyl groups or further branching decreases the activity, showing that the size of the molecule and distinct degree of steric hindrance of the quaternary nitrogen atom plays an important role.

Decrease of hydrophobicity by replacement of one of the ethyl groups by a hydroxyethyl (Table 2, No. 9 vs 1 and No. 10 vs No. 3) lowers the activity. Substitution of one ethyl group by benzyl substituent (Table 3, Nos. 2 and 3) or attachement of an heterocyclic system (Tables 4 and 5) to the beta carbon of one of the ethyl groups also has a mostly deteriorating effect on activity. This shows that the area occupied by the molecule and also a distinct degree of symmetry of the molecule are necessary to interact with the receptor at sympathetic ganglia. This factor possibly plays a part in compounds in which the aromatic nucleus is bound to the beta carbon by an ester or ether linkage (Tables 7–15). In spite of high activity of compounds Nos. 5 and 6 of the Table 9, (N-benzyl-N-phenylcarbamoyl derivatives of diethyldiisopropylammonium) they are significantly less active than the parent drug (Table 2, No. 2). The only one exception is compound No. 1 of Table 12, the metho salt of β-diisopropylaminoethyl N-(2-furfuryl)-N-phenylcarbamate.

Similar structure-activity relations were found in compounds in which the quaternary nitrogen atom is incorporated into a saturated heterocycle (Tables 16 and 17).

2. Symmetrical Bis-Quaternary Compounds

The structure-activity relations in the series of polymethylene-bis-trialkylammonium derivatives presented in Table 20 show that the length of the polymethylene chain connecting both quaternary nitrogen atoms has a key role in the degree of blocking activity of sympathetic ganglia. Further increasing of the number of methylene groups changes the blocking effect qualitatively. Decamethylene derivatives are very potent curariform agents. A second peak of ganglion-blocking activity was found in compounds having 15 to 17 methylene groups.

Much attention was paid to the relation of the distance between both cationic heads and the blocking activity in cholinergic receptors in different functional areas. This question, studied by several authors, was summarized by TRIGGLE (1965). The ganglion-blocking molecules must possess a range of interquaternary distances between limits of 6.0–7.8 Å. This requirement fulfills pentamethylene and hexa-methylene-bis-tri-methylammonium. The quality of alkyl substituents of both quaternary nitrogen atoms influence partially the distance probability distribution of the bis-quaternary compounds. Therefore, a compound with four carbon chain, tetramethylene-bis-diethylmethylammonium (Table 20, No. 3) is as active as hexamethonium (No. 9). Activity of the five carbon chain compound (No. 6) also indicates these relations. Validity of these considerations on the length of the methylene chain may be applied also to the symmetrical bis-quaternary heterocyclic derivatives (Tables 21–23) in which maximum activity was found in compounds with C_5–C_6 polymethylene chain. Compounds in which the central member of the poly-methylene chain is substituted by an oxygen atom (bis-quaternary oxapentane derivatives, Table 25) or by sulphur atom (thiapentane derivatives, Table 26) show similar relations. Maximum activity in the series of phenylalkane derivatives (Table 27) was also found in derivatives corresponding approximately to this rule.

The optimum length requirement for the polymethylene chain in symmetrical quaternary blocking agents, i.e. 5–6 carbon atoms, is not valid in asymmetrical bis-quaternary compounds in which one cationic head comprises a quaternary nitrogen containing heterocyclic system and the other one is formed by a trialkylammonium group (Table 29–34). The lack of systematic studies in asymmetrical quaternary compounds gives no possibility of formulating a more detailed rule in this series. In bis-quaternary compounds, in which one cationic head is formed by a quaternary heterocyclic nucleus and the other one by an trialkylammonium radical, the connection of both these sites in highly active substances can be provided by a chain of 2–6 methylene groups. This indicates that the distance of both quaternary sites plays a less important role in asymmetrical bis-quaternary compounds.

The ganglion-blocking activity is not bound only on the presence of one or two quaternary nitrogen atoms. Some of the polymethylene-bis-trialkylphosphonium, -bis-triarylphosphonium and -dialkylsulphonium derivatives are active blocking agents.

References

D'Arcy, P.F., Taylor, E.P.: Quaternary ammonium compounds in medicinal chemistry. I. J. Pharm. Pharmacol. *14*, 129–146 (1962)

Barlow, R.B., Ing, H.R.: Curare-like action of polymethylene bis-quaternary ammonium salts. Nature *161*, 718–719 (1948)

Barlow, R.B., Vane, J.R.: The ganglion-blocking properties of hexamethylene bisdialkylsul-phonium salts. Br. J. Pharmacol. *11*, 198–201 (1956)

Barlow, R.B., Zoller, A.: Some effects of long chain polymethylene bis-onium salts on junctional transmission in the peripheral nervous system. Br. J. Pharmacol. *23*, 131–150 (1964)

Bein, H.J., Meier, R.: Zur Pharmakologie des N,N,N′,N′-3-Pentamethyl-N,N′-diäthyl-3-aza-pentan-1,5-diammonium-dibromid (Ciba 9295), einer ganglionär hemmenden Substanz (Kurze Mitteilung). Experientia 6, 351–353 (1950)

Bickerton, R.K., Jacquart, M.L., Kinnard, W.J., Bianculli, J.A., Buckley, J.T.: Tetrahydroiso-quinoline and tetrahydroquinoline derivatives. J. Am. Pharm. Assoc. *49*, 183–186 (1960)

Brown, D.M., Turner, B.H.: The ganglionic blocking activity of a series of tertiary sulphonium quaternary ammonium salts. J. Pharm. Pharmacol. *11*, suppl. 95, 95–102 T (1959)

Buckley, J.P., Jacquart, M.L., Bickerton, R.K., Hudak, W.J., Schalit, F.M., Defeo, J.J., Bianculli, J.A.: An evaluation of certain hypotensive agents IV. Diquaternarized piperidine derivatives. J. Am. Pharm. Assoc. *49*, 586–589 (1960)

Cavallini, G., Mantegazza, P., Massarani, E., Tommasini, R.: Sull'attivita ganglioplegica di alcuni derivati alchilaminici dello stilbene e del difenily. Farmaco [Sci.] *8*, 2–16 (1953)

Cavallito, C.J., Gray, A.P.: Chemical nature and pharmacological actions of quaternary ammonium salts. In: Fortschritte der Arzneimittelforschung. Jucker, E. (ed.), Vol. II, 135–226 Basel, Stuttgart: Birkhäuser 1960

Cavallito, C.J., Gray, A.P., O'Dell, T.B.: Sites of action of some unsymmetric bis-quaternary hypotensive agents. Arch. Int. Pharmacodyn. Ther *101*, 38–48 (1955)

Chou, T.C., de Elio, F.J.: The anticurare activity of eserine on the superior cervical ganglion of the cat. Br. J. Pharmacol. *3*, 113–115 (1948)

Cook, D.L., Hambourger, W.E., Blanchi, R.G.: Pharmacology of a new autonomic ganglion blocking agent, 2,6-dimethyl-1,1-diethyl piperidinium bromide (SC–1950). J. Pharmacol. Exp. Ther. *99*, 435–443 (1950)

Cusic, J.W., Robinson, R.A.: Autonomic blocking agents. II. Alkamine esters and their quaternaries. J. Org. Chem. *16*, 1921–1930 (1951)

O'Dell, T.B., Napoli, M.D.: Pharmacology of some unsymmetrical bisquaternary hypotensive agents – substituted pyridine and piperidine derivatives. J. Pharmacol. Exp. Ther. *120*, 438–446 (1957)

O'Dell, T.B., Luna, C., Napoli, M.D.: Pharmacology of some new unsymmetrical bisquaternary hypotensive agents – carboline derivatives. J. Pharmacol. Exp. Ther. *114*, 306–316 (1965a)

O'Dell, T.B., Luna, C., Napoli, M.D.: Pharmacology of some new unsymmetrical bisquaternary hypotensive agents – isoquinoline derivatives. J. Pharmacol. Exp. Ther. *114*, 317–325 (1955b)

Della Bella, D.: Über ein ganglionlähmendes Sulphoniumderivat: das Hexamethylen-1,6-bis-Dimethylsulphonium. Arch. Exp. Pathol. Pharmakol. *226*, 335–339 (1955)

Fakstorp, J.T., Pedersen, J.G.A.: Ganglionic blocking activity of homologues and analogues of bis-choline ether salts. Acta Pharmacol. Toxicol. (Kbh) *13*, 359–367 (1957)

Fakstorp, J.T., Pedersen, J.G.A.: Ganglion-blocking action of some substituted choline phenyl ethers. Acta Pharmacol. Toxicol. (Kbh) *14*, 148–152 (1958)

Fakstorp, J.T., Pedersen, J.G.A., Poulsen, E., Schilling, M.: Ganglionic blocking activity of bis-trialkylammoniumethyl ether salts and their branched homologues. Acta Pharmacol. Toxicol. (Kbh) *13*, 52–58 (1957)

Ginzel, R.H., Klupp, H., Kraupp, O., Werner, G.: Ganglionärblockierende Wirkungen von Polymethylen-bis-Phosphonium-Verbindungen. Arch. Exp. Pathol. Pharmakol. *221*, 336–349 (1954)

Di Gregorio, G.J., Dipalma, J.R.: Some pharmacological actions of 2-phenylquinoline methiodide. Br. J. Pharmacol. *30*, 531–540 (1967)

Gyermek, L., Nádor, K.: Studies on cholinergic blocking substances. II. Correlations between structure and effect in antimuscarine, ganglion blocking and curare-like actions of mono- and bis-quaternary ammonium compounds. Acta Physiol. Hung. *3*, 183–193 (1952)

Gyermek, L., Nádor, K.: Studies on cholinergic blocking substances V. The pharmacology of monoquaternary tropeines acting on vegetative ganglia. Acta Physiol. Hung. *4*, 341–354 (1953)

Gyermek, L., Nádor, K.: The pharmacology of propane compounds in relation to their steric structure. J. Pharm. Pharmacol. *9*, 209–229 (1957)

Ing, H.R.: Structure-action relationships of hypotensive drugs. In: Hypotensive drugs. Harington, M. (ed.) 7–22, London, New York: Pergamon Press 1957

Jannasch, R.: Ganglienblocker. Pharm. Praxis. Beilage Nr. 7 zur Pharmazie *22*, 198–204 (1967)

Kharkevich, D.A.: Ganglionic agents. Moskva: Medgiz 1962

Lape, H.E., Hoppe, J.O.: The use of serial carotid occlusion, nictitating membrane, and cross-circulation technics in the investigation of the central hypotensive activity of ganglionic blocking agents. J. Pharmacol. Exp. Ther. *116*, 453–461 (1956)

Lape, H.E., Fort, D.J., Hoppe, J.O.: Observations on the ganglionic blocking properties of a series of bi-quaternary propane derivatives. J. Pharmacol. Exp. Ther. *116*, 462–468 (1956)

Mason, D.F.J., Wien, R.: The actions of heterocyclic bis-quaternary compounds especially of a pyrrolidinium series. Br. J. Pharmacol. *10*, 124–132 (1955)

Moe, G.K., Freyburger, W.A.: Ganglionic blocking agents. Pharmacol. Rev. *2*, 61–95 (1950)

Nádor, K.: Ganglionblocker. In: Fortschritte der Arzneimittelforschung. Jucker, E. (ed.), Vol. II, 297–416. Basel, Stuttgart: Birkhäuser 1960

Pallazo, G., Virno, M.: Farmaco [Sci.] *9*, 3 (1959); l.c. Nádor, K.: Ganglionblocker. In: Fortschritte der Arzneimittelforschung. Jucker, E. (ed.), Vol. II, 297–416. Basel, Stuttgart: Birkhäuser 1960

Paton, W.D.M.: The uses of the methonium compounds. J. R. Inst. Publ. Health Hyg. – February, 1953, pp. 1–20

Paton, W.D.M., Zaimis, E.J.: Curare-like action of polymethylene bis-quaternary ammonium salts. Nature *161*, 718–719 (1948)

Paton, W.D.M., Zaimis, E.J.: The pharmacological actions of polymethylene bistrimethyl-ammonium salts. Br. J. Pharmacol. *4*, 381–400 (1949)

Paton, W.D.M., Zaimis, E.J.: Paralysis of autonomic ganglia by methonium salts. Br. J. Pharmacol. *6*, 155–168 (1951)

Paton, W.D.M., Zaimis, F.J.: The methonium compounds. Pharmacol. Rev. *4*, 219–253 (1952)

Plummer, A.J., Trapold, J.H., Schneider, J.A., Maxwell, R.A., Earl, A.E.: Ganglionic blockade by a new bisquaternary series including chlorisondamine dimethochloride. J. Pharmacol. Exp. Ther. *115*, 172–184 (1955)

Protiva, M., Jílek, J.O., Exner, O.: Látky blokující sympatická ganglia I. Sulfoniová analoga nižších methoniumjodidů. Chem. Listy *47*, 580–583 (1953)

Robinson, R.A.: Autonomic blocking agents. I. Branched aliphatic quaternary ammonium and analogous cyclic ammonium salts. J. Org. Chem. *16*, 1911–1920 (1951)

Van Rossum, J. M.: Classification and molecular pharmacology of ganglionic blocking agents. Part II. Mode of action of competitive and non-competitive ganglionic blocking agents. Int. J. Neuropharmacol. *1*, 403–421 (1962)

Sharapov, I.M.: On the pharmacology of dioquine. Farmakol. Toksikol. *20*, no. 6, pp. 9–15 (1957)

Sharapov, I.M.: On the pharmacology of dicoline. Farmakol. Toksikol. *21*, No. 1, 19–24 (1958)

Standaert, F.G., Friess, S.L, Doty, R.O.: Comparative ganglion-blocking potencies of the geometric isomers of two cyclic 1,2-amino alcohols. J. Med. Pharm. Chem. *1*, 459–466 (1959)

Tommasini, R., Passerini, N.: Attivita gangioplegica di une serie di derivati mono-e bis-quaternari del 3-azabiciclo-(3.3 1)-nonano. Nota I. Farmaco [Sci.] *14*, 544–553 (1959)

Trčka, V., Lorencová, L.: Látky blokující sympatická ganglia V. Farmakologie nových derivátů několika typů. Čs. Farmacie *6*, 194–197 (1957)

Trčka, V., Vanček, M : Některé nové typy gangioplegik. Čs. Farmacie *8*, 316–325 (1959)

Trendelenburg, U.: Pharmacology of autonomic ganglia. Ann. Rev. Pharmacol. Toxicol. *1*, 219–238 (1961)

Triggle, D.J.: Cholinergic mechanisms: Blockade at ganglionic synapses. Chemical aspects of the autonomic nervous system. London, New York: Academic Press 1965

Triggle, D.J.: Analogs and antagonists of acetylcholine and norephinephrine: The relationships between chemical structure and biological activity. Neurotransmitter – receptor interactions. London, New York: Academic Press 1971

Vejdělek, Z.J.: Neue Typen synthetischer Verbindungen mit ganglienblockierender Wirkung. Arzneim. Forsch. *10*, 808–811 (1960)

Wien, R.: Relation of chemical structure of compounds to their action on autonomic ganglia. Arch. Int. Pharmacodyn. Ther. *97*, 395–406 (1954)

Wien, R., Mason, D.F.J.: The pharmacological actions of a series of phenyl alcane p-ω-bis(trialkylammonium) compounds. Br. J. Pharmacol. *8*, 306–314 (1953)

Wien, R., Mason, D.F.J., Edge, N.D., Langston, G.T.: The ganglion blocking properties of homologous compounds in the methonium series. Br. J. Pharmacol. *7*, 534–541 (1952)

Winbury, M.M.: Autonomic blocking compounds. I. Ganglion blocking action of some aliphatic quaternary ammonium salts, related alkyl piperidinium salts and 1,2,3,4-tetrahydroiso-quinolinium salts. J. Pharmacol. Exp. Ther. *105*, 327–336 (1952)

Winbury, M.M., Cook, D.L., Hambourger, W.E.: Autonomic blocking compounds II. Influence of secondary alkyl groups on ganglion blocking activity of various quaternary ammonium derivatives. Arch. Int. Pharmacodyn. Ther. *97*, 125–140 (1954)

Zaimis, E.J.: The interruption of ganglionic transmission and some of its problems. J. Pharm. Pharmacol. *7*, 497–511 (1955)

CHAPTER 4b

Relationship Between Chemical Structure and Ganglion-Blocking Activity
b) Tertiary and Secondary Amines

V. TRČKA

A. Introduction

The therapeutic effects of the first known quaternary ganglion-blocking agents in the treatment of hypertension (tetraethylammonium, hexamethonium) have stimulated a wide search for new drugs with similar effects. Several hundred quaternary and bis-quaternary derivatives have been synthesised and tested for ganglion-blocking activity. Several clinically successful drugs of this type have been found (Ansolysen, Pendiomide, Ecolide, etc.).

The relationship between the chemical structure of mono- and bis-quaternary ammonium compounds and their ganglion-blocking activity has been thoroughly discussed in a number of reviews (NÁDOR, 1960; KHARKEVICH, 1962, etc.). This chapter will therefore deal only with tertiary and secondary amines. The years 1955–1956, saw the appearance of the first reports on ganglion-blocking and hypotensive activity of mecamylamine (3-methylaminoisocamphane) (1) (MOYER et al., 1955; FREIS, 1955; FREIS and WILSON, 1955; SCHNECKLOTH et al., 1956, etc.). This substance was one of the first ganglion-blocking agents lacking a quaternary ammonium group.

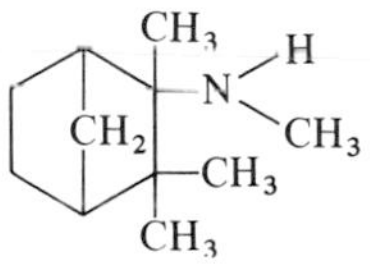

1.

Several non-quaternary substances with at least a partial ganglion-blocking effect had been described earlier. SYRNEVA (1950) found a weak ganglion-blocking activity of 2,6-dimethylpiperidine (nanophine), a substance isolated from Nanophyton erynaceum (2).

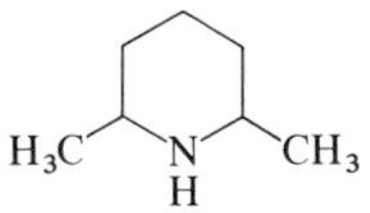

2.

Later, a similar activity of several tris-(dialkylaminoalkyl)-amines of general structural formula (3), in which R = methyl or ethyl and $n = 2$–4 were described by GYERMEK (1952), REITZE et al. (1953) and PLUMMER et al. (1954).

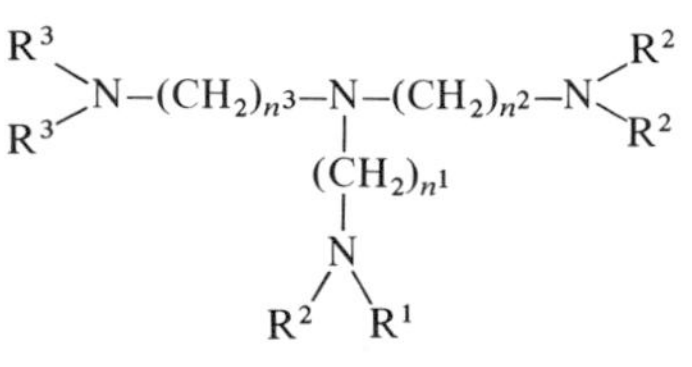

3.

The activity of mecamylamine in both clinical and experimental situations led to a search for further active compounds and to the study of structure-activity relationships in different mecamylamine congeners. It was established that ganglion-blocking activity was not bound up with bi-cyclic structure. The cyclohexylamine analogue of mecamylamine (4) showed higher activity than mecamylamine (Protiva et al., 1959; Vejdělek and Trčka, 1959; Trčka and Vaněček, 1959; Vejdělek et al., 1959).

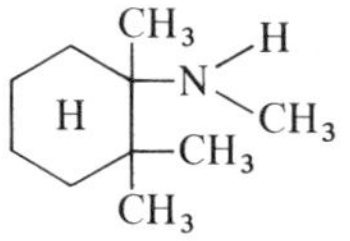

Since then, another very active compound, which is related to nanophine, i.e., 1,2,2,6,6-pentamethylpiperidine (pempidine) (5) (Spinks and Young, 1958; Lee et al., 1958; Harington et al., 1958), has been described:

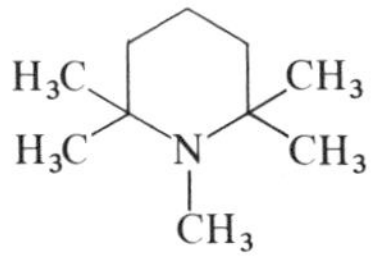

These findings, and the ganglion-blocking activity of several other secondary and tertiary amines, have led to the conclusion that this activity is connected with the presence of several methyl groups close to the nitrogen atom of a secondary or tertiary amine group (Spinks et al., 1968; Vejdělek and Trčka, 1959; Protiva et al., 1959). On the basis of this conclusion it was possible to assume that aliphatic compounds derived from mecamylamine and complying with the above assumption can exhibit ganglion-blocking activity. This idea was confirmed by synthesis of several highly active compounds with the general formula 6.

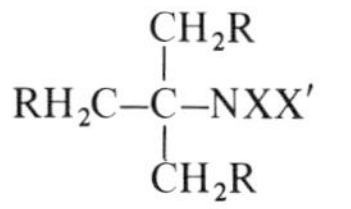

$$
\begin{array}{c}
CH_2R \\
| \\
RH_2C-C-NXX' \quad\quad 6. \\
| \\
CH_2R
\end{array}
$$

R represents methyl or another lower alkyl and NXX denotes a secondary or tertiary amino group (Vejdělek and Trčka, 1959; Trčka and Vaněček, 1959; Kochetkov et al., 1959; Hiltmann et al., 1960; Kharkevich, 1962a, etc.). However, several other lines of structure-activity relationships in non-quaternary ganglion-blocking agents were followed up. When interest in ganglion-blocking agents was at its height several extensive reviews on structure-activity relationships were published (Nádor, 1960; Vejdělek, 1960; Kharkevich, 1962). Most compounds treated in the present review were mentioned in the previous ones. Since then, only a limited number of new substances affecting sympathetic ganglia have been synthesised and tested. The aim of this review is to give a general survey of the effect of structural variations on the ganglion-blocking activity of non-quaternary drugs. The substances are tabulated according to their basic structure, quality, and number of substituents. The data on the activity of individual substances in the tables are based mainly on estimated values for ED_{50} in cat nicitating membrane (blockade of contractions elicited by preganglionic stimulation). Several compounds were evaluated by their antinicotinic activity (blockade of nicotinic convulsions in mice). These data are denoted by an asterisk in the tables. Papers dealing with secondary or tertiary amines structurally related to non-quaternary ganglion-blocking agents and in which other criteria of activity are indicated (e.g., hypotensive effect) are not included in this review.

To provide a uniform view on structure-activity relationships, the activity of all compounds was expressed in terms of the activity of mecamylamine. Data collected in studies in which hexamethonium or other ganglion-blocking agents were used as a standard were converted to the relative activity of mecamylamine. Estimation of relative activities has served as the basis of this transformation of original data: tetraethylammonium 40%, hexamethonium 80%, pempidine 240% (cat nictitating membrane). These relative activities were derived as approximate mean values from a series of data on relative activities of these drugs found by different authors (Table 1).

The values for relative activity given in the tables have to be considered as approximative, because several sources of inaccuracy are involved in a compilation of data from several papers.

The *methods of estimation* of ganglion-blocking activity used by different authors were not identical (e.g., different frequencies of preganglionic stimulation give different relative activities; MCISAAC et al., 1963).

Because the *dose-response curves* of hexamethonium and mecamylamine are not parallel, some differences in relative activities may occur when the activity of any of the series of compounds related to hexamethonium is compared with the activity of

Table 1. Relative activities of standard ganglion-blocking agents

Drug	Percentage activity (activity of mecamylamine $= 100\%$)	Ref.
Cat nictitating membrane		
Tetraethylammonium	39	SPINKS et al. (1958)
Hexamethonium	73	SPINKS et al. (1958)
	74	BAINBRIDGE and BROWN (1960)
	77	NADOR (1960)
	80	TRČKA and VANĚČEK (1959)
	82	CORNE and EDGE (1958)
	83	MCISAAK et al. (1963)
	83	EDGE et al. (1960)
	88	STONE et al. (1956)
	117	COOPER et al. (1971)
Pempidine	110	CORNE and EDGE (1958)
	239	SPINKS et al. (1958)
	253	NÁDOR (1960)
Nicotine convulsions in mice		
Hexamethonium	7	CORNE and EDGE (1958)
	34	STONE et al. (1956)
Pempidine	120	CORNE and EDGE (1958)

those related to mecamylamine. The ED_{50} is often given in milligrams per kilogram, regardless of the molecular weight of evaluated drugs.

The *potency* of mecamylamine in relation to hexamethonium or pempidine estimated from the data summarised in Table 1 is only a mean value of relative activities found by similar but not identical methods carried out under different conditions.

In spite of all these inconsistencies, transformed data reflect the change in relative activity induced by substitution of one chemical group by another substituent and allow comparison of the effects of similar structural changes in different types of compounds on ganglionic activity.

B. Structure-Activity Relationships in Different Structural Types of Non-Quaternary Ganglion-Blocking Agents

I. Substituted Aminoalkyl Derivatives

Ganglion-Blocking activity of different substituted alkylamines has been studied by several authors. Many monoamino derivatives have been described (Tables 2–4). Much less attention was paid to the diamino- and triaminoalkyl derivatives (Tables 5 and 6).

Most primary monoamines with a limited number of branchings of the alkyl chain display a ganglion-stimulating effect (Table 2, Nos. 12 and 19; Table 3, No. 1). Compounds with a larger alkyl residue may show a slight ganglion-blocking activity (Table 2, e.g., Nos. 29 and 32).

A stimulating effect on sympathetic ganglia in a large series of secondary and tertiary amines was found only in the case of compound No. 35 in Table 2. In all other derivatives of this type, the ganglion-blocking activity varied within the limits of 0 and 1000% of the activity of mecamylamine.

The monoaminoalkyl derivatives studied do not represent a sufficiently systematic series to allow the estimation of quantitative differences between the activity of secondary and tertiary methyl-, ethyl-, and isopropylamine derivatives.

The most active compound described is *N*-isopropyl-tert. butylamine (Table 2, No. 2). The corresponding *N*-sec. butyl- and *N*-sec. pentyl-derivatives (Table 2, Nos. 5 and 6) are less active. The activity is decreased by hydroxyalkyl groups (Table 2, Nos. 3, 4, and 11). Comparison of the relative activities of compounds 1 and 14 and of 9 and 15 in Table 2 suggests that the prolongation of the alkylamine residue by one methyl group does not substantially change the activity. The activity of secondary and tertiary amines increases, however, when the substituent R in the general formula in Table 2, is represented by the tert. butyl group (compare No. 13 with No. 23, or No. 8 with No. 25 in Table 2). The tert. butyl group reversed the ganglion-stimulating activity of the primary amine, No. 12 to ganglion-blockade (compound No. 22, Table 2). The methyl and ethyl groups substituting hydrogen atoms of the amino group are less active than the corresponding dimethylamines when the substituent R is represented by the tert. butyl group (compare No. 8 with No. 9 and No. 25 with No. 26).

Similar relationships can be found in the group of aminoalkyl derivatives with a higher number of carbon atoms in the side chain (Tables 3 and 4). The branching of the alkyl skeleton increases the activity only, to a definite degree (Table 3, No. 7 or 9

Table 2. Substituted aminoalkyl derivatives (A)

$$R-\underset{\underset{CH_3}{|}}{\overset{\overset{CH_3}{|}}{C}}-N\overset{R'}{\underset{R''}{<}}$$

Compound no.	R	R'	R''	Percentage activity (activity of mecamylamine = 100%)	References
1	CH_3	H	CH_2CH_3	70	KHARKEVICH, 1962
2	CH_3	H	$CH\overset{CH_3}{\underset{CH_3}{<}}$	200–1000	HILTMANN et al., 1960
3	CH_3	H	$CH\overset{CH_3}{\underset{CH_2OH}{<}}$	10	HILTMANN et al., 1960
4	CH_3	H	$CH\overset{CH_3}{\underset{CH_2OCH_3}{<}}$	20	HILTMANN et al., 1960
5	CH_3	H	$CH\overset{CH_3}{\underset{CH_2CH_3}{<}}$	100	HILTMANN et al., 1960
6	CH_3	H	$\underset{CH_2CH_3}{\overset{CH_3}{\underset{|}{\overset{|}{C}}}}-CH_3$	110 0	BRETHERICK et al., 1959 EASTON et al., 1966
7	CH_3	H	$\underset{CH=CH_2}{\overset{CH_3}{\underset{|}{\overset{|}{C}}}}-CH_3$	Active	EASTON et al., 1966
8	CH_3	CH_3	CH_3	6	KHARKEVICH, 1962
9	CH_3	CH_3	CH_2CH_3	30	KHARKEVICH, 1962
10	CH_3	CH_3	$CH\overset{CH_3}{\underset{CH_3}{<}}$	100	HILTMANN et al., 1960

Table 2. Substituted aminoalkyl derivatives (A) (continued)

Compound no.	R	R'	R''	Percentage activity (activity of meca- mylamine = 100%)	References
11	CH_2OH	CH_3	$CH\begin{smallmatrix}CH_3\\CH_3\end{smallmatrix}$	10	Hiltmann et al., 1960
12	CH_2CH_3	H	H	Stimul.[a]	Kharkevich, 1962
13	CH_2CH_3	H	CH_3	35	Kharkevich, 1962
14	CH_2CH_3	H	CH_2CH_3	60	Kharkevich, 1962
15	CH_2CH_3	CH_3	CH_2CH_3	40	Kharkevich, 1962
16	$(CH_2)_2CH_3$	H	CH_2CH_3	25	Kharkevich, 1962
17	$CH\begin{smallmatrix}CH_3\\CH_3\end{smallmatrix}$	H	CH_2CH_3	65	Kharkevich, 1962
18	$CH\begin{smallmatrix}CH_3\\CH_3\end{smallmatrix}$	CH_3	CH_3	20 / 20	Hiltmann et al., 1960 / Vejdělek et al., 1970
19	$(CH_2)_3CH_3$	H	H	Stimul.	Vejdělek et al., 1970
20	$(CH_2)_3CH_3$	H	CH_3	5	Vejdělek et al., 1970
21	$(CH_2)_3CH_3$	CH_3	CH_3	5	Vejdělek et al., 1970
22	$\overset{CH_3}{\underset{CH_3}{\overset{\vert}{C}-CH_3}}$	H	H	30 / 14	Kharkevich, 1962 / Trčka, 1961
23	$\overset{CH_3}{\underset{CH_3}{\overset{\vert}{C}-CH_3}}$	H	CH_3	150 / 110 / 85	Kharkevich, 1962 / Trčka and Vaneček, 1959 / Stone et al., 1962

Table 2. Substituted aminoalkyl derivatives (A) (continued)

Compound no.	R	R'	R''	Percentage activity (activity of meca-mylamine = 100%)	References
24	$\begin{array}{c} CH_3 \\ | \\ C-CH_3 \\ | \\ CH_3 \end{array}$	H	CH_2CH_3	35	KHARKEVICH, 1962
25	$\begin{array}{c} CH_3 \\ | \\ C-CH_3 \\ | \\ CH_3 \end{array}$	CH_3	CH_3	120 200	KHARKEVICH, 1962 TRČKA and VANĚČEK, 1959
26	$\begin{array}{c} CH_3 \\ | \\ C-CH_3 \\ | \\ CH_3 \end{array}$	CH_3	CH_2CH_3	60	KHARKEVICH, 1962
27	$\begin{array}{c} CH_3 \\ | \\ CH_2-C-CH_3 \\ | \\ CH_3 \end{array}$	H	CH_2CH_3	20	SPINKS and YOUNG, 1958
28	$\begin{array}{c} CH_3 \\ | \\ CH_2-C-CH_3 \\ | \\ CH_3 \end{array}$	CH_3	CH_3	10	SPINKS and YOUNG, 1958
29	$\begin{array}{c} CH_3 \\ | \\ C-CH_2CH_3 \\ | \\ CH_3 \end{array}$	H	H	10	VEJDĚLEK et al., 1970
30	$\begin{array}{c} CH_3 \\ | \\ C-CH_2CH_3 \\ | \\ CH_3 \end{array}$	H	CH_3	40	VEJDĚLEK et al., 1970
31	$\begin{array}{c} CH_3 \\ | \\ C-CH_2CH_3 \\ | \\ CH_3 \end{array}$	CH_3	CH_3	45	VEJDĚLEK et al., 1970
32	$\begin{array}{c} CH_3 \quad CH_3 \\ | \quad / \\ C-CH \\ | \quad \backslash \\ CH_3 \quad CH_3 \end{array}$	H	H	25	VEJDĚLEK et al., 1970

Table 2. Substituted aminoalkyl derivatives (A) (continued)

Compound no.	R	R'	R''	Percentage activity (activity of meca-mylamine = 100%)	References
33	$\begin{array}{c}CH_3\quad CH_3\\ |\quad\diagup\\ C{-}CH\\ |\quad\diagdown\\ CH_3\quad CH_3\end{array}$	H	CH_3	70	Vejdělek et al., 1970
34	$\begin{array}{c}CH_3\quad CH_3\\ |\quad\diagup\\ C{-}CH\\ |\quad\diagdown\\ CH_3\quad CH_3\end{array}$	CH_3	CH_3	120	Vejdělek et al., 1970
35	$\begin{array}{c}CH_3\\ |\\ C{-}\bigcirc\\ |\\ CH_3\end{array}$	H	CH_3	Stimul.	Vejdělek et al., 1970
36	$\begin{array}{c}CH_3\\ |\\ C{-}\bigcirc\\ |\\ CH_3\end{array}$	CH_3	CH_3	5	Vejdělek et al., 1970
37	$\begin{array}{c}CH_3\\ |\\ C{-}CH_2{-}\bigcirc\\ |\\ CH_3\end{array}$	H	CH_3	0	Vejdělek et al., 1970
38	$\begin{array}{c}CH_3\\ |\\ C{-}CH_2{-}\bigcirc\\ |\\ CH_3\end{array}$	CH_3	CH_3	0	Vejdělek et al., 1970

* Blockade of nicotinic convulsions in mice
[a] Stimul.: ganglionic stimulation

as against Table 4, No. 2 or 3). Tertiary methylamines are more active than the corresponding secondary ones (Table 3, No. 9, Table 4, No. 3 vs. Table 3, No. 7, Table 4, No. 2).

Generally, the activity of monoaminoalkyl derivatives depends on the total size of the molecule, on the length and branching of the alkyl residue, and on the number, size, and branching of the alkyl substituents in the amino group. The total number of carbon atoms and the of branchings of the alkyl residue has to be in equilibrium with the size of substituents of the amino group. If the main chain is represented by a larger, branched alkyl group, the methylamino or dimethylamino derivatives are the most active. Correspondingly, among the tert. butylamino derivatives, the highest

Table 3. Substituted aminoalkyl derivatives (B)

$$R-\underset{\underset{CH_2CH_3}{|}}{\overset{\overset{CH_3}{|}}{C}}-N\overset{R'}{\underset{R''}{\diagdown}}$$

Compound no.	R	R'	R''	Percentage activity (activity of meca-mylamine = 100%)	References
1	CH_2CH_3	H	H	Stimul.[a]	KHARKEVICH, 1962a
2	CH_2CH_3	H	CH_3	40	KHARKEVICH, 1962a
3	CH_2CH_3	H	CH_2CH_3	55	KHARKEVICH, 1962a
4	CH_2CH_3	CH_3	CH_3	35	KHARKEVICH, 1962a
5	CH_2CH_3	CH_3	CH_2CH_3	45	KHARKEVICH, 1962a
6	$\overset{\overset{CH_3}{|}}{\underset{\underset{CH_3}{|}}{C}}-CH_3$	H	H	Stimul.	TRČKA and VANĚČEK, 1959
7	$\overset{\overset{CH_3}{|}}{\underset{\underset{CH_3}{|}}{C}}-CH_3$	H	CH_3	200	TRČKA and VANĚČEK, 1959
8	$\overset{\overset{CH_3}{|}}{\underset{\underset{CH_3}{|}}{C}}-CH_3$	H	CH_2CH_3	40	KHARKEVICH, 1962a
9	$\overset{\overset{CH_3}{|}}{\underset{\underset{CH_3}{|}}{C}}-CH_3$	CH_3	CH_3	300	TRČKA and VANĚČEK, 1959
10	$CH_2CH_2CH_3$	H	CH_2CH_3	30	KHARKEVICH, 1962a

[a] Stimul.: ganglionic stimulation

Table 4. Substituted aminoalkyl derivatives (C)

$$R^2-\underset{\underset{R^3}{|}}{\overset{\overset{R^1}{|}}{C}}-N\overset{R'}{\underset{R''}{\diagup}}$$

Compound no.	R^1	R^2	R^3	R'	R''	Percentage activity (activity of meca-mylamine = 100%)	References
1	CH_3	$\overset{CH_3}{\underset{CH_3}{\overset{|}{C}}}-CH_3$	$\overset{CH_3}{\underset{CH_3}{\overset{\diagup}{CH}}}$	H	H	30	Trčka and Vaněček, 1959
2	CH_3	$\overset{CH_3}{\underset{CH_3}{\overset{|}{C}}}-CH_3$	$\overset{CH_3}{\underset{CH_3}{\overset{\diagup}{CH}}}$	H	CH_3	70	Trčka and Vaněček, 1959
3	CH_3	$\overset{CH_3}{\underset{CH_3}{\overset{|}{C}}}-CH_3$	$\overset{CH_3}{\underset{CH_3}{\overset{\diagup}{CH}}}$	CH_3	CH_3	125	Trčka and Vaněček, 1959
4	CH_2CH_3	CH_2CH_3	CH_2CH_3	H	H	20	Kharkevich, 1962a
5	CH_2CH_3	CH_2CH_3	CH_2CH_3	H	CH_3	55	Kharkevich, 1962a
6	CH_2CH_3	CH_2CH_3	CH_2CH_3	H	CH_2CH_3	140	Kharkevich, 1962a
7	CH_2CH_3	CH_2CH_3	CH_2CH_3	H	$\overset{CH_3}{\underset{CH_3}{\overset{\diagup}{CH}}}$	20	Hiltmann et al., 1960
8	CH_2CH_3	CH_2CH_3	CH_2CH_3	CH_3	CH_3	65	Kharkevich, 1962a
9	CH_2CH_3	CH_2CH_3	CH_2CH_3	CH_2CH_3	CH_2CH_3	45	Kharkevich, 1962a

activity is displayed by derivatives with larger alkyl groups substituting the hydrogen atom of the amino group. The isopropyl substituent seems to be optimum. With the increasing total number of carbon atoms, the number of methyl groups should increase to maintain high activity.

Diamino derivatives resembling the bis-quaternary ganglion-blocking agents of the penta- or hexamethonium type (Table 5) and tris-(dialkylaminoalkyl)-amines (Table 6) have only a limited effect on ganglia. Their effect seems to depend on the length of the alkyl chains.

Table 5. Diaminoalkylderivatives

$$\underset{R^1}{\overset{H}{\diagdown}}N-(CH_2)_n-N\underset{R^2}{\overset{H}{\diagup}}$$

Compound no.	R^1	R^2	n	Percentage activity (activity of meca-mylamine = 100%)	References
1	$C(CH_3)_3$	H	4	80	McCARTHY, 1965
2	$CH(CH_3)_2$	$CH(CH_3)_2$	4	Active	PANASHENKO, 1956
3	$(CH_2)_2CH(CH_3)_2$	H	5	Active	DOROZCEVA, 1955

Table 6. Tris–(dialkylaminoalkyl)–amines

$$\underset{R_2^2N(CH_2)_{n^2}}{\overset{R_2^1N(CH_2)_{n^1}}{\diagdown}}N(CH_2)_{n^3}-NR_2^3$$

R^1	R^2	R^3	n^1	n^2	n^3	Activity	References
C_2H_5	C_2H_5	C_2H_5	2	2	2	+++	PLUMMER et al., 1954
C_2H_5	C_2H_5	C_2H_5	3	2	2	++++	
C_2H_5	C_2H_5	C_2H_5	4	2	2	+++	
C_2H_5	C_2H_5	C_2H_5	5	2	2	0	
CH_3	C_2H_5	C_2H_5	3	2	2	+++	
C_3H_7	C_2H_5	C_2H_5	3	2	2	+	
C_4H_9	C_2H_5	C_2H_5	3	2	2	0	
C_2H_5	C_2H_5	C_2H_5	3	3	2	+	
C_2H_5	C_2H_5	C_2H_5	3	3	3	+	
CH_3	CH_3	CH_3	2	2	2	Active	GYERMEK, 1952

II. Alicyclic Amines

This type of blocking compounds is represented largely by a series of cyclohexylamine derivatives. Table 7 shows that the blocking activity depends on the number and localisation of methyl groups attached to the nucleus in the vicinity of the nitrogen atom of the amino group. The most active compounds, the 1,2,2-trimethylcyclohexylamines (Table 7, Nos. 10–12), display activity comparable to that of mecamylamine. This finding shows that the methylene bridge in the mecamylamine molecule is not an important factor in its activity. However, comparison of these compounds with cyclohexylamine derivatives Nos. 13–16 in Table 7 and compound No. 2, Table 8, indicates the decisive role of the three methyl groups surrounding the nitrogen atom of the amino group. Steric hindrance of the nitrogen atom seems to influence the activity more than a liphophil nature given by the number of methyl groups (compare No. 12, Table 7, and No. 2, Table 8).

The importance of the above-mentioned activity requirements can also be documented by substances of the monoamino and 1,4-diamino cyclohexane types (Table 9, Nos. 1–6). Primary and secondary amines are ganglionic stimulants. Only the tertiary amines (No. 3 and 6) display a weak blocking activity. The increased distance between the two amino groups in compound No. 7 in Table 9 may be responsible for its higher activity.

Cyclopentylamine derivatives (Table 10) show structure-activity relationship similar to those of cyclohexylamine derivatives. An active cyclobutylamine derivative (Table 20, No. 1) has also been described.

III. Derivatives of 3-Aminoisocamphane

The most active compounds of the 3-aminoisocamphane derivatives summarised in Table 11 are mecamylamine (compound No. 17) and dimecamine (No. 29).

Optical isomers of mecamylamine do not vary substantially in activity. The ganglion-blocking potency of the racemate and the *l*-form is the same, while *d*-mecamylamine exhibits activity about 20% lower (No. 17, Table 16).

The activity data for mecamylamine derivatives given in Table 11 clearly document the key role of the methyl groups close to the nitrogen atom. The lack of one methyl group in position 2 or 3 of aminoisocamphane (substituents R^1, R^2, R^3 in general formula in Table 11) decreases the activity. This can be demonstrated by comparing compounds 4, 13, and 17, for example. The lower activity of compound 4 than of No. 13 suggests that the absence of a methyl group in position 3 of aminoisocamphane (R^1) affects the activity more than withdrawal of a substituent in position 2 (R^2, R^3).

The activity is also influenced by the number and size of alkyl groups substituting hydrogen atoms of the amino group. As mentioned above, 3-methylamino- and 3-dimethylaminoisocamphane (Nos. 17 and 29) are the most active derivatives. Larger substituents than the methyl group decrease the activity (compare No. 17 with 18–28).

The data in Table 11 illustrate the decisive role of the number and size of substituents surrounding the nitrogen atom of 3-aminoisocamphane derivatives. These substituents bring about steric hindrance of the nitrogen atom as well as affecting lipophility of the molecule. Both factors seem to be at their optimum with four to five methyl groups in mecamylamine and dimecamine (Nos. 17 and 29, Table 11).

Table 7. Cyclohexylamine derivatives (A)

Compound no.	R^1	R^2	R^3	R'	R''	Configuration	Percentage activity (activity of mecamylamine = 100%)	References
1	H	CH_3	H	H	H	cis—	20—25	Trčka and Vaněček, 1959
2	H	CH_3	H	H	H	trans—	5	Trčka and Vaněček, 1959
3	H	CH_3	H	H	CH_3	cis—	10—15	Trčka and Vaněček, 1959
4	H	CH_3	H	H	CH_3	trans—	7—10	Trčka and Vaněček, 1959
5	H	CH_3	H	CH_3	CH_3	cis—	15—20	Trčka and Vaněček, 1959
6	H	CH_3	H	CH_3	CH_3	trans—	8—12	Trčka and Vaněček, 1959
7	H	CH_3	CH_3	H	H		10—15	Trčka and Vaněček, 1959
8	H	CH_3	CH_3	H	CH_3		15—20	Trčka and Vaněček, 1959
9	H	CH_2	CH_3	CH_3	CH_3		15—25	Trčka and Vaněček, 1959
10	CH_3	CH_3	CH_3	H	H		70—120	Trčka and Vaněček, 1959
11	CH_3	CH_3	CH_3	H	CH_3		80—140	Trčka and Vaněček, 1959
12	CH_3	CH_3	CH_3	CH_3	CH_3		120—250	Trčka and Vaněček, 1959
13	CH_3	H	H	H	H		Stimul.[a]	Trčka and Vaněček, 1959
14	CH_2CH_3	H	H	H	H		Very low activity	Kharkevich, 1962b
15	CH_3	H	H	H	CH_3		Stimul.	Trčka and Vaněček, 1959
							25	Kharkevich, 1962b
16	CH_3	H	H	CH_3	CH_3		25—50	Trčka and Vaněček, 1959
17	CH_2CH_3	H	H	H	CH_2CH_3		25	Kharkevich, 1962b
18	$(CH_2)_2CH_3$	H	H	H	$(CH_2)_2CH_3$		25	Kharkevich, 1962b

[a] Stimul.: gangloionic stimulation.

Table 8. Cyclohexylamine derivatives (B)

Compound no.	R^1	R^2	R'	R''	Percentage activity (activity of meca-mylamine = 100%)	References
1	H	CH_3	H	H	5	Trčka and Vaněček, 1959
2	H	CH_3	CH_3	CH_3	5–10	
3	CH_3	CH_3	H	H	12–15	

Table 9. Cyclohexylamine derivatives (C)

Compound no.	R'	R''	X	Percentage activity (activity of meca-mylamine = 100%)	References
1	H	H	H	Stimul.[a]	Trčka and Vaněček, 1959
2	H	CH_3	H	Stimul.	
3	CH_3	CH_3	H	5–10	
4	H	H	NH_2	Stimul.	
5	H	CH_3	$NHCH_3$	Stimul.	
6	CH_3	CH_3	$N(CH_3)_2$	5	
7	CH_3	CH_3	$(CH_2)_2N(CH_3)_2$	80	McMillan et al., 1956

[a] Stimul.: ganglionic stimulation

Table 10. Cyclopentylamine derivatives

Compound no.	R^1	R^2	R^3	R'	R''	Percentage activity (activity of meca-mylamine $= 100\%$)	References
1	CH_3	H	H	H	H	Very low activity	KHARKEVICH, 1962a and b
2	C_2H_5	H	H	H	CH_3	Very low activity	
3	CH_3	H	H	H	CH_3	25	
4	C_2H_5	H	H	H	C_2H_5	25	
5	C_2H_5	H	H	H	C_2H_5	25	
6	CH_3	CH_3	CH_3	H	CH_3	150	PROTIVA et al., 1965
7	CH_3	CH_3	CH_3	CH_3	CH_3	200	

Substitution in other positions of the 3-aminoisocamphane nucleus (Table 12, Nos. 1 and 2) or changes in the shape of the molecule led to decreased activity (Table 17, No. 3–10) in most instances.

IV. Piperidine Derivatives and Other N-Heterocyclic Compounds

The high ganglion-blocking potency and hypotensive activity of pempidine (1,-2,2,6,6-pentamethylpiperidine; Table 13, No. 18) stimulated synthesis and pharmacological study of many of its analogues. Structure-activity relationships in a series of piperidine derivatives substituted in positions 1, 2, and 6 are given in Table 13.

Piperidine (Table 13, No. 1) does not exhibit any ganglion-blocking activity. No distinct activity was found in 2-methylpiperidine (No. 2), and conflicting data have been published on 2,6-dimethylpiperidine (nanophine, no. 3). The activity rises with increasing numbers of methyl groups in positions 2 and 6 of the piperidine nucleus. 2,2,6,6-Tetramethylpiperidine (No. 5) reaches the activity of pempidine (penta-methylpiperidine, No. 19).

Substitution in position 1 seems to be less important than substitution in positions 2 and 6. Comparison of the activity data of compounds 1 and 8, No. 2 and 9, 3 and 10, and 5 and 19 (Table 13), shows only a very limited contribution of the methyl

Table 11. 3–Amino–isocamphane derivatives

Compound no.	R¹	R²	R³	R'	R''	Percentage activity (activity of meca-mylamine = 100%)	References
1	H	H	H	H	CH_3	(+)	Rubinstein et al., 1963
2	H	H	CH_3	H	CH_3	+++	Rubinstein et al., 1963
3	H	CH_3	CH_3	H	H	+	Rubinstein et al., 1963
4	H	CH_3	CH_3	H	CH_3	12	Edge et al., 1960
						60^a (d, l— —endo form)	Stone et al., 1962
						40^a (d, l— —exo form)	Stone et al., 1962
5	H	CH_3	CH_3	H	CH_2CH_3	+++	Rubinstein et al., 1963
6	H	CH_3	CH_3	H	$(CH_2)_2CH_3$	0	Rubinstein et al., 1963
7	H	CH_3	CH_3	H	$(CH_2)_3CH_3$	0	Rubinstein et al., 1963
8	H	CH_2CH_3	CH_2CH_3	H	CH_3	+++	Rubinstein et al., 1963
9	H	CH_3	CH_3	CH_3	CH_3	+++	Rubinstein et al., 1963
10	CH_3	H	H	H	CH_3	20	Edge et al., 1960
11	CH_2CH_3	H	H	H	CH_3	20	Edge et al., 1960
12	CH_3	H	CH_3	H	H	1	Edge et al., 1960
13	CH_3	H	CH_3	H	CH_3	30	Edge et al., 1960
14	CH_3	H	CH_3	H	CH_2-⬡	<1	Edge et al., 1960
15	CH_3	H	CH_3	CH_3	CH_3	40	Edge et al., 1960
16	CH	CH	CH	H	H	30	Trčka and Vaněček, 1959
						30^a	Stone et al., 1962
17	CH_3	CH_3	CH_3	H	CH_3	100 (dl—)	Edge et al., 1960, Stone et al., 1962, Trčka and Vaněček, 1959

Table 11. 3—Aminoisocamphane derivatives (continued)

Compound no.	R^1	R^2	R^3	R'	R''	Percentage activity (activity of mecamylamine = 100%)	References
						100 $(l-)$	TRČKA, 1961
						80 $(d-)$	TRČKA, 1961
						100[a] $(dl-)$	STONE et al., 1962
						85[a] $(d-)$	STONE et al., 1962
18	CH_3	CH_3	CH_3	H	CH_2CH_3	60[a]	STONE et al., 1962
19	CH_3	CH_3	CH_3	H	$(CH_2)_2CH_3$	12[a]	STONE et al., 1962
20	CH_3	CH_3	CH_3	H	$CH(CH_3)_3$	15[a]	STONE et al., 1962
21	CH_3	CH_3	CH_3	H	$(CH_2)_3CH_3$	Toxic	STONE et al., 1962
22	CH_3	CH_3	CH_3	H	$(CH_2)_4CH_3$	7[a]	STONE et al., 1962
23	CH_3	CH_3	CH_3	H	$(CH_2)_2C(CH_3)_3$	3[a]	STONE et al., 1962
24	CH_3	CH_3	CH_3	H	$CH_2CH=CH_2$	13[a]	STONE et al., 1962
25	CH_3	CH_3	CH_3	H	$(CH_2)_5CH_3$	3[a]	STONE et al., 1962
26	CH_3	CH_3	CH_3	H	$CH_2-\bigcirc$	2[a]	STONE et al., 1962
27	CH_3	CH_3	CH_3	H	$(CH_2)_2-\bigcirc$	5[a]	STONE et al., 1962
28	CH_3	CH_3	CH_3	H	$(CH_2)_3-\bigcirc$		STONE et al., 1962
29	CH_3	CH_3	CH_3	CH_3	CH_3	120	TRČKA and VANĚČEK, 1959
						110[a]	STONE et al., 1962
30	CH_3	CH_3	CH_3	CH_2CH_3	CH_2CH_3	24[a]	STONE et al., 1962
31	CH_3	CH_3	CH_3	CH_3	$CH_2-\bigcirc_N$	<10	TRČKA and VANĚČEK, 1959
32	CH_3	CH_3	CH_3	CH_3	$CO-\bigcirc_N$	<10	TRČKA and VANĚČEK, 1959
33	CH_3	CH_3	CH_3	CH_3	$(CH_2)_5-N\langle$	<10	TRČKA and VANĚČEK, 1959

[a] Blockade of nicotinic convulsions in mice.

Table 12. Isocamphane derivatives and related substances

Compound no.	Constitution		Percentage activity (activity of mecamylamine = 100%)	References
1		d, l—exo form	Active	RUBINSTEIN et al., 1958
			80*	STONE et al., 1962
		d, l—endo form	26	STONE et al., 1962
2			Active	RUBINSTEIN et al., 1958
3			12	EDGE et al., 1960

			R¹	R²	R³	R⁴		
4			CH_3	H	CH_3	CH_3	110	
5			CH_3	CH_3	CH_3	CH_3	80	
6			CH_3	CH_3	CH_3	H	45	EDGE et al., 1960
7			CH_3	CH_3	H	H	25	
8			C_2H_5	CH_3	H	H	15—20	

		R		
9		H	55	EDGE et al., 1960
10		CH_3	30	

* Blockade of nicotinic convulsions

Table 13. Piperidine derivatives (A)

Compound no.	R^1	R^2	R^3	R^4	R^5	Percentage activity (activity of mecamylamine = 100%)	References
1	H	H	II	H	H	0	SPINKS et al., 1958a
						Stimul.[a]	VIDAL– BERETERVIDE, 1966
2	CH$_3$	H	H	H	H	0	SPINKS et al., 1958a
						0,6	VIDAL– BERETERVIDE, 1966
3	H	CH$_3$	H	CH$_3$	H	0	SPINKS et al., 1958a
						2	TIKHONENKO, 1962b
						6	VIDAL– BERETERVIDE, 1966
						80	GYERMEK and NADOR, 1957
4	H	CH$_3$	CH$_2$	CH$_3$	H	40	SPINKS et al., 1958
						110	BRETHERICK et al., 1959
5	H	CH$_3$	CH$_3$	CH$_3$	CH$_3$	160	BRETHERICK et al., 1959
						170	TIKHONENKO, 1962a
							TIKHONENKO, 1962b
						180	VIDAL– BERETERVIDE, 1966
						200	SPINKS et al., 1958a
						Compund 19	PHILIPPOT et al., 1962
6	H	COO(CH$_2$)$_2$– –N(C$_2$H$_5$)$_2$	H	CH$_3$	H	15	RUBCOV et al., 1964
7	H	COO(CH$_2$)$_2$– –N(C$_2$H$_5$)$_2$	H	COO(CH$_2$)$_2$– –N(C$_2$H$_5$)$_2$	H	0	RUBCOV et al., 1964
8	CH$_3$	H	H	H	H	Stimul.	VIDAL– BERETERVIDE, 1966
						1	CUSIC and ROBINSON, 1951
9	CH$_3$	CH$_3$	H	H	H	1	SPINKS et al., 1958

Table 13. Piperidine derivatives (A) (continued)

Compound no.	R^1	R^2	R^3	R^4	R^5	Percentage activity (activity of meca-mylamine = 100%)	References
10	CH_3	CH_3	H	CH_3	H	8	Vidal–Beretervide, 1966
11	C_2H_5	CH_3	H	CH_3	H	10	
12	CH_3	$CH_2NH(CH_2)_2-N(C_2H_5)_2$	H	CH_3	H	80	Rubcov et al., 1964
13	CH_3	$CH_2N(C_2H_5)_2$	H	$CH_2N(C_2H_5)_2$	H	30	Rubcov et al., 1964
14	$(CH_2)_3OH$	CH_3	H	CH_3	H	Compound no. 3	Syrneva, 1961
15	$(CH_2)_3OCOCH_3$	CH_3	H	CH_3	H	Compound no. 3	Syrneva, 1961
16	$(CH_2)_3OCOC_2H_5$	CH_3	H	CH_3	H	Compound no. 3	Syrneva, 1961
17	$(CH_2)_3OCO$—⬡	CH_3	H	CH_3	H	Compound no. 3	Syrneva, 1961
18	$CO(CH_2)_2-N$	CH_3	H	CH_3	H	Compound no. 3	Syrneva, 1961
19	CH_3	CH_3	CH_3	CH_3	CH_3	110	Lee et al., 1958
						120	Tikhonenko, 1962a
							Tikhonenko, 1962b
						160	Bretherick et al., 1959
						250	Spinks et al., 1958
							Spinks and Young, 1958
20	CH_3	C CH	CH_3	CH_3	CH_3	Active	Easton et al., 1966
21	CH_2CH_3	CH_3	CH_3	CH_3	CH_3	70	Tikhonenko, 1962a
							Tikhonenko, 1962b
						160	Gyermek and Nador, 1957
						300	Spinks et al., 1958
22	$(CH_2)_2CH_3$	CH_3	CH_3	CH_3	CH_3	200	Spinks et al., 1958
23	nC_4H_9	CH_3	CH_3	CH_3	CH_3	150	Spinks et al., 1958
24	$CH_2CH=CH_2$	CH_3	CH_3	CH_3	CH_3	120	Spinks et al., 1958
25	$CH_2C_6H_5$	CH_3	CH_3	CH_3	CH_3	5	Tikhonenko, 1962a
							Tikhonenko, 1962b

Table 13. Piperidine derivatives (A) (continued)

Compound no.	R¹	R²	R³	R⁴	R⁵	Percentage activity (activity of mecamylamine = 100%)	References
						15	SPINKS et al., 1958
26	COCH₃	CH₃	CH₃	CH₃	CH₃	Compound 18	PHILIPPOT et al., 1962
27	NO	CH₃	CH₃	CH₃	CH₃	3	BRETHERICK et al., 1959
28	NH₂	CH₃	CH₃	CH₃	CH₃	110	BRETHERICK et al., 1959
29	NHCH₃	CH₃	CH₃	CH₃	CH₃	100	BRETHERICK et al., 1959
30	N(CH₃)₂	CH₃	CH₃	CH₃	CH₃	2	BRETHERICK et al., 1959
31	N=CH₂	CH₃	CH₃	CH₃	CH₃	140	BRETHERICK et al., 1959
32	N=CHCH₃	CH₃	CH₃	CH₃	CH₃	80	BRETHERICK et al., 1959

ª Stimul.: ganglionic stimulation.

group in position 1 to the activity. Larger substituents in the position 1 up to n-propyl or n-butyl group have a similar effect on activity to that of the methyl group (compare compound 19 with compounds 21–23) when positions 2 and 6 are substituted by methyl groups. Other substituents than lower alkyl groups in position 1 decrease the activity (Nos. 25–32). The methyl or dimethylaminopropyl group or a halogen atom in position 4 of the piperidine nucleus decreases the activity of pempidine to about half (Table 14). Other types of substitution in this position also have an unfavourable effect on activity (Table 15). A similar decline in activity was brought about by incorporation of a double bond into the piperidine ring (Table 16, No. 1; Table 18, No. 1), especially in combination with a substituent in position 4 (Table 16, Nos. 3 and 4). The low activity of the compounds presented in Table 17 seems to be due mainly to the absence of methyl groups in positions 2 and 6.

In summary, the ganglion-blocking activity of piperidine derivatives depends on the number of methyl groups in positions 2 and 6 (steric hindrance of the nitrogen atom), and on the quality of the substituent in position 1. As the number of methyl groups increases, the lipophility of the molecule rises. An additional increase of lipophility by means of a methyl or ethyl substituent on the nitrogen atom contributes to the activity.

The six-membered piperidine ring is not a condition for ganglion-blocking activity, as several pyrrolidine analogues of pempidine were found to be active (Table 18, e. g., Nos. 4–6 and 8). Structure-activity relationships in these compounds are similar to those in piperidine derivatives. Some activity was also seen in other N-heterocyclic compounds substituted by methyl groups on carbon atoms adjoining the nitrogen atom (Table 18, Nos. 9 and 10).

Table 14. Piperidine derivatives (B)

Compound no.	R^1	R^2	Percentage activity (activity of meca-mylamine = 100%)	References
1	H	CH$_3$	80	Vidal–Beretervide et al., 1966
2	CH$_3$	CH$_3$	90	Vidal–Beretervide et al., 1966
3	CH$_3$	(CH$_2$)$_3$N(CH$_3$)$_2$	80	McMillan et al., 1956
4	CH$_3$	Cl	80	Bretherick et al., 1959
5	CH$_3$	Br	80	Bretherick et al., 1959

Table 15. Piperidine derivatives (C)

Compound no.	R^1	R^2	Activity	References
1	H	=O	+	Simon and Vvedenskij, 1964
2	H		+	Philippot et al., 1962
3	H		+	Philippot et al., 1962
4	CH$_3$	=O	+	Philippot et al., 1962

Table 16. Piperidine derivatives (D)

Compound no.	R^1	R^2	Percentage activity (activity of meca-mylamine = 100%)	References
1	H	H	80	BRETHERICK et al., 1959
2	H	CH_3	80	
3	CH_3	H	180	
4	CH_3	C_2H_5	80	
5	CH_3	$(CH_2)_3N(CH_3)_2$	80	
6	CH_3	$C\equiv CH$	80	
7	NH_2	CH_3	80	
8	$NHCH_3$	H	80	

Among the quinuclidine derivatives presented in Table 19, only compound No. 2 showed significant activity.

The review of non-quaternary ganglion-blocking drugs includes several miscellaneous compounds tested for blocking activity on cat nictitating membrane (Table 20). Notable activity was described in one of the above-mentioned cyclobutyl derivatives (compound No. 1) and in 1,4-bis(dimethylaminomethyl)benzene (No. 2). The activity of other compounds in this table is low.

C. Conclusions

The common structural feature of highly active non-quaternary ganglion-blocking agents is that they are secondary or tertiary amines with a large number of methyl groups attached to the carbon atoms adjacent to the nitrogen atom of the amino group (SPINKS et al., 1958; VEJDĚLEK and TRČKA, 1959; PROTIVA et al., 1959; KOCHETKOV et al., 1959; HILTMANN et al., 1960; KHARKEVICH, 1962a). These methyl groups bring about a degree of steric hindrance of the nitrogen atom.

Table 17. Piperidine derivatives (E)

Compound no.	R^1	R^2	Percentage activity (activity of meca - mylamine = 100%)	References
1	H	$(CH_2)_2N(CH_3)_2$	<8	COLVILLE and FANELLI, 1956
2	H	$(CH_2)_2N$⬠	15	
3	H	$(CH_2)_2N$⬡	15	
4	H	$(CH_2)_2N$⬡O	<8	
5	CH_3	$(CH_2)_2N(CH_3)_2$	<8	
6	CH_3	$(CH_2)_2N$⬠	25	
7	CH_3	$(CH_2)_2N$⬡	8	
8	CH_3	$(CH_2)_2N$⬡O	<8	
9	CH_3	$(CH_2)_3N(CH_3)_2$	80	McMILLAN et al., 1956

| 10 | $(CH_2)_4N(CH_3)_2$ | | 80 | PHILLIPS, 1954 |

Table 18. Other N–heterocyclic compouns

Compound no.	Constitution		Percentage activity (activity of meca - mylamine = 100%)	References
1	H_3C, H_3C, N, CH_3, CH_3		110	BRETHERICK et al., 1959
2	H_3C, H_3C, N, H, CH_3		5	BRETHERICK et al., 1959
3		R = H	50	BRETHERICK et al., 1959
			0	EASTON et al., 1966
4	H_3C, H_3C, N, R, CH_3, CH_3	R = CH_3	50	BRETHERICK et al., 1959
			Active	EASTON et al., 1966
5		R = C_2H_5	200	BRETHERICK et al., 1959
6		R = C_3H_7	50	BRETHERICK et al., 1959
7	H_3C, CH_3, H_3C, CH_3, H_3C, N, H, CH_3		100	BRETHERICK et al., 1959
8	H_3C, H_3C, N, CH_2CH_3, CH_3, CH_3		75	BRETHERICK et al., 1959
9	H, N, H_3C, H_3C, N, CH_3, CH_3, CH_3		40	BRETHERICK et al., 1959
10	$(C_2H_5)_2NOC$, N, $CON(C_2H_5)_2$		0	RUBCOV et al., 1964

Table 19. Quinuclidine derivatives

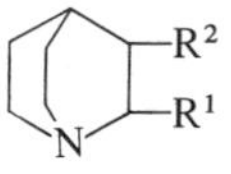

Compound no.	R¹	R²	Percentage activity (activity of mecamylamine = 100%)	References
1	COO(CH$_2$)$_2$N(C$_2$H$_5$)$_2$	H	Very weak	Sharapov, 1962
				Rubcov et al., 1964
2	CH$_2$NH(CH$_2$)$_2$N(C$_2$H$_5$)$_2$	H	80	
3	CH$_2$NH(CH$_2$)$_2$N(C$_2$H$_5$)$_2$	CH$_2$CH$_2$OH	Weak	

All active compounds include one of two closely related structural fragments (Vejdělek and Protiva, 1964) in aliphatic or alicyclic form:

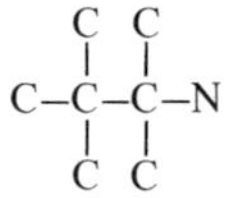

A 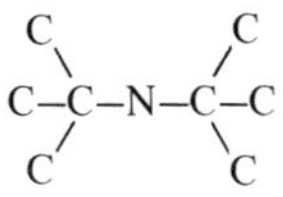   B

Fragment A can be found in compounds 1–4, for example:

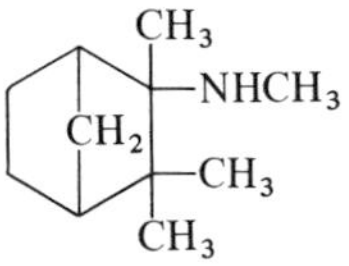

1. 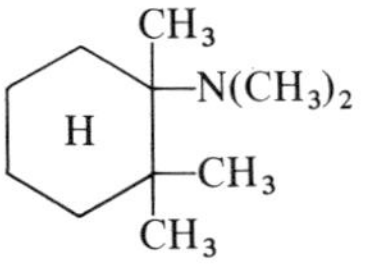   2. 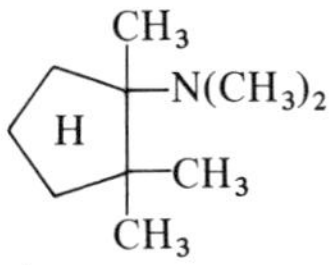   3. 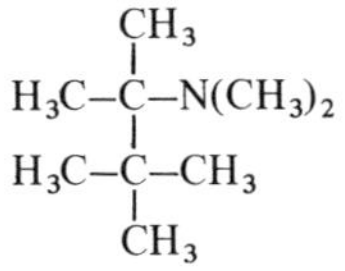   4.

Fragment B is represented by compound 5.:

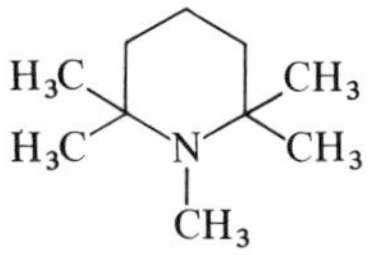

All these compounds have activity comparable to, or higher than, that of mecamylamine on cat nictitating membrane. They lower blood pressure by the blockade of sympathetic ganglia. Their antihypertensive effect has been proved clinically.

Analysis of the structure-activity relationships of the compounds summarised in Tables 2–20 shows certain specific requirements for the arrangement of a ganglion-blocking agent:

Table 20. Miscellaneous compounds

Compound no.		Percentage activity (activity of meca-mylamine = 100%)	References
1	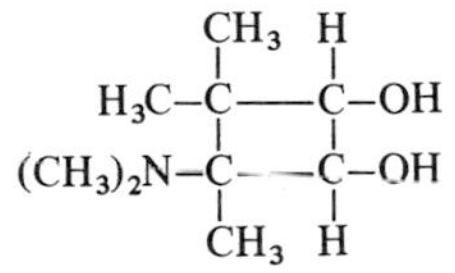 H₃C–C(CH₃)(—)–C(H)–OH ; (CH₃)₂N–C(CH₃)(—)–C(H)–OH	40	Pircio et al., 1966
2	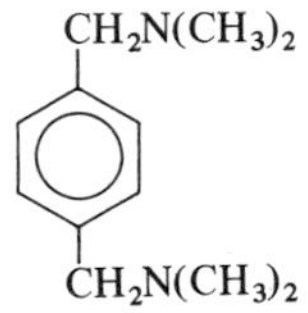 para-bis(CH₂N(CH₃)₂) benzene	80	McMillan et al., 1956
3	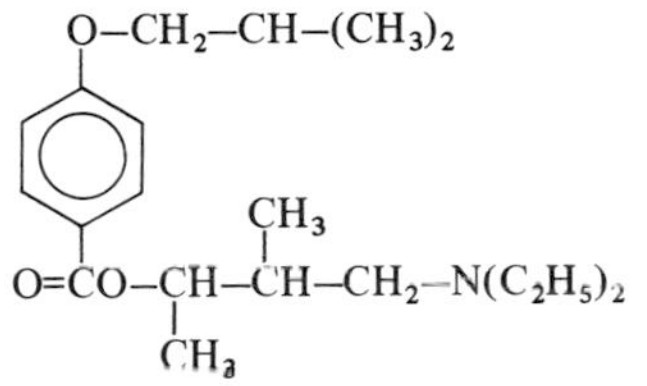 benzene with O–CH₂–CH–(CH₃)₂ and O=CO–CH(CH₃)–CH(CH₃)–CH₂–N(C₂H₅)₂	10–20	Akopyan, 1959
4	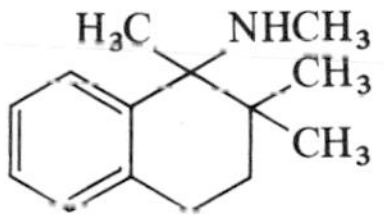 tetrahydronaphthalene derivative H₃C, NHCH₃, CH₃, CH₃	Very low activity	Vejdělek and Protiva, 1964
5	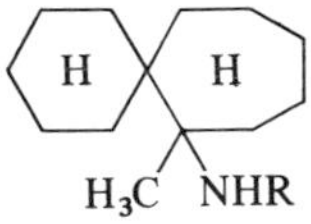 bicyclic H, H, H₃C, NHR	Very low activity	Protiva et al., 1965

Structures for Table 20:

Compound 1:
$$CH_3 \quad H$$
$$H_3C-C-\!\!-\!\!-C-OH$$
$$(CH_3)_2N-C-\!\!-\!\!-C-OH$$
$$CH_3 \quad H$$

Compound 2: benzene ring para-substituted with $CH_2N(CH_3)_2$ at top and $CH_2N(CH_3)_2$ at bottom.

Compound 3: benzene ring with $O-CH_2-CH-(CH_3)_2$ substituent and
$$O=\!\!\!\overset{CH_3}{\underset{CH_3}{CO-CH-CH-CH_2-N(C_2H_5)_2}}$$

Compound 4: H_3C, $NHCH_3$, CH_3, CH_3 substituted bicyclic ring.

Compound 5: bicyclic with H, H, H_3C, NHR.

1) The structure is represented by a saturated or partially unsaturated branched aliphatic, alicyclic, or heterocyclic system with a nitrogen atom forming an amino group;

2) The prerequisite for ganglion-blocking activity is a degree of steric hindrance of the nitrogen atom by methyl groups in its close vicinity;

3) Substitution of at least one hydrogen atom in the primary amino group by an alkyl group is a condition for ganglion-blocking activity: primary amines are usually ganglionic stimulants;

4) Methyl substitution of the amino group seems to be favourable in most cases, especially in tertiary amines. Secondary amines with an alkyl substituent higher than

in ethyl or isopropyl, and tertiary amines with residues higher than in methyl or ethyl display lower activity.

A rising number of methyl groups in the molecule is accompanied by increased lipophility, which is also an important factor in activity. The optimum ratio between steric hindrance of the nitrogen atom and lipophility cannot be derived from the summarised data, because of significant omissions from different series of compounds and some serious inconsistencies in the activities found by different authors.

The study of non-quaternary ganglion-blocking agents reached its peak between 1958 and 1962. The most active compounds were used in the therapy of hypertension for several years. Since the discovery of new drugs that lower blood pressure by other mechanisms (e.g., guanethidine, α-methyldopa etc.), interest in ganglion-blocking agents has decreased. Therefore only a few new agents affecting sympathetic ganglia have been described in last ten years. The reduced practical importance of these drugs probably explains why structure-activity relationships have not been studied by modern quantitative methods.

References

Akopyan, N. E.: Farmacological characteristics of ganglerone-chlorhydrate-α,β-dimethyl-diethyl-aminopropylic ether of p-isobutoxybenzoic acid. In: Ganglerone and experience of its clinical use. Mndjoyan, A.L. (ed.). Erevan: Izdatelstvo A. N. Armyanskoi SSR 1959 (Russ.)

Bainbridge, J.G., Brown, D.M.: Ganglion-blocking properties of atropine-like drugs. Br. J. Pharmacol. *15*, 147–151 (1960)

Bretherick, L., Lee, G.E., Lunt, E., Wragg, W.R., Edge, N.D.: Congeners of pempidine with high ganglion-blocking activity. Nature *184*, 1707–1778 (1959)

Colville, K.J., Fanelli, R.V.: The ganglion-blocking activity of a series of 4-aminoethylpiperidine derivatives. J. Am. Pharm. Assoc. Sci. Ed. *45*, 727–729 (1956)

Cooper, G.H., Green, D.M., Richard, R.L., Thompson, P.B.: The ganglion-blocking activity of diastereoisomeric dimethylaminobornyl acetates and their methiodides. J. Pharm. Pharmacol. *23*, 662–670 (1971)

Corne, S.J., Edge, N.D.: Pharmacological properties of pempidine (1:2:2:6:6-pentamethyl-piperidine), a new ganglion-blocking compound. Br. J. Pharmacol. *13*, 339–349 (1958)

Cusic, J.W., Robinson, R.A.: Autonomic blocking agents. II. Alkamine esters and their quaternaries. J. Org. Chem. *16*, 1921–1930 (1951)

Dorozceva, P.M.: On the correlation between the chemical structure and effect on vegetative ganglia of spherophyzine and *N*-isoamylkadaverine. Farmakol. Toksikol. *18*, No.6, 17–21 (1955) (Russ.)

Easton, N.R., Henderson, F.G., McMurray, W.I., Leonard, N.J.: Comparison of the hypotensive activities of highly hindered open-chain amines and their cyclic counterparts. J. Med. Chem. *9*, 465–468 (1966)

Edge, N.D., Corne, S.J., Lee, G.E., Wragg, W.R.: The ganglion-blocking activity of aminobicyclo [2,2,1] heptanes (congeners of mecamylamine) and bicyclo[3,2,1]azaoctanes (bridged congeners of pempidine). Br. J. Pharmacol. *15*, 207–214 (1960)

Freis, F.D.: Mecamylamine in hypertension. Lancet *1955 LLMXIX*, 977

Freis, E.D., Wilson, I.M.: Mecamylamine, eine neue, oral wirksame hypotensive Substanz. A.M.A. Arch. Intern. Med. *97*, 551–561 (1956)

Gyermek, L.: A "T52"-egy per os hatásos ganglionbénitó-pharmakologiája. Orv. Hetil. *94*, 381–382 (1952)

Gyermek, L., Nádor, K.: The pharmacology of propane compounds in relation to their steric structure. J. Pharm. Pharmacol. *9*, 209–229 (1957)

Harington, M., Kincaird, P., Milne, M.D.: Pharmacology and clinical use of pempidine in the treatment of hypertension. Lancet *1958 II*, 6–11

Hiltmann, R., Wollweber, H., Wirtt, W., Grönwald, R.: Einfache aliphatische Amine mit gan-glionplegischer und blutdrucksenkender Wirksamkeit. Angew. Chem. [Engl.] 72, 1001 (1960)

Kharkevich, D.A.: On ganglion-blocking activity of secondary and teriary aliphatic and alicyclic amines. Farmakol. Toksikol. 25, 151–160 (1962 a) (Russ.)

Kharkevich, D.A.: Ganglionic agents. Moskva: Medgiz 1962 b (Russ.)

Kochetcov, N.K., Khorlin, A.YA., Vorotnikova, L.A., Lopatina, K.I.: Amines with gangliolytic activity. II. Aliphatic amines with tertiary radicals. Zh. Obshch. Khim. 29, 3616–3619 (1959) (Russ.)

Lee, G.E., Wragg, W.R., Corne, S.J., Edge, N.D., Reading, H.W.: 1:2:2:6:6 pentamethyl-piperidine, a new hypotensive drug. Nature 181, 1717–1719 (1958)

McCarthy, D.A., Chen, G.M., Kaump, D.H., Potter, D., Holappa, K.K., Ensor, C.: The pharma-cologic and toxicologic evaluation of the ganglionic blocking agents, dibutadiamin. Arch. Intern. Pharmacodyn. 154, 263–282 (1965)

McIsaac, R.J., Millerschoen, N.R.: A comparison of the effect of mecamylamine and hexame-thonium on transmission in the superiore cervical ganglion of the cat. J. Pharmacol. 139, 18–24 (1963)

McMillan, F.H., Kun, K.A., McMillan, C.B., King, J.A.: Hexamethylene-l-6-bis-t-amines in which part of the six carbon chain is also part of a six-membered ring. J. Am. Chem. Soc. 78, 4077–4081 (1956)

Mndjoyan, A.L.: Ganglerone and experience of its clinical use. Erevan: Izdatelstvo A. N. Ar-myanskoi SSR 1959 (Russ.)

Moyer, J.H., Ford, R., Dennis, E., Handley, C.A.: Laboratory and clinical observations on mecamylamine as a hypotensive agent. Proc. Soc. Exp. Biol. Med. 90, 402–408 (1955 a)

Moyer, J.H., Dennis, E., Ford, R., Caplovitz, C.: Mecamylamine in the therapy of hypertension. Circulation 12, 751–755 (1955 b)

Nádor, K.: Ganglienblocker. In: Fortschritte der Arzneimittelforschung, Vol. II. Jucker, E. (ed.). Basel, Stuttgart: Birkhäuser 1960

Panashenko, A.D.: New active putrescine-like ganglion-blocking agents. Farmakol. Toxikol. 19, No.6, 17–22 (1956) (Russ.)

Panashenko, A.D., Ryabinin, A.A.: Derivatives of tetramethyl-endiamine (putrescine), the struc-ture and pharmacological activity. Farmakol. Toksikol. 18, No.6, 9–17 (1955) (Russ.)

Philippot, E., Denys, W., Dallemagne, M.J.: Action ganglioplégique de quelques dérivés de la 2,2,6,6,-tétraméthylpipéridine. Arch. Intern. Pharmacodyn. 135, 273–280 (1962)

Phillips, A.P.: Synthetic hypotensive agents. I. Some powerful new autonomic ganglionic block-ing agents derived from nicotine. J. Am. Chem. Soc. 76, 2211–2213 (1954)

Pircio, A.W., Parisek, P.J., Groskinski, E.J., Krementz, C.S.: A new series of cyclobutanolamines with hypotensive activity. Arch. Intern. Pharmacodyn. 163, 427–443 (1966)

Plummer, A.J., Schneider, J.A., Barrett, W.E.: A series of tris(dialkylaminoalkyl)amines with ganglionic-blocking activity. Arch. Intern. Pharmacodyn. 97, 1–12 (1954)

Protiva, M., Rajšner, V., Trčka, V., Vaněček, M., Vejdělek, Z.J.: Polymethylcyclohexylamine – neue hypotensiv wirksame Substanzen. Experientia 15, 54–55 (1959)

Protiva, M., Novák, L., Vejdělek, Z.J., Ernest, I.: Látky blokující sympatická ganglia. XIV. Synthesa několika nových alicyklických aminů. ČS. Farmacie 14, 346–351 (1965)

Reitze, W.R., Plummer, A.J., Barrett, W.E.: Properties of tris(2-diethylaminoethyl)amine trihy-drochloride, a ganglionic-blocking agent. Fed. Proc. 12, 360 (1953)

Rubcov, J.M., Šarapov, J.M., Măskovskij, M.D., Michlina, E.E., Nikitskaja, E.S., Vorobjeva, V.JA., Usovskaja, V.S.: Synthesa a farmakologický výzkum derivátů chinuklidinu, piperi-dinu a pyridinu. Čs. Farmacie 13, 299–315 (1964)

Rubinstein, K., Pedersen, J.G.A., Fakstorp, J., Rønnov-Jessen, V.: The edition of Acta Chem. Scand. in two parts (A and B) started in 1974 by the Vol.28. Hypotensive and ganglion-blocking action of methyl substituted 3-amino-norcamphanes. Experientia 14, 222–223 (1958)

Rubinstein, K., Elming, M., Fakstorp, J.: Ganglion-blocking aminobicyclo (2,2,1) heptanes. Acta Chem. Scand. 17, 2079–2082 (1963)

Schneckloth, R.E., Corcoran, A.C., Dustan, H.P., Page, I.H.: Mecamylamine in treatment of hypertensive disease. J. Am. Med. Assoc. 162, 868–875 (1956)

Shanor, S.P., Kinnard, V.J., Buckley, J.P.: Cardiovascular activity of mecamylamine, pempidine and several pempidine analogs. J. Pharm. Sci. *54*, 859–862 (1965)

Sharapov, I.M.: On the pharmacology of some 2-, 3-mono-, and 2,3-bis-substituted quinuclidine. Farmakol. Toksikol. *25*, 691–698 (1962) (Russ.)

Simon, I.B., Vvedenskij, V.P.: Synthesis of some derivatives of tetramethylpiperidine, II. Zh. Obshch. Khim. *34*, 4037–4039 (1964) (Russ.)

Spinks, A., Young, F.H.P.: Polyalkylpiperidines: a new series of ganglion-blocking agents. Nature *181*, 1397–1398 (1958)

Spinks, A., Young, E.H.P., Farrington, J.A., Dunlop, D.: The pharmacological actions of pempidine and its ethyl homologue. Br. J. Pharmacol. *13*, 501–520 (1958)

Stone, C.A., Torchiana, M.L., Navarro, A., Beyer, K.H.: Ganglionic-blocking properties of 3-methylaminoisocamphane hydrochloride (mecamylamine): a secondary amine. J. Pharmacol. Exp. Ther. *117*, 169–183 (1956)

Stone, C.A., Torchiana, M.L., Mecklenberg, K.L., Stavorski, J.: Chemistry and structure-activity relationship of mecamylamine and derivatives. J. Med. Pharm. Chem. *5*, 665–690 (1962)

Syrneva, Yu.I.: On the pharmacology of alkaloids of nanophyton. Farmakol. Toksikol. *13*, No.2, 26–28 (1950) (Russ.)

Syrneva, I.I.: On the relationship between the structure and the effects on choline-reactive systems of some 2,6-dimethylpiperidine derivatives. Farmakol. Toksikol. *24*, 304–309 (1961)

Tikhonenko, V.M.: On the pharmacology of some derivatives of polyalkylpiperidinic series. Farmakol. Toksikol. *25*, 698–705 (1962a) (Russ.)

Tikhonenko, V.M.: Zalezhnist farmakolohichnoi diyi khimichnoi budovy ganglioblokatoriv – pokhidnykh polialkilpiperydynu. Farm. Zh. *17*, No.1, 31–36 (1962b) (Ukr.)

Trčka, V.: Unpublished results 1961

Trčka, V., Vaněček, M.: Některé nové typy ganglioplegik. Čs. Farm. *8*, 316–325 (1959)

Vějdelek, Z.J.: Neue Typen synthetischer Verbindungen mit ganglien-blockierender Wirkung. Arzneim. Forsch. *10*, 808–811 (1960)

Vejdělek, Z.J., Protiva, M.: Ganglioplegica. VII. Derivate des 2-Aminoisocamphans. Coll. Czechoslov. Chem. Commun. *24*, 2614–2622 (1959)

Vejdělek, Z.J., Protiva, M.: Látky blokující sympatická ganglia. XII. 1,2,2-trimethyl-l-tetralylmethylamin. Čs. Farmacie *13*, 49–52 (1964)

Vejdělek, Z.J., Trčka, V.: Substituierte t-Hexylamine als neuer Typ hypotensiv wirksamer Verbindungen. Experientia *15*, 215–216 (1959)

Vejdělek, Z.J., Rajšner, M., Protiva, M.: Ganglioplegica. X. Derivate des Cyclohexylamines. Coll. Czechoslov. Chem. Commun. *25*, 245–253 (1960)

Vejdělek, Z.J., Trčka, V., Vaněček, M., Kakáč, B., Holubek, K.: Ganglionic-blocking agents. XV. Synthesis and activity of some tertiary hexylamines. Coll. Czechoslov. Chem. Commun. *35*, 2810–2830 (1970)

Vidal-Beretervide, K., Monti, M.J., Ruggia, R., Trinidad, H.: Ganglionic-blocking action of some methylpiperidines. J. Pharmacol. Exp. Ther. *152*, 181–185 (1966)

CHAPTER 5

Locus and Mechanism of Action of Ganglion-Blocking Agents

D.A. BROWN

A. Introduction

PATON and PERRY (1953) classified ganglion-blocking drugs "according to whether they act like acetylcholine or by preventing its action". They termed the former "depolarizing" and the latter "competitive" blocking drugs. They excluded "drugs such as local anaesthetics, which interfere with ganglionic transmission by preventing the release of acetylcholine", implying that true ganglion-blocking drugs have no such action (a thesis discussed further below).

The present review seeks to examine what refinements or modifications of this general concept, as stated or implied, may be warranted on the basis of more recent studies. For convenience, the same classification will be adhered to. Pertinent general reviews on the physiology and pharmacology of ganglionic transmission include those of KHARKEVICH (1962, 1967), VOLLE (1966, 1969), HAEFELY (1972), SKOK (1973), and NISHI (1974).

B. Competitive Blocking Agents

I. Effects on the Transmission of Single Impulses

Several investigators have monitored the effects of ganglion-blocking drugs on the transmission process with the aid of intracellular electrodes. Useful descriptions include those of ECCLES (1963) and LEES and NISHI (1972) (rabbit superior cervical ganglion); BLACKMAN et al. (1963) and RIKER (1964, 1965) (frog sympathetic ganglion); and BLACKMAN and PURVES (1969) and BLACKMAN et al. (1969) (guinea-pig sympathetic ganglia). Some observations are illustrated in Fig. 1. These (and the author's own unpublished) observations indicate the following sequence of events:

1) The *rate of rise of the excitatory postsynaptic potential (EPSP)* is slowed and its absolute amplitude is diminished. Even when still sufficient to generate a spike, the diminished EPSP can be inferred from the increased after-positivity following the spike (the latter being shunted by the high Na^+ conductance during a full EPSP). In multiply-innervated mammalian ganglion cells comparable effects result from a reduction of the orthodromic stimulus strength.

2) The *spike potential* is generated progressively later in the EPSP and eventually fails. In some ganglion cells, e.g., rabbit (ECCLES, 1963), frog (BLACKMAN et al., 1963), and rat (present author), the amplitude of the spike is also reduced. As suggested by BLACKMAN et al. (1963), this probably results from an enhanced degree of Na inactivation caused by the prolonged preceding depolarisation (cf. STONEY and MACHNE,

a   b

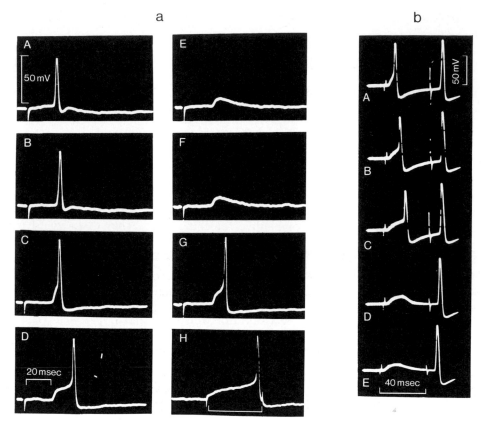

Fig. 1 a and b. Effect of competitive blocking agents on orthodromic transmission recorded intra-cellularly. **a** Action of d-tubocurarine (50 μg/ml^{-1}) on transmission in guinea-pig pelvic ganglion cells in vitro at 33–35 °C following hypogastric nerve stimulation (from Fig. 6 of BLACKMAN et al., 1969). A, control response; B-G, 10, 30, 35, 40, 50, and 60 min after adding d-tubocurarine. H, response to depolarising current pulse (indicated by horizontal bar). Note: (i) with addition of tubocurarine the orthodromic spike initially increases in amplitude, indicating appreciable "shunting" of the spike by the EPSP in A. (ii) The threshold for orthodromic spike generation in D is comparable to that for direct stimulation in H, suggesting that d-tubocurarine does not affect the spike threshold. **b** Progressive action of hexamethonium (0.7 mM) on responses of frog lumbar sympathetic neurone produced by orthodromic stimulation followed by anti-dromic stimulation (from Fig. 11 of BLACKMAN et al., 1963). In this cell the orthodromic spike became smaller with progressive delay in its generation (reflecting increased Na inactivation), but with no noticeable change in the excitable threshold

1969; ADAMS and BROWN, 1975). In guinea-pig ganglia, BLACKMAN et al. (1969) describe a clear *increase* in spike amplitude with progressive curarisation. These cells show high-frequency repetitive discharges in response to prolonged (50 ms) depolar-ising currents, with relatively little accommodation; Na inactivation during an EPSP may therefore be small, and insufficient to counteract the normal shunting of the orthodromic spike by the EPSP.

These observations have some bearing on interpretation of *extracellular* records of ganglionic and postganglionic action potentials. In such records the amplitude of the spike is usually taken as a measure of the number of neurones or axons firing. However, if the amplitudes of the individual ganglion cell spikes are altered as described above, this measure becomes unreliable. Further, the delayed spike generation would explain the apparent increase in "synaptic delay" and prolongation of the postganglionic action potential described by KHARKEVICH (1967).

3) The *voltage threshold for spike generation* by the EPSP does not appear to be appreciably elevated before failure, suggesting that the *excitability* of the cell is unchanged. (Some slight rise in voltage threshold might be anticipated when the spike is delayed, because of the increased Na inactivation referred to above.) With TEA the threshold is actually *reduced* (RIKER, 1965); this is discussed further below.

4) A *full spike* can still be elicited with direct stimulation (i.e., through passage of a depolarising current), without apparent elevation of current or voltage threshold. This confirms that excitability is not reduced. [Again, TEA renders the cell *more* sensitive to direct stimulation: RIKER (1964, 1965; see further below).]

5) *Invasion of the soma by antidromic spikes* is unaffected, indicating that conduction along postganglionic fibres is not blocked.

6) *Membrane potential, resistance*, and *time constant* are unchanged.

These effects are fully compatible with the suggestion of PATON and PERRY (1953) that competitive blocking drugs act by preventing the effect of acetylcholine in generating the EPSP, rather than, for instance, by exerting a (presumably site-selective) local anaesthetic action. The absence of any clear depression of excitability on antidromic invasion suggests that depression of presynaptic conduction and consequent impairment of transmitter release are unlikely to be the general mechanism of block. Nevertheless, the above experiments do not of themselves prove that the reduction in EPSP is postsynaptic in origin, and so cannot exclude presynaptic effects mediated through other than "local anaesthetic" actions; nor do they provide much information on the nature of acetylcholine antagonism. Information on these points deriving from other approaches is discussed below.

II. Presynaptic Effects

1. Acetylcholine Release

The effect of several ganglion-blocking agents on acetylcholine release by preganglionic nerves has been studied in the cat perfused superior cervical ganglion preparation. No clear depression of release was observed following the injection of full blocking amounts of *tubocurarine* or *hexamethonium* (BROWN and FELDBERG, 1936 b; PATON and ZAIMIS, 1951; MATTHEWS and QUILLIAM, 1964; MATTHEWS, 1966) or of high concentrations (block not assessed) of dihydro-β *erythroidine* or *mecamylamine* (MCKINSTRY and KOELLE, 1967 b). *Pempidine* appeared to produce a slight depression (CORNE and EDGE, 1958), which may have reflected the well-known diminution in release with continued perfusion in the absence of choline (cf. MATTHEWS, 1963; recovery was not apparent). *Tetraethylammonium* increases release (DOUGLAS and LYWOOD, 1961; MATTHEWS and QUILLIAM, 1964; see below). Some depression of acetylcholine release from the isolated rat phrenic nerve – diaphragm preparation has been reported, particularly at high stimulus frequencies (50 Hz) (BEANI et al., 1964); however, the concentrations used ($\geqslant 200\ \mu M$), even though insufficient to block neuromuscular transmission, are high compared with those required to block repetitive ganglionic transmission in vitro (see e.g., KOSTERLITZ et al., 1970).

Interpretation of changes in gross ACh release is hindered by an imprecise knowledge of the relationship between the measured ACh overflow and the degree of transmission. It could be argued, for example, that a very small reduction in overflow might reflect a significant reduction in transmission. The available evidence, however, rather suggests the contrary, namely that there is an appreciable "safety factor" for transmission at ganglionic synapses in terms of transmitter release (see, e.g., BROWN, 1954; SACCHI and PERRI, 1973).

In this context it may be pertinent to compare the effects of ganglion-blocking agents with those of local anaesthetics or other "non-specific" agents. Thus, MAT-THEWS and QUILLIAM (1964) measured the effects of a number of such agents on both ACh release and transmission (procaine, amylobarbitone, chloral hydrate, trichlore-thanol, methylpentynol and its carbamate ester, paraldehyde, and troxidone). With such agents, concentrations producing substantial (75%) but not complete block invariably reduced ACh release by at least 30%; in contrast, full blocking concentrations of hexamethonium failed to depress ACh release. This amply confirms the distinction drawn by PATON and PERRY (1953) and PATON (1954) between ganglion-blocking agents and local anaesthetics.

2. Choline Uptake

Adequate transmitter synthesis depends upon a ready supply of choline (BIRKS and MACINTOSH, 1961; METTHEWS, 1963). This is normally derived in large part from the hydrolysis of released acetylcholine (PERRY, 1953; COLLIER and MACINTOSH, 1969; BENNETT and MACLACHLAN, 1972b). The choline probably enters the preganglionic terminals via a carrier-mediated transport system (HODGKIN and MARTIN, 1965; DIAMOND and KENNEDY, 1969; YAMAMURA and SNYDER, 1973; PERT and SNYDER, 1974), although direct evidence for a choline carrier in preganglionic nerve terminals in the ganglion is, as yet, lacking (BOWERY and NEAL, 1975; KHATTAR and FRIESEN, 1975; SUSZKIW et al., 1976). Ganglion-blocking agents, including hexamethonium, tetraethylammonium and tubocurarine, have been reported to inhibit choline transport in erythrocytes (MARTIN, 1969), brain synaptosomes (DIAMOND and KENNEDY, 1969; HEMSWORTH et al., 1971), and rat diaphragm (ADAMIC, 1972); but the concentrations required exceeded 1 mM, so that such an action can be excluded as a contributory factor in their blocking action.

3. Acetylcholine Synthesis

Tertiary or secondary amines might enter the preganglionic fibres and inhibit acetylcholine synthesis in them. PARKINSON (1959) noted that neither pempidine nor mecamylamine inhibited acetylcholine synthesis by rabbit brain choline acetyltransferase at concentrations up to 6 mM and 60 μM respectively. (Higher concentrations of mecamylamine were precluded by interference with the bioassay. Since mecamylamine may concentrate in ganglion cells [see Sect. D] tests with higher concentrations and more modern radiochemical methods would be more definitive.) BHATNAGAR and MACINTOSH (1967) obtained evidence that quaternary ammonium agents (TEA, hexamethonium, tubocurarine) could inhibit ACh synthesis in brain tissue at 100 μM or more, TEA being the most potent. This effect of TEA can also be detected in intact ganglia (MATTHEWS, 1966; BHATNAGAR and MACINTOSH, 1967), but, since TEA increases ACh *release*, reduced synthesis is unlikely to contribute to ganglion block; effects of other quaternaries are probably unimportant since they would not normally penetrate to sites of synthesis.

4. Electrical Responses of Preganglionic Nerves and Their Terminals

QUILLIAM and SHAND (1964) made a useful comparison of the effects of ganglion-blocking agents and non-specific drugs on nerve conduction and synaptic transmission in the isolated rat superior cervical ganglion. The concentrations of hexamethonium, tetraethylammonium, or tubocurarine required to block conduction along the ascending (preganglionic) cervical sympathetic nerve trunk in the rat exceeded those required to block transmission in the superior cervical ganglion by a factor of at least 50; thus, even at full ganglion block the preganglionic action potential was not depressed by more than 25% (TEA actually increased the spike height). In contrast, procaine blocked preganglionic conduction at a concentration only 2.7 times the concentration that blocked transmission, so that the preganglionic spike was reduced by 83% at full transmission block. Comparison of the effect of a local anaesthetic agent with that produced by simply reducing the preganglionic stimulus strength led to the conclusion that the effect of a local anaesthetic on transmission through the ganglion was compatible with equal and additive depression of pre- and postganglionic nerve excitability. By contrast, it is clear that impaired conduction along nerve trunks per se does not contribute to the transmission block produced by C6, TEA or dTC, notwithstanding the fact that the fibres concerned are fine non-myelinated fibres in this species and therefore are presumably very sensitive to a local anaesthetic action.

These experiments are helpful in excluding local anaesthetic effects of quaternary blocking agents, and would have been even more useful for inclusion of tertiary or secondary amines. They do not, of course, exclude a more pronounced effect on fine nerve terminal branches (though, because of the small diameter of rat preganglionic trunk fibres, they suggest it to be rather unlikely) or a more specific interference with the release process. Some evidence against these two possibilities can be extracted from two other investigation.

DUNANT (1972) detected a component of the residual ganglionic potential after suppression of the postganglionic spike by mecamylamine, which could be attributed to action potentials in intraganglionic branches of the preganglionic fibres in the rat superior cervical ganglion. This spike was not depressed by acetylcholine, hemicholinium, or curare. The significance of this is diminished somewhat by the use of mecamylamine (which might have already exerted some presynaptic depression), but the point was made (DUNANT, 1972) that the residual spike could also be detected in the presence of 600 μM d-tubocurarine, 500 μM hexamethonium, or 200 μM pentolinium, and that addition of an excess of these agents did not further reduce the spike. GINSBORG (1971), recording the presynaptic spike in single fibres in frog sympathetic ganglia, noted that tubocurarine in concentrations sufficient to block transmission had no effect on the presynaptic spike, but that a reversible reduction sometimes occurred at $\geqslant 0.5$ mM.

A dramatic instance of the persistence of presynaptic excitability during ganglion block is provided by the observations of MARTIN and PILAR (1963) in chick ciliary ganglia. These show both electrical and chemical transmission: tubocurarine suppressed chemical transmission without affecting the electrical coupling signal.

5. Post-Tetanic Potentiation (PTP)

When the preganglionic nerves are stimulated repetitively at a high frequency (30–40 Hz), postganglionic action potentials generated by single orthodromic stimuli are enhanced; since there is no such enhancement of antidromic stimuli or of responses to orthodromic stimuli in another branch of the preganglionic imput, PTP in the ganglion appears to be a presynaptic phenomenon (LARRABEE and BRONK, 1974; JOB and LUNDBERG, 1952; MARTIN and PILAR, 1964 b). KHARKEVICH (1959; cf. 1967) reported that PTP is depressed (i.e., the percentage increment in single responses after the tetanus in reduced) to similar extents by hexamethonium, pendiomide, and mecamylamine, but is increased by TEA; barbiturates did not effect PTP. Taking the latter as the norm, it was suggested that the ganglion-blocking agents (excepting TEA, with its known enhancement of transmitter release, see above) might exert some presynaptic effect to reduce PTP. However, it is not clear that a barbiturate is the appropriate norm, since later is was shown that it clearly *does* affect presynaptic elements (cf. MATTHEWS and QUILLIAM, 1964). LEES and NISHI (1972), recording the intracellular EPSP in isolated rabbit ganglia, reported that hexamethonium and tubocurarine did not effect PTP but that mecamylamine had a very definite inhibitory effect that was strongly suggestive of a presynaptic action.

6. Repetitive Stimulation

It is a well-known phenomenon (described by PATON and ZAIMIS, 1949, 1951, and extensively documented by KHARKEVICH, 1962, 1967) that transmission of repetitive impulses is poorly sustained in the presence of competitive blocking agents. For example, whereas cat nictitating membrane normally shows a sustained contracture during 10-Hz stimulation, this contracture rapidly wanes after hexamethonium, with a corresponding diminution in the amplitude of the postganglionic action potential. The probable explanation for this (PATON, 1951) is that during the first few volleys of a tetanic train the amount of acetylcholine released per volley (PERRY, 1953; BIRKS and MACINTOSH, 1961) and the EPSP (BENNETT and MACLACHLAN, 1972) diminish exponentially toward a submaximal basal level; and that, since the average EPSP is diminished by the postsynaptic action of the blocker, so the EPSPs fall below the excitable threshold in an increasing proportion of cells. The tetanic failure itself is thus not indicative of a presynaptic action of the blocking agent. (This is not necessarily applicable to frequency-dependence of blockade under steady-state conditions, see below.) LEES and NISHI (1972) found that the tetanic run-down of the EPSP was much more pronounced in the presence of mecamylamine than in the presence of tubocurarine or hexamethonium. The normal tetanic run-down was attributed to a reduced quantal content *(m)* of the EPSP by about half from ~ 3.40 to ~ 1.90 (but see McLACHLAN, 1975); in the presence of mecamylamine, m was initially *greater* than normal (~ 650), but diminished more rapidly to a lower steady-state value (~ 200). This was interpreted as indicating an increased probability of release (p) of a quantum, counteracted by a decrease in the size of the available store (n) as though the actual quantal release rate were accelerated to a point where it exceeded transmitter mobilisation, so that the available transmitter became depleted. No such effects were detected with hexamethonium or tubocurarine; comparable investigations with other blocking agents such as TEA would be desirable.

The *steady-state* degree of block produced by hexamethonium or tetraethylammonium administered *during* on-going preganglionic stimulation also increases with increasing stimulus frequency RIKER and KOMALAHIRANYA, 1962; WINTERS and VOLLE, 1968). This would be easily explained (cf. PATON, 1951) if, in addition to the initial decline in acetylcholine release per volley during tetanic stimulation, the final steady-state release per volley were also to diminish with increasing frequency. Experiments by PERRY (1953) on ACh release in perfused cat ganglia and by NISHI et al. (1967) on isolated frog ganglia suggested that this was indeed the case. Thus, in PERRY'S (1953) experiments the final (steady-state) output per volley diminished with increasing stimulus frequency between 5 and 31 Hz, in such a manner as to give a constant output per unit time. This was interpreted as suggesting a constant fractional release per volley from a pool of transmitter showing a constant replenishment rate per unit time. However, in both sets of experiments, anticholinesterases were present to prevent ACh hydrolysis, without supplementary choline. Under these conditions, insufficient choline – normally yielded by hydrolysis of ACh – is available for sustained synthesis (BIRKS and MACINTOSH, 1961; MATTHEWS, 1963): when choline is added to the perfusion fluid the long-term volley output is *maintained* over the frequency range 4–16 Hz (BIRKS and MACINTOSH, 1961). Similarly the amplitude of the steady-state EPSP in the isolated guinea-pig ganglion, measured in the absence of anticholinesterase, remained constant over the frequency range 5–20 Hz (BENNETT and McLACHLAN, 1972b). These observations suggest that, under normal conditions the rate of transmitter synthesis is in fact closely geared to the stimulus frequency, to preclude the depletion of transmitter. It seems unlikely, therefore, that steady-state frequency-dependence results from a reduced transmitter release, and might be a postsynaptic phenomenon. One possibility is that with short-interval stimuli, the excitable threshold of the cell shows an accommodative rise (see, e.g., ECCLES, 1955, Fig. 7A; ERULKAR and WOODWARD, 1968, Fig. 7) that is insufficient to cause spike failure at rest but reduces the safety factor for transmission, so increasing the likelihood of failure when the EPSP is reduced. An alternative possibility is that agonist action might increase the effectiveness of the antagonist (see below and Addendum).

7. Presynaptic Acetylcholine Receptors

There is direct evidence that nerve terminals possess nicotinic acetylcholine receptors in frog and rat sympathetic ganglia: (i) application of ACh depolarizes these terminals, and this is prevented by nicotine (KOKETSU and NISHI, 1968); and (ii) carbachol transiently reduces the presynaptic terminal spike, and this is prevented by *d*-tubocurarine (GINSBORG, 1971). These receptors would provide a rationale for a presynaptic component to competitive ganglion block if a) the receptors were activated by synaptically released ACh and b) such activation participated in the transmission process. A hypothesis of precisely this nature was advanced by Koelle (1961), namely: The ACh first liberated at the terminals by the depolarizing action of the nerve action potential acts at the same terminals to maintain the depolarized state long enough to produce depolarization (mediated by further ACh release) at the postsynaptic site (Koelle, 1961b). The hypothesis was originally based on two observations: that acetylcholinesterase was localised presynaptically; and that preganglionic denervation reduced the postsynaptic response to carbachol and acetylcholine (after cholinesterase inhibition), suggesting a primarily presynaptic locus of action in the normally innervated ganglion (Volle and Koelle, 1961). Apart from the direct demonstration of presynaptic depolarisation by Koketsu and Nishi (1968) referred to above, two other subsequent observations appeared to support this view: (i) carbachol proved capable of releasing assayable amounts of ACh in perfused cat superior cervical ganglia (McKinstry et al., 1963; McKinstry and Koelle, 1967); and (ii) carbachol increased spontaneous mepp frequency at rat muscle end plates (Miyamoto and Volle, 1974). Notwithstanding these observations, the hypothesis now appears untenable on several grounds. 1. The *significance of the supporting evidence* has been questioned. (i) The effects of preganglionic denervation on ganglionic sensitivity are complex (Takeshige and Volle, 1963) and the original description of subsensitivity has not been fully confirmed (e.g. Brown, 1966a, 1969; McKinstry and Koelle, 1967; Hancock and Volle, 1970; but see Dun et al., 1976); (ii) the acetylcholine released by nicotinic agonists from perfused ganglia derives from the pool of "surplus" ACh generated in the presence of an anticholinesterase and *not* from the transmitter pool normally released by nerve impulses (Brown et al., 1970; Collier and Katz, 1970). [In any case, agonist-induced release is not prevented by ganglion-blocking agents: McKinstry and Koelle (1967b).] (iii) Unlike muscle, nicotinic agonists do not appear to increase spontaneous mEPSP frequency in ganglia (Ginsborg and Guerrero, 1964; Dennis et al., 1971). 2. Secondly, *quantal characteristics* of transmitter release at the ganglion, as pointed out by Katz (1969) accord with the views of non-interacting quantal events (Blackman et al., 1973b; Martin and Pilar, 1964a; Dennis et al., 1971; McLachlan, 1975). 3. Thirdly, *presynaptic depolarisation* would tend to reduce the release of transmitter by the succeeding impulse, by reducing spike amplitude – indeed, the observation of Ginsborg (1971) confirms such a reduction – whereas the available evidence suggests a facilitation of release by the preceding impulse (e.g., Martin and Pilar, 1964b).

Thus, even if a presynaptic feedback process occurred during transmission, negative rather than positive feedback would be anticipated; in which case, the suppression of feedback by a ganglion-blocking agent would *enhance* transmission rather than block it.

8. Conclusions

1) The *depression of transmission* produced by a *quaternary* ammonium blocking agent is entirely postsynaptic in origin. No presynaptic depression could be detected in terms of (i) total ACh release, (ii) quantal content of the EPSP, or (iii) preganglionic axon or terminal spike amplitude. (The effect of TEA in augmenting transmit-

ter release is exceptional, and stems from an occlusion of activated K^+ channels; see below.) The only rational basis for a presynaptic effect might reside in the presence of external presynaptic ACh receptors: however, it is most unlikely that these participate in the normal transmission process, and, even if they did, their properties are such as to imply that blockade would enhance release.

2) *Mecamylamine*, in contrast to quaternary agents, has been shown to be capable of exerting a presynaptic effect; This takes the form of an augmented run-down of transmitter release during tetanus, and an inhibition of post-tetanic potentiation (LEES and NISHI, 1972). This is not due to a "local anaesthetic" effect on the membrane, since the preterminal spike persists in the presence of mecamylamine. It may result from the ability of mecamylamine to penetrate cell mambranes and, by virtue of its basic character, to become concentrated in the nerve fibres (see Sect. D). Pempidine might be comparable in this respect. Two points need emphasising in connection with this effect: a) Presynaptic depression is not the sole cause of ganglion block by mecamylamine, since the postsynaptic response to ACh is also depressed. Further, steady-state ACh release measured in the perfused ganglion is unimpaired (McKINSTRY and KOELLE, 1967b). It may be that blockade of low-frequency transmission is largely postsynaptic in origin but that the presynaptic effect of mecamylamine enhances sensitivity to high-frequency transmission; b) Mecamylamine is exceptional and does not detract from the view expressed by LEES and NISHI (1972) that "inhibition of the release of acetylcholine is not an essential property of ganglion-blocking drugs"; this accords with the view of PATON and PERRY (1953).

III. Postsynaptic Effects

1. Neuronal Excitability

As pointed out above, transmission block by ganglion-blocking agents is not accompanied by a rise in the threshold for orthodromic or direct spikes. This implies that the electrical excitability of the neurones is unchanged. Results with two other experimental approaches accord with this view.

a) K^+ Stimulation

Under conditions where responses of the cat superior cervical ganglion to nicotinic agonists are blocked, responses to K^+ ions are largely unaffected by tubocurarine, tetraethylammonium or hexamethonium (BROWN and FELDBERG, 1936b; ACHESON and PEREIRA, 1946; TRENDELENBURG, 1959; BROWN and QUILLIAM, 1964; BROWN, 1966). The rationale behind these experiments is that the effect of increasing external $[K^+]$ is simply to depolarise the ganglion cell membrane through a reduction in E_K, thereby by-passing the stage of acetylcholine-receptor interaction. An impaired response would only be expected if (i) the membrane permeability to K^+ were reduced or (ii) the threshold depolarisation were raised. Two restrictions apply to these experiments. (i) K^+ ions also excite preganglionic fibres (BROWN and MACINTOSH, 1939) and release ACh from the perfused ganglion (BROWN and FELDBERG, 1936a). This may contribute to the postganglionic response, so that some reduction in the postganglionic response to K^+ ions is not incompatible with antagonism to acetylcholine (cf. BROWN and QUILLIAM, 1964), although the *major* action of K^+ at this site is undoubtedly postsynaptic (cf. Brown et al., 1970). (ii) Conversely, some greater resistance of K^+ excitation than ACh excitation to blockade is not incompatible with a 'local anaesthetic' action. Barbiturates and procaine may 'selectively' reduce ACh excitation (Exley, 1954; Brown and Quilliam, 1964), perhaps through an interaction with the activated ACh-receptor complex or with the ionic channel (Steinbach, 1968; Adams, 1974, 1975).

b) Antidromic Invasion

During blockade of the orthodromically generated ganglionic action potential the antidromically generated spike persists (extracellular recording: Quilliam and Shand, 1964; intracellular recording: Riker, 1964; Lees and Nishi, 1972). The concentration required to depress the (extracellular) antidromic potential in the rat superior cervical ganglion is 50–1000 times that necessary to reduce the orthodromic response – an order of "selectivity" comparable to that for preganglionic conduction block (Quilliam and Shand, 1964). Bearing in mind the unmyelinated nature of the postganglionic fibres and the rather poor safety factor for antidromic invasion of the soma, these experiments argue strongly against any change in postganglionic excitability through a "local anaesthetic" action in normal transmission-blocking concentrations. This conclusion applies not only to quaternary blocking agents but also to mecamylamine (Blackmann et al., 1963a; Lees and Nishi, 1972).

2. Action on Nicotinic Receptors

Paton and Perry (1953) classified blocking agents as "competitors" on the basis that they did not depolarise the ganglion but simply antagonised the action of acetylcholine. Lack of depolarisation has been amply confirmed (e.g., by Eccles, 1955; Shand, 1965). In addition, Pascoe (1956) and Brown et al. (1972) found that the depression of acetylcholine or carbachol depolarisation by hexamethonium in the isolated rat superior cervical ganglion closely resembled the effect of reducing the concentration of agonist. However, by comparison with skeletal muscle, information regarding the kinetics of agonist-antagonist interactions in ganglia is rudimentary, partly because of the less favourable anatomy for intracellular recording and drug application. For example, there have been no studies on the effect of antagonists on agonist dose-conductance curves or even on agonist dose-depolarisation curves, nor have there been any direct measurements of ligand-receptor binding. Some of the available information is summarised below. (See Addendum for more recent studies.)

a) Agonist Dose-Response Curves

Effects of antagonists on agonist dose-response curves have been measured by means of the contraction of isolated guinea-pig ileum in response to nicotine or DMPP (Trendelenburg, 1961; Van Rossum, 1962b), the contraction of cat nicitating membrane produced by close arterial injection of acetylcholine to the superior cervical ganglion (McIsaac and Millerschoen, 1963), or the acceleration of dog heart following injection of TMA or DMPP (Flacke and Fleisch, 1970). All these responses are very indirect indices of nicotinic receptor activation, thus limiting their interpretative power; in vivo experiments suffer from the further limitation of unknown and varying extracellular drug concentrations.

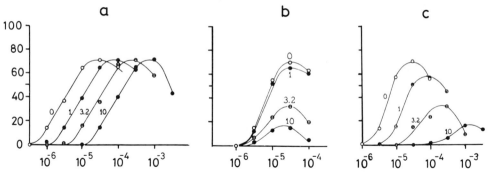

Fig. 2a–c. Antagonism of nicotine-induced contractions of the isolated guinea-pig jejunum by **a** hexamethonium **b** chlorisondamine, and **c** mecamylamine. (From VAN ROSSUM, 1962b.) *Ordinates:* contraction height, expressed as percentage of that produced by pyridine-3-methyltrimethyl-ammonium (see VAN ROSSUM, 1962a). *Abscissae:* molar concentration of nicotine. Numbers on graphs show concentration of antagonist used ($\times 10^{-6}$ M in a and c, $\times 10^{-7}$ M in b). Graphs are based on ascending (non-cumulative) nicotine doses

Using DMPP as agonist in guinea-pig ileum, TRENDELENBURG (1961) observed that hexamethonium produced a parallel shift of the agonist dose-contraction curve; that tetraethylammonium produced a parallel shift with a concentration-insensitive depression of the maximum contracture; that chlorisondamine depressed the contraction amplitude with little shift; and that mecamylamine produced both shift and depression. In this study, only hexamethonium appeared to act as a "competitive" antagonist – even then with some reservations, since the shift of the agonist dose-contraction curve with increasing hexamethonium concentration was less than that (0.95 $\log_{10}$ units per tenfold concentration increase) anticipated for simple competitive antagonism. (This might result from some additional effect of DMPP on the muscle itself at the high concentrations necessitated in the presence of hexamethonium, illustrating, perhaps, the limitations of this preparation.)

The more extensive studies of VAN ROSSUM (1962b) confirm and extend these conclusions. In essence, their observations (also on guinea-pig ileum, but using nicotine as the preferred agonist) can be summarised as follows (see Fig. 2 and Table 1). i) Hexamethonium, pentamethonium, azamethonium (Pendiomide), trimetaphan (Arfonad), and tetraethylammonium behaved as competitive antagonists. In these experiments the relationship between dose ratio and antagonist concentration over a limited (tenfold) concentration range accorded with true competition (Fig. 2a); ii) Chlorisondamine (Ecolid) pentacyne (Presidal) and trimethedine behaved as purely noncompetitive antagonists (Fig. 2b); iii) Mecamylamine and pempidine behaved as mixed competitive and noncompetitive antagonists, with a dissociation constant for competitive antagonism about ten times lower than that for noncompetitive antagonism (Fig. 2c); iv) Dissociation constants for competitive and non-competitive antagonists were both similar when tested against nicotine and DMPP, implying interaction with a single nicotinic receptor; v) Competitive antagonists of nicotine showed the same *type* of antagonism at acetylcholine receptors on smooth muscle (rat jejunum, furtrethonium as agonist) and skeletal muscle (frog rectus, suxamethonium), notwithstanding the higher antagonist concentrations required.

Table 1. Types of antagonism produced by ganglion-blocking agents at para-sympathetic ganglia, smooth muscle, and skeletal muscle. (After VAN ROSSUM, 1962b.) Values are apparent log K_I values derived from $pA_2(C)$ or $pD_2(N)$ measurements

Antagonist	Preparation		
	Parasympathetic ganglion[a]	Smooth muscle[b]	Skeletal muscle[c]
Pentamethonium	C − 5.8	C − 2.9	C − 4.1
Hexamethonium	C − 6.4	C − 2.9	C − 4.3
Azamethonium	C − 5.7	C − 4.1	C − 4.0
Trimetaphan	C − 5.8	C − 4.7	C − 4.8
Tetraethylammonium	C − 4.8	C	C − 2.7
Chlorisondamine	N − 6.2	C − > 2	N − 5.0
Pentacyne	N − 6.9	C − 5.5	N − 5.5
Cxg 213	N − 6.3	C − 5.5	N − 5.6
Trimethidine	N − 7.5	C − 5.7	N − 5.0
Mecamylamine	$M\begin{cases} -6.6(C) \\ -5.5(N) \end{cases}$		$M\begin{cases} -4.5(C) \\ -3.2(N) \end{cases}$
Pempidine	$M\begin{cases} -6.6(C) \\ -5.4(N) \end{cases}$		$M\begin{cases} -4.5(C) \\ -3.0(N) \end{cases}$

[a] Guinea-pig ileum (nicotine as agonist).
[b] Guinea-pig ileum (furtrethonium as agonist).
[c] Frog rectus (suxamethonium as agonist).
C: competitive; N: non-competitive; M: mixed (competitive + non-competitive)

On the other hand, non-competitive parasympathetic ganglion blockers acted non-competitively at muscle nicotinic receptors but competitively at smooth muscle muscarinic receptors, while mixed antagonists also showed mixed antagonism at these sites.

In guinea-pig ileum the dose-response curve for ganglion stimulants is bell shaped (see Fig. 2). Competitive antagonists shift both ascending and descending limbs in a parallel manner, implying that the bell shape arises from auto-inhibition of the *response* to receptor activation, rather than from auto-inhibition at the receptor itself (VAN ROSSUM, 1962a). The most likely explanation may be that, as the extent of ganglion cell depolarisation increases, the action potential discharge becomes pro-gessively briefer and may actually be suppressed by very large depolarisations (see GINSBORG and GUERRERO, 1964; HOLMAN et al., 1971), presumably reflecting an accommodative threshold rise (see below). However, the upper limit of frequency in intestinal parasympathetic ganglion cells is much higher than in most sympathetic neurones (see NISHI and NORTH, 1973).

A further suggested difference between the actions of hexamethonium and pempi-dine is provided by the observations of KOSTERLITZ et al. (1970) on the depression of the EPSP recorded in isolated rabbit superior cervical ganglia by means of the sucrose-gap technique. Whereas the slope for fractional inhibition of the EPSP by hexamethonium approximated to unity (compatible with competitive inhibition), that for inhibition by pempidine was very much shallower. However, this would *not* be predicted as a normal consequence of simple non-competitive inhibition as defined by (for example) SCHILD (1954) or ARIENS (1964, p. 149); rather, it may result from an additional presynaptic effect along the lines of that described for mecamylamine (LESS and NISHI, 1972).

MCISAAC and MILLERSCHOEN (1963) describe a parallel shift of the log agonist-effect curve (measured as the contraction of cat nictitating membrane produced by close arterial injections of acetylcholine to the superior cervical ganglion in the presence of atropine) following intravenous infusion of both hexamethonium and mecamylamine. FLACKE and FLEISCH (1970) also observed an apparently competitive inhibition of the cardio-accelerator effects of TMA and DMPP (given by close arterial injection to the right cardiac ganglion of dog in the presence of atropine) following intravenous injection of hexamethonium, tetraethylammonium, or mecamylamine. For hexamethonium a log (dose ratio -1) versus log (antagonist dose) plot was linear with slope 0.90 over a 30-fold antagonist concentration rage.

In general, therefore, it would appear from dose-response relationships that the simpler quaternary blocking agents behave overtly as expected for classic competitive antagonists, but that this may not be true for larger quaternary compound (such as chlorisondamine) or nonquaternary compounds. The above studies provide little additional information on the mechanism of noncompetitive antagonism. However, it is clear from the work of VAN ROSSUM (1962b) that this *cannot* be equated with non-specific antagonism, since the apparent K_I for non-competitive antagonism is sufficiently low to suggest that the antagonism is at the receptor level; nor (since non-competitive antagonism is not restricted to non-quaternary compounds) can it be simply attributed to an intracellular effect consequent upon cellular accumulation (cf. BENNETT et al., 1957).

One explanation for the combination of non-competitive antagonism with receptor specificity might be that the agonist produces a conformational change in the nicotinic receptor, such as to increase its affinity for certain antagonists. This effect (termed a metaphilic effect) has been demonstrated in skeletal muscle by RANG and RITTER (1969). Non-competitive antagonism would result because, with an increasing concentration of agonist, more of the receptor would be in the transformed (high-affinity) state, so allowing more receptor-antagonist binding. [This effect would be accentuated with sequential ascending agonist concentrations, as in the experiments of VAN ROSSUM (1962b).] A competitive antagonist would have a higher affinity for the resting (non-transformed) receptor, and a mixed antagonist would have a comparable affinity for both receptor states. (An alternative explanation, involving an interaction with agonist-opened ion channels is consider in the Addendum.)

There is one piece of research supporting such a possibility in ganglia, by ALKADHI and MCISAAC (1974). These investigators found that intermittent preganglionic nerve stimulation (40 Hz for 40 s every 10 min) increased the intensity of blockade produced in cat superior cervical ganglion by the non-competitive antagonists chlorisondamine and mecamylamine, but not that produced by the competitive antagonist hexamethonium. Further, the effect of preganglionic stimulation could be replicated by DMPP injections but not by methacholine injections or by antidromic postganglionic stimulation, suggesting a nicotinic-receptor phenomenon. The authors suggested an agonist-induced conformational change (but curiously without reference to the metaphilic effect).

Other authors have noted that a period of preganglionic nerve stimulation either before (PATON and ZAIMIS, 1951; WINTERS and VOLLE, 1968) or after (TRABER et al., 1967) administration of ganglion-blocking agents tends to increase the intensity of blockade, but in these studies no difference between competitive and non-competitive agents was described, and it is not clear how these might relate to the phenomenon described by ALKADHI and MCISAAC (1974). The dependence of ganglion block upon agonist activity and its relation to frequency dependence of blockade warrants further study.

b) Antagonist Interaction

HARVEY (1959) reported that the effects of tetraethylammonium and hexamethonium on transmission through the cat superior cervical ganglion were additive, as would be anticipated for a combination of competitive antagonists with not too dissimilar dissociation constants. However, MCISAAC and MILLERSCHOEN (1962) found that a combination of close arterial hexamethonium and mecamylamine were less than additive, and, further, that the addition of hexamethonium reduced the duration of blockade produced by mecamylamine. This suggests that hexamethonium lowered receptor occupancy by mecamylamine. GINSBORG and STEPHENSON (1974) provided a quantitative basis for such an action where (as is probably the case with hexamethonium and mecamylamine) the dissociation rate constants of the two antagonists differ appreciably. Further, under conditions when both agonist and antagonist receptor occupancy are high, and where the dissociation rate constant of the faster antagonist is not too slow compared with that of the agonist, a *reversal* of blockade by the faster antagonist is predicted. This appears to explain the well-known reversal of curare block by hexamethonium at the neuromuscular junction (FERRY and MARSHALL, 1973; BLACKMAN et al., 1975). No such reversal has been reported at ganglia, probably because the dissociation rate constant for hexamethonium at this site is too slow; such a reversal might best be tested with tetraethylammonium and mecamylamine. Bearing in mind the apparently different kinetics of block by hexamethonium and by mecamylamine (VAN ROSSUM, 1962b), there is an alternative explanation of nonadditive effects of these two agents, namely that if hexamethonium has a high affinity for the resting state of the receptor and mecamylamine a higher affinity for the transformed state, if these two states were in reversible equilibrium (cf. KATZ and THESLEFF, 1957; RANG and RITTER, 1970) binding of hexamethonium could shift the equilibrium in such a manner as to reduce the occupancy of mecamylamine. It would be interesting to have further information on the interaction of competitive and noncompetitive blocking agents under in vitro conditions.

c) Voltage-Dependence of Antagonist Action

BLACKMAN (1970) made the interesting observation that, in the presence of hexamethonium, membrane hyperpolarisation *reduced* the amplitude of the EPSP in guinea-pig sympathetic ganglion cells. Normally, such hyperpolarisation would be expected to *increase* the EPSP, by increasing the driving voltage, and this indeed occurred in the presence of tubocurarine. Thus, it appeared that membrane hyperpolarisation increased the blocking action of hexamethonium but not that of tubocurarine. The author suggested two possible explanations: That the binding of hexamethonium to the receptors was voltage-dependent; or that hexamethonium might also effect the ionic conductance change produced by the transmitter.

It may be of relevance to the latter interpretation that the blocking actions of local anaesthetics at the motor end plate are also voltage-dependent (STEINBACH, 1968; KORDAS, 1970; ADAMS, 1974, 1977). ADAMS (1977) attributed this to insertion (of procaine) into the ionic channel such that hyperpolarisation differentially increased the rate of binding and reduced the rate of dissociation. Since the rate constants for opening and closing of the ionic channels during transmitter action are themselves voltage-dependent, and are normally slowed by membrane hyperpolarisation (MAGLEBY and STEVENS, 1972), changing membrane potential can produce quite complex changes in drug action.

In the case of hexamethonium, it might be envisaged that insertion into the opened channel is favoured by its flexible structure, whereas the more rigid structure of tubocurarine would mitigate against such insertion. Since prior activation by transmitter would favour insertion, this could contribute to the tendency to increased block during tetanic stimulation. Further investigation of this aspect of hexamethonium action might be rewarding (see Addendum).

d) Denervation

PERRY and REINERT (1954) observed that, in the Locke-perfused cat superior cervical ganglion, certain ganglion-blocking agents, i.e., methonium compounds and azamethonium (Pendiomid), showed a *stimulant* action after chronic preganglionic denervation. This took the form of an overt contraction of the nictitating membrane or of an enhanced response to acetylcholine. In contrast, tubocurarine and tetraethylammonium retained their normal blocking action. The effects of denervation could be replicated by reducing the K^+ concentration of the perfusing solution from 2.7 to 0.34 mM or less (though transmission could still be blocked); conversely, raising $[K^+]$ partly reversed the effect of denervation. In a subsequent paper (PERRY and REINERT, 1955) it was reported that the effect of denervation could also be reversed by adding several amino acids to the perfusion fluid at a concentration of 1 mg/ml; glucose or intermediates of glucose metabolism showed no such effect. It was suggested that the effects stemmed from a fall in intracellular $[K^+]$, and that amino acids acted as K^+ carriers. As an extension of this, an intracellular action of the ganglion-blocking agents inhibiting aerobic metabolism was postulated. [Further information regarding the effect of ganglion-blocking agents on metabolism is given by KHARKEVICH (1967).] This interpretation of ganglion block is clearly at variance with that of a simple receptor antagonism, and challenges assumptions regarding the penetration of quaternary ammonium compounds. Unfortunately, no such effect of denervation is observed in blood-bathed ganglia or in vitro (see, e.g., MCISAAC and MILLERSCHOEN, 1962; BROWN et al., 1972), which rather hinders further analysis.

e) S-S Reduction

In eel electroplax (KARLIN and WINNIK, 1968) and chick beventer muscle (RANG and RITTER, 1971) reduction of S-S bonds with dithiothreitol converts the normally antagonistic action of hexamethonium to agonist. This does not occur in ganglia (BROWN and KWIATKOWSKI, 1975).

3. Action on Skeletal Muscle Receptors

As pointed out by VAN ROSSUM (1962b), the form of antagonism exhibited by different blocking agents at ganglia and that at the receptors of the frog rectus muscle are similar. However, the value of muscle receptors as models for analysing the action of ganglion-blocking agents must be limited by the very different affinity constants at the two sites (see Table 1).

There is, of course, abundant other evidence indication a substantial qualitative difference between acetylcholine receptors in ganglia and in skeletal muscle, including the following: (i) Decamethonium acts as an agonist on muscle, and an antagonist at ganglia (cf. PATON and PERRY, 1953); (ii) the snake venom α-bungarotoxin, which blocks the motor end plate (MILEDI and POTTER, 1971) has no action on transmission through sympathetic ganglia (MAGAZANIK et al., 1974; BROWN and FUMAGALLI, 1977); (iii) conversely, surugatoxin (the active principal of the mollusc *Babylonia japonica*) has a high affinity for ganglionic nicotinic receptors (10–60 nM) but does not affect skeletal muscle (HAYASHI and YAMADA, 1975; BROWN et al., 1976). From the viewpoint of future studies, acetylcholine receptors on certain invertebrate muscles, such as the "monoquaternary" receptor on leech dorsal muscle (cf. FLACKE and YEOH, 1968), show the greatest similarity to ganglionic receptors (KHROMOV-BORISOV and MICHELSON, 1966; BROWN and KWIATKOWSKI, 1976) and might prove suitable "models" for studying ganglion-type nicotinic ligands.

4. Action on Muscarinic Receptors

In addition to "nicotinic" receptors, sympathetic ganglion cells possess receptors analogous to peripheral "muscarinic" receptors. (See VOLLE, 1966a, b, 1969; TRENDELENBURG, 1967; HAEFELY, 1972; and NISHI, 1974 for detailed reviews.) Activation of these receptors by (for example) muscarine, pilocarpine, or methacholine produces a low-amplitude depolarisation capable of generating postganglionic action potentials; this effect is not prevented by hexamethonium but is blocked by atropine. The ionic mechanism for atropine-sensitive depolarisation of ganglion cells (NISHI et al., 1969; KOBAYSHI and LIBET, 1970–1974; WEIGHT and VOTAVA, 1970; KUBA and KOKETSU, 1974) differs from that for nicotinic depolarisation and also from that for peripheral muscarinic actions (cf. RANG, 1974), but may resemble that in central neurones (KRNJEVIC et al., 1971). Atropine-sensitive ganglion stimulation is also produced by two compounds without agonist activity on other peripheral muscarinic receptors, i.e., McN-A-343 (ROSKOWSKI, 1961) and AHR-602 (FRANKO et al., 1963). This might imply that ganglionic atropine-sensitive receptors differ from true muscarinic receptors, but it is not clear whether these compounds act in exactly the same way as other muscarinic stimulants on ganglia (JARAMILLO and VOLLE, 1967).

Ganglion-stimulant actions of muscarinic agonists are not blocked by hexamethonium or other nicotinic blocking agents in modest concentrations [nor by nicotinic depolarising blocking agents: JONES (1963)]. However, quantitative information on the relative affinities of nicotinic blocking agents for ganglionic nicotinic and muscarinic receptors is sparse. VAN ROSSUM (1962 b) compared the effects of several blocking agents on the responses of the guinea-pig ileum to nicotine and to McN-A-343 and pyridine-3-trimethylammonium (PTMT). [The last two were both judged to act on ganglia: VAN ROSSUM (1962 a)]. The agents listed in Table 1 showed 10–100 times more activity against nicotine than against either of the other two stimulants. [Interestingly, the antagonist affinities against McN-A-343 and PTMT were quite different (usually greater) than their affinities against the direct action of furtrethonium on smooth muscle receptors, which is in keeping with the view that ganglionic muscarinic receptors may differ from muscle receptors.] Recently we (BROWN et al., unpublished observations) have compared the effects of hexamethonium against carbachol-induced nicotinic depolarisation and muscarine-induced depolarisation of isolated rat ganglia: apparent affinity constants differed some 40-fold (7.6 μM against carbachol, 310 μM against muscarine). VAN ROSSUM (1962 b) detected a 10-fold difference in the hexamethonium affinity constant against nicotine and that against PTMT/McN-A-343.

Muscarinic receptors can also be activated by acetylcholine released from preganglionic fibres. Resistance of these receptors to ganglion-blocking agents then has the interesting consequence that during nicotinic receptor blockade a transmission "breakthrough" via the muscarinic receptors may occur (TRENDELENBURG, 1966; LEE and TRENDELENBURG, 1967; BROWN, A.M., 1967; FLACKE and GILLIS, 1968; CHEN, 1971). The essential requirement for this breakthrough is a high rate of preganglionic sympathetic stimulation ($\geqslant 10$ Hz); at sufficiently high rates transmission may be restored to its original level, with the difference that it is then resistant to further nicotinic blockade and blocked by atropine. One practical consequence of muscarinic breakthrough, raised by VOLLE (1966) and BROWN, A.M. (1967) is that it might contribute to the development of tolerance to ganglion-blocking drugs. Three factors could facilitate muscarinic transmission under these conditions:

1) The *preganglionic impulse frequency* may be reflexly increased above normal by the hypotension.

2) *Muscarinic transmission* during ganglion blockade is enhanced by anticholinesterase agents (HILTON, 1961; LONG and ECKSTEIN, 1961; LEVY and AHLQUIST, 1962; GILLIS et al., 1968), to the extent of fully reversing the block. [In contrast, normal transmission is not strongly facilitated by anticholinesterase drugs; see ZAIMIS, (1963).] Hence breakthrough tolerance would be encouraged by adjuvant anticholinesterase administration.

3) *Muscarinic receptors* appear to be sensitised following surgical denervation (AMBACHE et al., 1956; TAKESHIGE and VOLLE, 1963 b): pharmacological denervation may have a comparable effect. If tolerance did result from muscarinic breakthrough, one would expect atropine to reverse it: the author is unaware of any clinical reports to this effect. Further, it seems unlikely that the conditions necessary to "drive" muscarinic transmission experimentally will obtain clinically.

5. Action of Tetraethylammonium (TEA)

In ganglion-blocking concentrations (< 1 mM) TEA shows certain excitatory effects on ganglia that are not exhibited by other competitive blocking agents. In essence these comprise (a) an increased release of acetylcholine, and (b) increased ganglion cell excitability.

(a) DOUGLAS and LYWOOD (1961) reported that TEA (0.5–0.8 mM) increased the amount of acetylcholine released by preganglionic nerve stimulation from the perfused cat superior cervical ganglion. They showed that this effect differed from that of Ca^{2+} ions (cf. HARVEY and MACINTOSH, 1940; HUTTER and KOSTIAL, 1954) or Ba^{2+} ions (DOUGLAS et al., 1961) in that TEA did not restore acetylcholine release in Ca^{2+}-free solution (but see COLLIER and EXLEY, 1963), and suggested that the enhanced release following TEA was due to a prolonged preganglionic action potential (see below). This effect of TEA on the release of acetylcholine during nerve stimulation was also detected by MATTHEWS and QUILLIAM (1964). Subsequent experiments (MATTHEWS, 1966; BHATNAGAR and MACINTOSH, 1967) showed that in spite of this stimulant action on release, TEA exerted an *inhibitory* action on acetylcholine synthesis, which, like that of hemicholinium, was reversed by choline. It may be noted that there are no reports to the effect that TEA elicits the release of acetylcholine from an *un*stimulated ganglion.)

(b) RIKER (1964) reported three effects of TEA upon frog sympathetic ganglion cells. (i) In low concentrations (within the range blocking transmission, see below) TEA reduced the threshold for excitation by direct (depolarizing) current stimulation by some 7 mV. (ii) At higher concentrations (3–4 mM) TEA prolonged the ganglion cell spike and reduced the postive after-potential. (iii) At even higher concentrations (10–20 mM) TEA induced repetitive or "bursting" discharges of spikes in the ganglion cells. These effects were not accompanied by changes in cell membrane potential or input resistance. In a subsequent investigation (RIKER, 1965) on the action of TEA on synaptic transmission in the frog ganglion, the following further effects were revealed. (i) In ganglion-blocking concentrations (0.2–0.8 mM), TEA reduced the threshold for orthodromic spike generation (i.e., for a given EPSP amplitude the spike was generated at a lower level of depolarization). (ii) The synaptic delay in generation of the EPSP was lengthened by some 20% (from ~2.67 ms by 0.55 ± 0.04 ms), without any detectable change in conduction velocity along the preganglionic trunk fibres. (iii) The normal post-tetanic depression of transmission was prevented. It was suggested that the increased synaptic delay resulted from a decreased conduction velocity in the unmyelinated terminal portions of the preganglionic axons, and that the effect of TEA on ganglion cell excitability resulted from a displacement of Ca^{2+} from the membrane.

These effects of TEA on sympathetic ganglia show a resemblance to those described at other neurones and synapses.

a) Neuromuscular Junction

At the *neuromuscular junction* TEA increases twitch tension in response to motor-nerve stimulation when transmission has been depressed by curare (an "anti-curare" action: KENSLER, 1950; STOVNER, 1958). No such effect has been detected in ganglia: see ACHESON and PEREIRA (1946). KOKETSU (1958) analysed this effect in curarised frog muscle, using electrophysiological recording methods. At low concentrations (<1 mM), TEA augmented the end-plate potential but antagonised the response to exogenous (bath-applied) acetylcholine, suggesting a prejunctional effect. By recording extracellularly from intramuscular nerve terminals and intracellularly from intramuscular axons, KOKETSU (1958) detected a prolongation of the falling phase of the spike and an increased negative after-potential which, at higher concentrations (1–3 mM), generated repetitive discharges. Since there were no corresponding changes in the properties of the muscle fibre, KOKETSU (1958) suggested that the increased spike duration caused an increase in the amount of transmitter released by the motor nerve impulse, and that this accounted for the previously described ability of TEA to antagonise the blocking action of tubocurarine. COLLIER and EXLEY (1963) later showed that TEA did indeed augment acetylcholine release from phrenic nerves, and that this correlated reasonably well with its ability to antagonise curare. TEA also antagonised the depressant action of Ca^{2+} in reducing acetylcholine release and blocking transmission (cf. ganglia above).

b) Nerve

TEA has excitatory actions on *nerve*. Thus, COWAN and WALTER (1937) observed the following effects of 10 mM TEA on frog sciatic nerve: a prolonged negative afterpotential, repetitive discharges after a single shock, and spontaneous asynchronous activity at 15 mM or more. These were attributed to an increase in the timeconstant of accommodation and a reduced excitability threshold, as measured by the rheobase. The effects could be reversed by increasing external $[Ca^{2+}]$ to 7.2 mM. The authors concluded that TEA might displace Ca^{2+} ions from the "position that they normally occupy at the interface between the exterior of the nerve membrane and the surrounding solution".

Subsequently, effects of TEA on action potentials in a variety of nerve and muscle cell membranes were described, consisting predominantly of (i) a prolongation of the falling phase of the spike potential, with reduced membrane conductance, and (ii) at higher concentrations, repetitive spikes [crustacean muscle: FATT and KATZ (1953); crustacean nerve: BURKE et al. (1953); frog muscle: HAGIWARA and WATANABE (1955); squid axon: TASAKI and HAGIWARA (1957); frog spinal ganglion cells: KOKETSU et al. (1959)]. The last-named authors noted that TEA produced similar effects when applied exteriorly via the bathing medium or when injected intracellularly, and TASAKI and HAGIWARA (1957) noted that in squid axons TEA was effective *only* from the inside of the axon.

Studies on voltage-clamped squid axons and frog nerve nodes of Ranvier have revealed an appropriate ionic basis for these actions of TEA (see e.g., ARMSTRONG and BINSTOCK, 1965; ARMSTRONG, 1966, 1969; HILLE, 1967, 1970): it reduces the voltage-sensitive increase in K^+ conductance, g_K (delayed rectification) responsible for the falling phase of the spike, probably by "plugging" the K^+ channel opened during membrane depolarisation. Subsequent effects would then include a prolonged spike and negative after-potential, reduced positive after-potential (normally generated by a movement towards E_K during the period of high g_K), reduced excitable threshold and reduced accommodation (reflecting the fact that the increased g_K during depolarisation normally tends to stabilise the membrane potential) and a tendency towards oscillation of the membrane potential and repetitive discharges (HODGKIN and HUXLEY, 1952; HUXLEY, 1959).

Effects of TEA on ganglia may thus be interpreted as follows.

1) Presynaptically, TEA prolongs the spike duration. This leads to (i) an increased transmitter release, and (ii) a prolonged latency for EPSP generation (as in frog muscle: Koketsu, 1958), possibly because peak transmitter release is delayed until the end of the prolonged plateau of the TEA spike (Katz and Miledi, 1969).

2) Postsynaptically, the excitable threshold is lowered, the spike is prolonged, and eventually spontaneous discharges of postsynaptic origin are initiated, as indicated above.

3) Antagonism of the excitatory effects of TEA by Ca^{2+} ions might reflect the effect of the latter in reducing the inward Na^+ current (Frankenhaeuser and Hodgkin, 1957; Hille, 1968), so off-setting the increased excitability consequent upon K-channel occlusion.

It is noteworthy that the concentration of TEA required to affect g_K [half-maximal reduction in frog nodes at 0.4 mM: Hille (1970)] is almost precisely the same as is required to block transmission in frog ganglia (0.4 mM, cf. Fig. 1 of Riker, 1965). However, there is no reason to suppose that the effect on g_K results from an interaction with acetylcholine receptors. For example, equivalent concentrations of other quaternary ammonium compounds on g_K are (Hille, 1970): triethylpropylammonium, 2 mM; triethylmethylammonium, 15 mM; choline, 240 mM; tetramethylammonium, 500 mM. Accordingly, the excitatory actions of TEA represent the special circumstance in which a simple molecule has an equal (but quite modest) affinity for two functionally different receptors, and is not indicative of a general property of ganglion-blocking agents.

C. Depolarising Agents

Paton and Perry (1953) observed that the blocking action of acetylcholine, tetramethylammonium (TMA), or nicotine on cat superior cervical ganglion was accompanied (initially, at least) by depolarisation of the ganglion. They noted however, that the temporal relationship between depolarisation and transmission block was complex, particularly with nicotine. This and many subsequent investigations raised the question as to whether the block of transmission produced by depolarising agents results from the depolarisation itself, or from the interaction of the compound with the transmitter receptors, or from a combination of both.

Before examining the evidence relating to this question, it is necessary to make one point regarding the *measurement* of transmission during application of a depolarising agonist with extracellular electrodes. Unlike the situation in competitive block, during depolarisation the amplitude of the action potentials in the individual neurones is depressed, partly because the baseline is raised by the depolarisation itself and partly because the *height* of the action potential is reduced (Figs. 3–5, see also Ginsborg and Guerrero, 1964). Consequently, the amplitude of the extracellular action potential recorded from the ganglion no longer provides an index of the number of transmitting synapses; this may be more satisfactorily monitored by the action potential recorded from the postganglionic trunk at a point beyond the electrotonic spread of the depolarisation.

I. Depolarisation Block

1. Theory

The essential feature of depolarisation block is a reduction in the electrical excitability of the neurone such that the EPSP fails to reach the excitable threshold for spike generation. Although the amplitude of the EPSP itself may be reduced (see below), transmission block results in the first instance from the rise in excitable threshold. This is analogous to the mechanism of "depolarisation block" in muscle (cf. BURNS and PATON, 1951).

a) Effect on Excitability

A fall in excitability during the application of a depolarising agonist may be generated in two ways. *Firstly*, membrane depolarisation per se reduces excitability, by (i) inactivating the inward Na^+ current responsible for spike generation ("Na inactivation"), and (ii) increasing the outward K^+ current responsible for repolarisation ("delayed rectification") (see HODGKIN and HUXLEY, 1952). These effects can be replicated by prolonged depolarising currents and are equivalent to the process of accommodation. In a sympathetic ganglion cell, accommodation during membrane depolarisation may be detected as a reduced rate of rise of the action potential, a reduced positive overshoot, and (most significantly in the context of depolarisation block) a rise in the threshold membrane potential at which the spike is generated (STONEY and MACHNE, 1969; ADAMS and BROWN, 1975). *Secondly*, the increased membrane conductance produced by a nicotinic agonist (several-fold at high concentrations: cf. GINSBORG and GUERRERO, 1964, and Figs. 3 and 4) will further reduce the excitability, primarily through the increased K^+ conductance. A further consequence of a sustained conductance increase in sympathetic ganglion cells is a substantial change in Na^+ and K^+ gradients across the cell membrane (BROWN and SCHOLFIELD, 1974); the former will reduce the ionic driving force for spike generation.

b) Effect on the EPSP

The amplitude of the EPSP at the point of generation is given by

$$\Delta V = \frac{R_m}{R_m + R_t} (E_m - E_t)[1 - e^{-t/\tau}] ,$$

where R_m is the resting membrane resistance, R_t the resistance of the subsynaptic membrane during transmitter action, E_m the resting membrane potential, E_t the transmitter equilibrium potential, t the duration of the subsynaptic current, and τ the membrane time constant. Irrespective of whether the depolarising agonist actually affects transmitter-receptor interaction, it will reduce ΔV by the extent that R_m, E_m, and τ are reduced. Since t is approximately $0.2-0.4\tau$ and $R_t \leqslant R_m$ (SKOK, 1973; NISHI, 1974), ΔV will be reduced by 30–50% even if the effect of changing E_m is off-set by applied membrane current. This is of some importance when it comes to the question of assessing whether a depolarising agonist affects transmitter receptor interaction (see below). A further aspect of the conductance change is its effect on the electrotonic spread of the EPSP from the synapse to the point of spike generation. In amphibian ganglion cells, which have no dendrites, these two points are rather close, so spatial decrement can be ignored (see, e.g., MCMAHAN and KUFFLER, 1971; MATTHEWS, 1974). In mammals nearly all the synapses are located on dendrites (ELFVIN, 1963; FORSSMANN, 1964; TAXI, 1965; TAMARIND and QUILLIAM, 1971), whereas the spike is generated on the soma (ECCLES, 1963; SKOK, 1973) or in the initial segments of the axon (PERRI et al., 1970). The dendrites may be up to 150–200 μM long (MCLACHLAN, 1974; NISHI, 1974). Since the dendritic length constant is around twice this value (MCLACHLAN, 1974; NISHI, 1974) electrotonic attenuation of the EPSP between the synapse and the soma is normally quite small (<40%). If the membrane resistance is reduced, however, a more appreciable decrement might occur (e.g., ∼ 60% if the total transmembrane resistance is halved, assuming an infinite cylinder). Nevertheless, it should be stressed that while the *amplitude* of the EPSP may be depressed, since it is generated from a lower resting membrane potential, its absolute *height* would normally be increased. Thus, its ability to generate an action potential would not be affected unless there was a corresponding rise in the excitable threshold for spike generation.

2. Experimental Observations

a) Excitability Changes

The crucial test of whether the transmission block produced by a depolarising agent stems from its depolarising action is the demonstration of an appropriate change in neuronal excitability. In particular, such changes should extend to forms of excitation other than orthodromic activation alone (though with due allowance for spatial factors referred to above).

Three lines of experimental evidence suggest that this is indeed the case: i) TRENDELENBURG (1957) showed that the responses of cat superior cervical ganglion to both acetylcholine and K^+ injections were suppressed during transmission block produced by TMA and during the initial phase of nicotine block. ii) GINSBORG and GUERRERO (1964) observed a parallel reduction in both orthodromic and antidromic spike amplitudes in frog sympathetic ganglion cells during the onset and plateau of carbachol-induced depolarisation (Fig. 3a). iii) A parallel depression of orthodromic spikes and direct spikes is also elicited by depolarising current pulses in rat sympathetic ganglion cells during carbachol-induced depolarisation (ADAMS and BROWN, unpublished observations; Figs. 4 and 5). The effects recorded in Fig. 4 are fully in keeping with those anticipated for depolarisation block: the spike is slowed, the positive overshoot is reduced, and the voltage thresholds for orthodromic and direct spike generation are both elevated. It may be noted that the EPSP itself is not blocked, and that, although reduced in amplitude, at its peak the level of membrane depolarisation attained is well in excess of that originally attained prior to carbachol addition. Nevertheless, it is unable to generate a spike, presumably because the excitable threshold has risen to an even greater extent. (As pointed out above, a diminished EPSP amplitude is to be expected during an agonist-induced increase in depolarisation and conductance, even when transmitter-receptor interaction is unchanged. Thus, it is not easy to determine from Figs. 3–5 without further data whether transmitter-receptor interaction is impaired or not.)

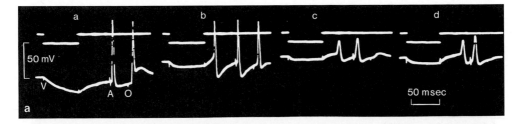

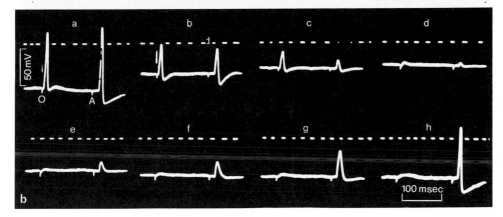

Fig. 3a and b. Effect of depolarising agonist on electrotonic responses to hyperpolarising current pulses (V), orthodromic spikes (O) and antidromic spikes (A) recorded from frog sympathetic ganglion cells in vitro. (From GINSBORG and GUERRERO, 1964.) **a** Responses recorded *a* before, and *b–d*, 10 s, 30 s, and 2 min 10 s after adding 150 μM carbachol. The input resistance was reduced from ~ 70 MΩ in *a* to ~ 5 MΩ in *c*, but shows partial recovery in *d*. Note that both orthodromic and antidromic spikes are depressed in parallel. (The extra spike in *b* in an "anode-break" spike.) **b** Responses recorded *a* before, and *b* 10 s, *c* 12 s, *d* 20 s, *e* 30 s, *f* 1 min, *g* 2 min 30 s, *h* 5 min 15 s after addition of 200 μM tetramethylammonium. *Broken line* indicates zero membrane potential. Note that the antidromic spike recovers before the orthodromic spike

b) Effect of Membrane Depolarisation

It might be anticipated that the effect of a depolarising agent would be imitated by depolarising the membrane electrically. There is some evidence both for and against this. (i) ECCLES (1956) noted that the change produced in the configuration of the extra-cellularly recorded orthodromic action potential in isolated rabbit superior cervical ganglion by nicotine could be imitated by extrinsic depolarising current. (ii) ADAMS and BROWN (1975, Fig. 7a) noted a comparable effect of depolarising current on the direct spike to that illustrated in Fig. 4a. (iii) RIKER (1968), however, was unable to block transmission in frog ganglion cells by depolarising the membrane 12 mV. The principal difficulty in evaluating these experiments is that membrane depolarisation alone would not be expected to exert such a profound effect on excitability as application of a nicotinic agonist, because it cannot fully replicate the component of increased membrane conductance (at least at modest levels of depolarisation). The experiments are therefore less conclusive than the excitability measurements illustrated in Figs. 3–5.

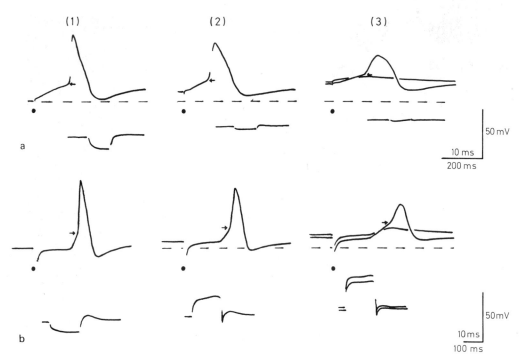

Fig. 4a and b. Effect of carbachol (180 μM in the presence of 2.9 μM hyoscine) on action potentials in rat superior cervical ganglion cells in vitro evoked by **a** depolarising current pulses and **b** preganglionic nerve stimuli at 0.5 Hz. (Unpublished observations of ADAMS and BROWN: see ADAMS and BROWN, 1975, for full experimental details.) Records are traced from a series of superimposed oscilloscope photographs taken *(1)* before and *(2)* and *(3)* during the development of carbachol-induced depolarisation. Spikes were recorded on the upper beam, electrotonic responses to constant-strength hyperpolarising current pulses on the lower beam, at a reduced sweep speed. [Apparent reversal of the electrotonic response in **b** is an artefactual consequence of the large conductance increase; see ADAMS and BROWN, (1975).] *Dashed lines* represent the resting membrane potential; *arrows* indicate the threshold for spike generation. The *dots* indicate the commencement of depolarising current pulse (in **a**) or the orthodromic stimulus (in **b**). *Vertical scale*, 50 mV. *Horizontal scales:* 10 ms (upper beam); 200 ms **a** and 100 ms **b** (lower beam). Note that carbachol produced a comparable rise in spike threshold for both direct and orthodromic stimulation

c) Effect of Restoring Membrane Potential

Attempts have been made to find out whether transmission blocked during exposure to depolarising agents is restored by hyperpolarising current. In frog sympathetic ganglia depolarised by some 12 mV with acetylcholine, RIKER (1968) was unable to restore the blocked orthodromic transmission by restoring the membrane potential. However, ADAMS and BROWN (1975) obtained partial restoration of the orthodromic spike in rat sympathetic ganglion cells by membrane hyperpolarisation. Two difficulties are presented in this type of experiment. Firstly, it is difficult to achieve complete repolarisation of a cell that has been strongly depolarised by a nicotinic agonist, because the low membrane resistance necessitates excessive current. Secondly, as pointed out in connection with electrical depolarisation, membrane hyperpolarisa-

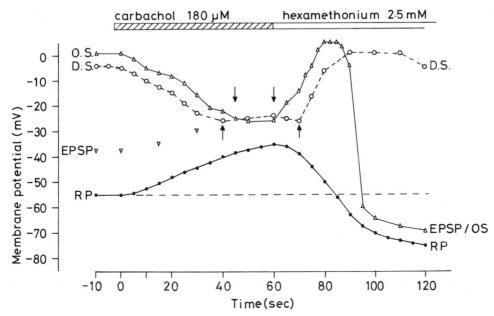

Fig. 5. Effect of 180 μM carbachol, followed at washout by 2.5 mM hexamethonium, on the orthodromic spike height *(O.S)*, direct spike height *(D.S)*, synaptic potential *(EPSP)* and resting potential *(RP)* recorded from a cell in an isolated rat superior cervical ganglion. (Unpublished observation of ADAMS and BROWN.) Plots were derived from a heated stylus recorder output, hence producing some spike attenuation. *Arrows* indicate points between which spike generation failed. Note that addition of hexamethonium initially *restored* the orthodromic spike *pari passu* membrane potential recovery, before itself blocking transmission. The hyperpolarisation in hexamethonium solution reflects electrogenic Na-pump activity (see BROWN et al., 1972); this eventually caused direct spike failure

tion will not reverse the high membrane conductance, which may be an additional cause of electrical inexcitability.

To some extent the experiment illustrated in Fig. 5 offers a partial solution to this problem, for both depolarisation and conductance increase were rapidly reversed by adding hexamethonium. It is noticeable that both orthodromic and direct excitability recovered at approximately the same rate, and that recovery occurred around the time that the membrane potential had returned to normal. Of course, hexamethonium itself eventually blocked transmission: the fact recovery occurred before block implies that the average receptor occupancy by depolarising agonist – and hence ease of block by hexamethonium – was less than the occupancy of subsynaptic receptors by transmitter (see below). Hexamethonium also precipitated an electrogenic hyperpolarisation, and this eventually suppressed direct spikes, as the depolarisation produced by current injection fails to reach threshold (the depolarising current pulses not being adjusted to ensure suprathreshold depolarisation.

d) Quantitative Relationship Between Depolarisation and Block

Using different concentrations of nicotine and TMA, SHAND (1965) obtained a fairly linear relationship between the magnitude of the ganglion depolarisation and the reduction in amplitude of the orthodromic spike potential. However, since this spike potential was recorded extracellularly through leads from the ganglion itself and the postganglionic nerve trunk, the change in amplitude of the ganglionic action potential is a measure not of the number of synapses blocked, but of the reduced spike amplitude of the individual neurones (as pointed out by GINSBORG and GUERRERO, 1964). Unfortunately there do not appear to have been any other comprehensive studies of this relationship in terms of dose sensitivity recorded by methods capable of avoiding this pitfall (e.g., by recording from the postganglionic trunk, or by intracellular recording). However, with one exception (that of RIKER, 1968), authors generally appear to agree that in the ganglion, transmission block only occurs after the administration of depolarising agents in concentrations producing appreciable depolarisation (GINSBORG and GUERRERO, 1964; GEBBER, 1968; HAEFELY, 1974a,b; ADAMS and BROWN, unpublished observations). RIKER (1968) found that a number of cells in frog ganglia were blocked by acetylcholine when the depolarisation produced was 5 mV or less, but also noted that all cells showing 20 mV or more depolarisation were blocked. Some dispersion in the sensitivity of transmission to depolarisation block must be expected, depending upon the degree to which the normal EPSP exceeds the excitable threshold. [It should be noted that in frog muscle, nicotine can reduce the end plate potential at concentrations well below those producing overt depolarisation: WANG and NARAHASHI, 1972. Lobeline (which exerts a nicotine-like action on the ganglion, albeit more prolonged: JARAMILLO and VOLLE, 1968; HAEFELY, 1974b) also inhibits both transmission and nicotinic depolarisation of frog muscle without producing overt end plate depolarisation (STEINBERG and VOLLE, 1972; VOLLE and REYNOLDS, 1973). These effects have not been detected in ganglia, which suggests that muscle is not always an appropriate model for drug action on ganglia.]

In apparent contradiction to most other results, KALLER (1956) observed that transmission block produced in rat superior cervical ganglion in vivo by intra-arterial infusions of depolarising agents (acetylcholine, nicotine, DMPP, TMA) was *not* preceded by overt stimulation as measured by eyelid responses. They did not attribute this to lack of depolarisation, but correctly interpreted it in terms of "a relatively high-rate of accommodation". It does indeed appear to be the case that accommodation to depolarisation is unusually rapid in rat ganglion. Thus, in the experiments illustrated in Figs. 4 and 5, rapid administration of carbachol to isolated rat ganglion via the bath fluid (exchange time 3–4 s, ADAMS and BROWN, 1975) failed to evoke spike potentials during the onset of depolarisation. In contrast, the administration of comparable doses of carbachol to frog ganglia usually induced trains of action potentials (GINSBORG and GUERRERO, 1964). *Iontophoretic* application of acetylcholine to rat ganglion cells readily elicits spikes (ADAMS and BROWN, unpublished observations), as in other ganglion cells (BLACKMAN et al., 1963; DENNIS et al., 1971; HOLMAN et al., 1971): with this mode of application the rate of depolarisation exceeds the rate of accommodation. It is important to recognise that ganglion cell depolarisation by exogenously applied agonist, even when of considerable magnitude, does not invariably result in the generation of action potentials, and that even when action potentials do result, their frequency and duration show a complex relationship to the depolarisation (cf. GINSBORG and GUERRERO, 1964; RIKER, 1967; HOLMAN et al., 1971). Thus, with low-amplitude depolarisation the discharge may persist for much longer than with larger depolarisations. Consequently, the sympathetic discharge produced by a nicotinic agonist is a poor index of the underlying depolarisation.

II. Dissociation of Depolarisation and Block

The above description suggests very strongly that the depolarising action of nicotinic agonists renders the cell inexcitable, and that this effect would be sufficient to account for the block of transmission observed during the depolarisation. Nevertheless, several lines of experimentation suggest that other factors may be involved, if not during the initial depolarisation, then at least afterwards. The principal experiments pointing in this direction are as follows.

1. Off-Set Rates in vivo

PATON and PERRY (1953) and LUNDBERG and THESLEFF (1953) reported that when nicotine was injected to cat ganglia in vivo, the block of transmission persisted after the ganglion depolarisation had subsided. This has been confirmed by other investigators (TAKESHIGEet al., 1963; GEBBER and VOLLE, 1966; GEBBER, 1968; HAEFELY, 1974 b). "Delayed" block is even more pronounced with lobeline (JARAMILLO and VOLLE, 1968; HAEFELY, 1974 b) but is less apparent with other nicotinic agonists (TMA, DMPP, choline esters) if administered in concentrations insufficient to generate a postactivation hyperpolarisation (see below). During this late phase of block, the ganglion becomes capable of direct excitation by (for example) K^+ (TRENDELENBURG, 1957) and shows reduced sensitivity to a nicotinic agonist (PATON and PERRY, 1953; HAEFELY, 1974 b). Further, the block becomes reversible with repetitive stimulation (LUNDBERG and THESLEFF, 1953). Thus, late nicotine block takes on certain characteristics associated with "competitive" block (PATON and PERRY, 1953). Since the concentration of depolarising agent at this time is presumably declining, receptor occupancy sufficent to antagonise the transmitter after depolarisation has subsided implies an equal or greater occupancy during depolarisation. In this case depolarisation might be regarded as a side effect of receptor occupation, the block being attributable to antagonism of the transmitter throughout rather than to the depolarisation. An observation of GEBBER (1968) that ganglion block *during* nicotine depolarisation is surmountable by repetitive preganglionic stimulation might be taken as support of a "competitive" element (though this can be explained in other ways; see below).

As pointed out earlier in connection with the depolarising action of carbachol (Figs. 3 and 4 above), the EPSP was not clearly depressed during depolarisation to an extent greater than that likely to result from the membrane potential and conductance change (though this has not been precisely quantitated in such a way as to preclude some depression), so that receptor occupancy by carbachol at the sites of transmitter action appears rather low. However, carbachol is a rather "strong" agonist, and it may be that nicotine acts as a "weaker" or " partial" agonist, so necessitating greater receptor occupancy per unit conductance increase (cf. STEPHENSON, 1956). In this case, grater "fade" of depolarisation would be anticipated on PATON's (1961) "rate theory" of drug action. An alternative view of receptor inactivation, perhaps more in keeping with current thought regarding the action of depolarising agents at skeletal muscle, is that the ganglionic receptors become "desensitised" during prolonged agonist action (see below). (It may be noted that desensitisation and partial agonism are not mutually exclusive.)

2. Postactivation Hyperpolarisation

Analysis of effects during off-set of ganglion cell depolarisation is complicated by the concurrent operation of an *electrogenic Na pump*. Because of their relatively small size, ganglion cells show a rapid net increase in intracellular Na^+ ion during agonist-induced depolarisation (BROWN and SCHOLFIELD, 1974). This is subsequently ex-truded electrogenically, to hyperpolarise the cell membrane (KOSTERLITZ et al., 1968; BROWN et al., 1972; LEES and WALLIS, 1974). Although analysed most intensively in vitro, this electrogenic hyperpolarisation has also been recorded after the injection of nicotinic agonists in vivo (GEBBER and VOLLE, 1966; JARAMILLO and VOLLE, 1968; MACHOVA and BOSKA, 1969; HAEFELY, 1972, 1974a,b). It must be recognised that even if it is insufficient to produce an overt hyperpolarisation, electrogenic Na exten-sion may hasten restoration of the resting potential. Its contribution at such a stage can be revealed by adding a rapidly acting competitive blocking agent, such as hexamethonium: reduction of the membrane conductance (increased by residual action of the nicotinic agonist) increases the hyperpolarising effect of the electrogenic Na^+ current and a rapid hyperpolarisation ensues (BROWN and SCHOLFIELD, 1970; BROWN et al., 1972; HAEFELY, 1972, 1974; see also Fig. 5). GEBBER and VOLLE (1966) showed that the electrogenic hyperpolarisation following the depolarisation pro-duced by TMA was capable of blocking transmission, and this has been confirmed for other nicotinic depolarising agents (JARAMILLO and VOLLE, 1968; MACHOVA and BOSKA, 1969; HAEFELY, 1974; see also Fig. 4). Moreover, since it is essentially a result of depolarisation, a depolarisation of sufficient magnitude produced by other ago-nists such as 5-hydroxytryptamine can produce a comparable phase of "postactiva-tion hyperpolarising block" (MACHOVA and BOSKA, 1969). [K^+-induced depolarisa-tion does not lead to a hyperpolarisation or subsequent transmission block, because the Na^+ influx is much less: BROWN (1966b) and GEBBER and VOLLE (1966).]

Transmission block during electrogenic hyperpolarisation probably occurs be-cause at the greater membrane potential, the EPSP fails to reach threshold: mem-brane hyperpolarisation beyond -60 mV does not alter the excitable threshold of the cell (ADAMS and BROWN, 1975 and unpublished observations) but will reduce the absolute level of membrane potential attained by the EPSP. During such hyperpolar-isation there appears to be no diminution in the amplitudes of either the EPSP or the depolarisation produced by nicotinic agonists – rather, they are augmented as ex-pected for the increased driving force (GEBBER and VOLLE, 1966; HAEFELY, 1974; ADAMS and BROWN, unpublished observation; see also Fig. 5). [Not surprisingly, hyperpolarisation-induced transmission block can be reversed by repetitive stimula-tion, which augments the EPSP; GEBBER and VOLLE (1966).]

Ganglion block associated with electrogenic hyperpolarisation following injec-tions of TMA, DMPP, or choline esters is separated from the transmission block occurring during the preceding depolarisation by a transient recovery period, giving a "tri-phasic" appearance to the transmission record (GEBBER and VOLLE, 1966; JARAMILLO and VOLLE, 1968; MACHOVA and BOSKA, 1969; HAEFELY, 1974). This

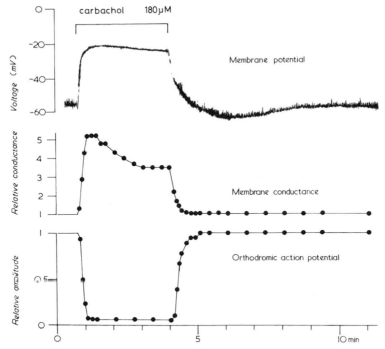

Fig. 6. Effect of a prolonged application of carbachol on membrane potential *(upper record)*, membrane conductance, measured from the electronic response to hyperpolarising current pulses *(middle record)* and orthodromic spike height *(lower record:* residual response is the EPSP) in an isolated rat sympathetic ganglion cell. Note that the conductance change diminishes in the continued presence of carbachol, suggesting some degree of desensitisation; notwithstanding, the orthodromic spike recovers very rapidly on removal of the carbachol (hexamethonium was not added to this preparation, cf. Fig. 5). (Unpublished observation of ADAMS and BROWN)

period of transient recovery can also be detected when the depolarisation in vitro is rapidly terminated by a competitive antagonist (see Fig. 5). Such effects constitute additional evidence that the block during the preceding depolarisation is intimately associated with the depolarisation (see below). Overt hyperpolarisation is less readily observed after nicotine injections (GEBBER and VOLLE, 1966; GEBBER, 1968; HAEFELY, 1974 b) and the intermission of transmission recovery in less pronounced, but may still be detected (see Fig. 6 in HAEFELY, 1974 b). No overt hyperpolarisation is detected after lobeline injections, unless a competitive inhibiter is added and transmission remains blocked both during and after the depolarisation (JARAMILLO and VOLLE, 1968; HAEFELY, 1974 b).

Since the hyperpolarisation is solely a consequence of previous Na influx, differences in the time course and magnitude of the subsequent hyperpolarisation produced by different agonists may seem rather surprising. This probably stems from the fact that the rate of recovery of depolarisation varies with different agonists, and that the slower the rate of recovery the less synchronised the hyperpolarisation becomes among the cell population. Hence, with extracellular recording, hyperpolarisation in one cell is shunted by continued depolarisation in another. One reason for the slow recovery and delayed or absent hyperpolarisation with nicotine is that, as a weak base, nicotine becomes concentrated within the cells of the ganglion (BROWN et al., 1971; BROWN and HALLIWELL, 1972). Its exit from them is slow (rate coefficient <0.1 min^{-1}), so that the cells form a slow-clearing "reservoir" of drug; further, there is some evidence that, during clearance, the immediately extraneuronal concentrations are sustained at a level capable of causing renewed receptor activation (BROWN and SCHOLFIELD, 1972; see also ADAMS, 1975). Such considerations would also apply to lobeline, but not to quaternary nonpenetrating agonists such as TMA or DMPP.

This line of reasoning has some bearing on the role played by electrogenic hyperpolarisation in the slow off-set of ganglionic blockade previously observed by PATON and PERRY (1953) and LUNDBERG and THESLEFF (1953). These authors did not detect a hyperpolarisation as such; however, it is quite conceivable that the apparent recovery of depolarisation may have reflected the algebraic sum of asynchronous depolarisation and on-going hyperpolarisation, to the extent that while some cells were still blocked through depolarisation, others were blocked through hyperpolarisation. In this context, it is noticeable that the time course of post-nicotine hyperpolarisation depicted by HAEFELY (1974b), which lasts about 10 min, is very similar to the time-course of postdepolarisation block illustrated by PATON and PERRY (1953) and LUNDBERG and THESLEFF (1953). Intracellular recording of these events in vivo would obviously assist in clarifying the situation.

3. Desensitisation

During prolonged application of nicotinic agonists to frog sympathetic ganglia in vitro, the conductance increase and membrane depolarisation produced by the agonist may diminish, and direct excitability, as measured by the antidromic spike, recovers but orthodromic transmission remains blocked (GINSBORG and GUERRERO, 1964). This type of nondepolarising block was observed with acetylcholine, carbachol and TMA. PILAR (1969, personal communication) has observed a comparable effect of acetylcholine in avian ciliary ganglion cells. Since intracellular recording was used in these studies and no hyperpolarisation was observed, this type of block cannot be attributed to postactivation hyperpolarisation. It more closely resembles the process observed in skeletal muscle and termed "desensitisation" (see, e.g., THESLEFF, 1955; KATZ and THESLEFF, 1957; RANG and RITTER, 1970; MAGAZANIK and VYSKOCIL, 1970, 1973; ADAMS, 1975).

The essence of desensitisation is that there is a transformation of the receptor and/or ionic channels from a sensitive/conducting to an insensitive/non-conducting state; on removal of the agonist, a gradual reversion to the sensitive/conducting state takes place. Consequently, during desensitisation the tissue becomes less sensitive to the transmitter in proportion to the number of receptors or channels inactivated. Block is thus of the non-competitive type, but not necessarily insurmountable so long as (i) not all receptors or channels are in the desensitised state and (ii) the amount of transmitter released is normally insufficient to saturate the local receptor population. In accordance with this, GINSBORG and GUERRERO (1964) found that after depolarisation in response to the first dose of agonist had subsided, a second application of agonist produced less effect and the sensitivity to transmitter was also reduced, as judged from the miniature EPSP amplitude; transmission block was not totally insurmountable, however, but could be relieved by tetanic stimulation.

The characteristics of this form of block resemble those described by PATON and PERRY (1953) and LUNDBERG and THESLEFF (1953) for that period of delayed recovery of transmission following subsidence of depolarisation after nicotine injections to cat ganglia in vivo. However, there are certain reservations to be made in equating the two processes. *Firstly,* GINSBORG and GUERRERO (1964) presented no information on the rate of recovery of desensitisation after washing out the agonists. On one model for desensitisation (KATZ and THESLEFF, 1957; RANG and RITTER, 1970), though the extents of desensitisation produced by different agonists vary, the rate constant for recovery would be expected to be the same for all agonists, whereas PATON and PERRY (1953) drew a clear distinction between the rates of recovery of transmission after different agonists. [This difficulty is not insuperable, since it may be explained by delayed agonist removal, as discussed above. Further, other models of desensitisation (e.g., ADAMS, 1975) involve no such constraint.] *Secondly,* it is not clear that desensitisation in mammalian ganglia is sufficiently pronounced or develops sufficiently rapidly to explain the in vivo observations. Certainly, in isolated rat ganglia desensitisation produced by a ganglion-blocking concentration of carbachol is quite modest (see Fig. 6) and recovery of transmission on removing carbachol can occur within seconds: it would be hard to explain the rapid restoration of transmission in the experiments illustrated in Figs. 5 and 6 if there were significant residual desensitisation to transmitter. Unfortunately, there is as yet no direct information on the amount of desensitisation produced in mammalian ganglia by nicotine, nor is there suitable information regarding the rates of onset and off-set of desensitisation at this site.

Perhaps the situation in which desensitisation may be of importance is that in which a high concentration of depolarising agent is maintained for some appreciable time – for instance, after repeated intravenous injections or infusions. Since this is the experimental circumstance in which persistent blockade by a depolarising agonist is most easily obtained, further analysis of desensitisation in ganglia may be important.

4. Differential Sites of Depolarisation and Transmission Block?

In addition to earlier-mentioned differences in rates of off-set, GEBBER (1968) discriminated between nicotine-induced depolarisation and block at cat superior cervical ganglia in the following ways: (i) Tubocurarine reversed depolarisation but intensified block. (ii) During transmission block there was a continuous asynchronous postganglionic discharge, blocked by tubocurarine. (iii) Whilst the nicotinic excitatory action of acetylcholine was reduced, muscarinic excitation by acetylcholine or methacholine and the excitatory effects of 5-hydroxytyptamine were enhanced. (iv) Tetanic stimulation relieved block during nicotine-induced depolarisation. On the grounds of these observations it was argued that blockade during nicotine depolarisation was not due to a reduced excitability. Competitive block was discounted on the basis of doubts about the degree of surmountability, and preganglionic block (see below) was discounted because of the reduced sensitivity to acetylcholine. It was suggested that depolarisation and transmission block were unrelated events mediated through different receptors, the former accounting for the enhanced sensitivity to 5-hydroxytryptamine and to muscarine. These arguments warrant further scrutiny, particularly where they relate to excitability changes.

The use of tubocurarine as a means of reversing depolarisation involves, of course, the complication that tubocurarine itself blocks transmission. Consequently, tubocurarine would be expected to restore transmission only if the concentration required to antagonise nicotine were less than that required to block subsynaptic acetylcholine receptors, or if the effects on the two receptors were temporally separated. These are rather critical requirements. They might obtain under conditions where the depolarising agent and transmitter were equally effective: in this case, because of uneven distribution of the transmitter, local subsynaptic receptor saturation during transmitter action might exceed the average receptor activation by the depolarising agonist (cf. HARTZELL et al., 1975; ADAMS, 1976), and might then be less "desaturated" by a competitive blocking agent. This type of effect could explain the transient restoration of transmission blocked by carbachol on the addition of hexamethonium (illustrated in Fig. 5), though here the experimental conditions are simplified. However, if nicotine were to have less efficacy than acetylcholine (as seems probable: VAN ROSSUM, 1962a) or were to dissociate less rapidly from the receptors, the necessary difference in receptor activation would be diminished.

The ability of nicotine to produce a continuous postganglionic discharge at a time when transmission is blocked is not unexpected and is in keeping with previous observations on the action of carbachol (GINSBORG and GUERRERO, 1964). Two points need emphasis (i) The ability of a synaptic potential to excite a spike during depolarisation is limited not only by the depolarisation itself but also by the conductance increase affecting both the amplitude and the electrotonic spread of the EPSP. The spike-generating action of exogenous nicotine will be less affected by this conductance increase, since it is more sustained and may be more diffuse in origin. (ii) Repetitive postganglionic firing will, of itself, occlude orthodromic spike generation. (It is also possible that nicotine might directly depolarise the initial segment or adjacent soma membrane.)

Muscarinic excitation and excitation by 5-hydroxytryptamine are quite different from that produced by normal transmitter action: the receptors concerned are undoubtedly not subsynaptic, and so are probably nearer to the point of spike generation [see (ii) above]; and muscarinic depolarisation would be expected to be augmented during membrane depolarisation, since it probably results from a reduced membrane conductance (see WEIGHT and VOTAVA, 1970).

Reversal of block by tetanic stimulation does not negate the concept of depolarisation block. The essence of depolarisation block is that the excitability of the neurone is reduced such that the EPSP is subthreshold; augmentation of the EPSP by tetanic stimulation would not itself further reduce excitability, because the transient depolarisations are too rapid, but could allow the EPSP to rise above the new threshold. Only if the depolarisation is such as to render the cell totally inexcitable would tetanic stimulation become ineffective.

Taken individually, therefore, the experiments of GEBBER (1968) do not invalidate the concept of depolarisation block, and so do not require the presence of separate depolarising and blocking receptors. Notwithstanding this, it is quite conceivable that nicotine-induced depolarisation arises from an action on extrasynaptic nicotinic receptors; however, focal iontophoretic experiments on frog parasympathetic ganglion cells do not show the presence of extrasynaptic receptors for acetylcholine (HARRIS et al., 1971).

5. Presynaptic Effects?

RIKER (1968) discriminated between depolarisation and transmission block produced by exogenous acetylcholine in frog ganglia in several ways. (i) In different cells there was no strong correlation between the amount of depolarisation and the incidence of block. (ii) Reversal of depolarisation by extrinsic current failed to restore transmission, leaving a greatly attenuated EPSP. (iii) Modest depolarisation by injected current failed to block transmission. The author concluded that "transmission-block by acetylcholine (1) is entirely independent of cell depolarisation, and (2) probably reflects on action at some site other than the ganglion cell", and went on to suggest that this other site is the preganglionic nerve terminal.

As pointed out earlier, the effects reported by RIKER (1968) are less convincing evidence against depolarisation block by acetylcholine than might at first appear, since they consider only the effect of changing membrane potential and do not take into account the effect of a conductance increase. Further, it is far from clear from these experiments why – even if not attributable to depolarisation per se – the block has to be placed at the presynaptic rather than postsynaptic side of the synapse.

Nevertheless, there is evidence from other investigations that nicotinic agonists *can* affect presynaptic terminals. KOKETSU and NISHI (1967), using an extracellular sucrose-gap technique, observed a depolarisation of presynaptic ganglia in vitro, which was reduced by tubocurarine. In the bullfrog ganglion acetylcholine and nicotine also reduced the amplitude of the "terminal" action potential. Acetylcholine failed to depolarise the preganglionic trunk fibres and did not induce antidromic responses. GINSBORG (1971) recorded electrical activity in individual preganglionic nerve terminals in frog sympathetic ganglia with extracellular glass microelectrodes (5–25 MΩ resistance). Acetylcholine or carbachol ($\geqslant 1\,mM$) transiently diminished or abolished the presynaptic spike; however, the spike recovered spontaneously in the continued presence of choline ester, and was refractory to a subsequent application. Spike blockade was antagonised by tubocurarine. It was suggested that spike depression resulted from terminal depolarisation, and that the terminal response showed rapid desensitisation. PILAR (1969 and personal communication), by direct intracellular recording from preganglionic terminals in avian ciliary ganglion, has confirmed that acetylcholine increases membrane conductance, depolarises the terminal, and reduces presynaptic spike amplitude, and that these effects show strong desensitisation. Acetylcholine also reduced the quantal content of the EPSP (as judged from coefficient of variance analysis), suggesting a reduced transmitter release.

The principal question arising from these observations is, of course, whether such presynaptic effects contribute to the blocking action of nicotinic agonists on transmission. The following observations suggest that their contribution is probably small.

1. *Presynaptic spike depression* was observed (GINSBORG, 1971) to begin *after* the postsynaptic response was reduced, and transmission to remain remain blocked long after the presynaptic spike had recovered. By raising $[K^+]$ GINSBORG and co-work-

ers also ascertained that quite substantial degrees of presynaptic spike depression (up to two-thirds) could occur without any impairment of the recorded postsynaptic response (though this safety factor would not apply during additional postsynaptic depression.

2. During *chemical transmission block* with acetylcholine, PILAR (personal communication) noted that the electrotonic coupling potential recorded in the ciliary ganglion cell (an index of presynaptic electrical activity in these electrically coupled synapses) was still detectable, and indeed was capable of sustaining electrical transmission. Although the postsynaptic conductance change limits the use of the coupling potential as an accurate measure of presynaptic response, its ability to generate electrical transmission suggests that the depression of chemical transmission was substantially postsynaptic in origin. In addition, rather rapid desensitisation of the presynaptic response to acetylcholine would preclude a material contribution to sustained transmission block.

3. When *nicotine* was *perfused through the cat superior cervical ganglion* in a concentration sufficient to block transmission (FELDBERG and VARTIAINEN, 1935) it neither evoked a release of acetylcholine nor reduced the amount released by cervical sympathetic stimulation. In addition, using radioactive labelling techniques to overcome the problem of separating endogenous and exogenous acetylcholine, COLLIER and KATZ (1970) found that a concentration of acetylcholine that blocked transmission failed to depress the release of ^{3}H-acetylcholine from the preganglionic nerve fibres in the perfused cat superior cervical ganglion.

6. Conclusions

To reiterate, depolarisation block as such may be envisaged as comprising (i) an elevated threshold for spike generation consequent upon both the membrane depolarisation – an accommodative response – and the conductance increase, and (ii) an attenuation of the EPSP (generated, in mammals, on dendrites) at the initial segment of the axon, consequent upon the increased conductance and reduced space constant of the soma-dendrite membrane. As a result, the EPSP fails to attain the threshold for spike generation.

There is clear evidence that an appropriate reduction in ganglion cell excitability occurs during application of a depolarising agent and that, during the initial phase of depolarisation, this is sufficient to account for the block of transmission. To this extent, therefore, true depolarisation block does occur.

Nevertheless, there is also evidence that block can persist or occur at a time when the initial depolarisation has subsided; by definition, this is no longer depolarisation block. This delayed phase of block is most pronounced (in mammalian ganglia at least) after nicotine or lobeline, and so is probably the principal type of block obtained when using such compounds to block transmission experimentally.

Several different explanations for this late phase of block have been suggested. The two that appear most plausible are (i) receptor desensitisation, associated with the *continued presence* of the depolarising agent, e.g., during infusions or repeated injections, and (ii) postactivation electrogenic hyperpolarisation, occurring *after removal* of the depolarising agent, and lasting some 5–15 min. Both processes appear to be associated with all nicotinic agonists on the ganglion (the amount of desensitisation might vary, but there is no experimental evidence concerning this). The prolonged duration of post-depolarising block after nicotine or lobeline might be explicable as a consequence of intracellular accumulation, such that a reservoir of drug is obtained whose slow clearance sustains the interstitial concentration. This would sustain desensitisation and delay postactivation hyperpolarisation. No unequivocal information exists to indicate how long desensitisation lasts, or whether the rate of recovery from desensitisation differs for different agonists, so the degree of overlap between the two processes is uncertain. Both processes have a superficial similarity in that they are (theoretically) surmountable, and hence reversible by repetitive stimulation, but can be readily distinguished in several other ways. To this extent, their relative significance is subject to experimental analysis.

Since the process of desensitisation begins at the time of agonist action, it could theoretically contribute to block during the depolarisation itself. This would be manifest as a greater reduction in the EPSP than predicted from the depolarisation and conductance increase itself. Some experiments (on frog ganglia) suggest that this happens; others (on rat ganglia) suggest not. Much depends on the rate and extent of desensitisation, and hence, in all probability, on the duration of exposure and nature of the depolarising agent. Experiments to clarify this point are needed. It should be borne in mind that if the excitable threshold is raised sufficiently, transmission will be blocked irrespective of the EPSP amplitude.

One final point: depolarising agents produce rapid net ionic changes in ganglion cells, so that membrane potential change alone is not a precise measure of receptor activation over prolonged contact times.

D. Intraganglionic Distribution of Ganglion-Blocking Drugs

Although there is a strong presumption that ganglion-blocking agents exert their primary action on the outside of the ganglion cell membrane (i.e., from the extracellular space), the point has been made above that accumulation in the intracellular space may indirectly affect their blocking action. Such accumulation has been substantiated for non-quaternary agents, but studies in other tissues suggest that the possibility of intracellular penetration of quaternary ammonium compounds cannot be excluded.

I. Non-Quaternary Agents

The penetration and cellular distribution of non-quaternary bases has been studied most extensively with nicotine. This compound rapidly penetrates the ganglion cell membrane, in such a way that its presence within the ganglion cell cytoplasm can be detected autoradiographically even after transient application of radiolabelled nicotine by close arterial injection (APPELGREN et al., 1963; BROWN et al., 1969). When sympathetic ganglia are incubated in radiolabelled nicotine solution in vitro, nicotine is progressively accumulated in the tissue until the overall intracellular concentration exceeds that in the surrounding medium by a factor of 5–8 (BROWN et al., 1971). The simplest explanation for this is that the cell membrane is readily permeant to a free nicotine base but not to protonated nicotine, so that the distribution of nicotine reflects the pH gradient between the extracellular fluid and the cytoplasm (cf. WEISS, 1968): thus, with a normal extracellular pH of 7.4 in 25 mM NaHCO$_3$-buffered medium, a cytoplasmic pH of 6.5–6.6 is indicated (BROWN and SCHOLFIELD, 1972). The probable correctness of this interpretation is indicated by the compatible distribution of certain other bases, such as atropine, morphine, and procaine, all of which attain an intracellular/extracellular concentration gradient of 5–7 (GARTH-WAITE, 1976). [It may be noted that this pH gradient appears incompatible with the distribution of weak acids, such as the conventional marker dimethyldiphenyl-oxazolidinedione (DMO). A plausible explanation may be forwarded in terms of different pH values of different cell compartments (BROWN and HALLIWELL, 1972), others, using different tissues, have favoured an intracellular binding or partitioning phenomenon for nicotine (PUTNEY and BORZELLECA, 1971; ALDERDICE and WEISS, 1974; WEISS and ALDERDICE, 1975), though it should be noted that such sites must be common to several bases.] Intracellularly accumulated nicotine, procaine, atropine, or morphine is washed out of the ganglion rather slowly: components of the exit curves may be detected with rate constants one or two orders of magnitude less than that predicted for simple extracellular clearance (BROWN and SCHOLFIELD, 1972; GARTHWAITE, unpublished observations).

It seems very likely that the intracellular accumulation and slow exit of nicotine, if determined simply by the membrane diffusibility of the free base and the trans-membrane pH gradient, will also apply to other non-quaternary blocking agents, such as lobeline, mecamylamine, and pempidine. There is indeed substantial evidence that the latter two drugs readily penetrate cell membranes (MILNE et al., 1957; HARINGTON et al., 1958) and that the degree of accumulation in cells is determined by the pH gradient, to the extent that a reduction in extracellular pH may precipitate a rapid exit of drug from intracellular storage sites (PAYNE and ROWE, 1957).

Two consequences arise from this distribution pattern. *Firstly*, intracellular accumulation and consequent protonation would tend to favour intracellular side effects. This may account for some of the complexities in their action, such as the modification of transmitter release produced by mecamylamine (LEES and NISHI, 1972) or (at the neuromuscular junction) by nicotine (STEINBERG and VOLLE, 1972). *Secondly*, by virtue of the relatively slow exit of intracellular base, intracellular accumulation forms a reservoir of drug, exit of which may sustain perineuronal concentrations and receptor activation long after extracellular material has cleared. Some evidence has been obtained to suggest that this makes a material contribution to the prolonged effect of nicotine (BROWN and SCHOLFIELD, 1972), and could explain certain differences between nicotine and lobeline on the one hand and quaternary depolarising agents on the other with respect to speed of recovery (see Sect. C).

1. Active Form of Non-Quaternary Compounds

Since non-quaternary bases can exist in two forms at equilibrium – free base and protonated base – the question has arisen as to which of these two forms is the active receptor ligand. On general grounds, it seems most likely that only the protonated form is active, since, at normal extracellular pH, the concentration of the protonated form of mecamylamine (pK_a 11.4), pempidine (pK_a 11.25), or nicotine (pK_a 8.01) exceeds that of the free base by factors of up to 10^4. Thus, the affinity constant for the free base would need to be very much higher than that of quaternary agents for it to exert any effect. Two lines of evidence (from experiments on muscle) tend to support this conclusion. (i) The effects of these compounds vary with extracellular pH as would be expected (from the degree of ionisation) if only the protonated form were active (BARLOW and HAMILTON, 1962; HAMILTON, 1963; BLACKMAN and RAY, 1964). (ii) The quaternary monomethiodide derivatives were of comparable potency to the ionised form of the parent compounds.

II. Quaternary Ammonium Compounds

There have been no direct studies on the distribution of quaternary ammonium bases within ganglia comparable to those of nicotine. In principle, as lipid-insoluble compounds, such agents would not be expected to penetrate neurones as readily as non-quaternary bases. However, there is some suggestion that hexamethonium may slowly penetrate cellular elements in ganglia in vivo, in that (i) if renal excretion is prevented, the tissue/plasma concentration ratio may rise to a value (0.634) somewhat higher than that (0.39, WOODWARD et al., 1969; ~0.45, BROWN et al., 1971) anticipated within the extracellular space and (ii) the clearance of ganglionic hexamethonium shows a component about twice as slow as the decline in plasma concentration (MCISAAC, 1962). Mechanisms of penetration (if any) into ganglion cells have not been determined experimentally, leaving inferences regarding possible mechanisms to be drawn solely from experiments on other tissues.

1. Diffusion

Simple diffusion across the membrane is unlikely, except, perhaps, with TEA: as pointed out in Sect. B. III. 5, this compound can be inserted into the voltage-dependent K^+ channels and so might conceivably penetrate through K^+ channels. (It should be noted that transmembrane diffusion of monoquaternary bases would generate, at equilibrium, an intracellular concentration 20–30 times that in the extracellular fluid – perhaps more in glial cells – in accordance with the transmembrane potential as predicted by the Nernst equation).

2. Receptor-Linked Penetration

CREESE and his associates (CREESE et al., 1963; TAYLOR et al., 1964; CREESE and MACLAGAN, 1970) have observed a concentrative accumulation of radiolabelled quaternary ammonium agonists (iodocholinium, decamethonium) into skeletal muscle which is suppressed by tubocurarine. The uptake process is slow [influx rate coefficient for decamethonium (at 5 μM external concentration) $= 1.24\,h^{-1}$, comparable to the resting Na^+ permeability: CREESE and ENGLAND (1970)]. Penetration in normal muscle fibres was restricted to the end plate region, but was greater and more widespread after denervation, corresponding to the spread of receptors (TAYLOR et al., 1965). Labelled decamethonium was retained firmly in the muscle fibre, and remained restricted to the end plate region up to 2 h after entry (TAYLOR et al., 1967; CREESE and MACLAGEN, 1970). The following conclusions can be drawn from other experiments.

1) The driving force for accumulation is the transmembrane potential, since accumulation is suppressed when the fibre is depolarised by K^+ ions.

2) Entry seems to be a consequence of acetylcholine-receptor interaction, since it is restricted to receptor regions and the inhibitor constant for tubocurarine is low (70 nM: CREESE and ENGLAND, 1970).

3) Entry is not due to depolarisation per se since K^+ depolarisation does not promote entry.

4) Influx is saturable, attaining a half-maximal velocity at 400 μM decamethonium (CREESE and ENGLAND, 1970). This was taken to suggest that it was mediated by a carrier rather than a consequence of a non-specific permeability increase. However, it should be noted that the fluxes of Na^+ ions in cultured muscle cells induced by carbachol also shows saturation kinetics (CATTERALL, 1975), as though receptor-induced ion flux involved a rate-limiting binding step, yet remaining passive in respect of electrochemical gradient.

5) As a consequence of receptor activation, such penetration is restricted to agonists: no comparable penetration of antagonists has been described.

3. Carrier-Mediated Entry

At least three carrier-systems for quaternary ammonium bases have been described in different tissues – the choline carrier (see Sect. B.2), an acetylcholine/carbachol carrier in brain, and a quaternarybase carrier in kidney.

a) Choline Carrier

Interaction of ganglion-blocking drugs with the choline carrier has been alluded to in Sect. II. B. II. Pertinent points with respect to ganglia are the following. (i) Of the ganglion-blocking agents interacting with the choline carrier, only TMA appears to act as a *substrate* – the remainder competitively *inhibit* choline influx in red cells (MARTIN, 1969). Thus, generalised entry through the choline carrier seems unlikely. (ii) The cellular location of the choline carrier(s) in the ganglion has not yet been defined (BOWERY and NEAL, 1975).

b) Brain Acetylcholine/Carbachol Carrier

(CREESE and TAYLOR, 1965, 1967 SCHUBERT and SUNDWALL, 1967 LIANG and QUASTEL, 1969 POLAK, 1969 TAYLOR et al., 1969).

This is driven by the membrane potential or Na gradient. It is inhibited by atropine, tubocurarine, morphine, physostigmine, and, among ganglion blocking agents, by TMA (K_I, 40 μM), TEA (K_I, 5 μM), hexamethonium (K_I, 12 μM), and nicotine (K_I, 6 μM) (LIANG and QUASTEL, 1969): it is not known whether these serve as substrates. As these values suggest, it is distinct from the choline carrier. Its cellular location (or presence in ganglia) is unknown.

c) Kidney

A number of quaternary ammonium bases are concentrated in renal tubular cells, including hexamethonium (MCISAAC, 1965), decamethonium, and TEA (HOLM, 1971). They probably serve as substrates for the organic cation secretory carrier

(PETERS, 1960). This carrier shows some similarity to the brain carrier (b) in inhibitor specificity. [A non-choline carrier for carbachol and decamethonium in red cells (MARTIN, 1969) may also be of the same species.]

Addendum

The suggestion by BLACKMAN (1970) that hexamethonium might block acetylcholine-operated ionic channels rather than acetylcholine receptors has recently received support from the experiments of MARTY et al. (1976) and ASCHER et al. (1978a) on voltage-clamped molluscan neurones. The blocking actions of both hexamethonium and tubocurarine were increased by membrane hyperpolarisation, the former showing about twice the voltage sensitivity of the latter. Such voltage sensitivity might result from the nature of the binding reaction or the effect of the electrical field in driving the antagonist into the channel.

ASCHER and his colleagues envisaged the following sequential scheme:

$$R \underset{k_{-A}}{\overset{k_{+A}}{\rightleftharpoons}} R_A \underset{k_{-B}}{\overset{k_{+B}}{\rightleftharpoons}} R_{AB} , \tag{1}$$

where R is the closed channel–receptor complex, R_A the open (conducting) channel, and R_{AB} the channel blocked by antagonist B. Exploiting the voltage-dependence of the block to apply voltage-jump relaxation methods, and combining these with steady-state current measurements, the authors adduced the following values for the rate constants k_{+B} and k_{-B} and the dissociation constant for the blocking reaction K_B $(=k_{-B}/k_{+B})$ at -80 mV transmembrane potential:

	Tubocurarine	Hexamethonium
k_{+B} $(M^{-1} s^{-1})$	4.4×10^5	7.5×10^5
k_{-B} (s^{-1})	0.1	0.5
K_B (M)	2.3×10^{-7}	6.7×10^{-7}

The authors excluded a significant competitive effect induced by antagonist binding to the closed channel–receptor complex (i.e., K'_B for the reaction $R \rightleftharpoons R_B$ greatly exceeds K_B), partly because the degree of block increased with agonist current even under conditions where the total proportion of channels in the open configuration was still small. (With a competitive receptor blocker, the degree of antagonism should *decrease* with increasing agonist dose, see below.)

The voltage-dependence of the binding constant, K_B, measured between -40 and -100 mV, accorded with the following expression:

$$K_B(V) = K_B(-80) \exp\left(\frac{-80+V}{v}\right), \tag{2}$$

where $V=$ membrane potential (in millivolts). The term v was about twice as large for hexamethonium and decamethonium than for tubocurarine or tetraethyl-ammonium, probably reflecting the divalent/monovalent nature of the blocking agents.

Subsequently, Ascher et al. (1978b) have reported that the essential features of hexamethonium block in molluscan neurones are also apparent in *rat parasympathetic ganglion cells*, though quantitative aspects have yet to be completed. This is an important advance, and might explain some of the more perplexing features of ganglion block referred to earlier.

For example, an essential feature of channel block is that blockade is facilitated by increasing the proportion of channels in the open state, or by increasing the total aggregate open time. This means that block is enhanced by increasing the agonist concentration or the duration for which it is applied. This could clearly contribute to the acute frequency-dependence of ganglion blockade or to sensitisation by a prior period of orthodromic stimulation.

Channel block might also explain why the measured potency of a ganglion-blocking agent, such as hexamethonium, is rather low notwithstanding its apparent specificity, since the full effect of the antagonist would only become manifest at receptor-saturating agonist concentrations. In effect, channel block is a form of "uncompetitive antagonism", so that the degree of inhibition (I) will increase with agonist concentration (A):

$$I = \frac{[A][B]}{1 + [A](1 + [B])} ,\tag{3}$$

where $[A] = A/K_A$ and $[B] = B/K_B$. Thus, only at infinitely high values of $[A]$ will $I = 0.5$ at $B = K_B$; at sub-saturation values of $[A]$, $I < 0.5$ at $B = K_B$, tending to zero as $[A]$ gets very low.

Underestimation of blockade will be exaggerated if an *indirect* measure of recording agonist action is used such that the measured response saturates at submaximal levels of receptor activation, e.g., agonist-induced membrane potential change. Thus, assuming a simple monomolecular agonist–receptor interaction, the conductance changes in the absence (ΔG) and presence ($\Delta G'$) of an uncompetitive channel-blocker would be given by

$$\Delta G / \Delta G_{max} = A/(A + K_A)\tag{4}$$

and

$$\Delta G' / \Delta G_{max} = A\beta^{-1}/(A + K_A\beta^{-1})\tag{5}$$

respectively, where $A =$ agonist concentration, $K_A =$ agonist dissociation constant and $\beta = (1 + B/K_B)$, B being the antagonist concentration. However, since the steady-state voltage deflexion (ΔV) is related to the conductance increase by the expression (Ginsborg, 1967):

$$\Delta V = E\left[\frac{\Delta G}{G + \Delta G}\right] ,\tag{6}$$

where E is the driving force for the agonist current and G is the resting cell conductance, Eqs. (4) and (5) transmute to:

$$\Delta V / \Delta V_{max} = A/(A + K^*) ,\tag{7}$$

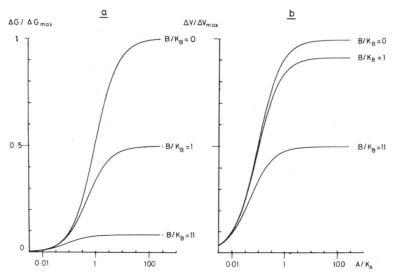

Fig. 7a and b. Conductance increases **a** and membrane depolarisation **b** produced by a nicotinic agonist A in the presence of an "uncompetitive" antagonist B, calculated from Eqs. (5) and (8). No allowance is made for voltage-dependence of block. (BROWN and VIJAYARAGHAVAN, unpublished)

where $K^* = K_A\left(\dfrac{G}{G+\Delta G_{max}}\right)$, and:

$$\Delta V'/\Delta V_{max} = Ax^{-1}/(A+K^*x^{-1}),\tag{8}$$

where $x = (\Delta G_{max} + \beta G)/(\Delta G_{max} + G)$ respectively.

Clearly, for any given value of B/K_B, x in Eq. (8) is much less than β in Eq. (5), so that the voltage response ΔV is more resistant to block that the conductance response ΔG. This is illustrated in Fig. 7 of this Addendum for the situation where $\Delta G_{max}/G = 10$ (an extreme situation, but perhaps not unreasonable for a receptor-saturating concentration of nicotinic agonist). Here, a concentration of antagonist sufficient to reduce the conductance response by half will only reduce the peak voltage response by some 16%; half-maximal reduction of the voltage response necessitates an 11-fold higher antagonist concentration. (It should be noted that this apparent discrepancy between antagonist potencies measured against voltage and conductance responses does *not* apply to pure *competitive* antagonists: in both cases the agonist dose-response curves are parallel and would be shifted in the presence of the antagonist by the same amount, $1 + B/K'_B$.)

On the other hand, the *form* of the voltage-displacement dose–response curve in the presence of a pure uncompetitive channel–blocker still shows evidence of un-competitive, rather than competitive, antagonism. Hence, the complexities intro-duced by indirect recording would not, of themselves, explain the apparent competitive shifts observed with hexamethonium (see above). Two further ex-planations are possible. (i) Since depolarisation will reduce the amount of channel block, the agonist-induced depolarisation might itself introduce some degree of surmountability (ASCHER, personal communication). (ii) Since voltage recording will underestimate K_B for channel block but not K'_B for receptor block (see above), a weak affinity for the receptors, undetectable with current recording in a voltage-clamp mode, would attain greater significance with voltage recording.

Acknowledgements. I thank Pergamon Press, the Physiological Society and the authors concerned for permission to reproduce Figs. 1–3. Previously unpublished work with Paul Adams was supported by grants from the American Medical Association Education and Research Foundation and the Medical Research Council.

References

Acheson, G.A., Pereira, S.A.: The blocking effect of tetraethylammonium ion on the superior cervical ganglion of the cat. J. Pharmacol. Exp. Ther. *87*, 273–280 (1946)

Adamic, S.: Effects of quaternary ammonium compounds on choline entry into the rat diaphragm muscle fibre. Biochem. Pharmacol. *21*, 2925–2929 (1972)

Adams, P.R.: The mechanism by which amylobarbitone and thiopentone block the end plate response to nicotinic agonists. J. Physiol. (Lond.) *241*, 41–42 P (1974)

Adams, P.R.: A study of desensitisation using voltage clamp. Pflügers Arch. *360*, 135–144 (1975a)

Adams, P.R.: A model for the procaine end plate current. J. Physiol. (Lond.) *246*, 61–62 P (1975b)

Adams, P.R.: A comparison of the time-course of excitation and inhibition by iontophoretic decamethonium in frog end plate. Br. J. Pharmacol. *57*, 1, 59–65 (1976)

Adams, P.R.: Voltage jump analysis of procaine action at frog end plate. J. Physiol. (Lond.) *268*, 291–318 (1977)

Adams, P.R., Brown, D.A.: Actions of γ-aminobutyric acid on sympathetic ganglion cells. J. Physiol. (Lond.) *250*, 85–120 (1975)

Alderdice, M.T., Weiss, G.B.: On ^{14}C-nicotine distribution and movements in slices from monkey cerebral cortex. Arch. Int. Pharmacodyn. *209*, 162–171 (1974)

Alkadhi, K.A., McIsaac, R.J.: Effect of preganglionic nerve stimulation on sensitivity of the superior cervical ganglion to nicotinic blocking agents. Br. J. Pharmacol. *51*, 533–539 (1974)

Ambache, N., Perry, W.L.M., Robertson, P.A.: The effect of muscarine on perfused superior cervical ganglia of cats. Br. J. Pharmacol. *11*, 442–448 (1956)

Appelgren, L.-E., Hansson, E., Schmiterlöw, C.G.: Localisation of radioactivity in the superior cervical ganglion of cats following injection of ^{14}C-labelled nicotine. Acta Physiol. Scand. *59*, 330–336 (1963)

Ariens, E.J.: Molecular pharmacology. Vol. I. New York: Academic Press 1964

Armstrong, C.M.: Time course of TEA$^+$-induced anomalous rectification in squid giant axons. J. Gen. Physiol. *50*, 491–503 (1966)

Armstrong, C.M.: Inactivation of g_K in squid axons. Biophys. J. *9*, A-248 (1969)

Armstrong, C.M., Binstock, L.: Anomalous rectification in the squid giant axon injected with tetraethylammonium chloride. J. Gen. Physiol. *48*, 859–872 (1965)

Ascher, P., Marty, A., Neild, T.O.: The mode of action of antagonists of the excitatory response to acetylcholine in *Aplysia* neurones. J. Physiol. (Lond.) *278*, 207–235 (1978a)

Ascher, P., Large, W.A., Rang, H.P.: The action of ganglion-blocking drugs studied by voltage-clamp. J. Physiol. (Lond.) *280*, 17P (1978b)

Barlow, R.B., Hamilton, J.T.: Effects of pH on the activity of nicotine and nicotine monomethiodide on the rat diaphragm. Br. J. Pharmacol. *18*, 543–549 (1962)

Beani, L., Bianchi, C., Bieber, G., Ledda, F.: The effect of some ganglion stimulants and blocking drugs on acetylcholine release from the mammalian neuromuscular junction. J. Pharm. Pharmacol. *16*, 557–560 (1964)

Bennett, G., Tyler, C., Zaimis, E.: Mecamylamine and its mode of action. Lancet *1957 II*, 218–222

Bennett, M.R., McLachlan, E.M.: An electrophysiological analysis of the storage of acetylcholine in preganglionic nerve terminals. J. Physiol. (Lond.) *22*, 657–668 (1972a)

Bennett, M.R., McLachlan, E.M.: An electrophysiological analysis of the synthesis of acetylcholine in preganglionic nerve terminals. J. Physiol. (Lond.) *221*, 669–682 (1972b)

Bhatnagar, S.P., MacIntosh, F.C.: Effect of quaternary bases and inorganic cations on acetylcholine synthesis in nervous tissue. Can. J. Physiol. Pharmacol. 45, 249–268 (1967)

Birks, R., MacIntosh, F.C.: Acetylcholine metabolism of a sympathetic ganglion. Can. J. Biochem. Physiol. 39, 787–827 (1961)

Blackman, J.G.: Dependence on membrane potential of the blocking action of hexamethonium at a sympathetic ganglionic synapse. Proc. Univ. Otago. Med. Sch. 48, 4–5 (1970)

Blackman, J.G., Purves, R.D.: Intracellular recordings from ganglia of the thoracic sympathetic chain of the guinea-pig. J. Physiol. (Lond.) 203, 173–198 (1969)

Blackman, J.G., Ray, C.: Actions of mecamylamine, dimecamine, pempidine and their two quaternary metho-salts at the neuromuscular junction. Br. J. Pharmacol. 22, 56–65 (1964)

Blackman, J.G., Ginsborg, B.L., Ray, C.: Synaptic transmission in the sympathetic ganglion of the frog. J. Physiol. (Lond.) 167, 355–373 (1963a)

Blackman, J.G., Ginsborg, B.L., Ray, C.: On the quantal release of the transmitter at a sympathetic synapse. J. Physiol. (Lond.) 167, 402–415 (1963b)

Blackman, J.G., Crowcroft, P.J., Devine, C.E., Holman, M.E., Yonemura, K.: Transmission from preganglionic fibres in the hypogastric nerve to peripheral ganglia of male guinea-pigs. J. Physiol. (Lond.) 201, 723–743 (1969)

Blackman, J.G., Gauldie, R.W., Milne, R.J.: Interaction of competitive antagonists: the anticurare action of hexamethonium and other antagonists at the skeletal neuromuscular junction. Br. J. Pharmacol. 54, 91–100 (1975)

Bowery, N.G., Neal, M.J.: Failure of denervation to influence the high affinity uptake of choline by sympathetic ganglia. Br. J. Pharmacol. 55, 278 P (1975)

Brown, A.M.: Cardiac sympathetic adrenergic pathways in which synaptic transmission is blocked by atropine sulphate. J. Physiol. (Lond.) 191, 271–288 (1967)

Brown, D.A.: Depolarisation of normal and pre-ganglionically denervated superior cervical ganglia by stimulant drugs. Br. J. Pharmacol. 26, 511–520 (1966a)

Brown, D.A.: Electrical responses of cat superior cervical ganglia in vivo to some stimulant drugs and their modification by hexamethonium and hyoscine. Br. J. Pharmacol. 26, 538–551 (1966b)

Brown, D.A.: Responses of normal and denervated cat superior cervical ganglia to some stimulant compounds. J. Physiol. (Lond.) 201, 225–236 (1969)

Brown, D.A., Fumagalli, L.: Dissociation of α-bungarotoxin binding and receptor block in the rat superior cervical ganglion. Brain Res. 129, 165–168 (1977)

Brown, D.A., Halliwell, J.V.: Intracellular pH in rat isolated superior cervical ganglia in relation to nicotine depolarisation and nicotine-uptake. Br. J. Pharmacol. 45, 349–359 (1972)

Brown, D.A., Kwiatkowski, D.: A note on the effect of dithiothreitol (DTT) on the depolarisation of isolated sympathetic ganglia by carbachol and bromo-acetylcholine. Br. J. Pharmacol. 56, 1, 128–130 (1976)

Brown, D.A., Quilliam, J.P.: Observations on the mode of action of some central depressant drugs on transmission through the cat superior cervical ganglion. Br. J. Pharmacol. 23, 257–272 (1964)

Brown, D.A., Scholfield, C.N.: Potentials in isolated rat superior cervical ganglia produced by nicotine. Br. J. Pharmacol. 40, 559–560 P (1970)

Brown, D.A., Scholfield, C.N.: Nicotine washout rates from isolated rat ganglia in relation to recovery from nicotine depolarisation. Br. J. Pharmacol. 45, 29–36 (1972)

Brown, D.A., Scholfield, C.N.: Changes of intracellular sodium and potassium ion concentrations in isolated rat superior cervical ganglia induced by depolarising agents. J. Physiol. (Lond.) 242, 307–319 (1974)

Brown, D.A., Hoffmann, P.C., Roth, L.J.: ^{3}H-nicotine in cat superior cervical and nodose ganglia after close-arterial injection in vivo. Br. J. Pharmacol. 35, 406–417 (1969)

Brown, D.A., Jones, K.B., Halliwell, J.V., Quilliam, J.P.: Evidence against a presynaptic action of acetylcholine during ganglionic transmission. Nature 226, 958–959 (1970)

Brown, D.A., Halliwell, J.V., Scholfield, C.N.: Uptake of nicotine and extracellular space markers by isolated rat ganglia in relation to receptor activation. Br. J. Pharmacol. 42, 100–113 (1971)

Brown, D.A., Brownstein, M.J., Scholfield, C.N.: Origin of the after hyperpolarisation that follows removal of depolarising agents from the isolated superior cervical ganglion of the rat. Br. J. Pharmacol. 44, 651–671 (1972)

Brown, D.A., Garthwaite, J., Hayashi, E., Yamada, S.: Action of surugatoxin on nicotinic receptors in the superior cervical ganglion of the rat. Br. J. Pharmacol. 58, 157–159 (1977)

Brown, G.L.: The effect of temperature on the release of acetylcholine from sympathetic ganglia. J. Physiol. (Lond.) 124, 26 P (1954)

Brown, G.L., Feldberg, W.: The action of potassium on the superior cervical ganglion of the cat. J. Physiol. (Lond.) 86, 290–305 (1936a)

Brown, G.L., Feldberg, W.: Differential paralysis of the superior cervical ganglion. J. Physiol. (Lond.) 86, 10 P (1936b)

Brown, G.L., MacIntosh, G.C.: Discharges in nerve fibres produced by potassium ions. J. Physiol. (Lond.) 96, 10–11 P (1939)

Burke, W., Katz, B., Machne, X.: The effect of quaternary ammonium ions on crustacean nerve fibres. J. Physiol. (Lond.) 722, 588–598 (1953)

Burns, B.D., Paton, W.D.M.: Depolarisation of the motor end plate by decamethonium and acetylcholine. J. Physiol. (Lond.) 115, 41–73 (1951)

Catterall, W.M.: Sodium transport by the acetylcholine receptor of cultured muscle cells. Proc. Natl. Acad. Sci. 250, 1776–1781 (1975)

Chen, S.S.: Transmission in superior cervical ganglion of the dog after cholinergic suppression. Am. J. Physiol. 221, 209–213 (1971)

Collier, B., Exley, D.A.: Mechanism of the antagonism by tetraethylammonium of neuromuscular block due to d-tubocurarine or calcium deficiency. Nature 199, 702–703 (1963)

Collier, B., Katz, H.S.: The release of acetylcholine by acetylcholine in the cat's superior cervical ganglion. Br. J. Pharmacol. 39, 428–438 (1970)

Collier, B., MacIntosh, F.C.: The source of choline for acetylcholine synthesis in a sympathetic ganglion. Can. J. Physiol. Pharmacol. 47, 127–135 (1969)

Corne, S.J., Edge, N.D.: Pharmacological properties of (1:2:2:6:6-pentamethylpiperidine), a new ganglion-blocking compound. Br. J. Pharmacol. 13, 339–349 (1958)

Cowan, S.L., Walter, W.G.: The effects of tetra-ethylammonium iodide on the electrical response and the accommodation of nerve. J. Physiol. (Lond.) 91, 101–126 (1937)

Creese, R., England, J.M.: Decamethonium in depolarised muscle and the effects of tubocurarine. J. Physiol. (Lond.) 210, 345–361 (1970)

Creese, R., MacLagan, J.: Entry of decamethonium in rat muscle studied by autoradiography. J. Physiol. (Lond.) 210, 363–386 (1970)

Creese, R., Taylor, D.B.: Entry of labelled carbachol in brain slices of the rat and the action of d-tubocurarine and strychnine. J. Pharmacol. Exp. Ther. 157, 406–419 (1967)

Creese, R., Taylor, D.B., Tilton, B.: The influence of curare on the uptake and release of a neuromuscular blocking agent labelled with radioactive iodine. J. Pharmacol. Exp. Ther. 139, 8–17 (1963)

Dennis, M.J., Harris, A.J., Kuffler, S.W.: Synaptic transmission and its duplication by focally applied acetylcholine in parasympathetic neurons in the heart of the frog. Proc. R. Soc. Lond. [Biol.] 177, 509–539 (1971)

Diamond, I., Kennedy, E.P.: Carrier-mediated transport of choline into synaptic nerve ending. J. Biol. Chem. 244, 3258–3263 (1969)

Douglas, W.W., Lywood, D.W.: The stimulant effect of TEA on acetylcholine output from the superior cervical ganglion: comparision with barium. Fed. Proc. 20, 324 (1961)

Douglas, W.W., Lywood, D.W., Straub, R.W.: The stimulant effect of barium on the release of acetylcholine from the superior cervical ganglion. J. Physiol. (Lond.) 156, 515–522 (1961)

Dun, N., Nishi, S., Karczmar, A.G.: Electrical properties of the membrane of denervated mammalian sympathetic ganglion cells. Neuropharmacology 15, 219–223 (1976)

Dunant, Y.: Some properties of the presynaptic nerve terminals in a mammalian sympathetic ganglion. J. Physiol. (Lond.) 221, 577–587 (1972)

Eccles, R.M.: Intracellular potentials recorded from a mammalian sympathetic ganglion. J. Physiol. (Lond.) 130, 572–584 (1955)

Eccles, R.M.: The effects of nicotine on synaptic transmission in the sympathetic ganglion. J. Pharmacol. Exp. Ther. 118, 26–38 (1956)

Eccles, R.M.: Orthodromic activation of single ganglion cells. J. Physiol. (Lond.) 165, 387–391 (1963)

Elfvin L.-G.: The ultrastructure of the superior cervical sympathetic ganglion of the cat. II. The structure of the preganglionic end fibres and the synapses as studied by serial sections. J. Ultrastruct. Res. 8, 441–476 (1963)

Erulkar, S.D., Woodward, J.K.: Intracellular recording from mammalian superior cervical ganglia in situ. J. Physiol. (Lond.) 199, 189–204 (1968)

Exley, K.A.: Depression of autonomic ganglia by barbiturates. Br. J. Pharmacol. 9, 170–181 (1954)

Fatt, P., Katz, B.: The electrical properties of crustacean muscle fibres. J. Physiol. (Lond.) 120, 171–204 (1953)

Feldberg, W., Vartiainen, A.: Further observations on the physiology and pharmacology of a sympathetic ganglion. J. Physiol. (Lond.) 83, 103–128 (1935)

Ferry, C.B., Marshall, A.R.: An anti-curare effect of hexamethonium at the mammalion neuromuscular junction. Br. J. Pharmacol. 47, 353–362 (1973)

Flacke, W., Fleisch, J.H.: The effect of ganglionic agonists and antagonists on the cardiac sympathetic ganglia of the dog. J. Pharmacol. Exp. Ther. 174, 45–55 (1970)

Flacke, W., Gillis, R.A.: Impulse transmission via nicotinic and muscarinic pathways in the stellate ganglion of the dog. J. Pharmacol. Exp. Ther. 163, 266–276 (1968)

Flacke, W., Yeoh, T.S.: Differentiation of acetylcholine and succinylcholine receptors in leech muscle. Br. J. Pharmacol. 33, 154–161 (1968)

Forssmann, W.G.: Studien über den Feinbau des Ganglion cervicale superius der Ratte. Acta Anat. (Basel) 59, 106–140 (1964)

Frankenhaeuser, B., Hodgkin, A.L.: The action of calcium on the electrical properties of squid axons. J. Physiol. (Lond.) 137, 218–244 (1957)

Franko, B.V., Ward, J.W., Alphin, R.S.: Pharmacologic studies of N-benzyl-3-pyrrolidylacetate methobromide (AHR-602), a ganglion stimulating agent. J. Pharmacol. Exp. Ther. 139, 25–30 (1963)

Garthwaite, J.: The uptake of weak acids and bases into isolated rat superior cervical ganglia in relation to intracellular pH. Br. J. Pharmacol. 56, 3, 353 P (1976)

Gebber, G.L.: Dissociation of depolarisation and ganglionic blockade induced by nicotine. J. Pharmacol. Exp. Ther. 160, 124–134 (1968)

Gebber, G.L., Volle, R.L.: Mechanisms involved in ganglionic blockade induced by tetramethylammonium. J. Pharmacol. Exp. Ther. 152, 18–28 (1966)

Gillis, R.A., Flacke, W., Garfield, J.M., Alper, M.H.: Actions of anticholinesterase agents upon ganglionic transmission in the dog. J. Pharmacol. Exp. Ther. 163, 277–286 (1968)

Ginsborg, B.L.: Ion movements in junctional transmission. Pharmacol. Rev. 19, 289–316 (1967)

Ginsborg, B.L.: On the presynaptic acetylcholine receptors in sympathetic ganglia of the frog. J. Physiol. (Lond.) 216, 237–246 (1971)

Ginsborg, B., Guerrero, S.: On the action of depolarising drugs on sympathetic ganglion cell of the frog. J. Physiol. (Lond.) 172, 189–206 (1964)

Ginsborg, B.L., Stephenson, R.P.: On the simultaneous action of two competitive antagonists. Br. J. Pharmacol. 51, 287–300 (1974)

Haefely, W.: Electrophysiology of the adrenergic neurone. In: Handbook of experimental pharmacology. Blaschko, H., Muscholl, E. (eds.), Vol. XXXIII, pp. 662–725. Berlin: Springer 1972

Haefely, W.: The effects of 1,1-dimethyl-4-phenyl-piperazinium (DMPP) in the cat superior cervical ganglion. Naunyn Schmiedebergs Arch. Pharmacol. 281, 57–91 (1974a)

Haefely, W.: The effects of various "nicotine-like" agents in the cat superior cervical ganglion in situ. Naunyn Schmiedebergs Arch. Pharmacol. 281, 93–117 (1974b)

Hagiwara, S., Watanabe, A.: The effect of tetraethylammonium chloride on the muscle membrane examined with an intracellular electrode. J. Physiol. (Lond.) 129, 513–527 (1955)

Hamilton, J.T.: The influence of pH on the activity of nicotine at the neuromuscular junction. Can. J. Biochem. 41, 283–289 (1963)

Hancock, J.C., Volle, R.L.: Stimulation by carbachol and tetramethylammonium ions of intact and denervated sympathetic ganglia. Life Sci. 9, 301–308 (1970)

Harington, M., Kincaid-Smith, P., Milne, M.D.: Pharmacology and clinical use of pempidine in the treatment of hypertension. Lancet 1958 II, 6–11

Harris, A.J., Kuffler, S.W., Dennis, M.J.: Differential chemosensitivity of synaptic and extrasynaptic areas on the neuronal surface membrane in parasympathetic neurons of the frog, tested by microapplication of acetylcholine. Proc. R. Soc. Lond. [Biol.] *177*, 541–553 (1971)

Hartzell, H.C., Kuffler, S.W., Yoshikami, D.: Post-synaptic potentiation: interaction between quanta of acetylcholine at the skeletal neuromuscular junction. J. Physiol. (Lond.) *251*, 427–464 (1975)

Harvey, A.M., MacIntosh, F.C.: Calcium and synaptic transmission in a sympathetic ganglion. J. Physiol. (Lond.) *97*, 408–416 (1940)

Harvey, S.C.: Combined effects of hexamethonium and tetraethylammonium. Arch. Int. Pharmacodyn. *114*, 232–242 (1958)

Hemsworth, B.A., Darmer, K.I., Jr., Bosman, H.B.: The incorporation of choline into isolated synaptosomal and synaptic vesicle fractions in the presence of quaternary ammonium compounds. Neuropharmacology *10*, 109–120 (1971)

Hille, B.: The selective inhibition of delayed potassium currents in nerve by tetraethylammonium ion. J. Gen. Physiol. *50*, 1287–1302 (1967)

Hille, B.: Charges and potentials at the nerve surface: divalent cations and pH. J. Gen. Physiol. *51*, 221–236 (1968)

Hille, B.: Ionic channels in nerve membranes. Prog. Biophys. Mol. Biol. *21*, 3–32 (1970)

Hilton, J.G.: The pressor response to neostigmine after ganglionic blockade. J. Pharmacol. Exp. Ther. *132*, 23–28 (1961)

Hodgkin, A.L., Huxley, A.F.: A quantitative description of membrane current and its application to conduction and excitation in nerve. J. Physiol. (Lond.) *117*, 500–544 (1952)

Hodgkin, A.L., Martin, K.: Choline uptake by giant axons of *Loligo*. J. Physiol. (Lond.) *179*, 26 *P* (1965)

Holm, J.: Effect of cholinergic and cholinergic blocking drugs on decamethonium uptake by slices of mouse kidney. Acta Pharmacol. Toxicol. (Kbh.) *30*, 81–88 (1971a)

Holm, J.: Effect of tetraethylammonium and N^1-methylnicotinamide on the uptake of decamethonium and carbamoylcholine by slices of mouse kidney. Acta Pharmacol. Toxicol. (Kbh.) *30*, 89–96 (1971b)

Holman, M.E., Muir, T.C., Szurszewski, J.H., Yonemura, K.: Effect of iontophoretic application of cholinergic agonists and their antagonists to guinea-pig pelvic ganglia. Br. J. Pharmacol. *41*, 26–40 (1971)

Hutter, O.F., Kostial, K.: Effect of magnesium and calcium ions on the release of acetylcholine. J. Physiol. (Lond.) *124*, 234–241 (1954)

Huxley, A.F.: Ion movements during nerve activity. Ann. N. Y. Acad. Sci. *81*, 221–245 (1959)

Jaramillo, J., Volle, R.L.: Non-muscarinic stimulation and block of a sympathetic ganglion by 4-(m-chlorophenylcarbamoyloxy)-2-butynyltrimethammonium chloride (McN-A 343). J. Pharmacol. Exp. Ther. *157*, 337–345 (1967)

Jaramillo, J., Volle, R.L.: A comparison of the ganglionic stimulating and blocking properties of some nicotinic drugs. Arch. Int. Pharmacodyn. *174*, 88–97 (1968)

Job, C., Lundberg, A.: On the significance of post- and presynaptic events for the facilitation and inhibition in the sympathetic ganglion of the cat. Acta Physiol. Scand. *28*, 14–28 (1952)

Jones, A.: Ganglionic actions of muscarinic compounds. J. Pharmacol. Exp. Ther. *141*, 195–205 (1963)

Kaller, H.: Die Erregbarkeit des Halsganglion der Ratte durch Pharmaka. Arch. Exp. Pathol. Pharmakol. *228*, 361–366 (1956a)

Kaller, H.: Pharmakologische Untersuchungen am oberen Halsganglion der Ratte bei intraarterieller Infusion. Arch. Int. Pharmacodyn. *105*, 337–348 (1956b)

Karlin, A., Winnik, M.: Reduction and specific alkylation of the receptor for acetylcholine. Proc. Natl. Acad. Sci. USA *60*, 668–674 (1968)

Katz, B.: The release of neural transmitter substances. Liverpool: Liverpool University Press 1969

Katz, B., Miledi, R.: Tetrodotoxin-resistant electrical activity in presynaptic terminals. J. Physiol. (Lond.) *203*, 459–487 (1969)

Katz, B., Thesleff, S.: A study of the "desensitisation" produced by acetylcholine at the motor end plate. J. Physiol. (Lond.) *138*, 63–80 (1957)

Kensler, C.J.: The anticurare activity of tetraethylammonium ion in the cat. Br. J. Pharmacol. *5*, 204–209 (1950)

Kharkevich, D.A.: Effects of the ganglion-blocking agents, Barbamyl, and novocain on the development of post-activation facilitation in sympathetic ganglia. Farmakol. Toksikol. *22*, 6, 493–499 (1959) (Russ.) (cf. Kharkevich, D.A., 1967)

Kharkevich, D.A.: Ganglionic agents. Moskva: Medgiz 1962 (Russ.)

Kharkevich, D.A.: "Ganglion-blocking and ganglion-stimulating agents". Oxford: Pergamon Press 1967 (translated from Russian edition, 1962)

Khatter, J.C., Friesen, A.J.D.: The effect of hemicholinium-3 on choline and acetylcholine levels in a sympathetic ganglion. Can. J. Physiol. *53*, 451–457 (1975)

Khromov-Borisov, N., Michelson, M.J.: The mutual dispositon of locomotor muscles, and the changes in their disposition in the course of development. Pharmacol. Rcv. *18*, 1051–1090 (1966)

Kobayashi, H., Libet, B.: Actions of noradrenaline and acetylcholine on sympathetic ganglion cells. J. Physiol. (Lond.) *208*, 353–372 (1970)

Kobayashi, H., Libet, B.: Is inactivation of potassium conductance involved in slow postsynaptic excitation of sympathetic ganglion cells? Effect of nicotine. Life Sci. *14*, 1871–1883 (1974)

Koelle, G.B.: A proposed dual neurohumoral role of acetylcholine: its functions at the pre- and postsynaptic sites. Nature *190*, 208–211 (1961a)

Koelle, G.B.: A new general concept of the neurohumoral functions of acetylcholine and acetylcholinesterase. J. Pharm. Pharmacol. *14*, 65–90 (1961b)

Koketsu, K.: Action of tetraethylammonium chloride on neuromuscular transmission in frogs. Am J. Physiol. *193*, 213–218 (1958)

Koketsu, K., Cerf, J.A., Nishi, S.: Effect of quaternary ammonium ions on electrical activity of spinal ganglion cells in frogs. J. Neurophysiol. *22*, 177–194 (1959)

Koketsu, K., Nishi, S.: Cholinergic receptors at sympathetic preganglionic nerve terminals. J. Physiol. (Lond.) *196*, 293–310 (1968)

Kordas, M.: The effect of procaine on neuromuscular transmission. J. Physiol. (Lond.) *209*, 689–699 (1970)

Kosterlitz, H.W., Lees, G.M., Wallis, D.I.: Resting and action potentials recorded by the sucrose-gap method in the rabbit superior cervical ganglion. J. Physiol. (Lond.) *195*, 39–53 (1968)

Kosterlitz, H.W., Lees, G.M., Wallis, D.I.: Synaptic potentials recorded by the sucrose-gap method from the rabbit superior cervical ganglion. Br. J. Pharmacol. *40*, 275–293 (1970)

Krnjevic, K., Pumain, R., Renaud, L.: The mechanism of excitation by acetylcholine in the cerebral cortex. J. Physiol. (Lond.) *215*, 247–268 (1971)

Kuba, K., Koketsu, K.: Ionic mechanism of the slow excitatory postsynaptic potential in bullfrog sympathetic ganglion cells. Brain Res. *81*, 338–342 (1974)

Larrabee, M.G., Bronk, D.W.: Prolonged facilitation of synaptic excitation in sympathetic ganglia. J. Neurophysiol. *10*, 139–154 (1947)

Lee, F.-L., Trendelenburg, U.: Muscarinic transmission of preganglionic impulses to the adrenal medulla of the cat. J. Pharmacol. Exp. Ther. *158*, 73–79 (1967)

Lees, G.M., Nishi, S.: Analysis of the mechanism of action of some ganglion-blocking drugs in the rabbit superior cervical ganglion. Br. J. Pharmacol. *46*, 78–88 (1972)

Lees, G.M., Wallis, D.I.: Hyperpolarisation of rabbit superior cervical ganglion cells due to activity of an electrogenic sodium pump. Br. J. Pharmacol. *50*, 79–93 (1974)

Levy, B., Ahlquist, R.P.: A study of sympathetic ganglion stimulants. J. Pharmacol. Exp. Ther. *137*, 219–228 (1962)

Liang, C.C., Quastel, J.H.: Uptake of acetylcholine in rat brain cortex slices. Biochem. Pharmacol. *18*, 1169–1185 (1969a)

Liang, C.C., Quastel, J.H.: Effect of drugs on the uptake of acetylcholine in rat brain cortex slices. Biochem. Pharmacol. *18*, 1187–1194 (1969b)

Long, J.P., Eckstein, J.W.: Ganglionic actions of neostigmine methyl sulphate. J. Pharmacol. Exp. Ther. *133*, 216–222 (1961)

Lundberg, A., Thesleff, S.: Dual action of nicotine on the sympathetic ganglion of the cat. Acta Physiol. Scand. *28*, 218–223 (1953)

Machová, J., Boška, D.: The effect of 5-hydroxytryptamine, dimethylphenyl-piperazinium, and acetylcholine on transmission and surface potential in the cat sympathetic ganglion. Eur. J. Pharmacol. 7, 152–158 (1969)

Magazanik, L.G., Vyskočil, F.: Dependence of acetylcholine desensitisation on the membrane potential of frog muscle fibre and on the ionic changes in the medium. J. Physiol. (Lond.) 210, 507–518 (1970)

Magazanik, L.G., Vyskočil, F.: Desensitisation at the motor end plate. In: Drug receptors. Rang, H.P. (ed.). London: MacMillan 1973

Magazanik, L.G., Ivanov, A.Ya., Lukomskaya, N.Ya.: The effect of snake venom polypeptides on cholinoreceptors in isolated rabbit ganglia. Neurofiziol. 6, 652–656 (1974) (Russ.)

Magleby, K.L., Stevens, C.F.: The effect of voltage on the time course of end plate currents. J. Physiol. (Lond.) 223, 151–171 (1972a)

Magleby, K.L., Stevens, C.F.: A quantitative description of end plate currents. J. Physiol. (Lond.) 223, 173–197 (1972b)

Martin, A.R., Pilar, G.: Dual mode of synaptic transmission in the avian ciliary ganglion. J. Physiol. (Lond.) 168, 443–463 (1963a)

Martin, A.R., Pilar, G.: Transmission through the ciliary ganglion of the chick. J. Physiol. (Lond.) 168, 464–475 (1963b)

Martin, A.R., Pilar, G.: Quantal components of the synaptic potential in the ciliary ganglion of the chick. J. Physiol. (Lond.) 175, 1–16 (1964a)

Martin, A.R., Pilar, G.: Presynaptic and post-synaptic events during post-tetanic potentiation and facilitation in the avian ciliary ganglion. J. Physiol. (Lond.) 175, 17–30 (1964b)

Martin, K.: Concentrative accumulation of choline by human erythrocytes. J. Gen. Physiol. 51, 497–516 (1968)

Martin, K.: Effects of quaternary ammonium compounds on choline transport in red cells. Br. J. Pharmacol. 36, 458–469 (1969)

Marty, A., Neild, T.O., Ascher, P.: Voltage-sensitivity of acetylcholine-currents in Aplysia neurones in the presence of curare. Nature (Lond.) 261, 501–503 (1976)

Mason, D.F.J.: A ganglion stimulating action of neostigmine. Br. J. Pharmacol. 18, 76–86 (1962a)

Mason, D.F.J.: Depolarising action of neostigmine at an autonomic ganglion. Br. J. Pharmacol. 18, 572–587 (1962b)

Matthews, E.K.: The effects of choline and other factors on the release of acetylcholine from the stimulated perfused superior cervical ganglion of the cat. Br. J. Pharmacol. 21, 244–249 (1963)

Matthews, E.K.: The presynaptic effects of quaternary ammonium compounds on the acetylcholine metabolism of a sympathetic ganglion. Br. J. Pharmacol. 26, 552–566 (1966)

Matthews, E.K., Quilliam, J.P.: Effects of central depressant drugs upon acetylcholine release. Br. J. Pharmacol. 22, 415–440 (1964)

Matthews, M.R.: Ultrastructure of ganglionic junctions. In: The peripheral nervous system. Hubbard, J.I. (ed.), pp. 111–150. New York: Plenum Press 1974

McIsaac, R.J.: The relationship between distribution and pharmacological activity of hexamethonium-N-methyl C^{14}. J. Pharmacol. Exp. Ther. 135, 335–343 (1962)

McIsaac, R.J.: The uptake of hexamethonium-C^{14} by kidney slices. J. Pharmacol. Exp. Ther. 150, 92–98 (1965)

McIsaac, R.J., Millerschoen, N.R.: A comparison of the effects of mecamylamine and hexamethonium on transmission in the superior cervical ganglion of the cat. J. Pharmacol. Exp. Ther. 139, 18–24 (1963)

McKinstry, D.N., Koelle, G.B.: Acetylcholine release from the cat superior cervical ganglion by carbachol. J. Pharmacol. Exp. Ther. 157, 319–327 (1967a)

McKinstry, D.N., Koelle, G.B.: Effects of drugs on acetylcholine release from the cat superior cervical ganglion by carbachol and by preganglionic stimulation. J. Pharmacol. Exp. Ther. 157, 328–336 (1967b)

McKinstry, D.N., Koenig, E., Koelle, W.A., Koelle, G.B.: The release of acetylcholine from a sympathetic ganglion by carbachol. Relationship to the functional significance of the localisation of acetylcholinesterase. Can. J. Biochem. Physiol. 41, 2599–2609 (1963)

McLachlan, E.: The formation of synapses in mammalian sympathetic ganglia reinnervated with preganglionic or somatic nerves. J. Physiol. (Lond.) 237, 217–242 (1974)

McLachlan, E.: An analysis of the release of acetylcholine from preganglionic nerve terminals. J. Physiol. (Lond.) 245, 447–466 (1975)

McMahan, U.T., Kuffler, S.W.: Visual identification of synaptic boutons or living ganglion cells and of varicosities in postganglionic axons in the heart of the frog. Proc. R. Soc. Lond. [Biol] 177, 485–508 (1971)

Miledi, R., Potter, L.T.: Acetylcholine receptors in muscle fibres. Nature 233, 599–603 (1971)

Milne, M.D., Rowe, G.G., Somers, K., Muehrcke, R.C., Crawford, M.A.: Observations on the pharmacology of mecamylamine. Clin. Sci. 16, 599–614 (1957)

Miyamoto, M.D., Volle, R.L.: Enhancement by carbachol of transmitter release from motor nerve terminals. Proc. Natl. Acad. Sci. USA 71, 1489–1492 (1974)

Muggleton, D.F., Reading, H.W.: Absorption, metabolism and elimination of pempidine in the rat. Br. J. Pharmacol. 14, 202–208 (1959)

Murayama, S., Unna, K.R.: Stimulant action of 4(-m-chlorophenyl carbomoyloxy)-2-butynyltrimethylammonium chloride (McN-A 343) on sympathetic ganglia. J. Pharmacol. Exp. Ther. 140, 183–192 (1963)

Nishi, S.: Ganglionic transmission. In: The peripheral nervous system. Hubbard, J.I. (ed.), pp. 225–256. New York: Plenum Press 1974

Nishi, S., North, R.A.: Intracellular recording from the myenteric plexus of guinea-pig ileum. J. Physiol. (Lond.) 231, 471–491 (1973)

Nishi, S., Soeda, H., Koketsu, K.: Release of acetylcholine from sympathetic preganglionic nerve terminals. J. Neurophysiol. 30, 114–134 (1967)

Nishi, S., Soeda, H., Koketsu, K.: Unusual nature of ganglionic slow EPSP studied by a voltage-clamp method. Life Sci. 8, 33–42 (1969)

Parkinson, J.: Effect of pempidine on the in vitro synthesis of acetylcholine. Nature 184, 554–555 (1959)

Pascoe, J.E.: The effects of acetylcholine and other drugs on the isolated superior cervical ganglion. J. Physiol. (Lond.) 132, 242–255 (1956)

Paton, W.D.M.: The pharmacology of decamethonium. Ann. N.Y. Acad. Sci. 54, 347–361 (1951)

Paton, W.D.M.: Types of pharmacological action at autonomic ganglia. Arch. Int. Pharmacodyn. 97, 267–281 (1954)

Paton, W.D.M.: A theory of drug action based on the rate of drug-receptor combination. Proc. R. Soc. Lond. [Biol.] 154, 21–69 (1961)

Paton, W.D.M., Perry, W.L.M.: The relationship between depolarisation and block in the cat's superior cervical ganglion. J. Physiol. (Lond.) 119, 43–57 (1953)

Paton, W.D.M., Zaimis, E.J.: The pharmacological actions of polymethylene bistrimethyl-ammonium salts. Br. J. Pharmacol. 4, 381–400 (1949)

Paton, W.D.M., Zaimis, E.J.: Paralysis of autonomic ganglia by methonium salts. Br. J. Pharmacol. 6, 155–168 (1951)

Payne, J.P., Rowe, G.G.: The effects of mecamylamine in the cat as modified by the administration of carbon dioxide. Br. J. Pharmacol. 12, 457–460 (1957)

Perri, V., Sacchi, O., Casella, C.: Electrical properties and synaptic connections of the sympathetic neurons in the rat and guinea-pig superior cervical ganglion. Pflügers Arch. 314, 40–54 (1970a)

Perri, V., Sacchi, O., Casella, C.: Synaptically mediated potentials elecited by the stimulation of post-ganglionic trunks in the guinea-pig superior cervical ganglion. Pflügers Arch. 314, 55–67 (1970b)

Perry, W.L.M.: Acetylcholine release in the cat's superior cervical ganglion. J. Physiol. (Lond.) 119, 439–454 (1953)

Perry, W.L.M., Reinert, H.: The effects of preganglionic denervation on the reactions of ganglion cells. J. Physiol. (Lond.) 126, 101–115 (1954)

Perry, W.L.M., Reinert, H.: On the metabolism of normal and denervated sympathetic ganglion cells. J. Physiol. (Lond.) 130, 156–166 (1955)

Pert, C.B., Snyder, S.H.: High affinity transport of choline into the myenteric plexus of guinea-pig intestine. J. Pharmacol. Exp. Ther. 191, 102–108 (1974)

Peters, L.: Renal tubular excretion of organic bases. Pharmacol. Rev. 12, 1–35 (1960)

Pilar, G.: Effect of ACh on pre- and postsynaptic elements of avian ciliary ganglion synapses. Fed. Proc. 28, 670 (1969)

Polak, R.L.: The influence of drugs on the uptake of acetylcholine by slices of rat cerebral cortex. Br. J. Pharmacol. *36*, 144–152 (1969)

Putney, J.W., Jr., Borzelleca, J.F.: On the mechanisms of ^{14}C-nicotine distribution in rat submaxillary gland in vitro. J. Pharmacol. Exp. Ther. *178*, 180–191 (1971)

Quilliam, J.P., Shand, D.G.: The selectivity of drugs blocking ganglionic transmission in the rat. Br. J. Pharmacol. *23*, 273–284 (1964)

Rang, H.P.: Acetylcholine receptors. Q. Rev. Biophys. 7, 283–400 (1974)

Rang, H.P., Ritter, J.M.: A new kind of drug antagonism: evidence that agonists cause a mulecular change in acetylcholine receptors. Mol. Pharmacol. *5*, 394–411 (1969)

Rang, H.P., Ritter, J.M.: On the mechanism of desensitisation at cholinergic receptors. Mol. Pharmacol. *6*, 357–382 (1970)

Rang, H.P., Ritter, J.M.: The effect of disulfide bond reduction on the properties of cholinergic receptors in chick muscle. Mol. Pharmacol. *7*, 620–631 (1971)

Riker, W.K.: Effects of tetraethylammonium chloride on electrical activities of frog sympathetic ganglion cells. J. Pharmacol. Exp. Ther. *145*, 317–325 (1964)

Riker, W.K.: Effects of tetraethylammonium on synaptic transmission in the frog sympathetic ganglion. J. Pharmacol. Exp. Ther. *147*, 161–171 (1965)

Riker, W.K.: The basis of the low-amplitude discharge produced by acetylcholine injection in sympathetic ganglia. J. Pharmacol. Exp. Ther. *155*, 203–210 (1967)

Riker, W.K.: Ganglion cell depolarisation and transmission block by ACh: independent events. J. Pharmacol. Exp. Ther. *159*, 345–352 (1968)

Riker, W.K., Komalahiranya, A.: Observations on the frequency dependence of sympathetic ganglion blockade. J. Pharmacol. Exp. Ther. *137*, 267–274 (1962)

Roszkowski, A.P.: An unusual type of sympathetic ganglion stimulant. J. Pharmacol. Exp. Ther. · *132*, 156–170 (1961)

Sacchi, O., Perri, V.: Quantal mechanism of transmitter release during progressive depletion of the presynaptic stores at a ganglionic synapse. J. Gen. Physiol. *61*, 342–360 (1973)

Schild, H.O.: Non-competitive drug antagonism. J. Physiol. (Lond.) *124*, 33–34 P (1954)

Schuberth, J., Sundwall, A.: Effects of some drugs on the uptake of acetylcholine in cortex slices of mouse brain. J. Neurochem. *14*, 807–812 (1967)

Shand, D.G.: The mode of action of drugs blocking ganglionic transmission in the rat. Br. J. Pharmacol. *24*, 89–97 (1965)

Skok, V.I.: Physiology of autonomic ganglia. Tokyo: Igaku Shoin 1973

Steinbach, A.B.: Alteraction by xylocaine (lidocaine) and its derivatives of the time-course of the end plate potential. J. Gen. Physiol. *52*, 144–161 (1968)

Steinberg, M.I., Volle, R.L.: A comparison of lobeline and nicotine at the frog neuromuscular junction. Naunyn Schmiedebergs Arch. Pharmacol. *272*, 16–31 (1972)

Stephenson, R.P.: A modification of receptor theory. Br. J. Pharmacol. *11*, 379–393 (1956)

Stoney, S.D., Machne, X.: Mechanisms of accommodation in different types of frog neurones. J. Gen. Physiol. *53*, 248–262 (1969)

Stovner, J.: Anti-curare affect of TEA. Acta Pharmacol. Toxicol. (Kbh.) *14*, 317–332 (1958)

Suszkiw, J.B., Beach, R.L., Pilar, G.R.: Choline uptake by cholinergic neuron cell somas. J. Neurochem. *26*, 1123–1131 (1976)

Takeshige, C., Volle, R.L.: Cholinoceptive sites in sympathetic ganglia. J. Pharmacol. Exp. Ther. *141*, 206–213 (1963 a)

Takeshige, C., Volle, R.L.: Asynchronous postganglionic firing from the cat superior cervical sympathetic ganglion treated with neostigmine. Br. J. Pharmacol. *20*, 214–220 (1963 b)

Takeshige, C., Pappano, A.J., DeGroat, W.C., Volle, R.L.: Ganglionic blockade produced in sympathetic ganglia by cholinomimetic drugs. J. Pharmacol. Exp. Ther. *141*, 333–342 (1963)

Tamarind, D.L., Quilliam, J.P.: Synaptic organisation and other ultrastructural features of the superior cervical ganglion of the rat, kitten and rabbit. Micron 2, 204–234 (1971)

Tasaki, I., Hagiwara, S.: Demonstration of two stable potential states in the squid giant axon under tetraethylammonium chloride. J. Gen. Physiol. *40*, 859–885 (1957)

Taylor, D.B., Creese, R., Scholes, N.W.: Effect of curare concentration, temperature and potassium ion concentration on the rate of uptake of a neuromuscular blocking agent labelled with radioactive iodine. J. Pharmacol. Exp. Ther. *144*, 293–300 (1964)

Taylor, D.B., Creese, R., Nedergaard, O.A., Case, R.: Labelled depolarising drugs in normal and denervated muscle. Nature 208, 901–902 (1965)

Taylor, D.B., Dixon, W.J., Creese, R., Case, R.: Diffusion of decamethonium in the rat. Nature 215, 989 (1967)

Taylor, D.B., Lu, T.C., Creese, R., Steinborn, J.: The uptake of methonium compounds by isolated slices of rat cerebral cortex. J. Neurochem. 16, 1173–1184 (1969)

Taxi, J.: Contribution à l'étude des connexions des neurones moteurs du systeme nerveux autonome. Ann. Sci. Nat. Zool. (12ᵉ series,) 7, 413–674 (1965)

Thesleff, S.: The mode of neuromuscular block caused by acetylcholine, nicotine, decamethonium and succinylcholine. Acta Physiol. Scand. 34, 218–231 (1955)

Traber, D.L., Carter, V.L., Jr., Gardier, R.W.: Regarding a necessary condition for ganglionic blockade with competitive agents. Arch. Int. Pharmacodyn. 168, 339–343 (1967)

Trendelenburg, U.: Reaktion sympathischer Ganglien während der Ganglienblockade durch Nicotin. Arch. Exp. Pathol. Pharmakol. 230, 448–456 (1957)

Trendelenburg, U.: Non-nicotinic ganglion-stimulating substances. Fed. Proc. 18, 1001–1005 (1959)

Trendelenburg, U.: Observations on the mode of action of some non-depolarising ganglion-blocking substances. Naunyn Schmiedebergs Arch. Exp. Pathol. Pharmacol. 241, 452–466 (1961)

Trendelenburg, U.: Transmission of preganglionic impulses through the muscarinic receptors of the superior cervical ganglion of the cat. J. Pharmacol. Exp. Ther. 154, 426–440 (1966)

Trendelenburg, U.: Some aspects of the pharmacology of autonomic ganglion cells. Ergebn. Physiol. 59, 1–83 (1967)

Van Rossum, J.M.: Classification and molecular pharmacology of ganglionic blocking agents. Part I. Mechanisms of ganglionic synaptic transmission and mode of action of ganglionic stimulants. Int. J. Neuropharmacol. 1, 97–110 (1962a)

Van Rossum, J.M.: Classification and molecular pharmacology of ganglionic blocking agents. Part II. Mode of action of competitive and non-competitive ganglion blocking agents. Int. J. Neuropharmacol. 1, 403–421 (1962b)

Volle, R.L.: Modification by drugs of synaptic mechanisms in autonomic ganglia. Pharmacol. Rev. 18, 839–869 (1966a)

Volle, R.L.: Ganglion blocking and stimulating agents. I. Muscarinic and nicotinic actions at autonomic ganglia. Oxford: Pergamon 1966b

Volle, R.L.: Ganglionic transmission. Annu. Rev. Pharmacol. 9, 135–146 (1969)

Volle, R.L., Koelle, G.B.: The physiological role of acetylcholinesterase in sympathetic ganglia. J. Pharmacol. Exp. Ther. 133, 223–240 (1961)

Volle, R.L., Reynolds, L.: Receptor desensitisation by lobeline and nicotine. Naunyn Schmiedebergs Arch. Pharmacol. 276, 49–54 (1973)

Wang, C.M., Narahashi, T.: Mechanisms of dual action of nicotine on end plate membranes. J. Pharmacol. Exp. Ther. 182, 427–441 (1972)

Weight, F., Votava, J.: Slow synaptic excitation in sympathetic ganglion cells: evidence for synaptic inactivation of potassium conductance. Science 170, 755–758 (1970)

Weiss, G.B.: Dependence of nicotine-C^{14} distribution and movements upon pH in frog sartorius muscle. J. Pharmacol. Exp. Ther. 160, 135–147 (1968)

Weiss, G.B., Alderdice, M.T.: Characterisation of [^{14}C]-nicotine accumulation and movements in slices from different rat brain areas. Neuropharmacology 14, 265–273 (1975)

Winters, A.D., Volle, R.L.: Relationship between frequency of stimulation and ganglionic blockade by drugs. Eur. J. Pharmacol. 2, 347–354 (1968)

Woodward, J.K., Bianchi, C.P., Erulkar, S.D.: Electrolyte distribution in rabbit superior cervical ganglion. J. Neurochem. 16, 289–299 (1969)

Yamamura, H.I., Snyder, S.H.: High affinity transport of choline into synaptosomes of rat brain. J. Neurochem. 21, 1355–1374 (1973)

Zaimis, E.J.: Actions at autonomic ganglia. In: Cholinesterase and anticholinesterase agents. Koelle, G.B. (ed.), pp. 530–569. Berlin: Springer 1963

CHAPTER 6

Action of Ganglion-Blocking Agents on the Cardiovascular System

D.M. AVIADO

A. Introduction

Until 15 years ago, the ganglion-blocking drugs were the most widely used drugs in the treatment of cardiovascular diseases. The haemodynamic action, consisting of hypotension and vasodilation, is highly desirable in the treatment of diseases such as essential hypertension, peripheral arterial insufficiency, pulmonary hypertension and pulmonary oedema.

At present in some countries, the ganglion-blocking drugs have been displaced by drugs developed in recent years, particularly the adrenergic neurone blockers and the beta-blockers or both, for essential hypertension. A retrospective review of the literature indicates that from the pharmacological standpoint, it has been premature to discard the ganglion-blocking drugs in favour of the recent selective blocking drugs. The adrenergic neurone blockers have to be supplemented with diuretics, and the accompanying cardiac stimulation has to be controlled by supplementary use of beta-blockers. In this era of awareness to the hazards of multiple drugs prescribed for patients, it is reasonable to question whether there should be a revival of ganglion-blocking drugs used alone in therapeutics. The hypotensive action of ganglion-blocking drugs is not accompanied by an increase in cardiac function of the intensity seen with adrenergic neurone blockers. Furthermore, the diuretic action of ganglion-blocking drugs would not necessitate the supplemental use of diuretics in all patients.

Another significant development in the field of ganglionic transmission is the identification of non-nicotinic receptors and drugs that are blocked by atropine. Although there has been persistent argument as to the physiological role of these receptors, it should be recalled that the pressor response to increased intracranial pressure involves both nicotinic and non-nicotinic receptors. However, the current search for the physiological significance has not pursued the original line, in which elevation of intracranial pressure was used as a pressor stimulus.

The purpose of this chapter is to recall the results of investigation on the cardio-vascular effects of ganglion-blocking drugs as they relate to the above-mentioned concepts, and to supply the basis for the continued therapeutic use of these drugs.

B. Hypotensive Action

The most conspicuous haemodynamic effect of the administration of ganglion-blocking drugs is the reduction in systemic arterial blood pressure. The hypotension is elicited in the treatment of essential hypertension or pulmonary oedema and for surgical operations. Experimental laboratory work has yielded observations that characterise the nature of the hypotensive action, specifically the influence on the hypotension of nervous mechanisms, humoral substances, and drugs.

I. Cardiovascular Reflexes and the Central Nervous System

Theoretically, ganglion blockade induced by drugs would be expected to result in complete isolation of the heart and blood vessels from central nervous and reflex control. Examination of the results of experiments indicates that this premise is not strictly accurate. STEINBERG and HILTON (1966a,b, 1967) and HILTON and STEINBERG (1966) reported that chlorisondamine did not completely block the pressor response to increased intracranial pressure and to occlusion of the common carotids to inactivate the baroreceptors in the carotid sinuses. The pressor response persisting after the injection of ganglion-blocking drugs was subsequently eliminated by the injection of atropine, presumably because the sympathetic outflow involving the non-nicotinic receptors was interrupted. PEDERSOLI (1970) has confirmed the ineffectiveness of hexamethonium alone and the necessity of injecting atropine to block the pressor effect of electrical stimulation of the central end of the vagus nerve. On the other hand, FADHEL and SEAGER (1969) were successful in blocking the pressor response by the application of a stimulus and drugs different from those used by the above-mentioned investigators. When veratrine was given by intracisternal injection, the resulting pressor response was blocked by doses of trimethaphan high enough to produce a severe depression of blood pressure. In the same investigation, FADHEL and SEAGER reported the incomplete blockade of the pressor response by intravenous injection of hexamethonium, thus showing a difference in effectiveness between two ganglion-blocking drugs. There has been no subsequent report comparing the completeness of blockade with trimethaphan to that obtained with other pressor-producing procedures, probably because of the limited interpretation possible from measurements of arterial blood pressure alone. Since arterial blood pressure is influenced by total systemic vascular resistance and cardiac output, the effectiveness of blockade by drugs may vary between the blood vessels and the heart.

II. Circulating Humoral Agents and Injected Drugs

Theoretically, ganglion blockade by drugs would also be expected to result in modulation of the pressor responses to injected drugs. More specifically, the injection of a vasoconstricting drug that elevates the arterial blood pressure would be expected to initiate reflex bradycardia and vasodilation through the carotid sinus and aortic arch baroreceptors: blockade of the autonomic ganglia would interrupt the reflexes so that the pressor effect of a vasoconstricting drug would be exaggerated. This expectation has been proved to be true following the intravenous injection of norepinephrine. However, the potentiation of the pressor response after hexamethonium is not only caused by the interruption of baroreceptor reflexes. EBLE et al. (1973), using the perfused leg of dog and blood-bathed organs for bioassay, reported that hexamethonium resulted in a delay in the inactivation of circulating norepinephrine. VANEVSKY and AZAROV (1973) observed an enhancement of the sensitivity of the mesoappendix blood vessels to norepinephrine and angiotensin following the administration of pentamine in rats. The potentiation of the pressor response also includes the direct response of the vascular smooth muscle to humoral vasoconstrictors, whether cathecholamine or polypeptide in structure.

The hypotensive action of ganglion-blocking drugs interacts with pressor drugs that stimulate the autonomic ganglia. The classic pressor agent is nicotine; one recent example is etoxadrol, a new dissociative anaesthetic with a pressor response that is blocked by hexamethonium (TRABER et al., 1973).

C. Cardiac Function

Like most other hypotensive drugs, ganglion-blocking drugs cause tachycardia when given by intravenous injection. However, the tachycardia characteristic of ganglion blockade, as against that caused by other hypotensive agents, is accompanied by varied effects on cardiac output, ventricular function, and coronary circulation.

I. Cardiac Output

The reported effects of intravenous injections of ganglion-blocking drugs on cardiac output are summarised in Table 1. There is a conspicuous reduction in systemic arterial blood pressure in several groups of subjects: normotensive and hypertensive patients and subjects with decompensated heart disease, cardiac asthma, mitral stenosis, pulmonary hypertension, and peripheral vascular disease, and those under general anaesthesia. The concomitant effects on cardiac output are variable.

1. Decreased Cardiac Output

The most usual response to ganglion-blocking agents is a significant reduction in cardiac output. It has not been possible to identify the cause of this reduction in cardiac output in man, but experiments in animals have suggested that the ultimate cause is a primary reduction in venous return brought about by pooling of blood in the dilated peripheral vessels. TRAPOLD (1956) was able to control cardiac output in anaesthetised dogs, and noted that hexamethonium, chlorisondamine and pentolinium decreased the return of blood from both venae cavae. A direct depression of the heart muscle can be excluded by the results from isolated heart experiments (LEE and SHIDEMAN, 1958). In the innervated heart, the change in the heart rate resulting from ganglion blockade will depend on whether the vagal or the sympathetic cardiac innervation is dominant prior to blockade. Since, in man, the heart is predominantly under vagal control, tachycardia with a reduction in stroke volume is the usual haemodynamic accompaniment of reduction in cardiac output.

2. Increased Cardiac Output

The patients who showed an increase in cardiac output as a result of ganglion-blocking drugs were those suffering from congestive heart failure, mitral stenosis, or cardiac asthma. Patients who had peripheral vascular disease without heart failure responded with an increase in output as measured by ballistocardiography, but confirmation by the Fick method is necessary in such patients. FREIS and his collaborators (1953) have explained the increase in cardiac output in patients with decom-

Table 1. Ganglion-blocking drugs and cardiac output

Drug (dose)	Clinical status (number of subjects)	Systemic art. BP %Δ	Cardiac output[a]	Systemic vasc. resist.	Ref.
Tetraethylammonium bromide or chloride (IV 2–6 mg/kg)	Normotensive (14)	−10	+ or −	−	FOWLER et al. (1950)
	Hypertensive (4)	−	−23	−	FRISK et al. (1948)
	Cardiopulm. dis. (10)	−	−32	−	FOWLER et al. (1950)
	Left heart failure (5)	−21	0	−28	HALMAGYI et al. (1953)
	Mitral stenosis (5)	−5	+12	−27	HALMAGYI et al. (1953)
	Mitral stenosis (6)	−	+ or −	+ or −	SCOTT et al. (1955)
	Peripheral vasc. dis. (11)	−5	+35 (BCG)	−	HORWITZ et al. (1949)
Hexamethonium bromide or chloride (IV 0.2–1 mg/kg)	Normotensive (10)	−20	+ or −	−17	RAKITA and SANCETTA (1953)
	Normotensive, anaesthetised (12)	−33	−15 (DYE)	−20	VAN BERGEN (1955)
	Hypertensive (5)	−25	−46	−60	GROB et al. (1953)
	Hypertensive (4)	−35	−10	−30	VARNAUSKAS (1955)
	Hypertensive, compensated (6)	−24	−22	0	FREIS et al. (1953)
	Hypertensive, decompensated (4)	−	+38	−47	FREIS et al. (1953)
	Pulmonary hypertensive (8)	−27	−16	−12	SANCETTA (1955)
	Mitral stenosis (19)	−	0	−32	SANCETTA (1957)
	Mitral stenosis (11)	−28	+ or −	−21	BALCHUM et al. (1957)
	Cardiac asthmas (21)	−	+44	−29	VINOGRADOV and TEIBERMAKHER (1966)
Penthamethonium bromide (IV 0.3–7 mg/kg)	Normotensive, anesthetised (6)	−	−53	−	SHACKMAN et al. (1952)
	Peripheral vasc. dis. (16)	−11	+29 (BCG)	−	NEEDLEMAN and HORWITZ (1953)
Pentolinium tartrate IV 0.03–0.04 mg/kg	Hypertensive (9)	−16	−21	0	CROSLEY et al. (1956)
	Hypertensive (5)	−36	−19	−20	SMITH et al. (1955)
Azamethonium bromide (IV 0.6–1.4 mg/kg)	Peripheral vasc. dis. (10)	−8	+23 (BCG)	−	NEEDLEMAN and HORWITZ (1953)
Trimethaphan camphor sulphonate (0.35–1.25 mg/min)	Normotensive pregnant (5)	−38	−19 (BCG)	−22	ASSALI et al. (1953)
	Hypertensive pregnant (3)	−33	−18 (BCG)	−22	ASSALI et al. (1953)
	Compensated (5)	−23	−17	−4	SOBOL et al. (1959)
	Decompensated (10)	−22	+17	−35	SOBOL et al. (1959)

[a] The percentage change represents the average value for the specified number of cases as measured by the Fick principle, expect in those lines indicated by: BCG=ballistocardiography, or DYE = dye dilution technique. The absence of figures for this column and the other columns is substituted by the directional change: (+) increased; (−) decreased; (0) unchanged.

pensated hearts in the following manner: The peripheral pooling of blood induced by ganglion-blocking agents would act like a venesection, reducing the loading pressure of the heart and thereby facilitating the recovery of the failing heart. In addition to this, the fall in aortic pressure would allow more complete emptying of the failing left ventricle. These proposed explanations depending on extracardiac mechanisms are plausible, but there is good evidence that the hypodynamic heart-lung preparation (dog) and the hypodynamic papillary muscle (cat) are stimulated directly by hexamethonium (LEE and SHIDEMAN, 1958). Such a positive inotropic action may contribute to the increase in cardiac output, but this can only be proved by direct coronary arterial injections in a dog with experimental cardiac failure. VINOGRADOV and TSIBERMAKLER (1966) have applied Starling's law to the heart in order give some insight into the increase in cardiac output after hexamethonium in the patient with heart disease. The reduction in ventricular after-load protects the infarcted heart on the basis of measurements of serum creatine phosphokinase in patients (SHELL and SOBEL, 1974) and histological changes in the rabbit with micro-focal cardiac necrosis (POKK, 1972).

II. Coronary Vascular Resistance

The available information on the human coronary circulation is limited to patients suffering from hypertension. GROB and his collaborators (1953) used the nitrous oxide method and observed the following after the administration of hexamethonium: The first patient manifested a reduction in coronary blood flow (-15%); the second patient had unchanged coronary blood flow but still showed a reduction in coronary vascular resistance (-40%). A more extensive study by CRUMPTON and his collaborators (1954), using hexamethonium in 16 normotensive and 7 renally hypertensive dogs, showed a marked reduction in coronary blood flow without a reduction in coronary vascular resistance. Cardiac work was also decreased, but myocardial oxygen consumption remained unchanged, so that cardiac efficiency was reduced. It is not possible to explain why this group of anaesthetised dogs did not show a reduction in coronary vascular resistance, whereas the two patients unanaesthetised) showed a reduction following hexamethonium. If additional studies reveal that the more consistent response is a reduction in coronary vascular resistance following hexamethonium, it will be admissible to conclude that the sympathetic nervous system can maintain some coronary vasomotor tone in some patients with hypertension.

D. Systemic Vascular Beds

Although ganglion-blocking drugs cause either a decrease or an increase in cardiac output, there is a consistent fall in systemic arterial pressure and also a fall in systemic vascular resistance. When both cardiac output and vascular resistance are reduced in the same patient, the latter is the more important cause of the hypotension. Most studies summarised in Table 1 show that the percentage reduction in vascular resistance is more intense than the percentage reduction in cardiac output. The percentage reduction in vascular resistance is probably an underestimation of the vascular effects of drugs because a reduction in cardiac output alone in anaesthetised dogs causes a passive increase in systemic vascular resistance (GREEN and KEPCHAR, 1959). TRAPOLD (1957) estimated that in dog the reduction in systemic arterial pressure produced by hexamethonium and chlorisondamine is dependent primarily (approximately 70%) upon a reduction in vascular resistance, and secondarily (30%) upon a reduction in venous return or cardiac output. The participation of the various vascular beds (other than the coronary) in bringing about a reduction in total systemic vascular resistance is considered below.

I. Cerebral Circulation

The most uniform result following the administration of hypotensive doses of any one of four ganglion-blocking drugs is a reduction in cerebral vascular resistance (Table 2). There is no information available on the effects of mecamylamine, pentolinium, pentamethonium and chlorisondamine, but there is no reason to suspect that these four agents will not induce the same cerebral haemodynamic pattern as the others. Almost all reports (except two) show a reduction in cerebral blood flow, but this is proportionately less than the reduction expected from a fall in systemic blood pressure alone. The ultimate cause of the reduction in cerebral vascular resistance is believed to be a local compensatory mechanism rather than a blockade of autonomic vasoconstrictor impulses. The basis for this explanation is that the human cerebral vessels do not appear to be controlled by the autonomic nervous system as much as by local changes in the blood tensions of oxygen and carbon dioxide. This local mechanism, causing cerebral vasodilation when pressure falls, is unique for vascular beds; the mechanism in other beds is just the opposite. Patients with hypertension and with symptoms of cerebral insufficiency are reported to behave in a similar manner to normotensive patients, with one exception. FINNERTY et al. (1954, 1957) noted that after the intravenous injection of hexamethonium and head up-tilting, patients may lose consciousness. The level of systemic arterial blood pressure at which consciousness was lost varied between 29 and 89 mm Hg, depending on the degree of vascular disease. Hypertensive patients fainted at a higher level of blood pressure than normotensive subjects, but in all cases consciousness was lost at about the same level of cerebral blood flow, i.e., at approximately 30–35 ml/100 g brain tissue/min. Reduction below this level of blood flow was explained by a reduction in cardiac output.

In dogs kept in a controlled state of hypotension induced by trimethaphan, there is a reduction in cortical blood flow measured by the thermal diffusion technique (CARTER and ATKINSON, 1973) or by means of a flow probe placed around the common carotids (MAGNESS et al., 1973). There is also a reduction in the height of the electrocortigram, representing a reduction of cerebral function. Unfortunately, these experiments were not extended to include recovery from trimethaphan.

II. Renal Circulation

The results obtained with five drugs are summarised in Table 3. There are no studies on human subjects with pentolinium, chlorisondamine, or mecamylamine, but studies in anaesthetised dogs show that the last two drugs cause a reduction in renal

Table 2. Ganglion-blocking drugs and cerebral circulation

Drug	Clinical status (number of subjects)	Cerebral blood flow[a] (C) %Δ	Cerebral vasc. resist.	Cerebral O$_2$ utilisation	Ref.
Tetraethylammonium chloride	Hypertensive (12)	(39) − 15	(3.8) − 36	(2.3) + 4	BESSMAN et al. (1952)
Hexamethonium bromide or chloride	Normotensive (9)	(57) − 30	(1.9) − 11	(3.2) − 12	MORRIS et al. (1953)
	Normotensive, young (7)	(46) − 33	(1.9) − 37	(2.8) + 4	FINNERTY et al. (1954)
	Normotensive, elderly (10)	(48) − 39	(1.7) − 31	(2.7) 0	FINNERTY et al. (1954)
	Normotensive (8)	(57) − 26	(1.8) − 17	(3.2) − 9	MOYER and MORRIS (1954)
	Normotensive, head up (10)	(53) − 11	(2.4) − 45	(3.3) + 3	STONE et al. (1955)
	Hypertensive, head up (9)	(50) − 40	(3.2) − 39		FINNERTY et al. (1957)
	Hypertensive, benign (8)	(48) − 39	(2.4) − 33	(2.8) − 4	FINNERTY et al. (1954)
	Hypertensive, malignant (7)	(60) − 42	(3.0) − 17	(3.5) − 11	FINNERTY et al. (1954)
	Hypertensive (13)	(55) − 16	(3.5) − 28	(3.6) − 3	CRUMPTON et al. (1955)
	Hypertensive (6)	(50) − 4	(3.2) − 27	(3.5) − 0	DEWAR et al. (1953)
	Cerebral insufficiency (5)	(35) + 6	(4.8) − 42	(2.3) +26	KLEH and FAZEKAS (1956)
Azemethonium bromide	Normotensive (5)	(51) − 8	(2.0) − 35	(2.8) + 7	MOYER and MORRIS (1954)
	Normotensive (9)	(53) +12	(1.5) − 20	(3.2) +10	BERNSMEIER and SIEMONS (1953)
Trimethaphan camphor sulphonate	Normotensive (6)	(52) − 32	(2.0) − 15	(3.1) − 10	MOYER and MORRIS (1954)
	Normotensive (5)	(50) − 6	(2.1) − 33	(2.9) 0	FAZEKAS et al. (1956)
	Hypertensive, moderate (4)	(57) − 12	(2.7) − 41	(3.0) + 3	FAZEKAS et al. (1956)
	Hypertensive, malignant (9)	(65) − 10	(3.0) − 37	(3.6) − 6	FAZEKAS et al. (1956)
	Renal-cerebral insuff. (12)	(49) − 2	(3.2) − 37	(2.7) 0	PARRISH et al. (1957)

[a] Cerebral blood flow is measured by the nitrous oxide method of KETY and SCHMIDT. For this and the other columns: (C) represents the average of control values for the specified number of subjects in the following units: Blood flow 2 ml/100 g/min; oxygen utilisation = ml/g100 g/min. The vascular resistance is expressed in terms of ratio of mean arterial blood pressure to cerebral blood flow value.

Table 3. Ganglion-blocking drugs and renal circulation

Drug	Clinical status (number of subjects)	Renal BF[a] %Δ	Renal vasc. resist.	Ref.
Tetraethylammonium bromide or chloride	Normotensive (8)	—	+	Aas and Blegen (1949)
Hexamethonium bromide or chloride	Normotensive (18) (Im)	−21	+10	Moyer et al. (1955)
	Normotensive (18) (Del)	−10	−30	Moyer et al. (1955)
	Hypertensive (5) −59	−59		Grob et al. (1953)
	Hypertensive (8)	−12		Redisch et al. (1954)
	Hypertensive (7)	+15		Ford et al. (1953)
	Hypertensive (10)	+ or −	−	Ullman and Diengott (1953)
	Decompensate (12)	+ or −	−	Ullman and Menczel (1956)
Pentamethonium bromide	Normotensive (2)	−18	+17	Mackinnon (1952)
	Hypertensive (6)	−27	+21	Mackinnon (1952)
	Anesthetised (10)	− 5	−	Miles et al. (1952)
Azamethonium bromide	Normotensive (9) (Im)	−15	+50	Moyer et al. (1955)
	Normotensive (9) (Del)	− 8	−12	Moyer et al. (1955)
Trimethaphan camphor sulphonate	Normotensive (9) (Im)	−32	+10	Moyer et al. (1955)
	Normotensive (9) (Del)	−55	+60	Moyer et al. (1955)
	Hypertensive (8)	−14	+ 4	Moyer et al. (1955)
	Renal insufficiency (12)	− 1	−	Parrish et al. (1957)

[a] The percentage change in real blood flow represents the average value for the specified number of cases as measured by the PAH clearance method. The absence of figures for this and the next column is substituted by directional change; (+) increased; (−) decreased. (Im) 10 min after injection; (Del): 1–2 h after injection.

blood flow (MOYER et al., 1955; PLUMMER et al., 1955). A reduction in renal blood flow by the other drugs has been reported in normotensive and hypertensive patients, but this was not a consistent finding. Some patients showed an increase in renal blood flow in spite of a reduction in blood pressure, indicating that renal vascular resistance was reduced. The patients who responded to ganglion blockade with a reduction in blood flow showed either a decrease or an increase in vascular resistance. MOYER and HANDLEY (1955) and MOYER et al. (1955) noted that hexamethonium, azamethonium or trimethaphan caused an initial increase in renal vascular resistance, followed by a prolonged decrease. The former coincided with the period of lowest blood pressure and was probably a passive response to this fall, i.e., the response differed from that of the cerebral bed. The delayed reduction in vascular resistance may be a manifestation of paralysis of sympathetic vasoconstrictor impulses to the renal vessels, but it is difficult to explain why its onset is delayed since these drugs are known to have an immediate onset of action. The immediate passive vasoconstriction is presumably transient.

In the anaesthetised dog, intravenous injection of trimethaphan caused a reduction in renal vascularity, as revealed by angiography (ELKIN and MENG, 1969). Pentolinium has been used as a tool to investigate the renal responses in animals following blockade of the autonomic nervous system. In the dog with experimental ascites induced by constriction of the inferior vena cava, pentolinium increased the excretion of sodium (FRANKO et al., 1963). In exercising rats, the accompanying elevation in plasma renin levels was reduced by the administration of pentolinium (BOZOVIC and CASTENFORS, 1967). These effects are desirable in the treatment of essential hypertension accompanied by renal problems. It is possible that these effects are unique for ganglion-blocking drugs and are not exerted by the new forms of adrenergic-blocking drugs that are currently used in the treatment of hypertension.

III. Pulmonary Circulation

The variability in the response of the pulmonary arterial mean pressure following intravenous injection of four ganglion-blocking agents is summarised in Table 4. There are no reports on the effects of chlorisondamine, mecamylamine, pentamethonium, and azamethonium. There are three explanations for the variability in response of pulmonary arterial pressure, namely:

1. A *rise or fall in cardiac output* may follow the administration of this group of drugs, and this may account for the rise and fall respectively of the pulmonary arterial pressure. There are several instances, indicated in Table 4, in which a fall in arterial pressure may occur in spite of a rise or no change in flow. This is an indication that alterations in blood flow cannot completely explain all the observed changes in pressure.

2. An *improvement in the performance of a failing left ventricle* has been described following ganglion blockade (see above). This has actually been verified in man by an observed reduction in pulmonary arterial wedged pressure, a measurement that has been regarded by many as a reasonable estimate of left atrial pressure. This reduction in pressure may account for some of the fall in arterial pressure, but the pressure

Table 4. Ganglion-blocking drugs and pulmonary circulation

Drug	Clinical status (number of subjects)	Pulm. art. BP %Δ	Pulm. BF	Total pulm. vasc. resist.[a]	Arteriolar vasc. resist.	Ref.
Tetraethylammonium bromide or chloride	Normotensive (9)	+ or –	+ or –	+ or –	+ or –	Fowler et al. (1950)
	Hypertensive (9)	–30	–23	–13		Frisk et al. (1948)
	Mitral stenosis (6)	P or –	+ or –	+ or –	+ or –	Scott et al. (1955)
	Mitral stenosis (5)	–26	+12	–35		Halmagy et al. (1953)
Hexamethonium bromide or chloride	Normotensive (10)	–	+ or –	+ or –		Rakita and Sancetta (1953)
	Hypertensive (6)	+ or –	0		+ or –	Werko et al. (1951)
	Hypertensive (4)	–	–10			Varnauskas (1955)
	Mitral stenosis (13)	–50	+ or –	–20	–36	Balchum et al. (1957)
	Mitral stenosis (19)	–18	0	–32	–14	Yu et al. (1958)
	Pulm. hypertensive (5)	–10	0		–5	Sancetta (1955)
	Pulm. hypertensive (4)	–30	+ or –	+ or –		Wilson and Keeley (1953)
	Heart disease (14)	–	–	0	0	Storstein and Tveten (1954)
Pentolinium tartrate	Hypertensive (9)	–20	–21	– 3		Crosley et al. (1956)
Trimethaphan camphor sulphonate	Hypertensive (7)	–	+ or –	+ or –		Eichna et al. (1956)

[a] The %Δ in total pulmonary vascular resistance is indicated as the average value for the specified number of cases by dividing the mean pulmonary arterial pressure by the pulmonary blood flow (cardiac output). The arterial vascular resistance uses the pressure gradient between artery and wedged artery pressures. Directional changes are represented as: (+) increased; (–) decreased; (0) unchanged.

gradient between the artery and the wedged artery is still reduced so that an actual reduction in pulmonary arterial resistance must be considered.

3. *Reduction in arterial resistance* caused by the blockade of sympathetic vaso-constrictors is a reasonable suggestion based on numerous reports that sympathetic nerves are capable of causing vasoconstriction of the pulmonary arteries (see references cited by AVIADO, 1965). Most of the reports deal with perfusion experiments of dog lungs, which also show that most ganglion-blocking drugs do not have any local dilator action independent of their blocking action. More recently, LANDYSHEVA et al. (1972) have used the inhalation route of administration for ganglion-blocking drugs to differentiate between organic and reversible components of pulmonary hypertension. This suggestion is a novel one and needs to be further investigated because the existing tests used for diagnosis are unsatisfactory.

IV. Splanchnic Circulation

There are only two studies on the splanchnic circulation in man, and both are limited to the effects of hexamethonium. Application of the bromsulphalein hepatic clearance method indicated that hepatic blood flow in 17 normotensive (REYNOLDS et al., 1953) and 6 hypertensive subjects (FREIS et al., 1953) is reduced by about 30%, proportionate to the reduction in systemic arterial pressure. The canine mesenteric vessels have been perfused by TRAPOLD (1956) with the following results: hexamethonium, pentolinium or chlorisondamine caused a definite decrease in vascular resistance, presumably by paralysing autonomic vasoconstrictor impulses. Without perfusion, the calculated resistance was either decreased or unchanged because of the passive effect of reduced pressure (increase of resistance, as in the kidney), causing the decrease in resistance initiated by blockade of vasoconstrictors.

The result is a reduction in portal venous pressure detected in patients with portal hypertension treated with trimethaphan (CINCOTTI and HUEMER, 1971) and in cats chronically treated with hexamethonium (GELMAN, 1973).

V. Limb Circulation

It is not possible to express the effects of drugs on blood flow to all the limbs in terms of percentage changes in total flow, because the clinical methods are limited to a segment of one extremity. Intravenous injections of tetraethylammonium (HOOBLER et al., 1949; HORWITZ et al., 1949), hexamethonium (FREIS et al., 1953; RESTALL and SMIRK, 1952; SCHNAPER et al., 1951), pentamethonium (NEEDLEMAN and HORWITZ, 1953), and azamethonium (MOYER and HANDLEY, 1955) have been reported to cause an increase in blood flow measured by means of plethysmography. Since blood pressure in such patients was either reduced or unchanged, it is safe to conclude that there is a reduction in vascular resistance. Some of the above reports concerned patients with peripheral vascular disease, whose lower extremities could respond to ganglion-blocking drugs as well as other known vasodilators. On the other hand, LEWIS and DESHMANKAR (1968) observed a reduction in blood flow in the upper extremities at the same time as an increased blood flow in the lower extremities in patients who received hexamethonium. The xenon clearance technique has not been applied to the study of limb blood flow, and if this were possible the results would presumably be comparable to those recorded in other organs.

E. Conclusions

A review of the haemodynamic effects of ganglion-blocking drugs has revealed an advance of our concepts on the control exerted by the autonomic neurones on the circulation. If the pulmonary circulation is excluded, the remaining problem is the allocation of cardiac output among the various systemic vascular beds. A reasonable estimate of the effects of ganglion-blocking drugs can be arrived at through a preliminary consideration of the haemodynamic situation in an hypothetical man described by BAZETT (1956). Table 5 summarizes the partition of cardiac output and oxygen consumption, with the following outstanding features:

1) The heart muscle, although weighing 0.5% of the total body mass, consumes 11.6% of the total body oxygen intake and receives 5% of the cardiac output. The oxygen consumed per unit mass of heart muscle is the highest and the arteriovenous oxygen difference is the largest.

2) The kidneys have the most abundant flow in terms of unit weight and they have the lowest arteriovenous oxygen difference.

3) The entire splanchnic bed receives the largest proportion of cardiac output and of oxygen use of any individual organ.

4) The brain ranks third to the heart muscle and kidneys in oxygen usage per unit weight and falls between both in terms of arteriovenous oxygen difference.

If the subjects who have been investigated and summarised in Tables 1–4 are assumed to have the same features as the above hypothetical man, it is possible to calculate the allocation of cardiac output to the various organs with the following suggested figures (AVIADO, 1960): The maximum reduction in vascular resistance for the coronary (−40%) and cerebral vessels (−40%), the maximum increase in the renal vessels (+60%), and unchanged splanchnic vascular resistance were used to calculate the distribution of cardiac output following the administration of hexamethonium. The outcome is favourable to the myocardium and brain (allocation increased to +8% and +23%, respectively). The kidneys suffer (by a reduction in allocation to −14%) since the extremities and splanchnic beds still receive the same percentages of cardiac output.

Table 5. Hypothetical man of Bazett following hexamethonium

Region	Mass (%)	O_2 consumption (%)	Control cardiac output: (% distribution)	Cardiac output after hexamethonium: (% distribution)
Heart muscle	0.5	11.6	5	8
Brain	2.2	18.4	14	23
Kidneys	0.5	7.2	23	14
Splanchnic bed	4.1	20.4	28	28
Skin	5.7	4.8	9	
Skeletal muscle	49.3	20.0	16; 30[a]	27[a]
Residual tissue	37.7	17.6	5	
Entire body	100 = 63 kg	100 = 250 ml	100 = 5.4 l/min	100 = 5.4 l/min

[a] The sum of values for skin, muscle, and residual tissues represents distribution to the limbs.

A more direct approach to the measurement of allocation of cardiac output is to measure output simultaneously with blood flow to one or more organs. Technically, such a design is difficult to execute in the same subject, but one report includes measurement of output and organ flow. FINNERTY and his collaborators (1957) have measured both in a group of patients and noted that the allocation to the brain increased by 15–18% of the control value after the administration of hexamethonium.

The use of hexamethonium in man has identified the interplay of autonomic nervous factors with non-nervous factors. Chemical blockade of the autonomic ganglia causes a fall in blood pressure that is not exclusively the result of a primary loss of vasoconstrictor tone or simple reduction of total systemic vascular resistance. Equally important is a reduction in circulatory blood volume, venous return, and cardiac output, provided the heart is not in failure. If the heart is in failure, a corresponding initial reduction in circulating blood volume from peripheral vasodilation is followed by an improvement in cardiac function and an increase in output.

The most surprising feature of the haemodynamic studies following hexamethonium is the improvement in allocation or distribution of cardiac output in favour of the heart and brain. Until this information became available in man, it was assumed from experiments on animals subjected to extensive sympathectomy or ablation of the spinal cord that the loss of autonomic nerves would mean a loss of the homeostatic nervous mechanism that would always shift the blood from the non-vital organs under powerful vasoconstrictor tone (kidney, intestines, extremities) to the vital organs under poor vasoconstrictor tone (brain and heart). The observations in man indicate that after the autonomic nervous system is blocked, the local regulatory mechanisms (such as the metabolic control of cerebral and coronary vessels) and the local unidentified vascular (autoregulatory) factors in the kidney and splanchnic bed come into play. These mechanisms that are independent of the autonomic nervous system are active in normotensive and hypertensive individuals and account for the relative safety of the use of ganglion-blocking drugs in antihypertensive therapy. Without these nonautonomic mechanisms, cerebral and coronary insufficiency manifested by fainting and cardiac arrhythmias would be more frequently encountered.

References

Aas, K., Blegen, E.: Effect of tetraethyl-ammonium bromide on the kidneys. Lancet *1949* *MMLVI*, 999–1001

Assali, N.S., Douglas, R.A., Suyemoto, R.: Observations on the hemodynamic properties of a thiophanium derivative, RO 2-2222 (Arfonad), in human subjects. Circulation *8*, 62–69 (1953)

Aviado, D.M.: Hemodynamic effects of ganglion-blocking drugs. Circ. Res. *8*, 304–314 (1960)

Aviado, D.M.: The lung circulation, Vol. I. Oxford, London, Edinburgh, New York, Paris, Frankfurt: Pergamon Press 1965

Balchum, O.J., Gensini, G., Blount, S.G., Jr.: Effect of hexamethonium upon the pulmonary vascular resistance in mitral stenosis. J. Lab. Clin. Med. *50*, 186–198 (1957)

Bazett, H.C.: The circulation. In: Medical physiology. Bart, P. (ed.). St. Louis: Mosby 1956

Bernsmeier, A., Siemons, K.: Der Hirnkreislauf bei der gesteuerten experimentellen Hypotension (Hypotension controllee). Schweiz. Med. Wochenschr. *83*, 210–212 (1953)

Bessman, A.N., Alman, R.W., Fazekas, J.F.: Effect of acute hypotension on cerebral hemodynamics and metabolism of elderly patients. Arch. Intern. Med. *89*, 893–898 (1952)

Bozovic, L., Castenfords, J.: Effect of ganglionic-blocking on plasma renin activity in exercising and pain-stressed rats. Acta Physiol. Scand. 70, 290–292 (1967)

Carter, L.P., Atkinson, J.R.: Cortical blood flow in controlled hypotension as measured by thermal diffusion. J. Neurol. Neurosurg. Psychiatry 36, 906–913 (1973)

Cincotti, J., Huemer, R.: Reduction of portal hypertension by ganglionic blockade. Dig. Dis. 16, 517–521 (1971)

Crosely, A.P., Jr., Brown, J.F., Tuchman, H., Crumpton, C.W., Huston, J.H., Rowe, G.G.: Acute hemodynamic and metabolic response of hypertensive patients to pentolinium tartrate. Circulation 14, 584–592 (1956)

Crumpton, C.W., Rowe, G.G., O'Brien, G., Murphy, Q.R., Jr.: Effect of hexamethonium bromide upon coronary flow, cardiac work and cardiac efficiency in normotensive and renal hypertensive dogs. Circ. Res. 2, 79–83 (1954)

Crumpton, C.W., Rowe, G.G., Capps, R.C., Whitmore, J.J., Murphy, Q.R.: Effect of hexamethonium upon cerebral blood flow and metabolism in patients with premalignant and malignant hypertension. Circulation 11, 106–109 (1955)

Dewar, H.A., Owen, S.G., Jenkins, A.R.: Effect of hexamethonium bromide on the cerebral circulation in hypertension. Br. Med. J. 1953 II, 1017–1018

Eble, J.N., Gowdey, C.W., Rudzik, A.D., Vane, J.R.: Study of the mechanisms of the modifying actions of hexamethonium on the cardiovascular response to norepinephrine. J. Pharmacol. Exp. Ther. 184, 649–655 (1973)

Eichna, L.W., Sobol, B.J., Kessler, R.H.: Hemodynamic and renal effects produced in congestive heart failure by the intravenous administration of a ganglionic blocking agent. Trans. A. Am. Physicians 64, 207–213 (1956)

Elkin, M., Meng, C.H.: Angiographic study of the effect of arfonad on renal vascularity in the dog. Am. J. Roentgenol. 107, 711–719 (1969)

Fadhel, N., Seager, L.D.: The influence of hexamethonium intracisternally and of hexamethonium and trimethaphan camphorsulfonate intravenously on the pressor responses to intracisternal veratrine. Proc. Soc. Exp. Biol. Med. 131, 1263–1269 (1969)

Fazekas, J.F., Albert, S.N., Alman, R.W.: Cerebral physiology of controlled hypotension. Arch. Surg. 73, 59–62 (1956)

Finnerty, F.A., Jr., Witkin, L., Fazekas, J.F.: Cerebral hemodynamics during cerebral ischemia induced by acute hypotension. J. Clin. Invest. 33, 1227–1232 (1954)

Finnerty, F.A., Jr. Guillaudeu, R.L., Fazekas, J.F.: Cardiac and cerebral hemodynamics in drug induced postural collapse. Circ. Res. 5, 35–39 (1957)

Ford, R.V., Moyer, J.H., Spurr, C.L.: Hexamethonium in the chronic treatment of hypertension; its effect on renal hemodynamics and on the excretion of water and electrolytes. J. Clin. Invest. 32, 1133–1139 (1953)

Fowler, N.O., Westcott, R.N., Hauenstein, V.D., Scott, R.C., McGuire, J.: Observations on autonomic participation in pulmonary arteriolar resistance in man. J. Clin. Invest. 29, 1387–1396 (1950)

Freis, E.D., Rose, J.C., Partenope, E.A., Higgins, T.F., Kelley, R.T., Schnaper, H.W., Johnson, R.L.: Hemodynamic effects of hypotensive drugs in man. III. Hexamethonium. J. Clin. Invest. 32, 1285–1298 (1953)

Frisk, A.R., Hammarstrom, S., Lagerlof, H., Werko, L., Bjorkenheim, G., Holmgren, A., Larsson, Y.: Effect of tetraethylammonium in arterial hypertension. Am. J. Med. 5, 807–814 (1948)

Gelman, S.I.: The effect of ganglionic block on hepatic circulation. Biull. Eksp. Biol. Med. 76, 9–11 (1973)

Green, H.D., Kepchar, J.H.: Control of peripheral resistance in major systemic vascular beds. Physiol. Rev. 39, 617–686 (1959)

Grob, D., Scarborough, W.R., Kattus, A.A., Jr., Langford, H.G.: Further observations on the effects of autonomic blocking agents in patients with hypertension. II. Hemodynamic, ballistocardiographic, and electrocardiographic effects of hexamethonium and pentamethonium. Circulation 8, 352–369 (1953)

Halmagy, D., Felkai, B., Ivanyi, J., Zsoter, T., Tenyi, M., Szucs, Z.S.: Role of the nervous system in the maintenance of pulmonary arterial hypertension in heart failure. Br. Heart. J. 15, 15–24 (1953)

Hilton, J.G., Steinberg, M.: Effects of ganglion- and parasympathetic-blocking drugs upon the pressor response elicited by elevation of the intracranial fluid pressure. J. Pharmacol. Exp. Ther. *153*, 285–291 (1966)

Hoobler, S.W., Malton, S.D., Ballantine, H.T., Cohen, S., Neligh, R.B., Peet, M.M., Lyons, R.H.: Studies on vasomotor tone. I. Effect of the tetraethylammonium ion on the peripheral blood flow of normal subjects. J. Clin. Invest. *28*, 638–647 (1949)

Horwitz, O., Montgomery, H., Longaker, E.D., Sayen, A.: Effects of vasodilator drugs and other procedures on digital cutaneous blood flow, cardiac output, blood pressure, pulse rate, body temperature, and metabolic rate. Am. J. Med. Sci. *218*, 669–682 (1949)

Kleh, J., Fazekas, J.F.: Effects of hypotensive agents on subjects with cerebral vascular insufficiency. J. Am. Geriatr. Soc. *4*, 18–23 (1956)

Landysheva, I.V., Zavolovskaya, L.I., Katyukhin, V.N.: Effect of hexonium and hexamethonium on the pulmonary circulation and the contractile function of the myocardium. Ter. Arkh. *44*, 54–60 (1972) (Russ.)

Lee, W.C., Shideman, F.E.: Inotropic action of hexamethonium. Circ. Res. *6*, 66–71 (1958)

Lewis, J.A., Deshmankar, B.S.: A reappraisal of vascular effects of hexamethonium. Can. J. Physiol. Pharmacol. *46*, 139–143 (1968)

Mackinnon, J.: Effect of hypotension-producing drugs on the renal circulation. Lancet *1952 MMLXIII*, 12–15

Magness, A., Yashon, D., Locke, G., Wiederholt, W., Hunt, W.E.: Cerebral function during trimethaphan-induced hypotension. Neurology *23*, 506–509 (1973)

Miles, B.E., Dewardener, II.E., Churchill Davidson, H.C., Wylie, W.D.: Effect on the renal circulation of pentamethonium bromide during anaesthesia. Clin. Sci. *11*, 73–79 (1952)

Morris, G.C., Jr., Moyer, J.H., Snyder, H.B., Haynes, B.W., Jr.: Vascular dynamics in controlled hypotension. Ann. Surg. *138*, 706–711 (1953)

Moyer, J.H., Handley, C.A.: Renal and cardiovascular hemodynamic response to ganglionic blockade with pendiomide and comparison with hexamethonium and arfonad. J. Pharmacol. Exp. Ther. *113*, 383–392 (1955)

Moyer, J.H., Morris, G.: Cerebral hemodynamics during controlled hypotension induced by the continuous infusion of ganglionic blocking agents (hexamethonium, pendiomide, and arfonad). J. Clin. Invest. *33*, 1081–1088 (1954)

Moyer, J.H., Ford, R., Dennis, E., Handley, C.A.: Laboratory and clinical observations on mecamylamine as a hypotensive agent. Proc. Soc. Exp. Biol. Med. *90*, 402–408 (1955)

Moyer, J.H., McConn, R., Morris, G.C.: Effect of controlled hypotension with pendiomide (as used in surgery) on renal hemodynamics and water and electrolyte excretion – a comparison with hexamethonium and arfonad and the effect of norepinephrine on these responses. Anesthesiology *16*, 355–364 (1955)

Moyer, J.H., McConn, R., Seibert, R.A.: Effect of blood pressure reduction with arfonad on renal hemodynamics and the excretion of water and electrolytes in patients with hypertension. Am. Heart J. *49*, 360–366 (1955)

Moyer, J.H., Morris, G., Seibert, R.A.: Renal function during controlled hypotension with hexamethonium and following norepinephrine. Surg. Gynecol. Obstet. *100*, 27–32 (1955)

Needleman, H.L., Horwitz, O.: Comparative study of the effects of three vasodilator drugs, pentamethonium bromide (C_5), Dilatol (SKF-1700-A) and pendiomide (BA-9295) on the digital cutaneous blood flow. Am. J. Med. Sci. *226*, 164–171 (1953)

Parrish, A.E., Kleh, J., Fazekas, J.F.: Renal and cerebral hemodynamics with hypotension. Am. J. Med. Sci. *233*, 35–39 (1957)

Pedersoli, W.H.: Effects of ganglionic and cholinergic blocking drugs on the pressor response to central vagal stimulation. Pharmacology *4*, 120–128 (1970)

Plummer, A.J., Trapold, J.H., Schneider, J.A., Maxwell, R.A., Earl, A.E.: Ganglionic blockade by a new bis-quaternary series including chlorisondamine dimethochloride. J. Pharmacol. Exp. Ther. *115*, 172–184 (1955)

Pokk, L.R.: Hexamethonium action on the development of myocardial necroses. Farmakol. Toksikol. *35*, 193–195 (1972)

Rakita, L., Sancetta, S.M.: Acute hemodynamic effects of hexamethonium in normotensive man. Circ. Res. *1*, 499–501 (1953)

Redisch, W., Wertheimer, L., Delisle, C., Steele, J.M.: Comparison of visceral and peripheral vascular beds in hypertensive patients. Circulation 9, 68–72 (1954)

Restall, P.A., Smirk, F.H.: Regulation of blood pressure levels by hexamethonium bromide and mechanical devices. Br. Heart J. 14, 1–12 (1952)

Reynolds, T.B., Paton, A., Freeman, M., Howard, F., Sherlock, S.: Effect of hexamethonium bromide on splanchnic blood flow, oxygen consumption, and glucose output in man. J. Clin. Invest. 32, 793–800 (1953)

Sancetta, S.M.: Acute hemodynamic effects of hexamethonium (C_6) in patients with emphysematous pulmonary hypertension. Am. Heart. J. 49, 501–506 (1955)

Sancetta, S.M.: Acute hemodynamic effects of total head-down body tilt and hexamethonium in normal and pulmonary emphysematous subjects. J. Lab. Clin. Med. 49, 684–693 (1957)

Schnaper, H.W., Johnson, R.L., Tuohy, E.B., Freis, E.D.: Effects of hexamethonium as compared to procaine or metacaine lumbar block on the blood flow to the foot of normal subjects. J. Clin. Invest. 30, 786–791 (1951)

Scott, R.C., Kaplan, S., Stiles, W.J.: Observations on the effect of tetraethylammonium chloride on the pulmonary vascular resistance in mitral stenosis. Am. Heart J. 50, 720–730 (1955)

Shackman, R., Graber, I.G., Melrose, D.G., Smith, J.: Hemodynamics of methonium hypotension during anaesthesia. Anaesthesia 7, 217–222 (1952)

Shell, W.E., Sobel, B.E.: Protection of jeopardized ischemic myocardium by reduction of ventricular afterload. N. Engl. J. Med. 291, 481–486 (1974)

Smith, J.R., Agrest, A., Hoobler, S.W.: Effect of acute and chronic administration of pentolinium tartrate on the blood pressure and cardiac output in hypertensive patients. Circulation 12, 777 (1955)

Sobol, B.J., Kessler, R.H., Rader, B., Eichna, L.W.: Cardiac, hemodynamic and renal functions in congestive heart failure during induced peripheral vasodilatation; relationship to Starling's law of the heart in man. J. Clin. Invest. 38, 557–578 (1959)

Steinberg, M., Hilton, J.G.: Site of action of atropine in blocking pressor response to increased intracranial pressure in chlorisondamine-treated dogs. Tex. Rep. Biol. Med. 24, 222–227 (1966a)

Steinberg, M., Hilton, J.G.: Effects of chlorisondamine and atropine on cardiovascular responses to stimulation of the carotid sinuses. Tex. Rep. Biol. Med. 24, 693–699 (1966b)

Steinberg, M., Hilton, J.G.: Effect of sympathectomy and adrenalectomy upon ganglion blockade. Pharmacol. Exp. Ther. 156, 215–220 (1967)

Stone, H.H., Mackrell, T.N., Wechsler, R.L.: Effect on cerebral circulation and metabolism in man of acute reduction in blood pressure by means of intravenous hexamethonium bromide and head-up tilt. Anesthesiology 16, 168–176 (1955)

Storstein, O., Tveten, H.: Effect of hexamethonium bromide on the pulmonary circulation. Scand. J. Clin. Lab. Invest. 6, 169–177 (1954)

Traber, D.L., Wilson, R.D., Priano, L.L.: The effect of autonomic blocking agents on the cardiovascular response to etoxadrol (CL 1848-C). 1. Ganglionic blockade. Arch. Int. Pharmacodyn. 204, 333–341 (1973)

Trapold, J.H.: Effect of ganglionic-blocking agents upon blood flow and resistance in the superior mesenteric artery of the dog. Circ. Res. 4, 718–723 (1956)

Trapold, J.H.: Role of venous return in the cardiovascular response following injection of ganglion-blocking agents. Circ. Res. 5, 444–450 (1957)

Ullmann, T.D., Diengott, D.: Effect of hexamethonium (C_6) on renal hemodynamics in man. Arch. Intern. Med. 92, 228–237 (1953)

Ullmann, T.D., Menczel, J.: Effect of a ganglionic blocking agent (hexamethonium) on renal function and on excretion of water and electrolytes in hypertension and in congestive heart failure. Am. Heart. J. 52, 106–120 (1956)

Van Bergen, F.H.: Hexamethonium-induced hypotension. Minn. Med. 38, 573–576 (1955)

Vanevsky, F.L., Azarov, V.I.: On the effect of vasoconstricting agents on hemodynamics under conditions of ganglionary blockade during the operation and general anesthesia. Vestn. Khir. 110, 80–83 (1973) (Russ.)

Varnauskas, E.: Studies in hypertensive cardiovascular disease with special reference to cardiac function. Scand. J. Clin. Lab. Invest. 7, 5–117 (1955)

Vinogradov, A.V., Tsibermakler, T.D.: Hemodynamic changes occurring in cardiac insufficiency under the influence of hexonium. Kardiologiia 6, 34–38 (1966) (Russ.)

Werko, L., Frisk, A.R., Wade, G., Ellasch, H.: Effect of hexamethonium bromide in arterial hypertension. Lancet 1951 II, 470–472

Wilson, V.H., Keeley, K.J.: Haemodynamic effects of hexamethonium bromide in patients with pulmonary hypertension and heart failure. S. Afr. J. Med. Sci. 18, 125–129 (1953)

Yu, P.N., Nye, R.E., Jr., Lovejoy, F.W., Jr., Schreiner, B.F., Yim, B.J.B.: Studies of pulmonary hypertension. IX. Effects of intravenous hexamethonium on pulmonary circulation in patients with mitral stenosis. J. Clin. Invest. 37, 194–201 (1958)

CHAPTER 7

Action of Ganglion-Blocking Agents on the Gastrointestinal Tract

D.F.J. MASON

A. Introduction

In their review in 1950, MOE and FREYBURGER found that tetraethylammonium reduced gastric motility, gastric secretion, and motility of the small intestine, also providing striking relief of pain in ulcer patients, but concluded that the effects produced by widespread autonomic blockade would preclude the general therapeutic exploitation of the effects. PATON discussed transmission and block in autonomic ganglia in 1954 and summarised the effects of ganglion-blockers in man by describing the "methonium man" in which he wrote. "... He dislikes speaking much unless helped with something to moisten his mouth and throat ... But he always behaves like a gentleman and never belches or hiccups ... peptic ulcer pass(es) him by. He is thin because his appetite is modest; he never feels hunger pains and his stomach never rumbles. He gets rather constipated so his intake of liquid paraffin is high ...".

Scattered through the literature are accounts of "paralytic ileus" – complete cessation of intestinal activity – produced by the administration of various ganglion-blocking compounds for the treatment of hypertension. Thus the compounds have adequate potency, but despite several attempts to introduce them into therapeutics for the treatment of disorders of the gastrointestinal tract, their use has been minimal, confirming the prediction of MOE and FREYBURGER. Partly because of this lack of therapeutic interest, our knowledge of the actions of these compounds on the gut has not progressed very far beyond the outline provided by PATON. Our knowledge of the physiology of the gastrointestinal tract is far from complete, but it is clear that both divisions of the autonomic nervous system are involved in its control, often in opposition, and either division will have different effects on different segments of the gut. Therefore, ganglion-blocking agents are not as valuable as specific parasympathetic or sympathetic inhibiting agents for use as tools to unravel the function of the autonomic nerves. These considerations are compounded by some species differences in the responses to these agents, thereby discouraging still further their use in experiments.

The major studies on the mode of action of ganglion-blocking agents have been on sympathetic ganglia. Parasympathetic ganglia are not so accessible, and therefore the actions on these ganglia have not been studied in the same detail. However, none of the studies where effects on parasympathetic and sympathetic ganglia have been compared, or where the effects on parasympathetic ganglia have been studied alone, has produced any evidence to suggest that the mode of action, or the potency of these compounds differs between the two types of ganglion (LUCO and MARCONI, 1949; WIEN and MASON, 1951; PERRY and WILSON, 1956; CORNE and EDGE, 1958; ALONSO-DE FORIDA et al., 1960; GARRETT, 1963).

B. Salivary Secretion

The secretion of saliva is dependent on the autonomic innervation (BURGEN and EMMELIN, 1961; HOLTON, 1973) and all studies in experimental animals and man have shown a reduction of salivary flow following the administration of ganglion-blocking compounds, thereby confirming the clinical reports of dry mouth in man. LYONS et al. (1947) used tetraethylammonium, MASON and WIEN (1955) used hexamethonium and pentolinium, while EMMELIN (1967) reported on the actions of tetraethylammonium, hexamethonium, chlorisondamine, and mecamylamine.

Stimulation of the preganglionic nerves of either division of the autonomic nervous system produces a flow of saliva, although the responses differ. Both responses are prevented by ganglion-blocking compounds. EMMELIN (1959) showed that the prolonged administration of chlorisondamine, and to a lesser extent hexamethonium, produced a similar supersensitivity towards adrenaline in the submaxillary gland to that produced by section of the *chorda tympani*. WELLS (1960) showed that the repeated administration of chlorisondamine to rats prevented the rapid growth of salivary glands that normally followed surgical stimuli, and suggested therefore that the autonomic nervous system controlled the size as well as the function of the salivary glands.

C. Oesophagus and Cardiac Sphincter

The structure of the oesophagus varies from one species to another, particularly in the relative preponderance of striated or smooth muscle (CHRISTENSEN, 1968) and hence in the extent to which autonomic nerves may be involved. MOE and FREYBURGER (1950) reported that tetraethylammonium had no effect on the oesophagus or cardia in man, where the lower third of the oesophagus is composed of smooth muscle in both layers. Carbaminoyl choline causes contraction of the longitudinal muscle from the oesophagus and this contraction is prevented by hexamethonium. CHRISTENSEN (1968) interprets this as indicating the existence of nicotinic receptors on ganglion cells in the oesophageal wall. Similarly, nicotine causes a relaxation of the circular muscle, which is sensitive to hexamethonium. These observations would be reconcilable with the earlier reports of MOE and FREYBURGER (1950) if the activity of the striated muscle masked any deficiency in activity of the smooth muscle due to the autonomic blockade, but normally the activities of the two types of muscle would need to be co-ordinated. TOYAMA et al. (1975) studied the effects of ganglion-blocking substances in dog. They chose this species because the oesophageal musculature is composed almost entirely of striated muscle. From the serosal surface they recorded electrical activity produced by stimulation of the vagus nerve. This activity was blocked by the neuromuscular blocking agents tubocurarine and suxamethonium, and it was also significantly reduced by hexamethonium or large doses of nicotine, while small doses of nicotine facilitated the response. The doses of hexamethonium ranged from 5 to 10 mg/kg body wt., which are lower than those normally producing neuromuscular block in this species, but the authors confirmed the point, since neuromuscular transmission in the diaphragm was not affected and therefore this action of hexamethonium was on ganglia.

The possibility that ganglion-blocking drugs might have an action on the cardiac sphincter has been little studied, perhaps because of the debate about the existence of a discrete sphincter.

In the cat, the lowest 2 cm of the oesophagus behaves like a sphincter, although histological study does not provide evidence of such a structure (CLARK and VANE, 1961). Distension of the oesophagus caused a relaxation of the sphincter, and this response could be prevented by vagotomy. Electrical stimulation of the peripheral end of the cut vagus also caused a relaxation that could be prevented by hexamethonium. Stimulation of the periarterial sympathetic nerves caused an increase in tone of the sphincter. Administration of hexamethonium to preparations with intact innervation resulted in a decrease in tone, which lasted about 5 min (CLARK and VANE, 1961). The direction of the change in tone produced by the ganglion-blocking drug will depend on the autonomic activity obtaining at that particular time.

By analogy with the effects of vagotomy, the ganglion-blocking agents may be expected to prevent a reflex relaxation, but not to completely prevent the passage of food, since after vagotomy material still passed the sphincter if the pressure in the oesophagus was raised from 12 to 18 cm of water. The ganglion blockers did not increase the reflux of gastric contents (INGELFINGER, 1958).

D. Gastric Motility

In an early study it was shown that tetraethylammonium was able to reduce the incidence of gastric ulcer that follows ligation of the pylorus in rats (LITTLE et al., 1947). This and other similar studies prompted many investigations into the action of each of the ganglion-blocking substances on the motility of the stomach. With hardly any exceptions, the investigators recorded a reduction or complete inhibition of gastric motility in man (e.g., ZWEIG et al., 1948; NELIGH et al., 1949; KAY and SMITH, 1950; SCOTT, et al., 1950; DOUTHWAITE and THORNE, 1951; MOHAY and GEHER, 1963; KLIN, 1965). Some of the studies were carried out in patients with ulcers and some improvement in their condition was seen.

When experiments were performed in experimental animals the results were not so consistant. LANE et al. (1949) were unable to demonstrate any great prolongation of the gastric emptying time in the dog after the administration of tetraethylammonium. This is the least potent of the ganglion blockers so GARG (1964, 1966) extended the experiments and found that chlorisondamine (0.3 mg/kg body wt.) had little effect, but pentolinium (0.5 mg/kg body wt.) reduced the movement of the test meal by 15–35% in dogs, rabbits, and guinea-pigs. The novement of the test meal was also slowed in dogs, rabbits and guinea-pigs by mecamylamine and pempidine.

In anaesthetised cats the immediate effect of hexamethonium is to stimulate the stomach to contract, while in rabbits there is relaxation (WIEN and MASON, 1951; PATON and ZAIMIS, 1952). Scattered through the literature there are several reports of onium ganglion-blocking substances producing a stimulation of one or another part of the gastrointestinal tract. The reports refer to different drugs and different species, and there is no clear evidence concerning the mechanism of the stimulation. In a report on the stimulant effect of hexamethonium and tetraethylammonium on cat ileum in vivo, PATON and ZAIMIS (1951) concluded that the contraction was due to a predominantly myogenic rhythmic activity, which was unmasked by the blockade of inhibitory impulses from the sympathetic and perhaps from the vagal nerves.

In other, isolated tissues there is also evidence of stimulant effects that could not be due to the inhibition of sympathetic tone.

Using the isolated nerve-stomach preparation of the rat, DELLA BELLA and ROG-NONI (1961) demonstrated the mutual antagonism of the responses to stimulation of the sympathetic and parasympathetic nerves. They showed that tetraethylammonium, hexamethonium, azamethonium, pempidine, and mecamylamine could block the stimulant effect of vagal stimulation.

E. Gastric Secretion

The study of gastrointestinal secretion, including gastric secretion, has advanced considerably during recent decades, with inevitable changes of opinion as new facets of the problem have been elucidated. The study has demanded rigourously controlled experiments to separate neural control from hormonal control, and then to establish the interrelations between the vagally controlled secretion, such as the "cephalic phase", the antral release of gastrin, as in the "gastric phase" and the "intestinal phase", with the various elements of positive and negative feedback (GREGORY, 1962; GROSSMAN, 1968; HOLTON, 1973).

By their nature, the ganglion-blocking agents have a general action on all ganglia and the result is perhaps more dramatic, but is less well defined than the effects seen in experiments where single nerves are divided or highly specific inhibitors employed.

In experimental animals and man the ganglion-blockers all reduce the volume, acidity, and peptic activity of the basal gastric secretions and of those evoked by test meals or by stimulation of the vagus nerves (ZWEIG et al., 1948; NELIGH et al., 1949; MACDONALD and SMITH, 1949; ROBERTSON et al., 1950; DOUTHWAITE and THORNE, 1951; WIEN and MASON, 1951). These compounds were also effective in blocking the increased secretion that was produced by an insulin-induced hypoglycaemia (NELIGH et al., 1949; ROBERTSON et al., 1950; PLUMMER et al., 1956; CLARK et al., 1964).

It is clear from these experiments that the compounds inhibit the neurally induced gastric secretion, but, although achlorhydria was produced in some instances, there is no evidence to show whether the antral release of gastrin or the responsiveness of the secretory cells to gastrin was modified.

The secretion due to histamine infusion was also reduced by the ganglion-blocking agents in most of the experiments. Where inhibition of the histamine-induced secretion was not seen the doses of the ganglion blockers were rather small. CLARK et al. (1964) have suggested that this reduction of the response indicated that histamine acts through the nerves.

NAKAJIMA and MAGEE (1970) also found that hexamethonium significantly reduced the secretion produced by the administration of the muscarinic ganglion-stimulating agent AHR 602 to dogs with Heidenhain pouches. They also confirmed the earlier observation of ODORI and MAGEE (1969) that the ganglion-blocking agents, pentolinium or hexamethonium did not reduce the response to pentagastrin administration.

F. Pancreatic Secretion

As with gastric secretion, the study of pancreatic secretion has not been greatly helped by the use of ganglion-blocking substances, and most of the analysis of the control of pancreatic secretion has been accomplished by the use of selective, controlled stimuli, highly selective blocking agents, and careful isolation of possible hormonal agents.

To quote GREGORY (1962): "The statement of MELLANBY that 'the enzyme content of the pancreatic juice is determined by the vagus nerve, whereas the quantity of bicarbonate solution in which the enzymes are contained is determined by secretin' only needs the addition of pancreozymin to complete the account". THOMAS (1968) concluded that the cephalic and gastric phases of pancreatic secretion are dependent on secretory nerves, while the intestinal phase is largely governed by hormones, but the release of the hormones from the intestine and their action on the pancreas may be partly dependent on neural mechanisms. PRESHAW (1968) considered the possible interaction of the neural and hormonal mechanisms, concluding that there might be a modest augmentation but that there was no evidence of any profound potentiation.

Therefore it might be expected that ganglion-blocking agents would inhibit the neurally controlled secretion, and by their action on motility reduce the local stimulus for the hormone control even if a direct neural step were not involved in the secretion or action of the hormone. THOMAS (1968) reported that ganglion-blockers did reduce pancreatic secretion. HONG et al. (1961) examined the influence of hexamethonium and some dietary factors on human pancreatic and biliary secretion. Both milk and *dl*-methionine, when administered by stomach tube, increased the volume output of pancreatic juice and bile. The respective concentrations of amylase, lipase, and cholic acid were also increased. Following a moderate dose of hexamethonium (25 mg) the pancreatic responses were not seen, but the biliary responses persisted unchanged. MAGEE et al. (1965) studied the effects of atropine and of pentolinium in the dog with a pancreatic fistula. Both drugs, and also section of the vagi, reduced the pancreatic response to intravenous secretin. Vagal section or ganglionic block also reduced the protein content of the secretion. The authors concluded that the parasympathetic innervation sensitised the gland to secretin.

G. Small Intestine

In man the ganglion-blocking compounds reduce or completely inhibit gastrointestinal motility when given in adequate doses. For example, DOUTHWAITE and THORNE (1951) found that 100 mg hexamethonium bromide given intramuscularly caused the duodenum to be dilated and immobile for up to 6 h. This property has been exploited in X-ray examination of the intestine. KLIN (1965) administered 5–10 mg pempidine orally before a barium meal and found that the movement of the radio-opaque material ceased temporarily and the small intestine was demonstrably dilated for 2–4 h. Attempts to administer the onium compounds by mouth in the treatment of hypertension provoked a series of eases of paralytic ileus (LOCKET, 1951), but this was not a toxic effect arising from the absorption of an abnormally high proportion of the dose, since Milne et al. (1957) report a case of paralylic ileus due to the administration of doses of mecamylamine that were regularly and completely absorbed. As will become apparent, the inhibition of motility or the paralytic ileus produced by the ganglion-blocking compounds is due to the inhibition of all autonomic activity, particularly the intrinsic peristaltic reflex. Hence it differs from the paralytic ileus that may follow surgery, where the cause may be an excessive sympathetic tone (Neely and Catchpole, 1971).

In experimental animals the effects of the ganglion-blocking substances, and particularly the onium compounds, are more variable. Bozler (1949) applied tetraethylammonium topically to the small intestine of anaesthetized rabbits and showed that both spontaneous and stimulated peristaltic waves were extinguished when they reached the point of application. Moe and Freyburger (1950) reported that tetraethylammonium potentiated the action of histamine on ileal Thiry-Vella loops in dogs, but caused a reduction of tone and depression of motility when administered alone. In anaesthetised dogs the motility was already depressed and the compound had no further effect, nor did it block the contractile response to vagal stimulation. Northrup et al. (1952) produced a significant depression of motility in the small intestine of unanaesthetised dogs with 20 mg tetraethylammonium/kg body wt. given subcutaneously. They measured motility in terms of the movement of a charcoal test meal. Paton and Zaimis (1951) found that both hexamethonium and tetraethylammonium caused vigorous localised activity of the circular muscle of the small intestine of cats. In their later review, Paton and Zaimis (1952) comment that these compounds depressed activity in the rabbit. Garg (1962) also found vigorous contractions of the circular muscle, but no increase in intestinal propulsion, when he administered hexamethonium or tetraethylammonium to dogs. Mecamylamine, pempidine, and pentolinium reduced the propulsive movement of the intestine as measured by the movement of a charcoal test meal (Garg, 1964, 1966). When chlorisondamine was administered to dogs there was no significant change in tone or motility, although the dose was large enough to produce hypotension (Plummer et al., 1956; Garg, 1964). These results are not easy to reconcile. Clearly the species affects the results, as does the presence of an anaesthetic, but there is not sufficient information to indicate the mechanism of the stimulant effect. Burks and Long (1967) isolated the circulation to lengths of dog small intestine, but left the neural connections intact. The vessels were perfused with Krebs solution. Intra-arterial injection of 100 µg hexamethonium caused a small, brief contracture and blocked the response to stimulation of the vagus. This suggests that the stimulant effect is due to an action on the intestine rather than elsewhere. Paton and Zaimis (1951) considered it to be due to an unmasked myogenic effect. Tetraethylammonium also has the property of increasing the release of acetylcholine from some cholinergic nerve endings (Douglas and Lywood, 1961; Mathews, 1961; Collier and Exley, 1963; Mathews and Quilliam, 1964), and this may also be a factor in the stimulant effect of tetraethylammonium.

In vitro experiments have concentrated largely on two areas, the ability of the ganglion-blocking compounds to inhibit the peristaltic reflex, and their effect on the responses of either longitudinal or circular muscle preparations to ganglion-stimulant substances. The possibility that the peristaltic reflex in isolated intestine could be used as a test for ganglion-blocking activity became apparent from the study of

FELDBERG and LIN (1949). They used the preparation originally described by TREN-
DELENBURG and showed that tubocurarine blocked the peristaltic reflex in isolated
segments of rabbit or guinea-pig ileum. They suggested that the initial contraction of
the longitudinal muscle following the rise in intraluminal pressure was a local muscle
response to stretch, and that subsequent contraction of the circular muscle and
relaxation of the longitudinal muscle were under nervous control. The site of action
of the tubocurarine was a synapse or synapses in the neural mechanism. KLINGE
(1951) used isolated cat ileum, reduced to tubular segments devoid of ganglion cells
and composed only of circular muscle and terminal nerve fibres. No spontaneously
propagated contractions were seen, but a wave of contraction could be induced with
acetylcholine. With this background, experiments examined the effects of ganglion-
blocking substances on the peristaltic reflex. MOE and FREYBURGER (1950) were
unable to block the reflex in isolated rabbit ileum with tetraethylammonium. In
isolated guinea-pig ileum the peristaltic reflex was readily blocked with hexamethonium or pentolinium (PATON and ZAIMIS, 1949; WIEN and MASON, 1951; MASON and
WIEN, 1955). Meanwhile, KOSTERLITZ and his co-workers continued to investigate
this intrinsic intestinal reflex elicited by raising the intraluminal pressure. They
concluded that the initial graded longitudinal contraction was not a muscle response
to stretch but was under nervous control and was initiated by radial stretch, but that
ganglion blockers did not modify this response althogh the nerve to the longitudinal
muscle appeared to be cholinergic. Studies using coaxial stimulation of the ileum
confirmed this interpretation (KOSTERLITZ and LEES, 1964; DZOLJIC, 1967). The contraction of the circular muscle, i.e., the emptying phase, was also under neural
control, but ganglion blockers (tubocurarine, hexamethonium, nicotine) could prevent this so that appropriate synaptic receptors must be present (KOSTERLITZ and
LEES, 1964).

The second experimental approach was to test the effect of the ganglion-blocking
drugs on the response of isolated ileum to ganglion-stimulant substances. FELDBERG
(1951) showed that the contraction of guinea-pig ileum elicited with nicotine could
be inhibited by ganglion-blocking substances, and if the response to nicotine were
interspersed with responses to other stimulant substances the specificity of the inhibition could be tested simultaneously. This method was used to examine the actions
of hexamethonium and of pempidine (PATON and ZAIMIS, 1949; WIEN and MASON,
1951; CORNE and EDGE, 1958).

When attempts were made to extend these experiments to other parts of the
intestine and to intestine from other species, it was found that the response to
nicotine was relaxation in the rabbit ileo-colic sphincter, human ileum and colon,
and rabbit colon, but these responses could be blocked by the ganglion-blocking
compounds (JARRETT, 1962; FISHLOCK and PARKES, 1966; DANIEL, 1968).

H. Colon

MOE and FREYBURGER (1950) described a depression of colonic activity following the
administration of tetraethylammonium to unanaesthetised dogs. Clinical experience
has confirmed that reduced activity of the colon, or constipation, was a recurrent
problem with the therapeutic application of the ganglion-blocking substances. The

"paralytic ileus" sometimes seen in patients included a depression of colonic activity (see also PATON, 1954). An exception to this was reported by PLUMMER et al. (1956). They studied the effects of chlorisondamine in anaesthetised dogs, and found that doses large enough to produce marked hypotension did not depress activity, but produced a marked increase in the motility of the colon. Hexamethonium had only a minimal, or no, stimulant effect. Thus, it seemed that apart from chlorisondamine the ganglion-blocking substances depressed motility and peristalsis in the colon as they did in the small intestine, and probably by an action on cholinergic synapses in the neural pathways of the intrinsic reflexes.

HUKUHARA and MUJAKE (1959) observed that peristalsis could be initiated in the denervated colon of anaesthetised dogs by mechanical stimulation of the mucosa, and that this response could be prevented by hexamethonium. CREMA (1970) obtained similar results with isolated cat colon. GARRY and GILLESPIE (1955) used isolated large intestine of rabbit, complete with the parasympathetic and sympathetic nerves. Stimulation of the pelvic nerves produced a contraction that could be blocked by hexamethonium or atropine. Stimulation of the sympathetic nerves inhibited the colon, but this could not be prevented by hexamethonium or atropine. LEE (1960) extended these studies by using isolated large intestine from guinea-pig as well as rabbit. In both species, stimulation of the pelvic nerves caused a contraction that could be prevented by hexamethonium, atropine, or nicotine. Stimulation of the sympathetic nerve usually inhibited peristalsis and relaxed the longitudinal muscle, but in a few experiments it produced a contraction, which was susceptible to block by atropine, hexamethonium, and nicotine, confirming an earlier observation by VARAGIC (1956). The same three agents abolished the peristalsis in guinea-pig colon, but even in high concentrations they failed to abolish peristaltic activity in rabbit colon, although peristalsis could be blocked in ileum from the same animals.

In an organ with responses as complex as those of the intestine it is valuable to confirm the observations and interpretations obtained with a blocking agent by using an appropriate agonist. GILLESPIE and MacKENNA (1960) found that high concentrations of nicotine caused contraction but low concentrations inhibited isolated rabbit colon, and this inhibition was blocked by hexamethonium. A similar relaxation, induced by nicotine and prevented by hexamethonium, has been demonstrated in the isolated rabbit ileo-colic sphincter, the guinea-pig *taenia coli*, the circular muscle of the human ileum and colon, and human *taenia coli* (JARRETT, 1962; WEISENTHAL et al., 1971; FISHLOCK and PARKS, 1963, 1966; BUCKNELL and WHITNEY, 1964). In experiments on the rabbit ileo-colic sphincter, JARRETT (1962) was able to show that doses of hexamethonium that just blocked the inhibition revealed a stimulant effect of nicotine, which was blocked with larger doses of hexamethonium. FISHLOCK and PARKS (1966) were only able to obtain relaxation in human colon and adjacent ileum, even in the presence of physostigmine. They concluded that none of the ganglion cells in this part of the intestine could be parasympathetic and discussed the possibility that the parasympathetic ganglion cells are sited remotely.

Studies in anaesthetised dogs showed that intravenous nicotine also caused a relaxation of the colon, but this was caused in part by the release of catecholamines from the adrenal medulla (WEISBRODT et al., 1970). Many of these studies were completed before the studies of NORBERG (1964) had shown that ideas about the interconnections of the autonomic nervous system in the gut wall needed to be revised. Similarly, very little of the evidence that led BURNSTOCK to postulate the existence of purinergic nerves involved in inhibitory reflexes that are part of the propulsive activity of the intestine (BURNSTOCK, 1972, 1975) had been found.

The observations of BURNSTOCK et al. (1966) and FURNESS (1970) indicated that the cell bodies of the nonadrenergic inhibitory nerves were located in Auerbach's plexus and that the presynaptic neurones were cholinergic, although BIANCHI et al. (1968) suggested a tryptaminergic link. In addition in most of the colon the extrinsic nerves do not control these inhibitory neurones. In many of the studies on the colon reviewed in this chapter, ganglion-blocking agents have been used as tools to elucidate some aspect of the physiology, because of their known specificity of action at certain accessible autonomic synapses. In the absence of proof, the use of ganglion-blocking agents as tools to block hitherto unknown synapses involves first the assumption that their mode of action is the same here as in the better-known synapses, and secondly that their potency is similar at all synapses. The observations of JARRETT (1962) might be regarded as suggesting a measure of differential sensitivity to nicotine and hexamethonium between the inhibitory and stimulant neural pathways. Such a differential sensitivity, if proved, could explain some of the unexpected findings of stimulant effects on the gastrointestinal tract following injections of ganglion-blocking substances.

Throughout the discussion of the action of ganglion-blocking substances on the gastrointestinal tract it has been implicit that these compounds have no trace of a direct effect (for example see PATON and ZAIMIS, 1952). When BULBRING (1955) examined the effect of hexamethonium on the membrane potential, spike discharge and tension in *taenia coli* of guinea-pig, she showed that high concentrations, 10^{-4} to 6×10^{-4}, increased the rate of discharge in five of six experiments, and lowered the membrane potential, while increasing the response to stretch, in four of the experiments. SUZUKI et al. (1963) observed a similar phenomenon with tetraethylammonium. Here again, the mechanism of the action is not clear, but the observations suggest the need for care in the use of these pharmacological tools.

References

Alonso-deForida, F., Cato, J., Ramirez, L., Pardo, E.G.: Effects of several blocking agents on sympathetic and parasympathetic action potentials. J. Pharmacol. Exp. Ther. *129*, 433–437 (1960)

Bianchi, C., Beani, L., Frigo, G.M., Orema, A.: Further evidence for the presence of non-adrenergic inhibitory structures in guinea-pig colon. Eur. J. Pharmacol. *4*, 51–62 (1968)

Bozler, E.: Myenteric reflex. Am. J. Physiol. *157*, 329–337 (1949)

Bucknell, A., Whitney, B.: A preliminary investigation of the pharmacology of the human isolated taenia coli preparation. Br. J. Pharmacol. *23*, 164–175 (1964)

Bulbring, E.: Correlation between membrane potential, spike discharge, and tension in smooth muscle. J. Physiol. (Lond.) *128*, 200–221 (1955)

Burgen, A.S.V., Emmelin, N.G.: Physiology of the salivary glands. London: Edward Arnold 1961

Burks, T.F., Long, J.P.: Release of 5-hydroxy-tryptamine from isolated dog intestine by nicotine. Br. J. Pharmacol. *30*, 229–239 (1967)

Burnstock, G.: Purinergic nerves. Pharmacol. Rev. *24*, 509–581 (1972)

Burnstock, G.: ATP and purinergic transmission. Neurotransmission, Vol. II, pp. 49–59. Proc. VI th Int. Cong. Pharmacol. Helsinki 1975

Burnstock, G., Campbell, G., Rand, M.J.: The inhibitory innervation of the taenia of the guinea-pig caecum. J. Physiol. (Lond.) *182*, 504–526 (1966)

Christensen, J.: Pharmacology of the oesophagus, Chap. 108, pp. 2325–2330. Handbook of physiology, Sect. 6, Alimentary canal, Vol. IV, Motility. Am. Physiol. Soc. 1968

Clark, C.G., Vane, J.F.: The cardiac sphincter of the cat. Gut *2*, 252–262 (1961)

Clark, C.G., Curnow, V.J., Murray, J.G., Stephens, F.D., Wylie, J.H.: Mode of action of histamine in causing gastric secretion in man. Gut *5*, 537–545 (1964)

Collier, B., Exley, K.A.: Mechanism of the antagonism by TEA of neuromuscular block due to *d*-tubocurarine or calcium deficiency. Nature (Lond.) *199*, 702–703 (1963)

Corne, S.J., Edge, N.D.: Pharmacological properties of pempidine (1:2:2:6:6:pentamethylene piperidine) a new ganglion-blocking compound. Br. J. Pharmacol. *13*, 339–349 (1958)

Crema, A.: On the polarity of the peristaltic reflex in the colon. In: Smooth muscle, pp. 342–348. Bulbring, E. et al. (eds.). London: Edward Arnold 1970

Daniel, E.E.: Pharmacology of the gastrointestinal tract, Chap. 108, pp. 2267–2324. Handbook of physiology, Sect. 6, Alimentary canal, Vol. IV, Motility. Am. Physiol. Soc. 1968

Della Bella, D., Rognoni, F.: Neurovegetative control of gastric motility in the isolated nerve-stomach preparation of the rat. J. Pharmacol. Exp. Ther. *134*, 184–189 (1961)

Douglas, W.W., Lywood, D.W.: The stimulant effect of tetraethylammonium on acetylcholine output from the superior cervical ganglion. Fed. Proc. *20*, 324 (1961)

Douthwaite, A.H., Thorne, M.G.: The effects of hexamethonium on the stomach. Br. Med. J. *1951 I*, 111–114

Dzoljic, M.: Stimulatory effect of tolazoline on smooth muscle. Br. J. Pharmacol. *30*, 203–212 (1967)

Emmelin, N.: Supersensitivity due to prolonged administration of ganglion-blocking compounds. Br. J. Pharmacol. *14*, 229–233 (1959)

Emmelin, N.: Pharmacology of the salivary glands. Chap. 39, pp. 669–678. Handbook of physiology, Sect. 6, Alimentary tract, Vol. II. Secretion. Am. Physiol. Soc. 1967

Feldberg, W.: Effects of ganglion-blocking substances on small intestine. J. Physiol. (Lond.) *113*, 483–505 (1951)

Feldberg, W., Lin, R.C.Y.: The action of local anaesthetics and *d*-tubocurarine on the isolated intestine of the rabbit and guinea-pig. Br. J. Pharmacol. *4*, 33–44 (1949)

Fishlock, D.J., Parks, A.G.: A study of human colonic muscle in vitro. Br. Med. J. *1963 II*, 666–667

Fishlock, D.J., Parks, A.G.: The action of nicotine on the circular muscle of the human ileum and colon in vitro. Br. J. Pharmacol. *26*, 79–86 (1966)

Furness, J.B.: An examination of the nerve mediated, hyoscine resistant excitation of the guinea-pig colon. J. Physiol. (Lond.) *207*, 803–822 (1970)

Garg, K.N.: Tetraethylammonium chloride and hexamethonium bromide on intestinal movements of dog. Indian. J. Physiol. Pharmacol. *6*, 137–140 (1962)

Garg, K.N.: Effects of chlorisondamine and pentolinium on the motility of small intestine. Indian. J. Med. Res. *52*, 49–51 (1964)

Garg, K.N.: Effects of mecamylamine and pempidine on the motility of small intestine in different species of animals. Indian. J. Med. Res. *54*, 1057–1059 (1966)

Garrett, J.: Selective blockade of sympathetic and parasympathetic ganglia. Arch. Int. Pharmacodyn. *144*, 381–391 (1963)

Garry, R.C., Gillespie, J.S.: The responses of the musculature of the colon of the rabbit to stimulation in vitro of the parasympathetic and sympathetic outflows. J. Physiol. (Lond.) *128*, 557–576 (1955)

Gillespie, J.S., MacKenna, B.R.: The inhibitory action of nicotine on the rabbit colon. J. Physiol. (Lond.) *152*, 191–205 (1960)

Gregory, R.A.: Secretory mechanism of the gastrointestinal tract. London: Edward Arnold 1962

Grossman, M.I.: Neural and hormonal stimulation of gastric secretion of acid, Chap. 47, pp. 835–863. Handbook of physiology. Sect. 6, Vol. II, Secretion. Am. Physiol. Soc. 1968

Holton, D.: Pharmacology of gastrointestinal motility and secretion, Vols. I and II. International encyclopedia of pharmacology and therapeutics. London: Pergamon Press 1973

Hong, S.S., Chin, D.S., Hur, K.B.: Influence of hexamethonium and some dietary factors on human pancreatic and bile secretion. J. Appl. Physiol. *16*, 810–814 (1961)

Hukuhara, T., Mujake, T.: Intrinsic reflexes in the colon. Jpn. J. Physiol. 9, 49–55 (1959)

Ingelfinger, F.J.: Esophageal motility. Physiol. Rev. 38, 533 (1958)

Jarrett, R.J.: Action of nicotine on the rabbit muscular organ (ileo-colic sphincter). Br. J. Pharmacol. 18, 397–404 (1962)

Kay, A.W., Smith, A.N.: Effect of hexamethonium iodide on gastric secretion. Br. Med. J. 1950 I, 460–463

Klin, V.A.: The use of a ganglion-blocking agent – Sinapleg (pempidine) in X-ray diagnosis of duodenal ulcer. Klin. Med. (Mosk.) 43, 66–69 (1965) (Russ.)

Klinge, F.W.: Behaviour of isolated intestinal segments without one or both plexuses. Am. J. Physiol. 164, 284–293 (1951)

Kosterlitz, H.W., Lees, G.M.: Pharmacological analysis of intrinsic intestinal reflexes. Pharmacol. Rev. 16, 301–339 (1964)

Lane, A., Robertson, C.R., Grossman, M.I.: Tetraethylammonium and gastric motility of the dog. Fed. Proc. 8, 91 (1949)

Lee, C.Y.: The effect of stimulation of extrinsic nerves on peristalsis and on release of 5-hydroxytryptamine in the large intestine of the guinea-pig and of the rabbit. J. Physiol. (Lond.) 152, 405–418 (1960)

Little, J.M., Ogle, B.C., Yeagley, J.D., Cager, D.: Effects of tetraethylammonium on experimental gastric ulceration in the rat. Science 106, 448–449 (1947)

Locket, S.: Paralytic ileus after hexamethonium. Br. Med. J. 1951 I, 1331–1332

Luco, J.V., Marconi, J.: Effects of tetraethylammonium bromide on the parasympathetic neuroeffector system. J. Pharmacol. Exp. Ther. 95, 171–176 (1949)

Lyons, R.H., Moe, G.K., Neligh, R.B., Hoobler, S.W., Campbell, K.N., Berry, R.L., Rennick, B.R.: The effects of blockade of the autonomic ganglia in man with tetraethylammonium. Am. J. Med. Sci. 213, 315–322 (1947)

MacDonald, J.R., Smith, A.N.: Effect of tetraethylammonium bromide on gastric secretion and motility. Br. Med. J. 1949 II, 620–622

Magee, D.F., Fragola, L.A., White, T.T.: Influence of parasympathetic innervation on the volume of pancreatic juice. Ann. Surg. 161, 15–20 (1965)

Mason, D.F.J., Wien, R.: The actions of heterocyclic bis-quaternary compounds especially of a pyrrolidinium series. Br. J. Pharmacol. 10, 124–132 (1955)

Mathews, E.K.: Central depressant drugs and acetylcholine release. Ph. D. Thesis, University of London, 1961

Mathews, E.K., Quilliam, J.P.: Effects of central depressant drugs upon acetylcholine release. Br. J. Pharmacol. 22, 415–440 (1964)

Milne, M.D., Rowe, G.G., Somers, K., Muehuke, R.C., Crawford, M.A.: Observations on the pharmacology of mecamylamine. Clin. Sci. 16, 599–614 (1957)

Moe, G.K., Freyburger, W.A.: Ganglion-blocking agents. Pharmacol. Rev. 2, 61–95 (1950)

Mohay, S., Geher, F.: Pharmacoradiographic studies of the stomach with pempidine. Ther. Hung. 11, 20–23 (1963)

Nakajima, S., Magee, D.F.: The effect of hexamethonium on gastric acid and pepsin response to pentagastrin, histamine, and AHR 602. Eur. J. Pharmacol. 10, 277–282 (1970)

Neely, J., Catchpole, B.: Ileus: the restoration of alimentary tract motility by pharmacological means. Br. J. Surg. 58, 21–28 (1971)

Neligh, R.B., Holt, J.F., Lyons, R.H., Hoobler, S.W., Moe, G.K.: Effects of tetraethylammonium chloride on the human gastrointestinal tract. Gastroenterology 12, 275–289 (1949)

Norberg, K.A.: Adrenergic innervation of the intestinal wall studied by fluorescence microscopy. Int. J. Neuropharmacol. 3, 379–382 (1964)

Northup, D.W., Stickney, J.C., Vanliere, E.J.: Effect of atropine tetraethylammonium, Banthine and Bantyl on motility of the small intestine. Am. J. Physiol. 171, 513–515 (1952)

Odori, Y., Magee, D.F.: The actions of some agents active at autonomic ganglionic sites on the secretory response of the Heidenhain pouch to various stimuli. Eur. J. Pharmacol. 8, 221–227 (1969)

Paton, W.D.M.: Transmission and block in autonomic ganglia. Pharmacol. Rev. 6, 59–68 (1954)

Paton, W.D.M., Zaimis, E.J.: The pharmacological actions of polymethylene bis-trimethylammonium salts. Br. J. Pharmacol. 4, 381–400 (1949)

Paton, W.D.M., Zaimis, E.J.: Paralysis of autonomic ganglia by methonium salts. Br. J. Pharmacol. *6*, 155–168 (1951)

Paton, W.D.M., Zaimis, E.J.: The methonium compounds. Pharmacol. Rev. *4*, 219–253 (1952)

Perry, W.L.M., Wilson, C.W.M.: The relative effects of ganglion-blocking compounds on the sympathetic and parasympathetic ganglia supplying the cat heart. Br. J. Pharmacol. *11*, 81–87 (1956)

Plummer, A.J., Barrett, W.E., Rutledge, R.: Some actions of chlorisondamine dimethochloride (Su 3088) (Ecolid) on the gastrointestinal tract. J. Pharmacol. *116*, 46 (1956)

Preshaw, R.M.: Integration of nervous and hormonal mechanisms for external pancreatic secretions, Chap. 56, pp. 997–1005. Handbook of physiology, Sect. 6, Alimentary canal, Vol. II, Secretion. Am. Physiol. Soc. 1968

Robertson, C.R., Blickenstaff, D., Grossman, M.I.: The effect of tetraethylammonium chloride on gastric secretion in the dog. J. Pharmacol. *100*, 194–199 (1950)

Scott, L.D.W., Kay, A.W., O'Hare, M.M., Simpson, J.A.: Hexamethonium in duodenal ulcer. Br. Med. J. *1950 II*, 1470–1472

Susuki, T., Nishiyama, A., Inomata, H.: Effect of tetraethylammonium ion on the electrical activity of smooth muscle cells. Nature (Lond.) *197*, 908–909 (1963)

Toyama, T., Yokoyama, I., Nishi, K.: Effect of hexamethonium and other ganglion-blocking agents on electrical activity of the oesophagus induced by vagal stimulation in the dog. Eur. J. Pharmacol. *31*, 63–71 (1975)

Thomas, J.E.: Neural regulation of pancreatic secretion, Chap. 54, pp. 955–968. Handbook of physiology, Sect. 6, Alimentary canal, Vol. II, Secretion. Am. Physiol. Soc. 1968

Varagic, V.: The effect of tolazoline and other substances on the response of the isolated colon of the rabbit to nerve stimulation. Arch. Int. Pharmacodyn. *106*, 141–150 (1965)

Weisbrodt, N.W., Hug, C.C., Schmiege, S.K., Bass, P.: Effect of nicotine and tyramine on contractile activity of the colon. Eur. J. Pharmacol. *12*, 310–319 (1970)

Weisenthal, L.M., Hug, C.C., Weisbrodt, N.W., Bass, P.: Adrenergic mechanisms in the relaxation of guinea-pig taenia coli in vitro. J. Pharmacol. *178*, 497–508 (1971)

Wells, H.: Inhibition by surgical procedures and drugs of the accelerated growth of salivary glands of rats. Am. J. Physiol. (Lond.) *199*, 1037–1040 (1960)

Wien, R., Mason, D.F.J.: Some actions of hexamethonium and certain homologues. Br. J. Pharmacol. *6*, 611–629 (1951)

Zweig, M., Steigmann, F., Meyer, K.A.: The effect of tetraethylammonium chloride on gastric motility and on the unstimulated, and histamine stimulated, gastric secretion. Gastroenterology *11*, 200–207 (1948)

CHAPTER 8

Absorption, Distribution, Fate, and Excretion of Ganglion-Blocking Compounds

D. F. J. MASON

A. Introduction

It has been said of the ganglion-blocking drugs that "many of the features of absorption, distribution and excretion of these drugs are predictable from a knowledge of their physical and chemical properties" (DOLLERY, 1964). While this may be true as a generalisation, there are still aspects that are incompletely understood. The non-depolarising ganglion-blocking compounds are divisible into two groups according to their physical and chemical properties and the major characteristics of their absorption, etc. Within each group the responses are essentially similar. The first is the onium group, which includes tetraethylammonium, hexamethonium, pendiomid, pentolinium, chlorisondamine and trimethaphan. These are compounds that are completely ionised in aqueous solution. The second group is represented by the secondary amine mecamylamine and the tertiary amine pempidine. Although this group of compounds all have high pKa values, so that at physiological pH they are very largely ionised, there is still some un-ionized compound present in aqueous solution.

B. Onium Compounds

I. Absorption

With the exception of the fate of trimethaphan and the mode of excretion of tetraethylammonium, the onium ganglion-blocking drugs appear to be similar in their absorption, distribution, and excretion so that conclusions drawn from experiments with one compound can be applied to other members of the group. Using the chemical assay procedure then available, RENNICK et al. (1947) were able to recover 64–68% of a parenterally administered dose of tetraethylammonium from the urine, while MILNE and OLEESKY (1951) were able to recover 74–104% of an intramuscular dose of hexamethonium. They concluded that the drug was readily absorbed, then excreted quantitatively, there being no important destructive process in the body. PATON and ZAIMIS (1952), HARRINGTON (1953), and BERDERKA et al. (1971) studied the absorption of drugs (including hexamethonium) administered intramuscularly and concluded that the limiting factor for absorption was the blood flow.

Once absorbed, hexamethonium is distributed evenly through the extracellular fluid, is not metabolised, and is excreted by glomerular filtration (MORRISON and PATON, 1953; MILNE and OLEESKY, 1951). It is on the basis of these conclusions that oral absorption was estimated by measuring the renal excretion of the compound.

Comparison of the oral LD_{50} and parenteral LD_{50} for all members of this group had yielded ratios that varied from 17 to 56, but were all large enough to suggest poor absorption by the oral route (BEIN and MEIER, 1951; PLUMMER et al., 1955; STONE et al., 1956). Only 4–16% of an oral dose of tetraethylammonium was excreted in the urine of normal man (RENNICK et al., 1947). Following oral administration to rabbit only 15–27% of a dose of hexamethonium was excreted in the urine (WIEN and MASON, 1951). In man, between 0.2 and 33.8% of an oral dose was excreted, as against 93% of an intramuscular dose, and 96% of a series of subcutaneous doses.

Similar results were obtained by other workers, using all the compounds in the group. The need to give much higher doses by the oral than by the parenteral route to produce comparable hypotensive effects confirmed these results.

The proportion of an oral dose that is absorbed is not so important as the regularity of that absorption. The absorption of the onium compounds from the gastrointestinal tract is notably variable. Several factors that affect the absorption have been identified. KAY and SMITH (1950), HARRINGTON (1953) and ROSENHEIM (1954) all showed that the absorption of hexamethonium varied according to the salt used. Oral administration of the bromide salt caused twice as much hexamethonium to appear in the urine as was found after the chloride, bitartrate or methane sulphate. The effectiveness and absorption of these compounds also varied widely with the relative timing of meals and doses. HARRINGTON (1953) found the fasting subject excreted 3–30 times more of the oral dose than a subject who had eaten 2 h before it, and this finding was confirmed by ROSENHEIM (1954) and SMIRK (1953). Most an of oral dose (average 75%) can be recovered from the faeces during the subsequent 48 h (HARRINGTON, 1953; MILNE and OLEESKY, 1951) while total recovery from urine and faeces ranged from 69–86%.

Although such a high proportion of the dose remained in the intestine, absorption seemed to be relatively brief in that maximal urinary excretion occurred at 2 h, while by 12 h excretion had fallen to a very low level, and none could be detected at 24 h. However, if gut movements ceased completely, there was continued absorption (ROSENHEIM, 1954).

LEVINE and her co-workers, studying the absorption of monoquaternary compounds from the intestine of the rat, found a similar rapid initial absorption, which soon declined. Total absorption over 24 h was 10–20% of the dose (LEVINE et al., 1955). Absorption was greatest in the segment of intestine closest to the pylorus. They concluded that the poor absorption was due to the formation of a nonabsorbable complex with mucin, but other substances administered concurrently could also reduce the absorption (LEVINE and PELIKAN, 1961; LEVINE, 1961). In their experiments, absorption of hexamethonium showed a similar pattern of rapid onset and then a decline, but it continued for longer.

It is usually assumed that absorption of foreign substances from the gastrointestinal tract only occurs with non-ionised lipid soluble forms (SCHANKER, 1971). However, these onium compounds are at least partly absorbed, although they are completely ionised and not lipid-soluble. In their studies with monoquaternary compounds, LEVINE and PELIKAN (1961) showed that absorption was not a simple function of dose, and some undefined process is involved, perhaps facilitated diffusion.

II. Distribution

The volume of distribution of the onium compounds corresponds closely to the volume of the extracellular fluid (YOUNG et al., 1951; PATON and ZAIMIS, 1952; MORRISON and PATON, 1953; MONGE et al., 1954). Examination of individual tissues from mice showed that initially, hexamethonium was distributed uniformly to most of the tissues including skeletal muscle and some adipose tissue, but not to brain. After an hour the concentration in muscle had declined to about 20% of the initial value, while the concentrations in the other tissues had declined little (LEVINE and CLARK, 1957; LEVINE, 1960).

McISAAC (1962) re-examined the distribution of hexamethonium to determine which of its aspects was related to pharmacological activity. Isotopically labelled hexamethonium, in a dose of 5 mg/kg body wt., was injected intravenously to cats. The compound rapidly entered most of the tissues but, except in the kidney, the distribution was primarily in the extracellular fluid. In nephrectomised preparations, or when the compound was continuously infused, the tissue-to-plasma concentration ratio did not reach unity but increased with time, suggesting that some drug had slowly moved into cells. The lowest concentrations were in brain, spinal cord, and cerebrospinal fluid, and the highest concentration was in the kidney. Autoradiographs of the kidney showed that the compound had entered the tubule cells of the cortex. The regression lines for the disappearance of the compound from ganglia and muscle could be resolved into two components. The first component was similar to that for plasma, but the second component was much slower. The disappearance of hexamethonium from kidney, brain, and liver was slow and the rate constants did not differ significantly from zero over a period of 8 h. No radioactivity was detected in the expired air and the total amount of hexamethonium recovered from the extracellular fluid, kidney, and urine represented 91.3% of the dose.

Chromatography of the recovered compound confirmed that it was similar to the starting material, suggesting that no significant metabolism of the drug had occurred. The author also compared the pharmacological response to the drug with the plasma concentration and concluded that there was a relationship. He could detect no relationship between pharmacological activity and the concentration of hexamethonium in the brain.

Almost since the earliest studies with ganglion-blocking compounds there had been suggestions that the locus of their hypotensive action was the central nervous system. Comparison of the traffic in the splanchnic nerve with the fall in blood pressure produced by a variety of quaternary ammonium compounds suggested that they were reduced concomitantly (DONATS and NICKERSON, 1956). However, using cross-circulation experiments, MURRAY et al. (1959) concluded that the administration of ganglion-blocking compounds (quaternary and non-quaternary) to the circulation to the head did not produce the characteristic fall in blood pressure, but this was readily produced if the drug was injected into the circulation to the body. All these experiments were acute and the period of observation limited. In clinical use the drugs are administered over long periods, and therefore some interest attached to the determination of the entry of the drugs into the central nervous system. This interest was sharpened by the observation of HALEY and McCORMICK (1957) that intracisternal injections of hexamethonium in the mouse caused Parkinsonian muscle tremors and vasodilatation, while FADHEL and SEAGER (1969) showed in dog that intracisternal injections of hexamethonium and trimethaphan prevented the pressor response to intracisternal veratrine.

LEVINE (1959) injected hexamethonium intravenously rats in a near-lethal dose of 75 mg/kg body wt. (in divided doses) and found that the ratio of concentrations in brain and blood was 0.19 at 30 min and 0.13 at 60 min. She suggested that sufficient hexamethonium was reaching the brain to produce the hypotensive effects. McISAAC (1962) used a dose of 5 mg/kg intravenously, which is nearer to the therapeutic or hypotensive dose, and showed that in cats a small amount of hexamethonium entered the brain, spinal cord, and cerebrospinal fluid quite quickly, but the rate of removal was negligible although recovery from the hypotensive response was complete in 2 h, as was recovery of the response to stimulation of the peripheral vagus and recovery from the block of transmission in the superior cervical ganglion.

While these studies made it seem unlikely that hexamethonium exerted its hypotensive effect through an action on the central nervous system, there was no definition either of the route by which the ionised compound had crossed the blood-brain barrier to reach the central nervous system, or of the fate of the compound.

SCHANKER et al. (1962) injected hexamethonium, decamethonium, and N^1-methylnicotinamide into the lateral cerebral ventricles of rabbits and found that these compounds left the cerebrospinal fluid more rapidly than could be accounted for by diffusion into the blood vessels and filtration through the arachnoid villi. Further, N^1-methylnicotinamide depressed the efflux of the other compounds, suggesting competition for a specific transport system. In vitro, the isolated rabbit choroid plexus took up the same three compounds against a concentration gradient and by a saturable process that could be inhibited by metabolic inhibitors. Both decamethonium and N^1-methylnicotinamide acted as competitive inhibitors of hexamethonium uptake. Similar transport processes were found in the choroid plexus of dog, cat, and guinea-pig, (TOCHINO and SCHANKER, 1965).

Thus, although the blood-brain and blood-cerebrospinal fluid barriers generally have the characteristics of lipoid membranes that are resistant to the passage of ionised substances, (RALL, 1971), it seemed possible that hexamethonium might reach the cerebrospinal fluid and perhaps the central nervous system, but was rapidly removed so that only a minimal concentration remained. GOSLING and LU (1969) injected four tritiated methonium compounds intramuscularly into rats, and after 4 h examined the brain, the cerebrospinal fluid, and the blood. The dose was 0.8 ml $10^{-2} M$ solution/kg body wt., which approaches the therapeutic dose for hexamethonium. The central nervous system had a higher affinity for the longer-chain compounds (hexa-, octa-, and decamethonium), which was unrelated to the plasma concentration measured 4 h after administration of the drug. Autoradiography of animals injected with hexa- and decamethonium showed that the radioactivity was associated with cells forming the choroid plexuses and the arachnoid. The authors pointed out that conclusive evidence of drug penetration into either cerebrospinal fluid or central nervous system had not been established. It also follows that the route by which these compounds reached these cells had not been established.

ROTH and BARLOW (1964) used autoradiography to demonstrate that quaternary compounds could be taken up into the central nervous system ASGHAR and ROTH (1971 a) re-examined the problem, using intravenous injections of 10–30 mg isotopically labelled hexamethonium/kg body wt., and examining the central nervous system at intervals of 5–60 min after injection. It was found that the compound penetrated various brain regions within 5 min in "pharmacologically significant amounts". Lower concentrations were found in the arachnoid pia and in the choroid plexus, but some of the radioactivity was also found to be associated with cellular elements of the central nervous system.

Thus, variations in technique, particularly dosage and interval after dosage, have generated series of data that are not easy to co-ordinate and several problems that are unanswered:

1. If hexamethonium does penetrate the central nervous system, by what route does it enter? ASGHAR and ROTH (1971a) suggested that one of the routes may be across the blood capillary-cerebrospinal fluid barrier located partly in the choroid plexus.

2. If hexamethonium does penetrate the central nervous system, is this property shared by other onium ganglion-blocking compounds? GOSLING and LU (1969) showed that some short-chain compounds are either not taken up or are rapidly removed from the central nervous system.

3. If hexamethonium does penetrate the central nervous system, does it exert any pharmacological effect at the concentration reached? The experiments of MURRAY et al. (1959) and of McISAAC (1962) suggest not.

In a second study concurrent with their studies on the central nervous system, ASGHAR and ROTH (1971b) showed that labelled hexamethonium accumulated in certain avascular cartilaginous tissues. There was little radioactivity in compact bone or in marrow of the femur. Cellular autoradiograms and histochemistry showed that the localisation was in areas rich in polysaccharides.

YOUNG (1952, 1953) studied the permeability of the rabbit placenta and showed that from day 23 to day 31, hexamethonium administered to the mother was transferred from the maternal to the foetal circulation. Equilibrium was never reached because the hexamethonium was excreted into the amniotic fluid, presumably through the foetal urine.

III. Excretion

After oral administration the majority of the dose was excreted in the faeces, and it was assumed that this material was unabsorbed drug, particularly as the majority of a parenterally administered dose was excreted in the urine. The possibility remained that some of the compound might be absorbed and then excreted in the bile. It fell to LEVINE and CLARK (1957) and LEVINE (1960) to demonstrate that no more than 3–4% of a parenterally administered dose of hexamethonium was excreted in the bile of rats. McISAAC (1962) confirmed that this is not an important route of elimination in the cat.

Many investigations have been made into the fate of the onium compounds, and all the investigators agree that, with the exception of trimethaphan, the compounds are eliminated by the kidney (e.g., RENNICK et al., 1947; ZAIMIS, 1950; MILNE and OLEESKY, 1951; WIEN and MASON, 1951; YOUNG et al., 1951; PATON and ZAIMIS, 1952; WIEN and MASON, 1953; HARRINGTON, 1953; ROSENHEIM, 1954; LEVINE, 1960). The bis-quaternary compounds are eliminated by glomerular filtration, since comparison of hexamethonium clearance with inulin clearance reveals a ratio of 1.1–1.2 in man, and comparison with creatinine clearance gives a ratio of 0.917 in cats (YOUNG et al., 1951; MCISAAC, 1962). However, this is not the only process occurring in the kidney. MCISAAC (1962, 1965) showed that hexamethonium was taken up by the kidneys of cats after an intravenous dose of 5 mg/kg. Autoradiography showed that the compound was retained in tubule cells of the renal cortex. In vitro, slices from the cortex of cat kidneys accumulated hexamethonium from the surrounding medium to give a tissue-to-medium ratio of 12. This uptake could be antagonised by metabolic inhibitors and by other quaternary compounds such as tetraethylammonium. Rabbit and rat kidney slices could not accumulate the compound in much above the concentration in the medium. A series of investigations reviewed by PETERS (1960) had shown that tetramethylammonium was secreted into the tubular urine of birds and mammals, probably by the cells of the proximal tubule (RENNICK and MOE, 1960) and this accounted for the brevity of its action (RENNICK et al., 1947). MCISAAC (1969) re-examined the problem, using renal cortex slices of rats, rabbits, chickens, dogs, and cats, and comparing the uptake of a series of bis-quaternary methonium compounds, tetraethylammonium, and N^1-methylnicotinamide. Great variability was found both in the uptake of different compounds, and in the uptake capacity of tissue from different species. He concluded that the bis-quaternary compounds were transported into renal cells by a mechanism involved in organic base transport, but that the rate of loss from the cells was low. It therefore seems likely that tubular secretion is not an important route for the elimination of onium compounds other than tetraethylammonium.

Trimethaphan is an exception to the pattern of elimination shown by the other onium compounds. This compound has a very brief action, indicating a very rapid elimination or metabolism. GERTNER et al. (1955) examined the urinary excretion of trimethaphan in seven patients receiving intravenous infusions of the drug and were only able to recover 31% of the total dose. They also showed in cats that neither intraportal administration nor exclusion of the liver or kidneys from the circulation altered the duration of action of the compound. They proposed a rapid destruction by some undetected extrahepatic and extrarenal mechanism. FRANCHI (1957) carried out similar experiments in rabbits and observed a prolongation of the action if either the liver or the kidneys were excluded from the circulation. AQUILAR and BOLDREY (1960) observed a toxic effect on the proximal tubules of monkeys when large doses of trimethaphan were administered. They postulated that this was related to a mechanism for the tubular secretion of the compound.

C. Secondary and Tertiary Amines

I. Absorption

This group of compounds is represented by the secondary amine mecamylamine, which has a pK_a of 11.3, and by the tertiary amine pempidine, with a pK_a of 10.4. The dissociation constant, and the lipid solubility of the un-ionised drug, are the most important determinants of the absorption of organic electrolytes. With a pK_a value of this order it might be expected that absorption would be slow and perhaps incomplete (SCHANKER, 1962, 1971).

Comparison of the toxicity by oral and parenteral routes and comparison of the doses that are effective by oral and parenteral routes suggested that both compounds were well, if not completely absorbed (STONE et al., 1956a; STONE et al., 1956b; FORD et al., 1956; CORNE and EDGE, 1958; SPINKS et al., 1958).

In a series of studies of gastrointestinal absorption in rat, it was confirmed that the gastrointestinal mucosa is predominantly a lipoid barrier; that acidic drugs are well absorbed from the stomach: that absorption from the intestine and colon is rapid for substances with pK_a values of 3–8 and much slower outside this range. In a further study on rates of absorption it was concluded that there was a slightly acidic environment at the intestine-blood barrier (SCHANKER et al., 1957, 1958; SCHANKER, 1959; HOGBEN et al., 1959).

When a solution of mecamylamine was passed once through the intestine, only 2–3% was absorbed, whatever part of the gastrointestinal tract was used. When the drug was perfused continuously through the intestine the absorption increased to 25% of the drug administered. In the dog, no mecamylamine was absorbed from Heidenhain pouches, but the compound was well absorbed from the small intestine (ZAWOISKI et al., 1958). When single doses of mecamylamine were administered orally to animals and man, renal elimination commenced quickly, reached a maximum in 2–4 h, and continued for more than 24 h. The total renal excretion varied from 50–75% of the dose administered (ALLENBY and TROUNCE, 1957; BAER et al., 1956). When the compound was administered by mouth daily over periods of up to 6 months, the urinary recovery averaged 60% of the drug administered (MILNE et al., 1957).

Studies in which pempidine was administered orally, and the renal elimination measured, also showed that a high proportion of the dose was absorbed. In rats the excretion was rapid and more complete than mecamylamine, with a urinary recovery of 40–45% of low doses and 70–80% of high doses (MUGGLETON and READING, 1959). In man a single oral dose was rapidly absorbed, with the plasma level reaching a maximum in 2 h and falling to a low value in 6 h (DOLLERY et al., 1960). After a single intravenous dose to man, 76% was recovered, as against 63% after an oral dose. No drug could be detected in the faeces after the oral dose. With continuous oral administration the recovery rate rose to 95% (HARRINGTON et al., 1958).

II. Distribution

The plasma concentrations of these compounds were very low, suggesting that the volume of distribution was greatly in excess of the extracellular fluid volume. After single doses both compounds were distributed throughout the tissues, with the highest concentrations in kidney, liver, and spleen, and the lowest concentrations in brain and skeletal muscle. The compounds penetrated into the cerebrospinal fluid, crossed the placenta to the foetus, and could be found in saliva and breast milk (MILNE et al., 1957; MUGGLETON and READING, 1959). These authors also concluded there was no evidence that the drugs were metabolised.

In dogs with Heidenhain pouches, mecamylamine accumulated in the gastric juice to give a concentration 20–40 times that in the plasma. No drug was secreted into the small intestine (STONE et al., 1956; ZAWOISKI et al., 1958).

In the blood the compounds were partly bound to protein (mecamylamine, 25%; pempidine, 1.2%) and partly taken up by erythrocytes. The erythrocyte-plasma concentration ratio was 1.15 for mecamylamine and 1.2 for pempidine.

The evidence that the compounds penetrate into cells has resulted in suggestions that, unlike the onium compounds, they are active at an intracellular site (BENNETT et al., 1957; VOLLE, 1969), although it has also been suggested that the mechanism of action of these compounds and that of the onium compounds is the same (MCISAAC and MILLERSCHOEN, 1963). If the compounds enter the cells by passive diffusion of the un-ionised form, as has been suggested for other biological membranes, the total intracellular concentration of the ionised and nonionised compound will depend in part upon the intracellular pH. BROWN and his colleagues have looked at a parallel problem, the intracellular uptake of nicotine. They found that in rat sympathetic ganglia the uptake differed significantly from the predicted value based upon the pK of nicotine and the intracellular pH of 7.33, which was derived from the ratio of the intracellular-to-extra cellular concentrations of a weak acid, 5,5-dimethyloxazolidine-2,4-dione. When the intracellular pH was calculated instead from the distribution of nicotine, a value of 6.63 was obtained if depolarisation of the ganglia was prevented with hexamethonium, or 6.54 in the absence of hexamethonium (BROWN and HALLIWELL, 1972). They proposed that the cell contained two compartments, an acid cytoplasm with an approximate pH of 6.6, and a more alkaline nucleus and mitochondria. Their colleague GARTHWAITE (1976) has studied the uptake into rat ganglion cells of a series of weak acids and bases, and has confirmed that two values can be derived for the intracellular pH, depending on whether the value is calculated from the intracellular-to-extracellular distribution ratio of an acid or a base. He comments that, "because of cell acidity, basic drugs may accumulate in these cells to a much higher concentration than in the surrounding medium. This may have implications for their pharmacology and toxicity".

One of the implications of the intracellular accumulation of mecamylamine and pempidine is the provision of a large reservoir of the compound, leading to a longer and smoother action of the compounds. This intracellular store can also be mobilised by procedures that alter the acid-base balance. PAYNE and ROWE (1957) showed that when respiratory acidosis was induced in cats by inhalation of 10% carbon dioxide, the actions of mecamylamine on blood pressure and neuromuscular transmission were increased. This was accompanied by an increase in the plasma level of mecamylamine from 13 to 18 µg/ml and a fall in the erythrocyte-to-plasma concentration ratio from 1.12 to 0.83.

The ability of these compounds to cross membranes and their presence in the central nervous system (BRODIE et al., 1960) raised the possibility that the hypotensive effect was due to a central action. DHAWAN and BHARGAVA (1960) administered pempidine intravenously to dogs and cats in doses (25 µg) too small to produce ganglion block, and in doses of 50 µg into the cerebral ventricles of dogs. The drug caused an increase of several reflex pressor responses, which the authors regarded as due to central facilitation by the drug. When they studied the effects of mecamylamine injected into the cerebral ventricle or into the vertebral arteries, they observed hypotension and a depression of certain reflexes that normally produce a pressor response (BHARGAVA and DHAWAN, 1963). The apparently different effects of these two compounds when injected into the central nervous system, despite their similar actions when injected peripherally, and the low concentration in the central nervous system following parenteral injection, suggest that their normal action was not on the central nervous system. This is in keeping with the observation of MURRAY et al. (1959), using cross-circulation experiments, that doses of up to 2 mg/kg mecamylamine in the circulation to the head failed to cause a fall in blood pressure.

III. Excretion

The renal elimination of mecamylamine and pempidine varies according to the pH of the urine (STONE et al. 1956a and b; HARRINGTON et al., 1958). In the dog rendered acidotic with ammonium chloride, the elimination of mecamylamine was 4.2 times the glomerular filtration rate. In the dog rendered alkalotic with sodium bicarbonate, the elimination was only 0.07 times the glomerular filtration rate (BAER et al., 1956 b). Similar changes were observed with pempidine when ammonium chloride and sodium bicarbonate were used concurrently. Since the administration of acetazolamide also reduced the excretion of these compounds it became clear that the pH of the urine was the determining factor and not the systemic acidoses or alkalosis. It had been shown earlier that tetraethylammonium was actively secreted in the proximal tubule and it was now suggested that mecamylamine was actively secreted or reabsorbed, but by pH-sensitive processes (BAER et al., 1956a). Careful experimentation under rigid control, so that passive diffusion could not affect the results, succeeded in demonstrating competition between mecamylamine and the transport of N^1-methylnicotinamide or tetraethylammonium (PETERS, 1960; VOLLE et al., 1960) and also between mepiperphenidol and mecamylamine or pempidine elimination (TORRETI et al., 1962). It was demonstrated that this mechanism was not the same as that for PAH and was not inhibited by probenecid. Experiments where passive diffusion was not controlled failed to show either a limitation or a saturation of renal elimination with increased load (BAER et al., 1956a; SCHRIBNER et al., 1959), and increasing the urine flow with an osmotic diuretic caused increased excretion of mecamylamine and pempidine, (SCHRIBNER et al., 1959). Both these responses suggest that under normal conditions the change in elimination with change in pH is due to a nonionic diffusion and that this completely masks the effect of any active transport. In patients receiving daily doses of mecamylamine, MILNE et al. (1957) showed that acidification of the urine first caused an increase in the proportion of the dose excreted from 60 to 78%, but despite continued acidification of the urine the percentage had fallen almost to the control value by the third day. Conversely, continuous administration of sodium bicarbonate reduced excretion to 38% but this had risen to 55% by the third day. Taking these observations with the results in the control of the blood pressure, the authors concluded that they represented an increase in the body content of mecamylamine following alkalinisation of the urine, and a reduction of the body content following acidification of the urine.

HARRINGTON and KINCAID-SMITH (1958) reported that the administration of chlorothiazide increased the hypotensive action of mecamylamine. Renal clearance of mecamylamine fell from 70% to less than 55% averaged over three days. The mechanism of this action remained uncertain. In studies with chlorothiazide and the onium compounds pentolinium or tetraethylammonium, DOLLERY et al. (1959) and DUSTON et al. (1959) found some potentiation of the hypotensive effect but concluded that this was a reflection of a reduction in the plasma volume. When similar studies were carried out with pempidine (DOLLERY et al., 1961) found that in the presence of chlorothiazide the hypotensive action of pempidine was increased and the plasma concentration of pempidine rose by a factor of 2–3. However, this rise in plasma level was greater than might have been expected from the increase in the hypotensive effect. The ratio of erythrocyte to plasma concentration stabilised at 1.2 with pempidine alone but was 0.7 after chlorothiazide. These changes were at least partly reconciled when the protein binding was examined. Pempidine alone did not react with serum albumin to any measurable extent. Chlorothiazide alone was extensively bound. Pempidine and chlorothiazide together resulted in considerable protein binding of pempidine without any change in the binding of chlorothiazide. Examination of the renal excretion of pempidine showed that this was unchanged in the presence of chlorothiazide but renal clearance fell to one-third of its previous value. It has subsequently been suggested that chlorothiazide acts as a bridge between the cationic pempidine and the albumin (cf. LA DU et al., 1971).

References

Allanby, K.D., Trounce, J.R.: Excretion of mecamylamine after intravenous and oral administration. Br. Med. J. *1957 II*, 1219

Aquilar, J.A., Boldrey, E.F.: Effect of Arfonad (trimetaphan) on monkey. Anesthesiology *21*, 3–12 (1960)

Asghar, K., Roth, L.J.: Entry and distribution of hexamethonium in the central nervous system. Biochem. Pharmacol. *20*, 2787–2795 (1971 a)

Asghar, K., Roth, L.J.: Distribution of hexamethonium and other quarternary ammonium compounds in cartilage. J. Pharmacol. Exp. Ther. *176*, 83–92 (1971 b)

Baer, J.E., Paulson, S.F., Russo, H.F., Beyer, K.H.: Renal elimination of 3-methylaminoisocamphane HCL (mecanylamine). Am. J. Physiol. *186*, 180–186 (1956 a)

Baer, J.E., Paulson, S.F., Russo, H.F., Beyer, K.H.: Renal elimination of 3-methylaminoisocamphane hydrochloride (mecamylamine). J. Pharmacol. Exp. Ther. *116*, 2–3 (1956 b)

Berderka, J., Takernori, A.E., Miller, J.W.: Absorption rates of various substances administered intramuscularly. Eur. J. Pharmacol. *15*, 132–136 (1971)

Bein, H.J., Meier, R.: Pharmacological investigation of pendiomid: a new ganglion-blocking agent. Schweiz. Med. Wochenschr. *81*, 446 (1951)

Bennett, G., Tyler, C., Zaimis, E.J.: Mecamylamine and its mode of action. Lancet *1957 II*, 218–222

Bhargava, H.P., Dhawan, K.N.: Depression of the vasomotor centre by mecamylamine, independent of its ganglion-blocking activity. Br. J. Pharmacol. *21*, 39–44 (1963)

Brodie, B.B., Kurtz, H., Schanker, L.S.: The importance of dissociation constant and lipid-solubility in influencing the passage of drugs into the C.S.F. J. Pharmacol. Exp. Ther. *130*, 20–35 (1960)

Brown, D.A., Halliwell, J.V.: Intracellular pH in rat isolated superior cervical ganglia in relation to nicotine-depolarisation and nicotine uptake. Br. J. Pharmacol. *45*, 349–359 (1972)

Corne, S.J., Edge, N.D.: Pharmacological properties of pempidine (1:2:2:6:6:pentamethylene piperidine) a new ganglion-blocking compound. Br. J. Pharmacol. *13*, 339–349 (1958)

Dhawan, K.N., Bhargava, K.P.: Central vasomotor effects of a new ganglion-blocking agent, 1:2:2:6:6:pentamethylpiperidine (pempidine). Br. J. Pharmacol. *15*, 215–218 (1960)

Dollery, C.T.: Absorption, distribution and excretion of drugs used to treat bypertension. In: Absorption and distribution of drugs. Binns, T.B. (ed.), pp. 157–164. Edinburgh, London: E and S Livingstone 1964

Dollery, C.T., Harrington, M., Kaufman, G.: The mode of action of chlorothiazide in hypertension: with special reference to potentiation of ganglion blockers. Lancet 1959 I, 1215

Dollery, C.T., Emslie-Smith, D., Muggleton, D.F.: Plasma pempidine concentration in hypertensives. Br. Med. J. 1960 I, 521–523

Dollery, C.T., Emslie-Smith, D., Muggleton, D.F.: Action of chlorothiazide on the distribution, excretion, and hypotensive effects of pempidine in man. Br. J. Pharmacol. 17, 488–506 (1961)

Dontas, A.S., Nickerson, M.: Central and peripheral components of the actions of "ganglionic" blocking agents. J. Pharmacol. Exp. Ther. 120, 147–159 (1956)

Duston, H.P., Comming, G.R., Corcoran, A.C., Page, I.H.: A mechanism of chlorothiazide enhanced effectiness of antihypertensive ganglioplegic drugs. Circulation. 19, 360–365 (1959)

Fadhel, N., Seager, L.D.: Influence of hexamethonium intracisternally and hexamethonium and trimethaphan camphorsulfonate intravenously on the pressor response to intracisternal veratrine. Proc. Soc. Exp. Biol. Med. 131, 1263 (1969)

Ford, R.V., Madison, J.C., Moyer, J.M.: Pharmacology of mecamylamine. Am. J. Med. Sci. 232, 120–143 (1956)

Franchi, G.: The effect of hepatectomy and nephrectomy on the hypotension caused by trimetaphan camphorsulphonate. Minerva. Anestesid. 23, 194 (1957)

Garthwaite, J.: The uptake of weak acids and bases into isolated rat superior cervical ganglia in relation to intracellular pH. Br. J. Pharmacol. 56, 3, 353 P (1976)

Gertner, S.B., Little, D.M., Bonnycastle, D.D.: Urinary excretion of Arfonad by patients undergoing "controlled hypertension" during surgery. Anaesthesiology 16, 495–501 (1955)

Gosling, J.A., Lu, T.C.: Uptake and distribution of some quaternary ammonium compounds in the central nervous system of the rat. J. Pharmacol. Exp. Ther. 167, 56–62 (1969)

Haley, T.J., McCormick, W.G.: Pharmacological effects produced by intracerebral injection of drugs in the conscious mouse. Br. J. Pharmacol. 12, 12–15 (1957)

Harrington, M.: The absorption and excretion of hexamethonium salts. Clin. Sci. 12, 185–198 (1953)

Harrington, M., Kincaid-Smith, P.: Effect of chlorothiazide on the hypotensive action of mecamylamine and on its urinary excretion. Lancet 1958 I, 403–404

Harrington, M., Kincaid-Smith, P., Milne, M.D.: Pharmacology and clinical use of pempidine in the treatment of hypertension. Lancet 1958 II, 6–11

Hogben, C.A.M., Tocco, D.J., Brodie, B.B., Schanker, L.S.: On the mechanism of intestinal absorption of drugs. J. Pharmacol. Exp. Ther. 125, 275–282 (1959)

Kay, A.W., Smith, A.N.: Effects of oral hexamethonium salts on gastric secretion. Br. Med. J. 1950 II, 807–809

La Du, B.N., Mandel, H.G., Way, E.L.: Fundamentals of drug metabolism aand drug dispositon. Baltimore: Williams and Wilkins 1971

Levine, R.R.: Presence of certain onium compounds in brain tissue following intravenous administration to rats. Nature (Lond.) 184, 1412–1414 (1959)

Levine, R.R.: The physiological disposition of hexamethonium and related compounds. J. Pharmacol. Exp. Ther. 129, 296–304 (1960)

Levine, R.R.: The influence of the intraluminal intestinal milieu on the absorption of an organic cation and an anionic agent. J. Pharmacol. Exp. Ther. 131, 328–333 (1961)

Levine, R.R., Blair, M.R., Clark, B.B.: Factors influencing the intestinal absorption of certain monoquaternary anticholinergic compounds with special reference to benzomethamine N-diethylaminoethyl N^1-methyl benzilamide methobromide (M.C. 3199). J. Pharmacol. Exp. Ther. 114, 78–86 (1955)

Levine, R.R., Clark, B.B.: Physiologic disposition of hexamethonium and chemically related compounds. Fed. Proc. 16, 317 (1957)

Levine, R.R., Pelikan, E.W.: The influence of experimental procedures and dose on the intestinal absorption of an onium compound, benzomethamine. J. Pharmacol. Exp. Ther. 131, 319–327 (1961)

McIsaac, R.J.: The relationship between diposition and pharmacological activity of hexamethonium-N-methyl C^{14}. J. Pharmacol. Exp. Ther. 135, 335–343 (1962)

McIsaac, R.J.: The uptake of hexamethonium C^{14} by kidney slices. J. Pharmacol. Exp. Ther. 150, 92–98 (1965)

McIsaac, R.J.: The binding of organic bases to kidney cortex slices. J. Pharmacol. Exp. Ther. *168*, 6–12 (1969)

McIsaac, R.J., Millerschoen, N.R.: A comparison of the effects of mecamylamine and hexamethonium on transmission in the superior cervical ganglion of the cat. J. Pharmacol. Exp. Ther. *139*, 18–24 (1963)

Milne, G.E., Oleesky, S.: Excretion of the methonium compounds. Lancet *1951 I*, 889–890

Milne, M.D., Rowe, G.G., Somers, K., Muehrcke, R.C., Crawford, M.A.: Observations on the pharmacology of mecamylamine. Clin. Sci. *16*, 599–614 (1957)

Monge, C.C., Corcoran, A.C., del Greco, F., Page, I.H.: Volume of distribution of hexamethonium in nephrectomized dog. Am. J. Physiol. *178*, 256–258 (1954)

Morrison, B., Paton, W.D.M.: Effects of hexamethonium on normal individuals in relation to its concentration in the plasma. Br. Med. J. *1953 I*, 1299–1305

Muggleton, D.F., Reading, H.W.: Absorption, metabolism, and clearance of pempidine in the rat. Br. J. Pharmacol. *14*, 202–208 (1959)

Murray, R., Beck, L., Rondell, P.A., Bohr, D.F.: A study of the central action of ganglionic blocking agents. J. Pharmacol. Exp. Ther. *127*, 157–163 (1959)

Paton, W.D.M., Zaimis, E.J.: The methonium compounds. Pharmacol. Rev. *4*, 219–253 (1952)

Payne, J.P., Rowe, G.G.: The effects of mecamylamine in the cat as modified by the administration of carbon dioxide. Br. J. Pharmacol. *12*, 457–460 (1957)

Peters, L.: Renal tubular excretion of organic bases. Pharmacol. Rev. *12*, 1–35 (1960)

Plummer, A.J., Trappold, J.H., Schneider, J.A., Maxwell, R.A., Earl, A.R.: Ganglion blockade by a new bioquaternary series including chlorisondamine dimethochloride. J. Pharmacol. Exp. Ther. *115*, 173–184 (1955)

Rall, D.P.: Drug entry into brain and cerebrospinal fluid. In: Concepts in biochemical pharmacology, Part I, handbook of experimental pharmacology, Vol. XXVIII/1. Brodie, B.B., Gillette, J.R. (eds.). Berlin: Springer 1971

Rennick, B.R., Moe, G.K.: Stop-flow localisation of renal tubular excretion of tetraethylammonium. Am. J. Physiol. *198*, 1267–1270 (1960)

Rennick, B.R., Moe, G.K., Lyons, R.H., Hoobler, S.W., Neligh, R.: Absorption and renal excretion of the tetraethylammonium ion. J. Pharmacol. Exp. Ther. *91*, 210 (1947)

Rosenheim, M.L.: The treatment of severe hypertension. Br. Med. J. *1954 II*, 4898, 1181

Roth, L.J., Barlow, C.F.: Isotopes in experimental pharmacology, p.49. Chicago: University of Chicago Press 1964

Schanker, L.S.: Absorption of drugs from the rat colon. J. Pharmac. Exp. Ther. *126*, 283–290 (1959)

Schanker, L.S.: Passage of drugs across body membranes. Pharmacol. Rev. *14*, 501–530 (1962)

Schanker, L.S.: Absorption of drugs from the gastrointestinal tract. In: Concepts in biochemical pharmacology, Part I, handbook of experimental pharmacology, Vol. XXVIII/1. Brodie, B.B., Gillette, J.R. (eds.). Berlin: Springer 1971

Schanker, L.S., Shore, P.A., Brodie, B.B., Hogben, C.A.M.: Absorption of drugs from the stomach I. The Rat. J. Pharmacol. Exp. Ther. *120*, 528–539 (1957)

Schanker, L.S., Tocco, D.J., Brodie, B.B., Hogben, C.A.M.: Absorption of drugs from the rat small intestine. J. Pharmacol. Exp. Ther. *123*, 81–87 (1958)

Schanker, L.S., Prokop, L.D., Schou, J., Sisodia, P.: Rapid efflux of some quaternary ammonium compounds from cerebrospinal fluid. Life Sci. *1*, 515–521 and Erratum 659–611 (1962)

Schribner, B.H., Crawford, M.A., Dempster, W.J.: Urinary excretion by non-ionic diffusion. Am. J. Physiol. *196*, 1135–1140 (1959)

Smirk, F.H.: Action of a new methonium compound in arterial hypertension. Lancet *1953 I*, 457

Spinks, A., Young, E.H.P., Farrington, J.A., Dunlop, D.: The pharmacological actions of pempidine and its ethylhomologue. Br. J. Pharmacol. *13*, 501–520 (1958)

Stone, C.A., Baer, J.E., Zawoiski, E.J., Beyer, K.H.: Pharmacology and physiological disposition of 3-methylaminoisocamphane (mecamylamine): a secondary amine ganglion-blocking agent. Am. J. Med. Sci. *232*, 115 (1956a)

Stone, D.A., Torchiana, M.L., Navarro, A., Beyer, K.H.: Ganglionic-blocking properties of 3-methylamino-isocamphane hydrochloride, (mecamylamine) a secondary amine. J. Pharmacol. Exp. Ther. *117*, 169–183 (1956b)

Tochino, Y., Schanker, L.S.: Active transport of quaternary ammonium compounds by the choroid plexus, in vitro. Am. J. Physiol. *208*, 666–673 (1965)

Torretti, J., Weiner, I.M., Mudge, G.H.: Renal tubular secretion and reabsorption of organic bases in the dog. J. Clin. Invest. *41*, 793–804 (1962)

Volle, R.: Ganglionic transmission. Annu. Rev. Pharmacol. *9*, 135–146 (1969)

Volle, R., Green, R.E., Peters, L.: Renal tubular transport relationships between N^1-methylnicotinamide (NMN), mecamylamine, quinine, quinidine, and quinacrime in the avian kidney. J. Pharmacol. Exp. Ther. *129*, 388–393 (1960)

Wien, R., Mason, D.F.J.: Some actions of hexamethonium and certain homologues. Br. J. Pharmacol. *6*, 611–629 (1951)

Wien, R., Mason, D.F.J.: The pharmacological action of a series of phenyl alkaneβ-ω bis(trialkylammonium) compounds. Br. J. Pharmacol. *8*, 306–314 (1953)

Young, I.M.: The placental transfer of hexamethonium bromide in the rabbit and its appearance in the amniotic fluid. J. Physiol. (Lond.) *116*, 4 *P* (1952)

Young, I.: The placental transfer of hexamethonium bromide and the origin of amniotic fluid in the rabbit. J. Physiol. (Lond.) *122*, 93–101 (1953)

Young, I.M., de Wardener, H.E., Miles, B.E.: Mechanism of the renal excretion of methonium compounds. Br. Med. J. *1951 II*, 1500–1501 (1951)

Zaimis, E.J.: The synthesis of methonium compounds, their isolation from urine, and their photometric determination. Br. J. Pharmacol. *5*, 424 (1950)

Zawoiski, E.J., Baer, J.E., Braunschweig, L.W., Paulson, F., Shermer, A., Beyer, K.H.: Gastrointestinal secretion and absorption of 3-methylaminoisocamphane hydrochloride (mecamylamine). J. Pharmacol. Exp. Ther. *122*, 442–448 (1958)

CHAPTER 9

Nicotinic Ganglion-Stimulating Agents

R.L. VOLLE

A. Introduction

The classic subgrouping of cholinoceptive sites proposed by DALE is based on the different pharmacological properties of muscarine and nicotine. Stated in the simplest terms, a drug is said to be a nicotinic agonist when it causes the general biphasic pattern of excitation and depression of excitable tissues that is produced by nicotine. More rigorous definitions of nicotinic agonists include susceptibility to blockade by specific antagonists, of which hexamethonium and d-tubocurarine can be regarded as prototypical drugs. It is generally understood that the responses to nicotinic agents are resistant to blockade by atropine or adrenergic blocking drugs. It is in this context that the term nicotinic agent is used in this chapter.

The distribution of nicotinic receptive sites is widespread in the peripheral nervous system. Moreover, the nicotinic receptors are not always associated with synapses or junctions, and the distribution of nicotinic receptors, and hence the responsiveness of tissues to nicotinic agents, may bear little relationship to cholinergic transmission. In addition to the well-known localisation of nicotinic receptive sites on the postjunctional membrane of autonomic ganglia and the neuromuscular junction, it is well established that nicotine and related drugs activate receptive sites in non-myelinated vagal C-fibres, postanglionic sympathetic neurones and a large number of sensory nerve endings. At each of these non-synaptic sites the nicotinic agents cause excitation of the tissues manifest in depolarisation of the cells, the initiation of action potentials, or the blockade of axonal conduction. At each of these sites, the actions of the nicotinic drugs are prevented by hexamethonium given in concentrations that have no effect on the normal physiological activities of those tissues. It is of some importance that no difference exists in the dose of the nicotinic drugs required for producing threshold stimulation at sensory and ganglionic sites (VOLLE and KOELLE, 1975).

Like the peripheral neurones, various nerve terminals are also sensitive to the actions of nicotine. There is good evidence to show that preganglionic nerve terminals, adrenergic nerve endings, and motor nerve terminals possess cholinoceptive sites that can be activated by the nicotinic drugs *(vide infra)*. Whether or not the presynaptic receptors for acetylcholine and nicotinic agents are activated under physiological conditions by the transmitter is moot. However, there can be little doubt that they contribute to the overall pharmacological action of the nicotinic drugs. Therefore, in autonomic ganglia the actions of the nicotinic drugs may alter transmission by affecting transmitter release, the activation of subsynaptic nicotinic receptors, the activation of extrajunctional nicotinic receptors and depolarisation of the postganglionic axon.

Several thorough reviews have been published in recent years on various aspects of ganglionic transmission and ganglionic responses to drugs (KHARKEVICH, 1962, 1967; VOLLE, 1966 a, b, 1969, 1975; GYERMEK, 1967; TAUC, 1967; TRENDELENBURG, 1967; HAEFELY, 1972; KOSTERLITZ, 1972). The review by HAEFELY is of particular note.

B. Pharmacological Ambiguities of Ganglionic Receptors

In the traditional view, ganglionic transmission occurs *via* the activation of nicotinic receptors. The classification is based on the observation that drugs related to nicotine imitate, in a superficial way, a number of characteristics of ganglionic transmission. For example, like transmission, the stimulation of ganglion cells by the nicotinic drugs is prevented by drugs related to hexamethonium and *d*-tubocurarine. It has also been known for some time that drugs related to muscarine also stimulate mammalian sympathetic ganglia, and that, unlike the nicotinic drugs, the muscarinic drugs stimulate ganglion cells by mechanisms insensitive to blockade by hexamethonium but extremely sensitive to blockade by atropine. Included among the muscarinic drugs are muscarine, methacholine and pilocarpine (this Volume, Chap. 10).

Under normal conditions, small doses of atropine have no effect on transmission in mammalian sympathetic ganglia or on the response of the ganglia to the nicotinic drugs. Conversely, doses of hexamethonium or *d*-tubocurarine that depress ganglionic transmission do not block the firing evoked by muscarinic drugs.

In view of the foregoing, it is of some interest that several studies indicate either a lack of specificity of action for the ganglion-stimulating agents or an interaction between nicotinic and muscarinic ganglionic receptors. The depolarisation of frog ganglion cells produced by methacholine is blocked by either atropine or hexamethonium (GINSBORG, 1965). The muscarinic compound pilocarpine blocks transmission in frog ganglia but fails to stimulate or depolarise the ganglion cells. Although GINSBORG (1965) interprets these findings as an indication that there are no muscarinic receptors in sympathetic ganglia, the alternative interpretation that the blocking drugs do not discriminate between nicotinic and muscarinic receptors is also worth consideration. A similar lack of discrimination by the blocking agents is found in cat sympathetic ganglia (GEBBER and SNYDER, 1968) when tetramethylammonium is administered to the superior cervical ganglia by infusion at a constant rate. The firing produced by tetramethylammonium is blocked either by small doses of atropine or by hexamethonium. In a similar way, the ganglion-stimulating actions of choline are antagonised by both hexamethonium and atropine (KRSTIĆ, 1972), which has led to the suggestion that the cholinoceptive sites in the superior cervical ganglia are of an intermediate type with pharmacological characteristics of both nicotinic and muscarinic receptors. A number of α-, β-, and γ-substituted pyridylmethyltrimethylammonium ions stimulate both nicotinic and muscarinic receptors in the superior cervical ganglion of the cat (HAMILTON and RUBINSTEIN, 1968). The ratio of nicotinic to muscarinic activity varies within the series of compounds studied. Nonetheless, the findings are consistent with the notion that a clear distinction between nicotinic and muscarinic receptors in ganglia is not always possible. A similar conclusion was reached by BELESLIN and MALOBABIĆ (1974), who reported that cholinoceptive sites of intramural ganglia of guinea-pig ileum are of an intermediate type with properties of both sub-groups.

The conversion of muscarinic receptors to those sensitive to blockade by hexamethonium can be demonstrated in rat sympathetic ganglia perfused in situ with Locke's solution. The discharge evoked by acetylcholine in rat sympathetic ganglia with normal circulation contains two components. The first component occurring is depressed by hexamethonium and the late component is prevented by atropine. The combination of hexamethonium and atropine is required to prevent the total response to acetylcholine (HANCOCK and VOLLE 1970a). In ganglia perfused with Locke's solution, acetylcholine causes a bi-modal pattern of firing similar to that of normal ganglia. Small doses of atropine block the late, low-amplitude component of the response. In contrast to the results obtained with normal ganglia, however, hexamethonium also blocks the late component of the responses to acetylcholine.

ROSZKOWSKI (1961) described the stimulation of sympathetic ganglia caused by McN-A-343 as being unaffected by large doses of hexamethonium but depressed completely by small doses of atropine. JARAMILLO and VOLLE (1967b) demonstrated that the postganglionic discharge evoked by McN-A-343 in cat sympathetic ganglia contains two components, one sensitive to low doses of atropine and the other resistant to both atropine and hexamethonium. In the intact rat superior cervical ganglion, McN-A-343 causes a pattern of firing similar to that observed in the cat. Large doses of hexamethonium do not alter the pattern of firing caused by McN-A-343 and small doses of atropine partially block the McN-A-343-evoked discharge. The response to McN-A-343 remaining after atropine is not blocked either by the subsequent administration of hexamethonium in doses sufficient to abolish transmission or by higher doses of atropine (HANCOCK and VOLLE, 1970a). The pattern of the postganglionic discharge caused by McN-A-343 in perfused ganglia is indistinguishable from that occurring in the normally circulated ganglia. In perfused ganglia, however, the discharge is blocked completely by either atropine or hexamethonium (HANCOCK and VOLLE, 1970a).

The postganglionic discharges evoked by oxotremorine in cat are blocked by low doses of atropine and unaffected by hexamethonium (DE GROAT and VOLLE, 1963; JARAMILLO and VOLLE, 1967a). In the normally circulated ganglia of the rat, atropine completely blocks the firing caused by oxotremorine, whereas hexamethonium is without effect on the firing. By contrast, the oxotremorine-induced firing in perfused ganglia (Fig. 1) is blocked by either atropine or hexamethonium (HANCOCK and VOLLE, 1970a).

The finding that firing produced in perfused ganglia of the rat by muscarinic drugs is sensitive to blockade by either hexamethonium or atropine is difficult to explain. AMBACHE et al. (1956) reported that the response of perfused cat sympathetic ganglia to muscarine is sensitive to blockade by either hexamethonium or small doses of atropine. It is unlikely that the difference between perfused ganglia and ganglia with intact circulations can be attributed to differences in the delivery of drugs to the ganglia. Comparisons of ganglionic responses to hexamethonium and the nicotine-like drugs indicate that there are no differences in the amounts of the drugs required to cause a block of transmission or to cause firing in the two types of ganglia. The amounts of muscarine-like drugs required to cause firing in perfused ganglia are also indistinguishable from those of the normal ganglia. The additional

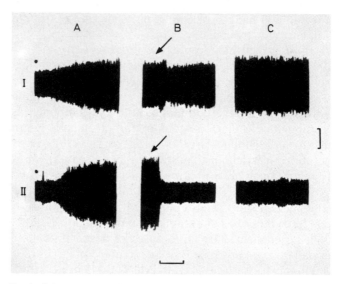

Fig. 1. Postganglionic firing produced in rat superior cervical ganglia by the muscarinic substance oxotremorine. The top row (I) shows the response to oxotremorine in a normal ganglion before, during (at *arrow*), and after the administration of a large dose of hexamethonium (1 mg). The bottom row (II) of records were obtained in a ganglia perfused with Locke's solution. Oxotremorine-induced firing was sensitive to blockade by a small dose of hexamethonium (0.1 mg). The vertical and horizontal calibrations are 20 μV and 5 s, respectively. The intervals between *A* and *B* and between *B* and *C* are 45 s (HANCOCK and VOLLE, 1970a)

finding that the firing produced by McN-A-343 is resistant to blockade by extremely large doses of hexamethonium in the normal ganglion but is quite sensitive to hexamethonium in perfused ganglia is difficult to explain on the basis of a differential delivery of drugs to the receptor. For reasons that are not clear, it appears that the process of perfusion induces changes in the muscarinic receptors, making them sensitive to blockade by hexamethonium. Clearly, care must be exercised in interpreting receptor classification in autonomic ganglia since the specificity of blockade by prototypical agents may be compromised by the experimental conditions used.

C. Postjunctional Responses to Acetylcholine and Nicotinic Agents

I. The Acetylcholine Potential

The primary electrical signs of the ganglionic transmission process have been characterised in rather precise studies of transmission in amphibian and mammalian sympathetic ganglia (e.g., ECCLES, 1955; NISHI and KOKETSU, 1960; BLACKMAN et al., 1963). In autonomic ganglia, adequate preganglionic stimulation gives rise to a graded, relatively long-lasting synaptic potential (EPSP) that is sensitive to blockade by hexamethonium and related drugs.

The finding that acetylcholine applied by the iontophoretic method evokes a postjunctional depolarisation with electrical and pharmacological properties similar to those of the EPSP may be taken as further evidence for the view that acetylcholine

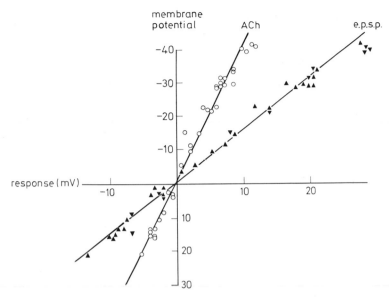

Fig. 2. Reversal potential for the transmitter *(e.p.s.p.)* and the acetylcholine *(ACh)* potential. The graph shows that the reversal potential was the same for both the transmitter and iontophoretically applied acetylcholine (DENNIS et al., 1971)

is the primary transmitter in autonomic ganglia (BLACKMAN et al., 1963; DENNIS et al., 1971). By the judicious application of acetylcholine, it is possible to match the amplitude and time course of the acetylcholine-evoked depolarisation with that of the EPSP and, even, the spontaneous miniature EPSPs. More important, it appears that the equilibrium potential for the response to acetylcholine and the EPSP are identical (NISHI et al., 1969; DENNIS et al., 1971), indicating a common underlying ionic mechanism for transmitter and applied acetylcholine (Fig. 2). The reversal potential falls between 0 and -12 mV for frog cardiac vagal ganglion cells (DENNIS et al., 1971) and ranges from -7 to -14 mV for frog and toad paravertebral ganglia (NISHI and KOKETSU, 1960; NISHI et al., 1969). At a normal resting membrane potential, the application of acetylcholine or preganglionic stimulation produces a net inward flow of ions. When the inside of the cell is made positive by extrinsic currents, the flow of ions produced by acetylcholine is in the outward direction. At the equilibrium potential, however, acetylcholine and the transmitter produce no net flow of ionic currents. A common reversal potential for a putative transmitter substance and the transmitter is good evidence that the permeability changes in the postsynaptic region are produced by the activation of the same receptor-ionophore complex.

Thus, the simulation by applied acetylcholine of the transmitter consists of (1) a wave form of depolarisation comparable in its temporal characteristics to the synaptic potential, (2) a common reversal potential with the synaptic potential, (3) blockade by drugs known to interact competitively with the nicotinic receptor, and (4) densensitisation by acetylcholine of the responsiveness of the subsynaptic receptor to the transmitter *(vide infra)*. Collectively, the data comprise strong evidence to show that applied acetylcholine has the capacity to stimulate the receptor activated by the transmitter and to cause the same ionic permeability changes in the postsynaptic membrane.

The primary electrogenic event underlying the acetylcholine potential appears to be an increase in sodium conductance. Activation of the nicotinic receptor by acetylcholine or the transmitter leads to an inward movement of ions and depolarisation of the ganglion cell. Calcium ions are effective substitutes for sodium and maintain the depolarising response to acetylcholine (PAPPANO and VOLLE, 1966; KOKETSU et al., 1968). Like the depolarisation produced by acetylcholine in the presence of sodium ions, that produced in the presence of calcium ions is blocked by ganglion-blocking agents.

In contrast to calcium ions, lithium ions are unable to support ganglionic depolarisation by acetylcholine (KLINGMAN, 1966; PAPPANO and VOLLE, 1967). Perfusion of ganglia with solutions containing lithium chloride as a complete replacement for sodium chloride results in complete failure of transmission, acetylcholine-induced firing, and acetylcholine-induced depolarisation. Since ganglionic depolarisation by acetylcholine originates in the ganglion cells, the parallel decline of transmission and the acetylcholine-induced activity in ganglia perfused with lithium chloride indicates a primary postsynaptic locus for the ganglion block produced by lithium ions. As indicated above, the ability of acetylcholine to depolarise the ganglion results mainly from an increase in membrane permeability to sodium ions. Accordingly, the failure of lithium to substitute more effectively for sodium could arise either because lithium cannot penetrate the cell as well as sodium or because the accumulation of lithium within the cell alters the membrane potential and the chemical gradient across the cell for the ion.

The finding that repetitive preganglionic stimulation accelerates the rate of onset of the failure of transmission and the responses to injected acetylcholine in ganglia perfused with lithium chloride is compatible with the latter possibility. Whereas 20 min are required for failure of transmission and the acetylcholine-induced responses when the ganglion is stimulated at a rate of 0.5 Hz, only 10–12 min are required when preganglionic stimulation at a rate of 2.0 Hz is used (PAPPANO and VOLLE, 1967). The most reasonable explanation for the inverse relationship between the frequency of preganglionic stimulation and the time required for ganglionic blockade is an increase in the rate of intracellular accumulation of lithium. In amphibian skeletal muscle fibres, the extrusion of lithium occurs at a rate only about 10% that of sodium (KEYNES and SWAN, 1959). In spinal motoneurones the sodium-pump mechanism extrudes lithium at one-half the rate of sodium (ARAKI et al., 1965). The depression by lithium ions of post-tetanic hyperpolarisation of mammalian unmyelinated fibres is attributed to the inability of the fibres to extrude lithium as rapidly as sodium (RITCHIE and STRAUB, 1957). Thus, it is reasonable to postulate that lithium fails to support ganglionic transmission and depolarisation by acetylcholine, because of an intracellular accumulation of the ion (WOODWARD et al., 1969). Unfortunately, little information is available at present about the sodium-pump mechanism in sympathetic ganglion cells.

The inability of lithium to act as a more suitable substitute for sodium in the synapses of mammalian sympathetic ganglia is in sharp contrast to its known ability to do so in peripheral nerve and muscle (HODGKIN and KATZ, 1949; KEYNES and SWAN, 1959). The discrepancy may be due to the time allowed for the exposure of the tissues to lithium ions. When used for short periods, lithium can serve as an adequate replacement for sodium ions in sympathetic ganglia. However, prolonged periods of exposure to lithium may result in the intracellular accumulation of the ion and the abolition of the processes involved in the generation of synaptic potentials and action potentials.

Parenthetically, periods of spontaneous firing occurs in some ganglia perfused with lithium solutions (PAPPANO and VOLLE, 1967). A similar observation has been made at the neuromuscular junction, where it was found that lithium causes a delayed, but marked, increase in the frequency of spontaneously occurring miniature end plate potentials (ONODERA and YAMAKAWA, 1966; KELLY, 1968; BENOIT et al., 1973; BRANISTEANU and VOLLE, 1975). The increased rate of transmitter discharge caused by lithium is due probably to the accumulation of lithium by the nerve terminals.

Relatively little direct evidence is available to show whether or not the stimulation of nicotinic sites by nicotinic agents other than acetylcholine results in the activation of the same electrogenic process as that activated by the transmitter. It has been shown in frog sympathetic ganglia that bath-applied carbachol, tetramethylammonium, and nicotine cause a dose-dependent depolarisation of the cells and the generation of action potentials (GINSBORG and GUERRERO, 1964; RIKER, 1967). The excitatory actions of these drugs is prevented or interrupted by d-tubocurarine. In addition, membrane resistance is decreased during the ganglion-cell depolarisation produced by the drugs (GINSBORG and GUERRERO, 1964; RIKER, 1967; KOKETSU, 1969). There is no information, however, about the equilibrium potential for the nicotinic drug-induced depolarisation. Peak depolarisation by the drugs takes the membrane potential to -10 to $-20\,mV$, within the range of values for the equilibrium potential, and this may indicate a commonality of mechanisms. Since receptor desensitisation is known to occur consistently with bath-applied nicotinic agents, the extent of peak depolarisation may be an underestimate. In view of the known differences between the activation of ionic channels at the end plate by nicotinic drugs and the transmitter (KATZ and MILEDI, 1971; COLQUHOUN et al., 1975) it is reasonable to expect that the nicotinic ganglion-stimulating agents may not imitate precisely the effects of the transmitter.

II. Surface or Demarcation Potentials

Earlier studies using surface recording electrodes to measure the ganglionic demarcation potential obtained results with nicotinic drugs that were remarkably similar to those obtained later from single cells by means of intracellular recording (PATON and PERRY, 1953; LUNDBERG and THESLEFF, 1953; ECCLES, 1956; PASCOE, 1956). With this method it was shown that a variety of nicotinic agents decrease the demarcation potential between the body of the ganglion and the crushed end of a postganglionic nerve but do not depolarise the postganglionic nerve trunk. A discharge of postganglionic firing coincides with the surface wave of depolarisation (TAKESHIGE et al., 1963, Fig. 3). Both the discharge and the depolarisation are depressed by hexamethonium.

The pattern of depolarisation produced by several nicotinic agents differs in contour and effect. Whereas dimethylphenylpiperazinium and tetramethylam-

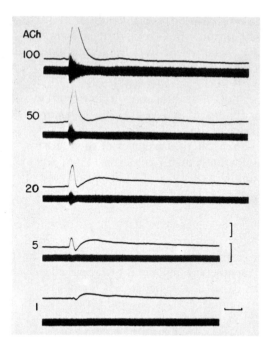

Fig. 3. Surface potentials and postganglionic discharges evoked by graded doses (μg) of acetylcholine given intra-arterially to the cat superior cervical ganglion. Depending upon the dose of acetylcholine used, the surface potential consisted sequentially of depolarisation, hyperpolarisation, and depolarisation. Postganglionic firing coincided with the initial phase of depolarisation. The top vertical calibration is 400 μV and applies to the surface potential; the bottom calibration is 20 μV and applies to the firing. The horizontal calibration is 4 s (TAKESHIGE and VOLLE, 1964 c)

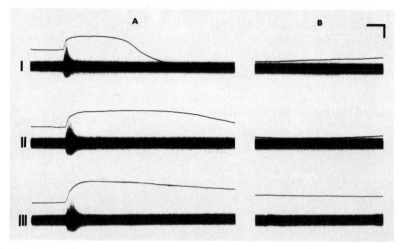

Fig. 4. Surface potentials and postganglionic firing recorded simultaneously from cat superior cervical ganglia after the intra-arterial administration of dimethylphenylpiperazinium (I: 5 μg), tetramethylammonium (II: 10 μg), and lobeline (III: 2 μg). The interval between A and B is 2 min. The vertical calibration is 1 mV when applied to the surface potential and 10 μV when applied to the firing. The horizontal calibration is 10 s (JARAMILLO and VOLLE, 1968 a)

monium cause a bi-phasic pattern of depolarisation and hyperpolarisation, lobeline does not (JARAMILLO and VOLLE, 1968a; HAEFELY, 1974b; Fig. 4). Each of the agents causes postganglionic firing that is antagonised by hexamethonium. More will be said later about the postexcitatory period of ganglionic hyperpolarisation.

The depolarisation produced by the nicotinic ganglion-stimulating agents subsides in the continued presence of the drugs (GINSBORG and GUERRERO, 1964) until the membrane potential returns to near-normal values. As might be expected, the decrease in membrane resistance produced by the drugs subsides at the same rate as does the depolarisation of the cells. Little is understood about the mechanisms whereby the fade of depolarisation occurs. An analogous situation exists at the neuromuscular junction, where the process has been studied in great detail. Adaptation to cholinomimetic depolarising agents at the end plate is attributed to receptor desensitisation involving a deformation of the receptor (THESLEFF, 1955; KATZ and THESLEFF, 1957; MAGAZANIK, 1969; RANG and RITTER, 1969). The deformed receptor, while still able to combine with acetylcholine or nicotinic drugs, is unable to activate electrogenic processes. There is an uncoupling of the receptor and the membrane ionophore, and time is required in the absence of the drug for the deformed receptor to revert to its normal status. Desensitisation of the nicotinic receptor causes a decrease in synaptic efficiency because of the inability of the transmitter to activate the receptor ionophore complex. It is likely that a similar process accounts for the fade of depolarisation and blockade of transmission observed in autonomic ganglia during the continued presence of nicotinic drugs.

D. Blockade of Transmission by Nicotinic Drugs

Nicotinic drugs are known to block ganglionic transmission by two different, but related mechanisms. The first phase of blockade coincides with depolarisation of the ganglion and the second phase occurs in the presence of the nicotinic agents at a time when the depolarisation has subsided (PATON and PERRY, 1953; ECCLES, 1956; GINSBORG and GUERRERO, 1964; Fig. 5). For some drugs, the second phase of blockade coincides with ganglionic hyperpolarisation.

I. Depolarisation Blockade

When depolarised by nicotinic agents, the ganglion cells are unresponsive to all types of stimulation. During depolarisation, ganglion cell action potentials activated by either ortho- or antidromic stimulation are blocked and the amplitudes of miniature EPSPs are reduced (Fig. 5). In addition, ganglion cell discharges produced by non-nicotinic agents such as potassium ions, histamine, and 5-hydroxytryptamine are prevented during the period of depolarisation. The responsiveness of the cells to these agents and to antidromic stimulation is restored as cell depolarisation subsides and membrane resistance increases (TRENDELENBURG, 1959; GINSBORG and GUER-RERO, 1964). Presumably the non-specific blockade occurring during depolarisation is due to the inactivation of sodium conductance in the ganglion cell membrane area adjacent to subsynaptic and extrajunctional nicotinic receptors.

An apparent dissociation between ganglion cell depolarisation and blockade by nicotinic drugs can be demonstrated. A partial antagonism of the blockade of gan-

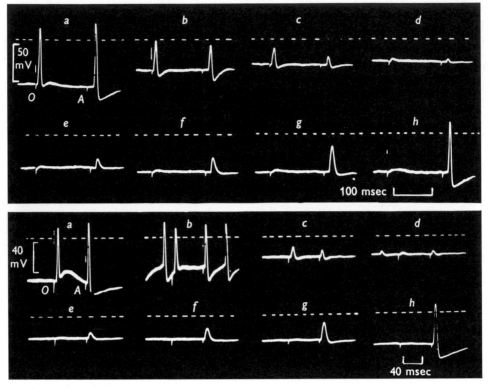

Fig.5. Effects of nicotinic agents on frog ganglion cell response to ortho- (O) and antidromic (A) stimulation. Dashed line shows zero potential between bath and microelectrode in the bathing solution. Top panel shows response to tetramethylammonium $(2 \times 10^{-4} M)$ added to bath between *(a)* and *(b)*. Records taken at: *b*, 10 s; *c*, 12 s; *d*, 20 s; *e*, 30 s; *f*, 1 min; *g*, 2 min 30 s; *h*, 5 min 15 s. Bottom panel shows response of another ganglion cell to nicotine $(5 \times 10^{-4} M)$. Records taken at: *b*, 14 s; *c*, 18 s; *d*, 30 s; *e*, 1 min; *f*, 1 min 30 s; *g*, 2 min; *h*, 6 min 30 s (GINSBORG and GUERRERO, 1964)

glionic transmission by nicotinic drugs occurs when either calcium ions or barium ions are administered during the period of depolarisation blockade. These ions cause no change in the amplitude of the drug-induced depolarisation, but increase the amplitude of the ganglionic action potential produced by preganglionic stimulation and recorded during the period of depolarisation (TAKESHIGE and VOLLE, 1964a, b). There is no easy way to account for this finding. Obviously, surface recording systems detect the activity of a large population of fibres and, for this reason, results obtained by this method are not easy to interpret. On the other hand, the divalent cations are known to delay sodium inactivation, thus allowing for spike generation to occur at lower resting membrane potentials. It may be by this mechanism that calcium and barium ions cause the apparent separation of depolarisation from blockade.

That the blockade of transmission by nicotine may be unrelated to depolarisation of the ganglion has been suggested also by GEBBER (1968), who found that (a) tetanic preganglionic stimulation applied during the period of depolarisation by nicotine antagonizes the blockade of transmission, (b) d-tubocurarine prevents the depolarisation but enhances the blockade, (c) ganglionic responses to non-nicotinic ganglion-stimulating agents are enhanced by nicotine, and (d) postganglionic firing by nicotine infusions is maintained during transmitter blockade. The technique used by GEBBER involved the simultaneous recording of surface potentials and postganglionic discharges of the cat superior cervical ganglion. As mentioned earlier, one of the difficulties in accepting the idea that depolarisation and ganglionic blockade can be separated as causal events is the use of a recording system that monitors a large cell population. Equally important, the actions of nicotine and related drugs to block transmission are complex. When drugs are applied slowly by perfusion or intra-arterial injection, it is likely that the process of receptor blockade has already progressed so that depolarisation and blockade occur simultaneously. It may be for this reason that d-tubocurarine can be shown to enhance blockade by nicotine at a time when depolarisation is depressed and that tetanic preganglionic stimulation causes an antagonism of blockade.

Using intracellular recording methods in frog sympathetic ganglia, RIKER (1968) studied the blockade of transmission produced by acetylcholine and concluded that acetylcholine causes ganglionic blockade by an effect on the unmyelinated presynaptic nerve terminals and not by depolarisation of the ganglion cells. This conclusion was based on four observations:

1) Acetylcholine depresses the orthodromic spike in doses that have no effect on the antidromic spike

2) Relief of acetylcholine-induced depolarisation by extrinsic hyperpolarising currents fails to restore transmission

3) There is no obvious relationship between the dose of acetylcholine required to block transmission and the extent of depolarisation

4) Extrinsic depolarising current fails to block the orthodromic spike.

There is little doubt that these findings represent an interesting array of data to show the separation of ganglionic depolarisation and blockade of transmission.

Several factors should be kept in mind when these experiments are considered. First, the data do not preclude depolarisation blockade by acetylcholine. The classic demonstration (TRENDELENBURG, 1959) that large doses of acetylcholine and other nicotinic drugs prevent ganglionic responses to both specific and non-specific (e.g., potassium) stimulants is explained best in terms of ganglionic cellular depolarisation. GINSBORG and GUERRERO (1964) showed that acetylcholine depresses the antidromic spike activity, and it is reasonable to attribute the blockade to the coincidental depolarisation of the cell soma. Second, there is no evidence to show that the block is due to acetylcholine and not to choline. In RIKER's experiments, large amounts of acetylcholine are perfused slowly over the ganglia and there is ample time for a breakdown of large quantities of acetylcholine to form choline. It is well known that choline has prominent ganglionic activity (GEBBER and VOLLE, 1965; KRSTIĆ, 1972). In the superior cervical ganglion of the rabbit studied by the sucrose-gap method, acetylcholine reaches the ganglion primarily as choline (KOSTERLITZ et al., 1968). Finally, it is not possible in sympathetic ganglia to identify with certainty a presynaptic locus of inhibition with the technique of intracellular recording as used by RIKER. Inactivation of the subsynaptic acetylcholine receptor by doses of acetylcholine too small to cause depolarisation may occur. If so, it is not possible to distin-

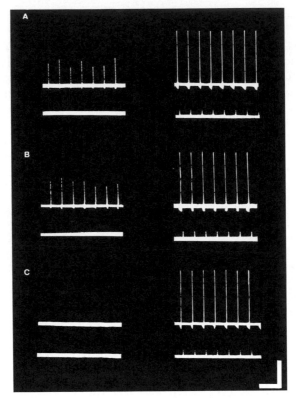

Fig.6. End plate potentials *(left)* and acetylcholine potential *(right)* of frog sartorius muscle bathed in magnesium Ringer solution. Top row *(A)* shows response to nerve stimulation (0.5 Hz) and iontophoretic potential (0.5 Hz) of untreated end plate. Middle row *(B)* shows the responses of the same end plate after DMAE $(4 \times 10^{-6}\ M)$. Bottom row *(C)* shows effects of carbachol $(2 \times 10^{-5}\ M)$ on DMAE-treated end plate. Carbachol blocked the end plate potential but not the acetylcholine potential. After DMAE, carbachol did not cause depolarisation of end plate (not shown). Resting potential of cell was -88 mV. The vertical and horizontal calibrations are 10 mV and 4 s, respectively (Volle and Henderson, 1975)

guish between presynaptic blockade and subsynaptic receptor inactivation. As found by Ginsborg and Guerrero (1964), the decrease by acetylcholine in the amplitude of miniature synaptic potentials indicates a depression of postjunctional sensitivity of the chemoreceptive sites.

Some insight into the complexities of ganglion blockade by nicotinic agents is provided by a substance that blocks the excitatory actions of nicotine when used in concentrations far below those required to block ganglionic transmission. The compound is DMAE [α,α'-bis(dimethylammoniumacetaldehyde diethylacetal)*p,p'*-diacetylbiphenyldibromide], an analog of hemicholinium-3 (Wong and Long, 1967, 1968). Ganglionic stimulation by nicotine, tetramethylammonium, and dimethylphenylpiperazinium is quite sensitive to blockade by DMAE. Since the compound blocks nicotine-induced stimulation at a time when transmission is unaffected, it is a useful agent for the study of nicotine-induced blockade of transmission (Volle and

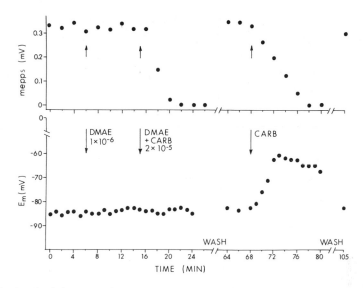

Fig. 7. Blockade of miniature end plate potentials (mepps) and depolarisation of frog sartorius muscle end plate by carbachol (2×10^{-5} M) during and after exposure to DMAE. Carbachol depressed mepp at a time when depolarisation by carbachol was blocked by DMAE (VOLLE and HENDERSON, 1975)

HENDERSON, 1975). JARAMILLO (1968) studied the effects of DMAE on ganglionic transmission in the cat superior cervical ganglion, using surface and postganglionic recording systems. The main finding is that DMAE prevents ganglionic depolarisation and postganglionic firing produced by tetramethylammonium and dimethylphenylpiperazinium, but enhances the blockade of transmission produced by the drugs. The second phase of blockade (presumably due to receptor desensitisation) produced by the drugs is prevented by DMAE, so that it is unlikely that the actions of DMAE can be explained by an unmasking of or enhancement of the desensitisation process. These facts seem to point to a dissociation between nicotinic drug-induced firing and depolarisation and nicotinic drug blockade of transmission.

The anti-nicotinic actions of DMAE were studied at the frog neuromuscular junction, where nicotinic agents are known to cause blockade of neuromuscular transmission by both end plate depolarisation and receptor desensitisation (VOLLE and HENDERSON, 1975). The advantage of using the frog neuromuscular junction depends upon the relative technical simplicity of recording from single end plates and applying drugs directly, by iontophoretic means, to the nicotinic receptors on the end plate. With this system it was found, as expected, that carbachol, when applied in the bathing Ringer solution, causes depolarisation of the end plate and a blockade of (a) the end plate potentials (EPPs), (b) the miniature EPPs (mepps), and (c) the end plate potential produced by iontophoretic acetylcholine. DMAE, in concentrations having no effect on the EPPs, mepps, or iontophoretic acetylcholine potential, prevents the depolarisation of the end plate produced by carbachol and the blockade by carbachol of the acetylcholine potential. However, the blockade of EPPs and mepps by carbachol is enhanced by DMAE (Figs. 6 and 7). These findings suggest that carbachol has actions not only on the end plate, but also on the motor nerve terminal.

Clearly, the ability of DMAE to antagonise depolarisation of the end plate by carbachol and the blockade by carbachol of the iontophoretic acetylcholine potential results from the postjunctional actions of both carbachol and DMAE. The reason for the discrimination by DMAE between the depolarisation of the end plate by bath-applied carbachol and that produced by iontophoretically applied acetylcholine is not understood. Since the parameters of activating ionic channels differ widely for various nicotinic substances and may depend upon the rate of application (KATZ and MILEDI, 1971; COLQUHOUN et al., 1975), the differential blocking action of DMAE may be accounted for on this basis.

Nicotinic drugs are known to depress transmitter release at the frog neuromuscular junction (EDWARDS and IKEDA, 1962; STEINBERG and VOLLE, 1972). It follows that an action of carbachol on the motor nerve terminals to depress transmitter release would explain the failure of DMAE to antagonise the carbachol-induced depression of the EPPs at a time when the carbachol-induced depolarisation has been prevented. A prejunctional site of action for carbachol also accounts for the blockade by carbachol of EPPs at a time when the blockade by carbachol of the iontophoretic acetylcholine potential has been prevented by DMAE. However, the blockade of mepps by carbachol is difficult to explain in terms of a prejunctional site of action. Nicotinic drugs depress evoked transmitter output, presumably as a consequence of nerve terminal depolarisation and reduction in the amplitude of the incoming nerve terminal action potential. Although depolarisation of the nerve terminals by carbachol causes an increase in the frequency of mepps (MIYAMOTO and VOLLE, 1974), there is no evidence to show that a reduction in the size of the mepps is associated with nerve terminal depolarisation. In the absence of DMAE, the decreased amplitude of mepps produced by nicotinic drugs is related to postjunctional depolarisation.

It is worth noting that DMAE has important prejunctional actions. At some end plates, DMAE depresses EPPs but not the iontophoretic acetylcholine potential. In addition to the differential blocking action of DMAE on EPPs and the iontophoretic acetylcholine potential, DMAE depresses transmitter release by a frequency-dependent process (VOLLE, 1973; BRANISTEANU et al., 1975). Concentrations of DMAE that have no effect on the amplitude of EPPs evoked by low-frequency stimulation (0.5 Hz) cause a marked blockade when the frequency of stimulation is increased to 5 or 10 Hz. The blockade occurring under these conditions is due to a decrease in the number of quanta of transmitter release by the nerve impulse. The possibility exists, therefore, that carbachol enhances the prejunctional blocking actions of DMAE and, in this regard, is similar to repetitive nerve stimulation. This mechanism would account for the depression by carbachol of both the EPPs and the mepps.

II. Prolonged Ganglionic Blockade

PATON and PERRY (1953) showed that the depolarisation of the ganglion by nicotine persists for a shorter period than does the blockade of transmission. They concluded that the blockade of transmission occurring at a time when repolarisation of the ganglion has taken place is due to a competitive blockade of the nicotinic receptors much in the same way as transmission is blocked by hexamethonium. The two phases of blockade can be distinguished on the basis of alterations of ganglionic sensitivity to nicotinic and non-nicotinic agents. Like transmission, ganglionic response to nicotinic drugs is blocked during both phases of the actions of nicotine. However, non-nicotinic ganglion-stimulating agents (e.g., potassium ions, 5-hydroxytryptamine, histamine, etc.) are blocked only during the period of ganglionic depolarisation (TRENDELENBURG, 1959). It is reasonable to conclude, therefore, that the persistent transmission blockade produced by nicotinic drugs is due to a specific blockade of nicotinic receptors.

Observations similar to those made by PATON and PERRY (1953) have been made by GINSBORG and GUERRERO (1964) with intracellular recording from frog ganglion cells (Fig. 5). They were able to show that the blockade of transmission outlasts the depolarisation of the ganglion cell caused by nicotine and related drugs and that during the late period of blockade the responsiveness of the ganglion cells to antidromic stimulation is restored. Although it can be concluded that a prolonged blocking action is due to a reduction in the chemosensitivity of the membrane, no evidence is available to show whether the action is due to a competitive (hexamethonium-like action) effect or not.

There is some reason to think that the persistent blockade may be unrelated to the stimulating actions of the nicotinic drugs. RIKER (1968) has reported that transmission in frog ganglion cells is often blocked by acetylcholine applied in concentrations having no detectable effect on the resting membrane potential. Although RIKER (1968) interprets these findings to mean that ganglionic blockade by acetylcholine is due to a presynaptic effect, the alternative possibility that acetylcholine reduces the chemosensitivity of subsynaptic receptors has not been tested and, therefore, cannot be ruled out.

It is of some interest that blockade of transmission at the neuromuscular junction occurs for doses of nicotine too small to depolarise the end plate (WANG and NARAHASHI, 1972). Similarly, lobeline, a drug known to have actions on sympathetic ganglia much like those of nicotine (JARAMILLO and VOLLE, 1968a; HAEFELY, 1974b), causes a blockade of neuromuscular transmission by a non-competitive mechanism and this is different from that produced by d-tubocurarine (STEINBERG and VOLLE, 1972; HANCOCK and HENDERSON, 1972; VOLLE, 1974). Lobeline does not depolarise the end plate or alter the release of the transmitter (STEINBERG and VOLLE, 1972). These observations (RIKER, 1968; WANG and NARAHASHI, 1972) raise the interesting question about receptor activation as a prerequisite for the second-phase blockade of transmission or receptor desensitisation to occur. The process of receptor desensitisation may not require the activation of electrogenic mechanisms.

The same pattern of blockade by nicotinic drugs occurs at nonsynaptic tissues. For example, conduction of impulses in vagal non-medullated fibres in situ is transiently blocked by nicotine and related drugs. Since the blockade by nicotine is antagonised, in turn, by hexamethonium it can be assumed that nicotinic receptors exist in the vagal fibres. The assumption is made that the blockade of conduction results from depolarisation of the nerve fibres. However, in the continued presence of nicotine, nerve conduction is restored. If a second application of a larger dose of nicotine is given, conduction blockade does not occur (Fig. 8). The continued presence of nicotinic drugs has no effect on conduction blockade by local anaesthetics or

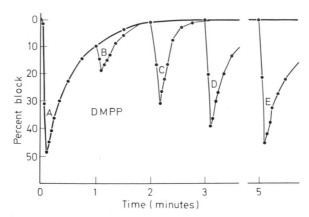

Fig. 8. Conduction blockade in vagus-nodose ganglion of the cat by dimethylphenylpiperazinium (DMPP) and the anti-nicotinic effect of DMPP. Curve *A* shows the time course of conduction blockade caused by a single injection of DMPP (20 μg, IA). Curves *B* (1 min), *C* (2 min), *D* (3 min), and *E* (5 min) show the blockade produced by a second dose of DMPP (20 μg) (Hancock and Volle, 1969a)

potassium chloride. Conversely, blockade of conduction by potassium ions does not alter the blockade caused by nicotinic drugs. With time, in the absence of nicotine, the blockade of axonal conduction by nicotine reappears. Thus, in vagal C fibres the receptors for nicotine are present and display all the pharmacological characteristics of the ganglionic nicotinic receptor (Hancock and Volle, 1969a; see also Armett and Ritchie, 1961).

It has been observed that perfusion of the vagus nerve in situ with Lock's solution prevents the development of the anti-nicotinic action of the nicotinic drugs (Hancock and Volle, 1969a). Conduction in the perfused vagal fibres is blocked by nicotinic drugs, which are, in turn, blocked by hexamethonium. Thus, both the nicotinic agents and hexamethonium have their usual and expected effects. But the anti-nicotinic action of nicotine could not be demonstrated (Fig. 9). A second dose of the nicotinic agent given quickly after the first always causes conduction blockade. Obviously, this means either that the anti-nicotinic effect does not occur on that the conditions for its demonstration are not present.

The observation bears on the mechanism of the persistent anti-nicotinic action of nicotinic drugs. Inasmuch as hexamethonium retains its anti-nicotinic action in perfused vagal fibres, it is reasonable to conclude that if the nicotinic drugs have a hexamethonium-like action, it should be possible to detect such action. By extrapolation to autonomic ganglia, it may be concluded that the prolonged blockade produced by nicotinic drugs is not due to a hexamethonium-like action as proposed originally by Paton and Perry (1953). The findings with perfused vagal fibres are more consistent with the view that the anti-nicotinic action is due to receptor desensitisation (Thesleff, 1955) and that, for some unexplained reason, replacement of the normal circulation with Locke's solution prevents desensitisation of the receptor from taking place. It is consistent also with the finding by Alkadhi and McIsaac (1974) that repeated administrations of dimethylphenylpiperazinium enhances gan-

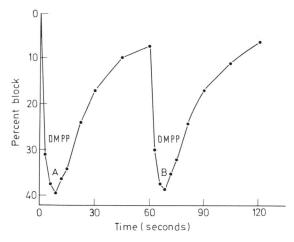

Fig. 9. Conduction blockade by dimethylphenylpiperazinium (5 μg) in perfused cat vagus-nodose ganglion. Second dose of DMPP caused same blockade as the first (HANCOCK and VOLLE, 1969a)

glion blockade by competitive blocking agents. Receptor desensitisation is known to enhance the interaction between the receptor and some antagonists (RANG and RITTER, 1969).

III. Postexcitatory Ganglionic Hyperpolarisation

PASCOE (1956), using isolated rat superior cervical ganglia, showed that a marked increase in the demarcation in potential is produced when nicotinic drugs are removed from the bathing solution. He noted that d-tubocurarine, but not hexamethonium, selectively prevents nicotine-induced ganglionic hyperpolarisation. It now appears that the nicotinic drugs produce the hyperpolarising response as a consequence of the activation of an electrogenic sodium pump in the ganglion cells. The electrolyte disturbance produced as a consequence of cellular depolarisation and discharge is repaired by the extrusion of sodium and the uptake of potassium.

Ganglionic depolarisation and firing evoked by acetylcholine, tetramethylammonium and dimethylphenylpiperazinium are followed by hyperpolarisation (TAKESHIGE and VOLLE, 1964c; GEBBER and VOLLE, 1966; GUMULKA and SZRENIAWSKI, 1968; JARAMILLO and VOLLE, 1968b; HANCOCK and VOLLE, 1969b; MACHOVA and BOSKA, 1969; KOSTERLITZ et al., 1970; BROWN et al., 1972; HAEFELY, 1974a). Coincidental with the hyperpolarisation are a decrease in the amplitude of the ganglionic spike and an increase in the amplitude of the negative after-potential of the spike (Fig. 10). Some evidence has been obtained to show that the decrease in spike amplitude is unrelated to ganglionic hyperpolarisation and is due most probably to desensitisation of the receptor. The increase in the amplitude of the negative after-potential (or persistent synaptic potential) is an expected consequence of ganglionic cellular hyperpolarisation.

The first indication that the hyperpolarisation differed from the ganglionic inhibitory potential or hyperpolarisation produced by either catecholamines or musca-

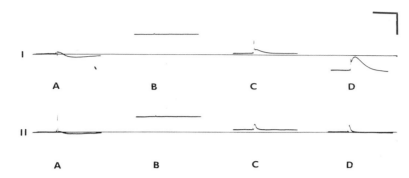

Fig. 10. Ganglionic blockade and hyperpolarisation produced by dimethylphenylpiperazinium in cat superior cervical ganglia before *(I)* and during *(II)* perfusion with lithium Locke solution. Ganglion was stimulated at a rate of 0.3 Hz. Records *A*, action potential before DMPP; records *B*, 1 min after DMPP, records *C* and *D* are 3 and 5 min after DMPP. Vertical and horizontal calibrations are 1 mV and 250 ms, respectively. Solid line is resting demarcation potential so that upward displacement indicates depolarisation and downward displacement, hyperpolarisation. Note striking change in contour of ganglionic action potential in record *D* of row *1* (JARAMILLO and VOLLE, 1968 b)

rinic ganglionic stimulation was the finding that ouabain selectively prevents the hyperpolarisation produced by the nicotinic drugs (GEBBER and VOLLE, 1966; HAEFE-LY, 1974 a). It is reasonable, therefore, to suspect that the hyperpolarisation is conditional upon a metabolically dependent exchange of sodium and potassium ions similar to that underlying the positive potential produced by rapid stimulation of non-myelinated fibres (RANG and RITCHIE, 1968).

This proposal was tested in perfused ganglia by replacing part of the sodium content of the Locke's solution with lithium ions (JARAMILLO and VOLLE, 1968 b). The inability of lithium ions to be extruded from intracellular sites has been demonstrated in a number of excitable tissues (KEYNES and SWAN, 1959; WOODWARD et al., 1969). In ganglia perfused with solutions containing lithium as a partial substitute for sodium, ganglionic hyperpolarisation by dimethylphenylpiperazinium is abolished (Fig. 10). It follows logically that the depression of the hyperpolarisation observed in ganglia perfused with lithium-Locke's solution can be explained by postulating that the hyperpolarisation is due to the rapid exchange of intracellular cations for extracellular potassium ions by the ganglion cells and that lithium ions impair the process. That the decreased hyperpolarisation is not due to a reduction in the concentration of sodium ions in the perfusion fluid is indicated by the fact that partial replacement of sodium by equivalent amounts of sucrose has no effect on the response to dimethylphenylpiperazinium.

Although somewhat less effective than either potassium or rubidium ions, caesium ions accelerate the efflux of sodium ions from intracellular sites within the peripheral nerve of invertebrates, enhance oxygen consumption in invertebrate neurones, and stimulates neuronal adenosine triphosphatase activity (SJODIN and BEAUGE, 1968; BAKER and CONNELLY, 1966). Therefore, caesium ions would be expected to have marked effects on DMPP-induced hyperpolarisation if a) the hyperpolarisation is due to a metabolically dependent sodium-potassium exchange, and b) the action of caesium ions on mammalian ganglion cells is the same as its actions on invertebrate neurones.

Striking effects of caesium are obtained when the ion is given during the hyperpolarisation that occurs after preganglionic stimulation with supramaximal impulses at a rate of 10–30 Hz for 30 s. Caesium causes a marked increase in the amplitude of the post-tetanic hyperpolarisation. In like manner, caesium given during the hyperpolarisation produced by nicotinic drugs causes an increase in the hyperpolarisation. When given before or during the period of depolarisation, caesium has no effect on the ganglionic hyperpolarisation produced by dimethylphenylpiperazinium (HANCOCK and VOLLE, 1969b). These findings have been confirmed by HAEFELY (1974a).

Similar evidence for an electrogenic pump mechanism to explain the hyperpolarisation following nicotinic agents has been described by KOSTERLITZ et al. (1970), who found that the hyperpolarisation depends upon extracellular potassium. In the sucrose-gap arrangement of recording from mammalian superior cervical ganglia, acetylcholine causes a depolarisation in potassium-free solution that is maintained for many minutes and subsides gradually over many more minutes to a small hyperpolarisation. When potassium is added to the bathing solution, an abrupt, large hyperpolarisation occurs. The situation is much the same as that observed by RANG and RITCHIE (1968) when vagal non-myelinated fibres are stimulated rapidly in potassium-free solutions. In this situation, the restoration of potassium results in a marked increase in the amplitude of post-tetanic hyperpolarisation, presumably because of the activation of an electrogenic pump in the vagal fibres.

The cellular origin of the postexcitatory hyperpolarisation is of some interest. As expected, HAEFELY (1974a) found that tetrodotoxin prevented the cellular discharge produced by dimethylphenylpiperazinium but had no effect on ganglion cellular depolarisation produced by the drug. In addition, tetrodotoxin had no effect on the postexcitatory hyperpolarisation. The surface potentials produced by the nicotinic drug in tetrodotoxin-treated ganglia are identical with those of otherwise untreated ganglia. This observation suggests that the hyperpolarisation is not due to repetitive spike activity but is due to ganglion cell depolarisation. BROWN and SCHOLFIELD (1974a, b) have shown in isolated rat sympathetic ganglia that carbachol and nicotine increase intracellular sodium and decrease intracellular potassium ions. Ouabain, metabolic inhibitors, and low temperature reduce the rate at which the electrolyte imbalance is corrected following removal of the drug. A sodium-pump mechanism in ganglia can account for these findings.

Not all nicotinic ganglion-stimulating agents cause the postexcitatory period of hyperpolarisation. Lobeline, an alkaloid with most of the pharmacological properties of nicotine, causes ganglionic depolarisation and firing but not ganglionic hyperpolarisation (Fig.4; JARAMILLO and VOLLE, 1968a; HAEFELY, 1974b). The blockade of transmission produced by lobeline persists beyond the period of ganglionic depolarisation. It is now known that lobeline possesses considerable local anaesthetic activity (HAEFELY, 1974b; VOLLE, 1974). On frog sartorius muscle, for example, lobeline is only slightly less active than butacaine in causing membrane depolarisation of muscles in chloride-free Ringer solution and blocking potassium ion exchange. The suggestion has been made that the local anaesthetic action of lobeline contributes to its ability to block neuromuscular transmission and to cause a decrease in chemosensitivity similar to that caused by receptor desensitisation (VOLLE,

1974). A similar process may occur in sympathetic ganglia to obscure the expected post-depolarisation period of hyperpolarisation. Hyperpolarisation may not be apparent when ion exchange is reduced.

It is unlikely that the postexcitatory hyperpolarisation contributes greatly to the blockade of synaptic transmission. In ganglia perfused with lithium-containing Locke's solution, the hyperpolarisation, but not the blockade of transmission, caused by dimethylphenylpiperazinium is prevented (Fig. 10; JARAMILLO and VOLLE, 1968 b). Conversely, caesium enhances the hyperpolarisation, but reduces the blockade of transmission produced by dimethylphenylpiperazinium (HANCOCK and VOLLE, 1969 b). However, as pointed out by HAEFELY (1974 a), the amplitude of a ganglionic spike recorded from the surface of the ganglion in relation to the demarcation potential is not a reliable estimate of the true status of ganglionic transmission and, therefore, divergences between spike amplitude and the demarcation potential of the type reported above with lithium and caesium must be evaluated with caution. GINSBORG and GUERRERO (1964) make a similar comment when comparing their observations made in single cells with those made by PATON and PERRY (1953) in whole ganglia. It is probable that ganglionic hyperpolarisation reduces the excitable state of the ganglion cells to some extent. However, when compared to the loss of excitability produced by receptor desensitisation, the depression of excitability is not great.

IV. Presynaptic Nerve Terminals

Insofar as can be determined, electrophysiological and neurochemical events in the preganglionic nerve terminals are similar to those of other junctions where transmission occurs by chemical means. Ganglion-blocking drugs related to hexamethonium have little or no direct effect on events in the nerve terminals and do not have any appreciable effect on transmitter release (BLACKMAN et al., 1963; MATTHEWS, 1966). By contrast, nicotinic agents appear to have significant effects on conduction in the nerve terminals and on transmitter release (KOKETSU and NISHI, 1968; PILAR, 1969; GINSBORG, 1971).

The most direct evidence of a presynaptic site of action for nicotinic drugs has been obtained in the avian ciliary ganglion, where it is possible, because of their relatively large size, to impale the presynaptic nerve terminals with microelectrodes (MARTIN and PILAR, 1964). The chemical component of transmission in the chick ciliary ganglion is mediated by acetylcholine. Acetylcholine applied to the ciliary ganglion in the presence of anticholinesterase agents causes a decrease in nerve terminal membrane conductance, depolarisation of the terminals, and a blockade of nerve terminal conduction (PILAR, 1969). Although the effects of hexamethonium and related substances on the acetylcholine-induced depolarisation of the nerve terminals have not been tested, it has been shown that repetitive application of acetylcholine at short intervals results in a reduced responsiveness of the terminals to acetylcholine. Thus, desensitisation to acetylcholine can be demonstrated in the nerve terminal, and provides reasonable evidence for the existence in the nerve terminal of an acetylcholine receptor.

Bullfrog and rat sympathetic ganglia arranged in the sucrose-gap method so that presynaptic events can be studied give somewhat indirect, but real evidence of presynaptic depolarisation by nicotine and acetylcholine (KOKETSU and NISHI, 1968). Nerve terminal depolarisation by acetylcholine is blocked by nicotine or d-tubocurarine, and is unaffected by atropine. Action potentials in the nerve terminals are depressed by the nicotinic drugs. Of considerable interest, because it bears on the question of whether or not endogenous acetylcholine can activate presynaptic nerve terminal receptors, is the finding that the nerve terminals are depolarised following repetitive stimulation. Anti-cholinesterase drugs potentiate and nicotine blocks the presynaptic nerve terminal depolarisation evoked by repetitive nerve stimulation. Therefore, the possibility must be entertained that the slow depolarisation is due to the activation of presynaptic acetylcholine receptors by acetylcholine subsequent to its release from the nerve terminals.

The findings of KOKETSU and NISHI (1968) have been supported by GINSBORG (1971), who used single preganglionic fibres so that the ambiguities of recording from a population of fibres can be eliminated. It was found with single fibres that acetylcholine or carbachol depolarises the nerve terminal and blocks nerve terminal conduction by d-tubocurarine-sensitive mechanism. Unlike the results of KOKETSU and NISHI (1968) and GINSBORG (1971), those obtained by DUNANT (1972) indicate that acetylcholine has no effect on the presynaptic nerve terminals of the rat. However, because of limitations inherent in the recording system, effects lasting less than 2 min cannot be detected (DUNANT, 1972) and this methodological limitation is sufficient to account for the discrepancy in the data, since there is good evidence to show that desensitisation to acetylcholine occurs rapidly in the nerve terminals.

The nerve terminals of the neuromuscular junction are also depolarised by nicotinic drugs and it is probable that the depolarisation leads to decreased release of transmitter (CIANI and EDWARDS, 1963; HUBBARD et al., 1965; STEINBERG and VOLLE, 1972). The precise mechanism underlying the depression by nicotine of transmitter release is not known. However, there is ample evidence available to suggest that the depression of transmitter release caused by nicotine is related to depolarisation of the unmyelinated motor nerve terminals. First, nicotine can directly depolarise non-myelinated nerve fibres in mammals (ARMETT and RITCHIE, 1961) and preganglionic nerve terminals in amphibia (KOKETSU and NISHI, 1968). It is reasonable to suppose that motor nerve terminals are also depolarised directly by nicotine. Although it is conceivable that terminal depolarisation may occur indirectly through the release of potassium from depolarised muscle fibres (HENDERSON and HANCOCK, 1971), such an effect would be expected to be associated with an increase, rather than a decrease, in transmitter release (TAKEUCHI and TAKEUCHI, 1961). Second, depolarising current applied to motor nerve terminals in both amphibian and mammalian systems decreases the amplitude of evoked EPPs (VLADIMIROVA, 1963; HUBBARD and WILLIS, 1968). Thus, it is possible that nicotine-induced terminal depolarisation is the cause of the decrease in transmitter output, perhaps mediated by an alteration in the nerve action potential duration or amplitude (TAKEUCHI and TAKEUCHI, 1962; DUDEL, 1971). On the other hand, terminal depolarisation is apparently not necessarily required to obtain a decrease in transmitter release upon exposure to acetylcholine (HUBBARD et al., 1865). Presumably depolarisation at a site proximal to the terminals is sufficient to interfere with invasion of the nerve terminals by the nerve action potential. The present data do not provide any means for distinguishing between depolarisation by nicotine of the terminals or of sites proximal to the terminals.

The question of why nerve terminal depolarisation in ganglia and at the nerve muscle junctions does not lead to increased transmitter release needs to be raised (GINSBORG and GUERRERO, 1964; HUBBARD et al., 1965). At the adrenergic neuro-effector junction, nicotine, acetylcholine, and related drugs cause the release of norepinephrine (FERRY, 1963; BURN and RAND, 1965). Therefore, either cholinergic nerve terminals differ in a fundamental way from adrenergic nerve terminals or the methods for demonstrating a presynaptic excitatory action of nicotinic drugs are inadequate.

NISHI (1970) reported that high concentrations of acetylcholine cause only a slight increase in the frequency of miniature ganglionic EPSPs (3 of 16 cells tested), an action which would be expected with depolarisation of the nerve terminals. A similar lack of effect of acetylcholine on spontaneous transmitter release has been reported for the neuromuscular junction (HUBBARD et al., 1965). However, when the mepp frequency of frog sartorius muscle end plates is increased by elevating the extracellular potassium, it can be shown that carbachol causes a striking increase in mepp frequency (MIYAMOTO and VOLLE, 1974). KATZ and MILEDI (1972) have noted that acetylcholine occasionally increases the frequency of mepps, and relate the variability of the response to acetylcholine to the initial level of the resting potentials of the nerve terminals. If the assumption that mepps reflect the release of acetylcholine from storage sites is valid, then the increase in mepp frequency caused by carbachol clearly indicates the ability of nicotinic agents to cause acetylcholine release from the motor nerve terminals.

The possibility that the increase in mepp frequency produced by carbachol can be explained by potassium ions released from the carbachol-depolarised end plate must be considered (KATZ, 1962). Direct evidence for or against this mechanism is not available. However, there are strong arguments against the involvement of potassium ions released from muscle in the prejunctional effects of cholinomimetic agents (ECCLES, 1964; KATZ, 1969). Whereas anticholinesterase agents cause antidromic discharges in the motor nerve (RIKER and STANDAERT, 1966), potassium ions do not. Furthermore, at sympathetic ganglia, intense tetanic stimulation of postganglionic cells, which would be expected to release potassium ions, does not cause presynaptic depolarisation (KOKETSU and NISHI, 1968; NISHI, 1970). Finally, it appears highly unlikely that such depolarisations of nerve endings by nicotinic agents would occur by way of a mechanism different from that at other nerves, e.g., vagal C fibres, where a role for potassium release from other sites in untenable.

The overall effects of nerve terminal depolarisation on transmitter release are not clear, however, for depolarisation by potassium increases both mepp frequency and evoked quantal release (HUBBARD et al., 1969). It may be that low levels of depolarisation caused by nicotinic agents or potassium ions increase calcium conductance and facilitate evoked release, whereas higher levels of depolarisation cause a depression of release by reduction in the size of the action potential. Depending on the amount of depolarisation, then, either an increase or a decrease in release might be seen.

There is some neurochemical evidence to show that nicotinic drugs cause the release of acetylcholine from presynaptic endings. Using perfused ganglia and assaying for released acetylcholine, McKINSTRY et al. (1963) found that carbachol causes the release of acetylcholine into the perfusion stream. This observation was confirmed subsequently by others (e.g., COLLIER and KATZ, 1970). However, there is an important issue remaining to be considered, concerning the radiotracer studies at sympathetic ganglia, which show that carbachol fails to promote acetylcholine release from transmitter storage sites (BROWN et al., 1970; COLLIER and KATZ, 1970). As mentioned before, carbachol (MIYAMOTO and VOLLE, 1974) and acetylcholine (KATZ and MILEDI, 1972) cause an increase in mepp frequency. Since mepps reflect transmitter release from nerve terminal storage sites, the nicotinic drugs appear to cause release from such sites. The failure to provide direct evidence of drug-induced transmitter release by the radiotracer method may be due to several factors. It should be noted that there is evidence for receptor desensitisation at nerve terminals, since the application of high doses of nicotinic agents results in only a transient depolarisation (see above). It is conceivable, therefore, that the high doses of carbachol used in the radiotracer studies with perfused ganglia cause a rapid desensitisation and repolarisation of the nerve terminals, so that transmitter release occurs for only a brief period. Because of the relatively long sampling time needed for the assay, the increase in acetylcholine release by carbachol may not be detected. With lower doses of carbachol used in the electrophysiological studies, a smaller, but more prolonged depolarisation would be expected to occur and a more persistent release of transmitter observed.

There are additional complexities. It appears that different ganglionic stores of acetylcholine are acted upon by nicotinic drugs and by the preganglionic action potential. For example, hexamethonium abolishes the release of acetylcholine evoked by carbachol but not that caused by nerve impulses. Conversely, elevation of extracellular calcium in the perfusion stream enhances transmitter release during nerve stimulation and depresses the release evoked by carbachol (McKINSTRY and KOELLE, 1967). COLLIER and KATZ (1970) have obtained good evidence to show that acetylcholine causes the release of "surplus" acetylcholine but not "depot" acetylcholine. Since there is good reason to suppose that mEPSPs reflect transmitter release from "depot" stores, the failure of acetylcholine to cause a prominent increase in the frequency of mEPSPs (NISHI, 1970) can be reconciled with the neurochemical findings. The release of acetylcholine from "surplus" stores would not be expected to be easily detected by electrophysiological means. The mechanism whereby acetylcholine causes the release of acetylcholine from nerve terminal "surplus" stores is not understood and needs to be studied further. Virtually nothing is known about how drugs can cause release from the pool of transmitter unavailable for release by the nerve impulse. Some experiments have shown that the release of acetylcholine from the surplus pool does not involve an exchange reaction with exogenous acetylcholine or applied nicotine (COLLIER and KATZ, 1975). In addition, it has been shown that pilocarpine causes release from the surplus pool by a mechanism sensitive to atropine. Thus, both nicotinic and muscarinic agents release acetylcholine from ganglia treated with anticholinesterase agents (COLLIER and KATZ, 1975).

Although clear evidence of receptors for acetylcholine on preganglionic and other cholinergic nerve terminals exists, it is not certain that they play any role in the transmission process. For a good discussion of this aspect of presynaptic acetylcholine receptors see KATZ (1969). The presynaptic terminals are, however, a site of action for nicotinic drugs to block ganglionic transmission.

E. Denervated Ganglia

A number of conflicting observations has been made on the effects of chronic dener-vation on the responses of sympathetic ganglia to nicotinic and muscarinic stimulat-ing agents. The contradictory findings are largely due to difficulties in assessing the sensitivity of the ganglion cells to applied drugs in a precise quantitative way. Most commonly, whole ganglia or multifibre preparations are used to determine threshold values or maximum levels of stimulation caused by nicotinic drugs. Because of obvious inherent technical problems with multifibre preparations, their use for this purpose may provide limited information. Moreover, any assessment of ganglionic stimulation may be altered by the simultaneous development of receptor desensitisa-tion, the sensitivity of the system then being a function of opposing actions. Finally, the presence in ganglia of both nicotinic and muscarinic receptors complicates mat-ters further. Some studies were made before a general awareness of the different ganglionic receptors existed.

Nonetheless, chronic denervation causes marked changes in the responsiveness of the ganglion cells to cholinomimetic drugs. In 1954, Perry and Reinert observed that hexamethonium fails to block the response of denervated ganglion cells of cat to acetylcholine, as measured by contraction of the nictitating membrane. The block-ade by hexamethonium of responses to tetramethylammonium and nicotine is unaf-fected by chronic preganglionic denervation.

Although it is well established that denervation enhances ganglionic responses to muscarinic drugs, there is some question about whether or not chronic denervation affects ganglionic activation by nicotinic drugs. Pascoe (1956) showed that the de-marcation potential of isolated ganglia is decreased to the same extent by nicotinic drugs in normal and denervated ganglia. This finding was confirmed later by Brown (1966, 1969). A similar observation was made by Lukomskaya (1967) and Vickerson and Varma (1969), who used contraction of the nictitating membrane as an index of ganglionic stimulation by nicotinic and muscarinic drugs. Responses to muscarinic drugs are enhanced, whereas responses to nicotinic drugs are unaffected by chronic preganglionic denervation.

In contrast, others have reported that denervation of sympathetic ganglia results in subsensitivity to nicotinic drugs. Volle and Koelle (1961) measured the thresh-old doses of carbachol required to cause postganglionic firing in normal and dener-vated ganglion, and found that denervation results in a marked increase in the threshold dose for postganglionic firing. However, no difference in the threshold dose for firing is noted when tetramethylammonium (Volle and Koelle, 1961) or acetylcholine are used (Takeshige and Volle, 1963). Because of the differences between these results with carbachol and those obtained by Brown (1966, 1969), the effects of chronic denervation on ganglionic responses to nicotinic drugs were re-examined in rat sympathetic ganglia with intact preganglionic nerves and ganglia denervated either acutely or chronically (Hancock and Volle, 1970b). When com-pared with acutely denervated ganglia, chronically denervated ganglia have identical thresholds for carbachol-induced firing. This finding is at variance with the earlier report by Volle and Koelle (1961) describing subsensitivity to carbachol in cat superior cervical ganglia. However, when compared to intact ganglia, both the acutely and chronically denervated ganglia are more sensitive to carbachol.

It is unlikely that the same processes are involved in the increased sensitivity of acutely and chronically denervated ganglia to carbachol. Since the major difference between acutely denervated ganglia and ganglia with intact preganglionic nerves lies in the surgical procedures used to isolate the cervical sympathetic trunk, it is reasonable to suggest that the process of tying and cutting the preganglionic nerve and the manipulation required to separate the preganglionic nerve from adjoining tissues sensitises the ganglia to carbachol. In accordance with this proposal is the observation that repetitive preganglionic stimulation markedly enhances the postganglionic response to carbachol (VOLLE, 1962). If the foregoing is valid, it then follows that acutely denervated ganglia, having been sensitised by the surgical process, do not reflect a normal state insofar as carbachol-induced firing is concerned. A better estimate of the effect of chronic denervation on the responsiveness of the ganglion cells to carbachol can be obtained by comparing responses in chronically denervated ganglia with those obtained in ganglia with the preganglionic nerve intact. When this is done, the threshold dose of carbachol is found to be five-fold lower in chronically denervated ganglia. This comparison is in keeping with earlier reports that chronic denervation usually leads to enhanced ganglionic responses to muscarinic compounds. Part of the ganglionic firing produced by carbachol is mediated by way of muscarinic receptors.

Unlike that for carbachol, the threshold dose of tetramethylammonium required to cause postganglionic firing is the same in intact, acutely denervated, and chronically denervated ganglia (HANCOCK and VOLLE, 1970b). This observation accords with earlier findings showing no change in the sensitivity of chronically denervated ganglia to nicotinic drugs (PASCOE, 1956; TAKESHIGE and VOLLE, 1963). Moreover, the observation is consistent with the finding that tetanic stimulation lowers the threshold dose of firing for carbachol but has no effect on the threshold dose of firing for tetramethylammonium (VOLLE, 1962). The differences between carbachol and tetramethylammonium in denervated ganglia and post-tetanic stimulation is due to the muscarinic component present in the response to carbachol.

To date, the most consistent picture to emerge concerning nicotinic responses in chronically denervated ganglia is that denervation has no effect on the response to nicotinic drugs (PASCOE, 1956; VOLLE and KOELLE, 1961; TAKESHIGE and VOLLE, 1963; BROWN, 1966, 1969; LUKOMSKAYA, 1967; VICKERSON and VARMA, 1969; HANCOCK and VOLLE, 1970b). In addition, there is general agreement that denervation enhances ganglionic responses to muscarinic ganglion-stimulating agents.

There are, however, some studies showing subsensitivity of the ganglion to nicotinic agents. GREEN (1969), using the superior cervical ganglion-nictitating membrane system, found that ganglia treated with anticholinesterase agents and methoscopolamine show reduced responsiveness to acetylcholine 2 weeks after denervation of the ganglia. The ganglia are also less responsive to potassium ions and to carbachol. In a similar study, KRSTIĆ (1972) found that chronic denervation results in reduced ganglionic responsiveness to choline and dimethylphenylpiperazinium. In normal ganglia, choline is known to cause ganglionic depolarisation and firing by mechanisms similar to acetylcholine (GEBBER and VOLLE, 1965); however, in denervated ganglia the response to choline, but not to dimethylphenylpiperazinium, is blocked by atropine (KRSTIĆ, 1972). Thus, there appears to be a muscarinic component in the ganglion responses to choline.

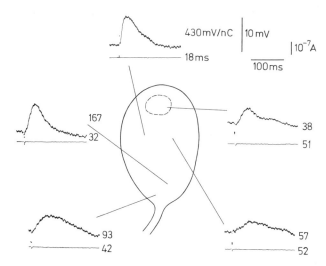

Fig. 11. Variability in acetylcholine responses evoked from different spots on the neuronal surface of denervated frog vagal ganglion cells. Acetylcholine was released from a micropipette by a 1 ms current pulse, monitored on the lower sweeps. Sample records from 5 spots on the surface of a cell. With each record is a number indicating the sensitivity (mV/nC) and, below this, the time to peak of the response (ms) measured at that spot. No synaptic boutons were identified on this cell, and the spots were randomly selected. At each spot the "current response" could be obtained by increasing the intensity of the current pulse through the acetylcholine electrode (HARRIS et al., 1971)

   In an interesting preliminary report, DUN and NISHI (1974) described subsensitivity to nicotine and acetylcholine (in the presence of atropine) in single cells of the rabbit superior cervical ganglion. Although there are no changes in the resting membrane potential or the passive electrical properties of the membrane, there is a reduced response to the nicotinic drugs and an enhanced response to muscarinic drugs. These experiments need to be repeated and extended.

   KUFFLER et al. (1971) have made a detailed study of the distribution of acetylcholine-sensitive sites in the vagal ganglion cells of the frog heart. In normally innervated cells, the chemosensitive sites are limited to subsynaptic regions; in denervated ganglion cells the entire cell surface shows varying degrees of sensitivity to iontophoretically applied acetylcholine (Fig. 11). The findings in ganglia correspond to those made in denervated muscle (GINETZINSKY and SHAMARINA, 1942; AXELSSON and THESLEFF, 1959; MILEDI, 1960). There is no information about the pharmacological properties of the newly formed chemosensitive sites in frog vagal ganglion cells. They may or may not be sensitive to blockade by atropine.

F. Conclusions

The varied actions of nicotinic drugs on autonomic ganglia are described graphically in Fig. 12 (HAEFELY, 1974a). Most of the nicotinic agents cause a bi-phasic sequence of depolarisation followed by hyperpolarisation of the ganglion cells. The hyperpolarisation is eliminated when the electrogenic sodium-pump mechanism is sup-

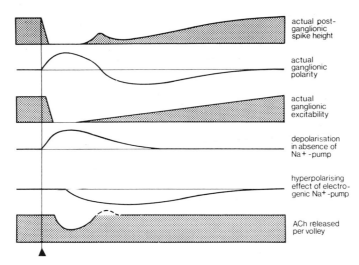

actual post-
ganglionic
spike height

actual
ganglionic
polarity

actual
ganglionic
excitability

depolarisation
in absence of
Na + -pump

hyperpolarising
effect of electro-
genic Na+ -pump

ACh released
per volley

Fig. 12. The effects of dimethylphenylpiperazinium as a representative nicotinic drug on the superior cervical ganglion. See text for discussion (HAEFELY, 1974a)

pressed. Ganglionic excitability and action potential amplitude are depressed during both phases of the ganglionic response to the drugs. However, it is probable that receptor desensitisation accounts for most of the reduced excitability during the late phase of transmission blockade. Finally, the nicotinic agents affect transmitter release from the preganglionic nerve terminals. Whereas evoked transmitter release is depressed, spontaneous release may be enhanced, albeit briefly, by the nicotinic drugs.

References

Alkadhi, K.A., McIsaac, R.J.: Effect of preganglionic nerve stimulation on the sensitivity of the superior cervical ganglion to nicotine blocking agents. Br. J. Pharmacol. 51, 533–539 (1974)

Ambache, N., Perry, W.L.M., Robertson, P.A.: The effect of muscarine on perfused superior cervical ganglia of cats. Br. J. Pharmacol. 11, 442–448 (1956)

Armett, C.J., Ritchie, J.M.: The action of acetylcholine and some related substances on conduction in mammalian non-myelinated nerve fibres. J. Physiol. (Lond.) 155, 372–384 (1961)

Axelsson, J., Thesleff, S.: A study of supersensitivity in denervated mammalian skeletal muscle. J. Physiol. (Lond.) 147, 178–193 (1959)

Baker, P.F., Connelly, C.M.: Some properties of the external activation site of the sodium pump in crab nerve. J. Physiol. (Lond.) 185, 270–297 (1966)

Beleslin, D.B., Malobabić, Z.S.: Cholinoceptive sites in the ganglia of myenteric plexus subserving the peristaltic reflex of guinea-pig isolated ileum. Neuropharmacology 13, 1091–1094 (1974)

Benoit, P.N., Audibert-Benoit, M.L., Peyrot, M.: Importance des effets presynaptiques dans le blocage de la jonction neuromusculaire de grenouille par substitution du lithium au sodium dans le milieu de survie. Arch. Ital. Biol. 3, 323–335 (1973)

Blackman, J.G., Ginsborg, B.L., Ray, C.: Synaptic transmission in the sympathetic ganglion of the frog. J. Physiol. (Lond.) 167, 355–373 (1963)

Branisteanu, D.D., Volle, R.L.: Modification by lithium of transmitter release at the neuromuscular junction of the frog. J. Pharmacol. Exp. Ther. 194, 362–372 (1975)

Branisteanu, D.D., Miyamoto, M.D., Volle, R.L.: Quantal release parameters during fade of end plate potentials. Naunyn Schmiedebergs Arch. Pharmacol. 288, 323–327 (1975)

Brown, D.A.: Depolarisation of normal and preganglionically denervated superior cervical ganglia by stimulant drugs. Br. J. Pharmacol. 26, 511–520 (1966)

Brown, D.A.: Responses of normal and denervated cat superior cervical ganglia to some stimulant compounds. J. Physiol. (Lond.) 201, 225–236 (1969)

Brown, D.A., Scholfield, C.N.: Movements of labelled sodium ions in isolated rat superior cervical ganglia. J. Physiol. (Lond.) 242, 321–351 (1974a)

Brown, D.A., Scholfield, C.N.: Changes of intracellular sodium and potassium ion concentrations in isolated rat superior cervical ganglia induced by depolarising agents. J. Physiol. (Lond.) 242, 307–319 (1974b)

Brown, D.A., Jones, K.B., Halliwell, J.V., Quilliam, J.P.: Evidence against a presynaptic action of acetylcholine during ganglionic transmission. Nature (Lond.) 226, 958–959 (1970)

Brown, D.A., Brownstein, M.J., Scholfield, C.N.: Origin of the after-hyperpolarisation that follows removal of depolarising agents from the isolated superior cervical ganglion of the rat. Br. J. Pharmacol. 44, 651–670 (1972)

Burn, J.H., Rand, M.J.: Acetylcholine in adrenergic transmission. Annu. Rev. Pharmacol. 5, 163–182 (1965)

Ciani, S., Edwards, C.: The effect of acetylcholine on neuromuscular transmission in the frog. J. Pharmacol. Exp. Ther. 142, 21–23 (1963)

Collier, B., Katz, H.S.: The release of acetylcholine by acetylcholine in the cat's superior cervical ganglion. Br. J. Pharmacol. 39, 428–438 (1970)

Collier, B., Katz, H.S.: The synthesis, turnover, and release of surplus acetylcholine in a sympathetic ganglion. J. Physiol. (Lond.) 214, 537–552 (1971)

Collier, B., Katz, H.S.: Studies upon the mechanism by which acetylcholine releases surplus acetylcholine in a sympathetic ganglion. Br. J. Pharmacol. 55, 189–197 (1975)

Colquhoun, D., Dionne, V.E., Steinbach, J.H., Stevens, C.F.: Conductance of channels opened by acetylcholine-like drugs in muscle end plate. Nature (Lond.) 253, 204–206 (1975)

DeGroat, W.C., Volle, R.L.: Ganglionic actions of oxotremorine. Life Sci. 8, 618–623 (1963)

Dennis, M.J., Harris, A.J., Kuffler, S.W.: Synaptic transmission and its duplication by locally applied acetylcholine in parasympathetic neurons in the heart of the frog. Proc. R. Soc. London [Biol.] 177, 509–539 (1971)

Dudel, J.: The effect of polarising current on action potential and transmitter release in crayfish motor nerve terminals. Pflügers Arch. 324, 227–248 (1971)

Dun, N., Nishi, S.: Electrophysiological investigations of the denervated sympathetic ganglion. Fed. Proc. 33, 299 (1974)

Dunant, Y.: Some properties of the presynaptic nerve terminals in a mammalian sympathetic ganglion. J. Physiol. (Lond.) 221, 577–587 (1972)

Eccles, J.C.: The physiology of synapses, p. 130. New York: Springer 1964

Eccles, R.M.: Intracellular potentials recorded from a mammalian sympathetic ganglion. J. Physiol. (Lond.) 130, 572–584 (1955)

Eccles, R.M.: The effect of nicotine on synaptic transmission in the sympathetic ganglion. J. Pharmacol. Exp. Ther. 118, 26–38 (1956)

Edwards, C., Ikeda, K.: Effects of 2-PAM and succinylcholine on neuromuscular transmission in the frog. J. Pharmacol. Exp. Ther. 138, 322–328 (1962)

Ferry, C.B.: The sympathomimetic effect of acetylcholine on the spleen of the cat. J. Physiol. (Lond.) 167, 487–504 (1963)

Gebber, G.L.: Dissociation of depolarisation and ganglionic blockade induced by nicotine. J. Pharmacol. Exp. Ther. 160, 124–134 (1968)

Gebber, G.L., Volle, R.L.: Ganglionic stimulating properties of aliphatic esters of choline and thiocholine. J. Pharmacol. Exp. Ther. 150, 67–74 (1965)

Gebber, G.L., Volle, R.L.: Mechanisms involved in ganglionic blockade induced by tetramethylammonium. J. Pharmacol. Exp. Ther. 152, 18–28 (1966)

Gebber, G.L., Snyder, D.W.: Observations on drug-induced activation of cholinoceptive sites in a sympathetic ganglion. J. Pharmacol. Exp. Ther. 163, 64–74 (1968)

Ginetzinsky, A.G., Shamarina, N.M.: The tonomotor phenomenon in denervated muscle. Usp. Sovrem. Biol. 15, 283–294 (1942) (Russ.)

Ginsborg, B.L.: The actions of McN-A-343, pilocarpine and acetyl-β-methylcholine on sympathetic ganglion cells of the frog. J. Pharmacol. Exp. Ther. *150*, 216–219 (1965)

Ginsborg, B.L.: On the presynaptic acetylcholine receptors in sympathetic ganglia of the frog. J. Physiol. (Lond.) *216*, 237–246 (1971)

Ginsborg, B.L., Guerrero, S.: On the action of depolarising drugs on sympathetic ganglion cells of the frog. J. Physiol. (Lond.) *172*, 189–206 (1964)

Green III, R.D.: The effect of denervation on the sensitivity of the superior cervical ganglion of the pithed cat. J. Pharmacol. Exp. Ther. *167*, 143–150 (1969)

Gumulka, W., Szreniawski, Z.: The effect of 1,1-dimethyl-4-phenylpiperazinium iodide on transmission in the superior cervical ganglion of the cat. Int. J. Neuropharmacol. 7, 511–515 (1968)

Gyermek, L.: Ganglionic stimulant and depressant agents. In: Drugs affecting the peripheral nervous system. Burger, A. (ed.), Vol. I, pp. 149–326. New York: Marcel Dekker 1967

Haefely, W.: Electrophysiology of the adrenergic neuron. In: Catecholamines. Blaschko, H., Muscholl, E. (eds.), pp. 661–725. Berlin, Heidelberg, New York: Springer 1972

Haefely, W.: The effects of 1,1-dimethyl-4-phenyl-piperazinium (DMPP) in the cat superior cervical ganglion in situ. Naunyn Schmiedebergs Arch. Pharmacol. *281*, 57–91 (1974a)

Haefely, W.: The effects of various "nicotine-like" agents in the cat superior cervical ganglion in situ. Naunyn Schmiedebergs Arch. Pharmacol. *281*, 93–117 (1974b)

Hamilton, J.T., Rubinstein, H.M.: Nicotinic and muscarinic activity of benzyltrimethylammonium and its α-, β-, and γ-substituted pyridylmethyltrimethylammonium analogs. J. Pharmacol. Exp. Ther. *160*, 112–123 (1968)

Hancock, J.C., Henderson, E.G.: Antinicotinic action of nicotine and lobeline on frog sartorius muscle. Naunyn Schmiedebergs Arch. Pharmacol. *272*, 307–324 (1972)

Hancock, J.C., Volle, R.L.: Blockade of conduction in vagal fibres by nicotinic drugs. Arch. Int. Pharmacodyn. *178*, 85–98 (1969a)

Hancock, J.C., Volle, R.L.: Enhancement by cesium ions of ganglionic hyperpolarisation induced by dimethylphenylpiperazinium (DMPP) and repetitive preganglionic stimulation. J. Pharmacol. Exp. Ther. *169*, 201–210 (1969b)

Hancock, J.C., Volle, R.L.: Cholinoceptive sites in the rat superior cervical ganglion. Arch. Int. Pharmacodyn. *184*, 111–120 (1970a)

Hancock, J.C., Volle, R.L.: Stimulation by carbachol and tetramethylammonium ions of intact and denervated sympathetic ganglia. Life Sci. 9, 301–308 (1970b)

Henderson, E.G., Hancock, J.C.: Nicotine-induced depolarisation and stimulation of potassium efflux in striated muscle. J. Pharmacol. Exp. Ther. *177*, 377–388 (1971)

Hodgkin, A.L., Katz, B.: The effect of sodium ions on the electrical activity of the giant axon of the squid. J. Physiol. (Lond.) *108*, 37–77 (1949)

Hubbard, J.I., Willis, W.D.: The effects of depolarisation of motor nerve terminals upon the release of transmitter by nerve impulses. J. Physiol. (Lond.) *194*, 381–405 (1968)

Hubbard, J.I., Schmidt, R.F., Yokota, T.: The effect of acetylcholine upon mammalian motor nerve terminals. J. Physiol. (Lond.) *181*, 810–829 (1965)

Hubbard, J.I., Llinás, R., Quastel, D.M.J.: Electrophysiological analysis of synaptic transmission. Baltimore: Williams and Wilkens 1969

Jaramillo, J.: Ganglionic actions of α,α'-bis-(dimethylammoniumacetylaldehyde diethylacetal)-p-p'-diacetylbiphenyl dibromide (DMAE). J. Pharmacol. Exp. Ther. *162*, 30–37 (1968)

Jaramillo, J., Volle, R.L.: Ganglion blockade by muscarine, oxotremorine and AHR-602. J. Pharmacol. Exp. Ther. *158*, 80–88 (1967a)

Jaramillo, J., Volle, R.L.: Nonmuscarinic stimulation and block of a sympathetic ganglion by 4-(m-chlorophenylcarbamoyloxy)-2-butyryltrimethylammonium chloride (McN-A-343). J. Pharmacol. Exp. Ther. *157*, 337–345 (1967b)

Jaramillo, J., Volle, R.L.: A comparison of the ganglionic stimulating and blocking properties of some nicotinic drugs. Arch. Int. Pharmacodyn. *174*, 88–97 (1968a)

Jaramillo, J., Volle, R.L.: Effects of lithium on ganglionic hyperpolarisation and blockade by dimethylphenylpiperazinium. J. Pharmacol. Exp. Ther. *164*, 166–175 (1968b)

Katz, B.: The transmission of impulses from nerve to muscle, and the cellular unit of synaptic action. Proc. R. Soc. Lond. [Biol.] *155*, 455–477 (1962)

Katz, B.: The release of neural transmitter substances. Liverpool: University Press 1969

Katz, B., Miledi, R.: Further observations on acetylcholine noise. Nature (Lond.) *232*, 124–126 (1971)

Katz, B., Miledi, R.: The statistical nature of the acetylcholine potential and its molecular components. J. Physiol. (Lond.) *224*, 665–699 (1972)

Katz, B., Thesleff, S.: A study of the "desensitisation" produced by acetylcholine at the motor end plate. J. Physiol. (Lond.) *138*, 63–80 (1957)

Kelly, J.S.: The antagonism of Ca^{2+} by Na^+ and other monovalent ions at the frog neuromuscular junction. Q. J. Exp. Physiol. *53*, 239–249 (1968)

Keynes, R.D., Swan, R.C.: The permeability of frog muscle fibres to lithium ions. J. Physiol. (Lond.) *147*, 626–638 (1959)

Kharkevich, D.A.: Ganglionic agents. Moskva: Medgiz 1962 (Russ.)

Kharkevich, D.A.: Ganglion-blocking and ganglion-stimulating agents. Oxford: Pergamon Press 1967 (translated from Russian edition, 1962)

Klingman, J.D.: Effects of lithium ions on the rat superior cervical ganglion. Life Sci. *5*, 365–373 (1966)

Koketsu, K.: Cholinergic synaptic potentials and the underlying ionic mechanisms. Fed. Proc. *28*, 101–112 (1969)

Koketsu, K., Nishi, S.: Cholinergic receptors at sympathetic preganglionic nerve terminals. J. Physiol. (Lond.) *196*, 293–310 (1968a)

Koketsu, K., Nishi, S., Soeda, H.: Calcium and acetylcholine-potential of bullfrog sympathetic ganglion cell membrane. Life Sci. *7*, Part I, 955–963 (1968b)

Kosterlitz, H.W., Lees, G.M.: Interrelationships between adrenergic and cholinergic mechanisms. In: Catecholamines. Blaschko, H., Muscholl, E. (eds.). Berlin, Heidelberg, New York: Springer 1972

Kosterlitz, H.W., Lees, G.M., Wallis, D.I.: Resting and action potentials recorded by the sucrose-gap method in the superior cervical ganglion of the rabbit. J. Physiol. (Lond.) *195*, 39–53 (1968)

Kosterlitz, H.W., Lees, G.M., Wallis, D.I.: Further evidence for an electrogenic pump in a mammalian sympathetic ganglion. Br. J. Pharmacol. *38*, 464–465 P (1970)

Kristić, M.K.: The action of choline on the superior cervical ganglion of the cat. Eur. J. Pharmacol. *17*, 87–96 (1972)

Kuffler, S.W., Dennis, M.J., Harris, A.J.: The development of chemosensitivity in extrasynaptic areas of the neuronal surface after denervation of parasympathetic ganglion cells in the heart of the frog. Proc. R. Soc. Lond. [Biol.] *177*, 555–563 (1971)

Lukomskaya, N.Ya.: Change in cholinergic sensitivity after denervation of the superior cervical ganglion of the cat. Zh. Evol. Biokhim. Fiziol. *5*, 65–73 (1969) (Russ.)

Lundberg, A., Thesleff, S.: Dual action of nicotine on the sympathetic ganglion of the cat. Acta Physiol. Scand. *28*, 218–223 (1953)

Machová, J., Boška, D.: The effect of 5-hydroxytryptamine, dimethylphenylpiperazinium and acetylcholine on transmission and surface potential in the cat sympathetic ganglion. Eur. J. Pharmacol. *7*, 152–158 (1969)

Magazanik, L.G.: Mechanism of desensitisation of the postsynaptic membrane of the muscle membrane. Biofizika *13*, 199–214 (1969) (Russ.)

Martin, A.R., Pilar, G.: Quantal components of the synaptic potential in the ciliary ganglion of the chick. J. Physiol. (Lond.) *175*, 1–16 (1964)

Matthews, E.K.: The presynaptic effects of quaternary ammonium compounds on the acetylcholine metabolism of a sympathetic ganglion. Br. J. Pharmacol. Chemother. *26*, 552–566 (1966)

McKinstry, D.N., Koelle, G.B.: Acetylcholine release from the cat superior cervical ganglion by carbachol. J. Pharmacol. Exp. Ther. *157*, 319–327 (1967)

McKinstry, D.N., Koenig, E., Koelle, W.A., Koelle, G.B.: The release of acetylcholine from a sympathetic ganglion by carbachol. Relationship to the functional significance of the localisation of acetylcholinesterase. Can. J. Biochem. Physiol. *41*, 2599–2609 (1963)

Miledi, R.: The acetylcholine sensitivity of frog muscle fibres after complete or partial denervation. J. Physiol. (Lond.) *151*, 1–23 (1960)

Miyamoto, M.D., Volle, R.L.: Enhancement by carbachol of transmitter release from motor nerve terminals. Proc. Natl. Acad. Sci. USA *71*, 1489–1492 (1974)

Nishi, S.: The cholinergic and adrenergic receptors of presynaptic nerves of sympathetic ganglia. Fed. Proc. *29*, 1956–1965 (1970)

Nishi, S., Koketsu, K.: Electrical properties and activities of single sympathetic neurones in frogs. J. Cell. Comp. Physiol. 55, 15–30 (1960)

Nishi, S., Soeda, H., Koketsu, K.: Influence of membrane potential on the fast-acetylcholine potential of sympathetic ganglion cells. Life Sci. 8, Part I, 499–505 (1969)

Onodera, K., Yamakawa, K.: The effects of lithium on the neuromuscular junction of the frog. Jpn. J. Physiol. 16, 541–550 (1966)

Pappano, A.J., Volle, R.L.: Observations on the role of calcium ions in ganglionic responses to acetylcholine. J. Pharmacol. Exp. Ther. 152, 171–180 (1966)

Pappano, A.J., Volle, R.L.: Actions of lithium ions in mammalian sympathetic ganglia. J. Pharmacol. Exp. Ther. 157, 346–355 (1967)

Pascoe, J.E.: The effects of acetylcholine and other drugs on the isolated superior cervical ganglion. J. Physiol. (Lond.) 132, 242–255 (1956)

Paton, W.D.M., Perry, W.L.M.: The relationship between depolarisation and block in the cat's superior cervical ganglion. J. Physiol. (Lond.) 119, 43–57 (1953)

Perry, W.L.M., Reinert, H.: The effects of preganglionic denervation on the reactions of ganglion cells. J. Physiol. (Lond.) 126, 101–115 (1954)

Pilar, G.: The physiology of preganglionic terminals. NATO Advanced Study Institute 46–61 (1969)

Rang, H.P., Ritchie, J.M.: On the electrogenic sodium pump in mammalian non-myelinated nerve fibres and its activation by various external cations. J. Physiol. (Lond.) 196, 183–221 (1968)

Rang, H.P., Ritter, J.M.: A new kind of drug antagonism: Evidence that agonists cause a molecular change in acetylcholine receptors. Mol. Pharmacol. 5, 394–411 (1969)

Riker, W.K.: The basis of the low-amplitude discharge produced by acetylcholine injections in sympathetic ganglia. J. Pharmacol. Exp. Ther. 155, 203–210 (1967)

Riker, W.K.: Ganglion cell depolarisation and transmission block by ACh: independent events. J. Pharmacol. Exp. Ther. 159, 345–352 (1968)

Riker, W.F. Jr., Standaert, F.G.: The action of facilitatory drugs and acetylcholine on neuromuscular transmission. Ann. N.Y. Acad. Sci. 135, 163–176 (1966)

Ritchie, J.M., Straub, R.: The hyperpolarisation which follows activity in mammalian nonmedullated fibres. J. Physiol. (Lond.) 136, 80–97 (1957)

Roszkowski, A.P.: An unusual type of sympathetic ganglionic stimulant. J. Pharmacol. Exp. Ther. 132, 156–170 (1961)

Sjodin, R.A., Beauge, L.A.: Coupling and selectivity of sodium and potassium transport in squid giant axons. J. Gen. Physiol. 51, 152–161 S (1968)

Steinberg, M.I., Volle, R.I.: A comparison of lobeline and nicotine at the frog neuromuscular junction. Naunyn Schmiedebergs Arch. Pharmacol. 272, 16–31 (1972)

Takeshige, C., Volle, R.L.: Bimodal response of sympathetic ganglia to acetylcholine following eserine or repetitive preganglionic stimulation. J. Pharmacol. Exp. Ther. 138, 66–73 (1962)

Takeshige, C., Volle, R.L.: Cholinoceptive sites in denervated sympathetic ganglia. J. Pharmacol. Exp. Ther. 141, 206–213 (1963a)

Takeshige, C., Volle, R.L.: Asynchronous postganglionic firing from the cat superior cervical sympathetic ganglion treated with neostigmine. Br. J. Pharmacol. 20, 214–220 (1963b)

Takeshige, C., Volle, R.L.: Similarities in the ganglionic actions of calcium ions and atropine. J. Pharmacol. Exp. Ther. 145, 173–180 (1964a)

Takeshige, C., Volle, R.L.: The effects of barium and other inorganic cations on sympathetic ganglia. J. Pharmacol. Exp. Ther. 146, 327–334 (1964b)

Takeshige, C., Volle, R.L.: Modification of ganglionic responses to cholinomimetic drugs following preganglionic stimulation, anticholinesterase agents and pilocarpine. J. Pharmacol. Exp. Ther. 146, 335–343 (1964c)

Takeshige, C., Pappano, A.J., DeGroat, W.C., Volle, R.L.: Ganglionic blockade produced in sympathetic ganglia by cholinomimetic drugs. J. Pharmacol. Exp. Ther. 141, 333–342 (1963)

Takeuchi, A., Takeuchi, N.: Changes in potassium concentration around motor nerve terminals, produced by current flow, and their effects on neuromuscular transmission. J. Physiol. (Lond.) 155, 46–58 (1961)

Takeuchi, A., Takeuchi, N.: Electrical changes in pre- and postsynaptic axons of the giant synapse of Loligo. J. Gen. Physiol. 45, 1181–1193 (1962)

Tauc, L.: Transmission in invertebrate and vertebrate ganglia. Physiol. Rev. 47, 521–593 (1967)

Thesleff, S.: The mode of neuromuscular block caused by acetylcholine, nicotine, decamethon-
    ium, and succinylcholine. Acta Physiol. Scand. *34*, 218–231 (1955)
Trendelenburg, U.: Non-nicotinic ganglion-stimulating substances. Fed. Proc. *18*, 1001–1005
    (1959)
Trendelenburg, U.: Some aspects of the pharmacology of autonomic ganglion cells. Ergeb.
    Physiol. *59*, 1–85 (1967)
Vickerson, F.H.L., Varma, D.R.: Effects of denervation on the sensitivity of the superior cervical
    ganglion of the cat to acetylcholine and McN-A-343. Can. J. Biochem. Physiol. *47*, 255–259
    (1969)
Vladimirova, I.A.: The effect of electrical polarisation of the motor nerve endings on the trans-
    mission through them of single impulses. Bull. Exp. Biol. Med. *56*, 1180–1183 (1963) (Russ.)
Volle, R.L.: Enhancement of postganglionic responses to stimulating agents following repetitive
    preganglionic stimulation. J. Pharmacol. Exp. Ther. *136*, 68–74 (1962)
Volle, R.L.: Muscarinic and nicotinic stimulant actions at autonomic ganglia. International
    encylopedia of pharmacology and therapeutics, Sect. 12, Vol. I. London: Pergamon Press
    1966 a
Volle, R.L.: Modification by drugs of synaptic mechanisms in autonomic ganglia. Pharmacol.
    Rev. *18*, 839–869 (1966 b)
Volle, R.L.: Frequency dependent decrease of quantal content in a drug-treated neuromuscular
    junction. Naunyn Schmidebergs Arch. Pharmacol. *278*, 271–284 (1973)
Volle, R.L.: Blockade by lobeline of potassium exchange in skeletal muscle. Relationship to
    receptor desensitisation at the end plate. Naunyn Schmiedebergs Arch. Pharmacol. *282*,
    335–347 (1974)
Volle, R.L.: Cellular pharmacology of autonomic ganglia. In: Cellular pharmacology of excitable
    tissues. Narahashi, T. (ed.), pp. 89–140. Springfield: Charles C. Thomas 1975
Volle, R.L., Henderson, E.G.: Pre- and postjunctional neuromuscular blockade by carbachol.
    Naunyn Schmiedebergs Arch. Pharmacol. *291*, 4, 359–370 (1975)
Volle, R.L., Koelle, G.B.: The physiological role of acetylcholinesterase in sympathetic ganglia. J.
    Pharmacoe. Exp. Ther. *129*, 223–240 (1961)
Volle, R.L., Koelle, G.B.: Ganglionic stimulating and blocking agents. In: The pharmacological
    basis of therapeutics, 5 th ed., Goodman, L.S., Gilman, A., (eds.), pp. 565–574. New York:
    Macmillan 1975
Wang, C.M., Narahashi, T.: Mechanisms of dual action of nicotine on end plate membranes. J.
    Pharmacol. Exp. Ther. *182*, 427–441 (1972)
Wong, S., Long, J.P.: Potentiation of action of catecholamines by a derivative of hemicholinium.
    J. Pharmacol. Exp. Ther. *156*, 469–482 (1967)
Wong, S., Long, J.P.: Antagonism of ganglionic stimulants by α,α'-bis-(dimethylammoni-
    umacetaldehyde diethylacetal)-p-p'-diacetylbiphenyl bromide (DMAE). J. Pharmacol. Exp.
    Ther. *164*, 176–184 (1968)
Woodward, J.K., Bianchi, C.P., Erulkar, S.D.: Electrolyte distribution in rabbit superior cervical
    ganglion. J. Neurochem. *16*, 289–299 (1969)

CHAPTER 10

Non-Nicotinic Chemical Stimulation
of Automatic Ganglia

W.E. HAEFELY

A. Introduction

This chapter deals with agents (a) that are able to induce the generation of action potentials in autonomic ganglion cells and/or to facilitate the generation of action potentials in response to orthodromic or direct electrical stimulation or to chemical stimulation and (b) whose sites of action in the membrane of ganglion cells are not on the nicotinic acetylcholine receptor (nAChR)[1]. The ganglionic effects of non-nicotinic ganglion-stimulating agents are mediated by (a) specific receptors different from the nAChR, (b) non-specific alterations of the properties of the ganglion cell membrane, or (c) changes in the ionic distribution between the interior and the exterior of ganglion cells.

Several earlier reviews on this topic exist (KHARKEVICH, 1967; VOLLE, 1966a,b; TRENDELENBURG, 1967), that by TRENDELENBURG (1967) comprehensively covering the literature on non-nicotinic stimulants up to 1966 and containing excellent introductions into the history of muscarinic stimulants, histamine, 5-hydroxytryptamine, and polypeptides, which the interested reader should consult. The reviews by VOLLE (1966a,b) and by HAEFELY (1972) are mainly concerned with electrophysiological aspects of ganglionic transmission. During the past few years, research in ganglionic pharmacology has led to the discovery of only a few novel ganglion-stimulating agents; it has been directed mainly towards a better understanding of non-nicotinic ganglionic stimulation and towards definition of the conditions under which this stimulation occurs.

The aim of the present review is not to cite all papers in which a non-nicotinic ganglion-stimulating agent is mentioned, but to put emphasis on those studies that provide quantitative information and possible explanations for previous observations of non-nicotinic ganglionic stimulation.

While all autonomic ganglion cells investigated so far have been found to be consistently excited by acetylcholine (ACh) through nAChR, there is a bewildering variability in the sensitivity of individual ganglion cells and whole ganglia to non-

---

[1] Abbreviations used in this chapter
ACh, acetylcholine; AChR, acetylcholine receptor; nAChR, nicotinic acetylcholine receptor; mAChR, muscarinic acetylcholine receptor; AChE, acetylcholine esterase; AHR-602, *n*-benzyl-3-pyrrolidyl acetate methobromide; C_6, hexamethonium; cAMP, adenosine 3',3'-monophosphate; DMPP, 1,1-dimethyl-4-phenyl-piperazinium iodide; *d*-TC, *d*-tubocur-arine; 5-HT, 5-hydroxytryptamine; cGMP, guanosine 3',5'-monophosphate; McN-A-343, 4-(*m*-chlorophenylcarbamoyloxy)-2-buty-nyltrimethylammonium chloride; EPSP, excitatory postsynaptic potential; IPSP, inhibitory postsynaptic potential; TEA, tetraethylammonium; TMA, tetramethylammonium.

nicotinic stimulants. Autonomic ganglia are often made up of a very inhomogeneous population of cells with respect to size, synaptic connections, projections, transmitter, etc. So far no systematic study has been made of the sensitivity to non-nicotinic stimulants of sympathetic and parasympathetic ganglia, of identical ganglia in different species, or of different ganglia in the same individual. Great care must, therefore, be taken to avoid any unjustified generalisations.

The agents to be discussed below have only one property in common: their stimulant effects of ganglion cells are resistant to classic ganglion-blocking drugs like *d*-tubocurarine (*d*-TC), hexamethonium (C_6), mecamylamine, and tetraethyl-ammonium (TEA) in doses that markedly depress or abolish the ganglion-stimulating effect of nicotine. This statement contains an important aspect of the problem of drug interaction experiments. In fact, it would be naïve to believe that the above-mentioned anti-nicotinic agents exhibit an absolute pharmacological specificity. There will be a dose with any compound which, besides blocking nAChR, also affects other receptors or non-specific properties of neuronal elements. The same is certainly true for anti-muscarinic agents, antihistamines and 5-hydroxytryptamine antagonists. Not every ganglionic stimulation abolished by atropine is per se a muscarinic response; the two optical isomers of atropine, *l*- and *d*-hyoscyamine, are equipotent in blocking transmission in the rat superior cervical ganglion (NILWISES and SCHMIDT, 1965), although the anti-muscarinic activity of atropine resides entirely in the natural *l*-hyoscyamine. It is imperative in most situations not to use maximally effective doses of an antagonist in order to differentiate drug receptors, but rather to determine precisely in each experiment the degree of antagonism actually achieved.

Non-nicotinic ganglion stimulants known so far can be divided into three classes.

Endogenous compounds and their derivatives or analogues make up the first class. They produce their effects by combining with specific pharmacological receptors in the membrane. Operationally, these receptors can be defined as macromolecules that undergo conformational changes upon binding an agonist molecule. These changes result in altered membrane properties such as the degree or selectivity of ionic conductance or the operation of active ion transport either directly – if the receptor molecules are ionophores or ion pumps – or indirectly by transferring signals to membrane ionophors or constituents of membrane pumps. The receptor molecules have a "receptive site," which recognises and binds molecules that are able to induce the required conformational change (agonists) or to selectively prevent this effect (antagonists). The various receptors can be characterised by their affinity for different agonists and antagonists in a way analogous to that used to distinguish different enzymes by their affinities for substrates and inhibitors. Examples are the muscarinic cholinergic receptor or ACh receptor (mAChR), the 5-hydroxytryptamine (5-HT) receptors, histamine receptors, etc.

The second class is made up of *compounds that affect membrane properties in a similar way* to representatives of the first class. However, the onset of their effect is usually slow and, once fully developed, slowly reversible by wash-out of the compound. Examples are the inhibitors of Na^+ and K^+ ATPase, such as cardiac glycosides, and some veratrum alkaloids, which alter the resting ionic conductance and the time course of the conductance changes that underly the action potential.

Inorganic cations, which as charge carriers either alter primarily some membrane properties or change the ionic concentration gradients between the cell interior and exterior that are responsible for the trans-membrane potential, make up the third class. The potassium ion (K^+) is the classic representative.

This classification of non-nicotinic ganglion stimulants may not be definitive, but it is felt to represent the current state of knowledge.

B. Muscarinic Ganglion Stimulants

I. General Information

Most of our knowledge on muscarinic cholinoceptors or cholinergic receptors (mAChRs) is derived from smooth muscle, especially of the intestine. Although mAChRs have not yet been isolated in a pure form and chemically characterised, they are real entities, most probably integral macromolecules of cell membranes. They have spots on which low-molecular ligands bind reversibly and thereby induce conformational changes. These ligands are called muscarinic agonists (Fig. 1). The relative potencies of a series of agonists for inducing changes in the receptor molecule, and consequently a measurable functional response of a cell or a whole organ, characterises the receptor from the agonist point of view. Typical and highly selective muscarinic agonists are, e.g., muscarine, methacholine, pilocarpine. The "activation" of the receptor molecule by agonists can be prevented by antagonist molecules that attach themselves either also to the binding site for agonists – but obviously in a less perfect manner – or to other spots on the receptor molecule, whereby the spatial arrangement of the agonist-binding site is modified. Typical muscarinic antagonists are atropine and hyoscine. The cellular response to the activation of one kind of receptor, e.g., the mAChR, may be quite different from the response induced by the activation of another receptor, e.g., of a nAChR, or the activation of two different receptors may result in an identical response of the target cell. The pharmacology of autonomic ganglia has been confusing for many decades because the names of the receptors on ganglion cells were coined according to the whole ganglionic response they mediated rather than according to the affinities of agonists and antagonists.

1. Acetylcholine (ACh)

The action of ACh on autonomic ganglia can be investigated by two different approaches. Firstly, ACh can be applied by one of several ways (addition to the blood or an artificial electrolyte solution irrigating a ganglion in situ, incubation of an isolated ganglion and microiontophoretic application) to a ganglion preparation ("exogenous" ACh). Several drawbacks are inherent in this approach. In fact, it is quite obvious that ACh applied to a ganglion from the outside, even with a micropipette, will never mimic in all respects the ACh released from preganglionic nerve endings into the synaptic space. It is, therefore, important to observe due reservations when comparing findings with "exogenous" ACh and observations on the effect of ACh released during preganglionic nerve activity ("endogenous ACh").

An introduction to the problem of muscarinic ganglionic stimulation is provided by the following very illustrative example (Fig. 2B and D). FLEISCH et al. (1969) injected ACh into the blood supply of the *dog sympathetic stellate ganglion in situ* and recorded the positive chronotropic responses of the heart. The effect of ACh was

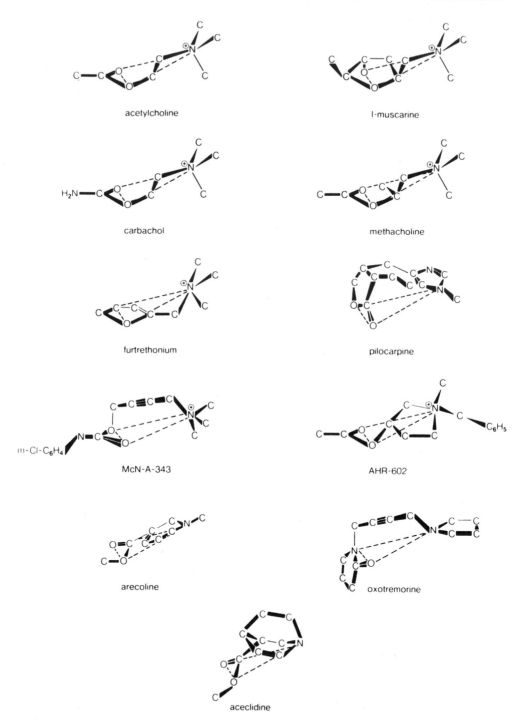

Fig. 1. Main muscarinic ganglion-stimulating agents with possible conformations to fit an hypothetical three-point receptor site

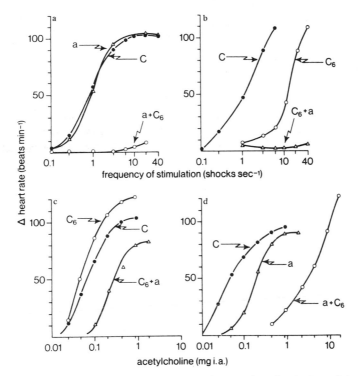

Fig. 2a–d. Effects of C_6, atropine and their combination on the stimulation of the dog stellate ganglion in situ by endogenous **(a, b)** and exogenous **(c, d)** ACh. On the ordinate is plotted the increase of the heart rate as the index of ganglionic stimulation, on the abscissa the frequency of stimulation of the preganglionic nerves **(a, b)** or of the doses of ACh injected close-arterially **(c, d)**. *c* pre-drug control values, *a* indicates atropine i.v. (0.03–3 mg/kg in *A*, 0.03 mg/kg in **b**, 1–3 mg/kg in **c**, 3 mg/kg in **d**). C_6 was given in doses of 4–10 mg/kg in **a**, in doses of 10–30 mg/kg in **b** and **c**, and 100 mg/kg in **d**. The curves are based on the results of FLACKE and GILLIS (1968) **(a, b)** and FLEISCH et al. (1969) **(c, d)**

unaffected by even high doses of C_6, d-TC, mecamylamine, and chlorisondamine. On the other hand, atropine (1–3 mg kg^{-1}) shifted the dose-response curve of ACh to the right by a factor of 3. Higher doses of atropine were no more effective. After an ineffective dose of C_6 (10–30 mg kg^{-1}), however, increasing doses of atropine (0.01–1 mg kg^{-1}) produced a step-wise shift of the dose-response curve to the right; the pA_2 value calculated from these shifts was 8.44. Conversely, when atropine (3 mg kg^{-1}) was given first, then subsequent doses of C_6 also resulted in a shift to the right with a calculated pA_2 value of 5.57.

The following findings were obtained with "endogenous" ACh (FLACKE and GIL-LIS, 1968) (Fig. 2 A, B): The curve relating the frequency of preganglionic stimulation to the heart rate response was shifted to the right by C_6 and the C_6-resistant responses were abolished by a low dose of atropine. Atropine alone did not affect the curve, but in its presence C_6 now abolished the responses to preganglionic stimulation. The unavoidable conclusion, that both exogenous and endogenous ACh were able to stimulate the stellate ganglion by either nicotinic or muscarinic receptors, is fully supported by an increasing number of observations on the same and other ganglia. In marked contrast to the findings in cat stellate ganglion, no trace of a C_6-resistant stimulation by exogenous and endogenous ACh was observed in the *cat parasympathetic ciliary ganglion in situ* (SCHAFFNER, 1973; SCHAFFNER and HAEFELY, 1974).

Between these two extreme situations represented by the sympathetic stellate ganglion of dog and the parasympathetic ciliary ganglion of cat, respectively, a large number of observations on more or less marked muscarinic stimulation can be ranged. There would be little sense in citing all the accidental observations of a muscarinic stimulant effect of ACh scattered through the literature. Only those experiments will be discussed that provide insight into the operation of muscarinic ganglionic stimulation.

As already pointed out, the dog stellate ganglion is an example of a ganglion with very powerful muscarinic excitatory mechanisms (FLACKE and GILLIS, 1968; FLEISCH et al., 1969). Since it is easy in the dog stellate ganglion preparation to study either the nicotinic or the muscarinic pathway of transmission separately, GILLIS et al. (1968) were able to clarify the controversy about the facilitation of ganglionic transmission and the reversal of transmission block by anticholinesterases. Both eserine and diisopropylfluorophosphate potentiated the transmission of preganglionic impulses during blockade of nAChRs, but had no effect on the purely nicotinic effects of preganglionic stimulation. These findings were extended to the situation in which transmission was depressed by hemicholinium-3. BROWN, A.M. (1967), working with dogs and cats, recorded the electrical activity in postganglionic fibres to the heart in response to preganglionic stimuli. During the i.v. infusion of high amounts of C_6, the synchronous mass action potentials recorded in the cardiac nerves in response to preganglionic stimulation at 20/s for 10 s disappeared and were replaced by a continuous low-amplitude asynchronous firing that persisted 0.5–4 min after the end of the stimulation period. These discharges were abolished by 30 μg/kg of atropine i.v. The fundamentally different pattern of postganglionic firing in the normal state and during blockade of nAChR will become understandable below in the discussion on the slow synaptic potential of the ganglion.

In the *cat superior cervical ganglion*, the most frequently used ganglion preparation, nictitating membrane contractions in response to preganglionic stimuli have never been reported after blockade with C_6, despite the fact that electrophysiologists have long known that this blocking agent does not abolish all electric responses in cells (for the history of slow synaptic potentials in autonomic ganglia see HAEFELY, 1972). However, when TRENDELENBURG (1966 b) investigated transmission through the cat superior cervical ganglion in situ during the late phase of nicotine-induced blockade, trains of preganglionic stimuli at a rate of 25/s produced small contractions of the nictitating membrane, while i.a. injections of nicotine were ineffective. The responses to preganglionic stimuli had a longer latency than responses in the unblocked condition, and lasted at least five times longer. They were readily blocked by atropine and reduced by morphine.

The analysis of the C_6-sensitive and the atropine-sensitive ganglion-stimulating effects of ACh requires the use of electrophysiological methods (Fig. 3). The close-arterial injection of ACh in normal ganglia usually produces a simple short-lasting depolarisation, which is accompanied by a brisk discharge in postganglionic nerves,

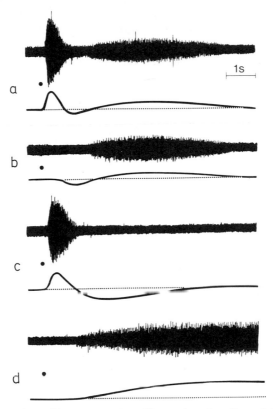

Fig.3a–d. Half-schematic oscilloscope tracings illustrating the effect of ACh and pilocarpine injected into the arterial blood supply of the cat superior cervical ganglion in situ on the electrical activity in a postganglionic nerve (upper traces of the pairs) and on the ganglionic surface potential (bottom traces of the pairs). **a** the effect of ACh in the absence of other drugs, **b** the effect of the same dose of ACh after a dose of C_6 that abolished orthodromic action potentials, **c** after recovery from C_6 and after a low dose of hyoscine. **d** shows the initial phase of the long lasting ganglionic stimulation induced by pilocarpine. Dots indicate the time of intra-arterial injections

as first described by TAKESHIGE and VOLLE (1963b). After very high doses, the initial depolarisation was followed by prolonged hyperpolarisation. In rare cases, a more complex sequence of events was observed. The initial transient depolarisation was followed by a delayed one of lower amplitude but longer duration. A faint discharge sometimes occurred during this late depolarisation. This complex response was regularly observed after several procedures such as chronic denervation, repetitive preganglionic stimulation (TAKESHIGE and VOLLE, 1962, 1963a, 1964c) and after drugs such as anticholinesterases (TAKESHIGE and VOLLE, 1963b), isoprenaline (DE GROAT and VOLLE, 1966), and KCl (TAKESHIGE and VOLLE, 1963b). The bi-modal stimulation could be clearly ascribed to activation of nAChRs and mAChRs, since the early depolarisation and discharge were blocked by C_6 and similar drugs, whereas the late depolarisation and firing were abolished by atropine or hyoscine. The two phases were separated by a short intermediary phase characterised by a relative or absolute hyperpolarisation and a postganglionic silence. This inhibitory phase is also abolished by atropine and is due either to activation of a special kind of mAChR (inhibitory mAChR) or to the intraganglionic release of catecholamines. The multiphasic events elicited by exogenous ACh under the special conditions mentioned above ("sensitisation") have a counterpart in the events observed in a ganglion partially blocked by C_6 in response to short trains of preganglionic stimuli, or even to a single preganglionic impulse under optimal sensitising conditions (HAEFELY, 1974c). They consist of an early depolarisation (the N wave), an intermediate hyperpolarisation (P wave) and the late depolarisation (LN wave).

The N wave is abolished by high doses of C_6, whereas the other two waves and the asynchronous discharge coinciding with the LN wave are sensitive to atropine. A large body of evidence elaborated in other sympathetic ganglia permits the identification of the three waves as the sum of the extracellularly recorded synaptic potentials, the fast (nicotinic) EPSP, the (muscarinic or catecholaminergic) IPSP, and the (muscarinic) slow EPSP.

It has also been established that the transmission of preganglionic impulses during blockade of nicotinic receptors is accomplished by the summation of individual slow EPSPs during and after a train of preganglionic tetanic stimulation. The dual stimulant action of ACh explains findings obtained in isolated ganglia, in which the time course of the ACh effect, so clearly seen with bolus injections into the blood supply in situ, is absent. Thus, BROWN, D.A. (1966a) was able to reduce the ACh-induced depolarisation in isolated kitten ganglia by C_6 and to abolish it by the addition of hyoscine. The dual stimulant action of ACh is probably the clue to the old controversy of whether chronic denervation of the ganglion changes its sensitivity to the transmitter. Three recent investigations of this problem published within the same year yielded apparently contradictory results (GREEN, 1969; BROWN, D.A., 1969; VICKERSON and VARMA, 1969). Besides the difficulty of finding an appropriate parameter of "ganglionic stimulation" (depolarisation? postganglionic discharge? nictitating membrane contraction?), possible opposite changes in the reactivity of nicotinic and muscarinic mechanisms offer a number of pitfalls.

After elimination of the problem of cholinesterase, GREEN (1969) showed convincingly that the nicotinic stimulant potency of ACh was decreased. Whether the more pronounced effect of ACh through mAChRs in the denervated ganglion fully or incompletely compensates for the reduced nicotinic stimulant mechanism cannot be answered definitively. An interesting observation of GEBBER and SNYDER (1968) illustrates the rapid changes that can occur in nicotinic and muscarinic reactions. In a normal ganglion, a bolus injection of ACh produced a discharge that could be blocked by C_6. The i.a. infusion of constant amounts of ACh produced a postganglionic firing that became virtually resistant to C_6 after only 2 min of infusion, but was completely abolished by atropine. The marked shift of the action of ACh from purely nicotinic stimulation to purely or predominantly muscarinic stimulation in the experiments of GEBBER and SNYDER (1968) is probably related to the fact that the most effective "sensitisation" of the cat superior cervical ganglion to muscarinic responses occurs in the late phase of block by nicotine, which is due to a desensitisation of nAChRs (HAEFELY, 1974b,c). The combination of a slight ganglionic depolarisation and a desensitisation of nAChRs made it possible to obtain P and LN waves in the cat superior cervical ganglion as well as a late discharge in response to a single preganglionic volley (HAEFELY, 1974c).

In the isolated *rat superior cervical ganglion* (DOLIVO and KOELLE, 1970) atropine abolished the discharges induced by adding ACh to the bathing solution. Similarly, asynchronous discharges occurring in eserinised ganglia following repetitive preganglionic stimulation was abolished by atropine but enhanced by *d*-TC (DUNANT and DOLIVO, 1967; DOLIVO and KOELLE, 1970). The depolarisation of the rat superior cervical ganglion incubated in a solution containing ACh was reduced by either C_6 or atropine, and virtually abolished by the combination of the two agents (BROWN, D.A., 1966 a). Close-arterial injection of ACh (5–10 µg) produced a bi-modal firing in the rat superior cervical ganglion in situ, the first phase being sensitive to C_6 and the second one to low doses of atropine (HANCOCK et al., 1969). Bi-modal firing was also induced in the ganglion perfused in situ; in this case, however, the second phase could be blocked by either C_6 or atropine. The authors concluded that perfusion of the ganglion altered the specificity of nAChRs and mAChRs.

The identical nature of the LN wave and the late depolarisation in response to exogenous ACh has been discussed above in connection with the cat superior cervical ganglion. It must be emphasised, however, that the present views on synaptic muscarinic events in autonomic ganglia are largely the result of studies performed on rabbit and frog sympathetic ganglia in the laboratories of LIBET (LIBET, 1967; LIBET et al., 1968; LIBET and KOBAYASHI, 1969) and of KOKETSU et al., 1968 a, b; KOKETSU, 1969). The results obtained by these two groups of investigators have been presented in detail in an earlier review (HAEFELY, 1972). Only some aspects that are of particular interest for the pharmacologist and are related to the ionic mechanisms of muscarinic stimulation will, therefore, be mentioned below.

The *isolated rabbit superior cervical ganglion* was used recently to study the controversial effect of chronic denervation on nicotinic and muscarinic responses (DUN et al., 1976 a). Intracellular recording was used to obtain dose-response curves for the depolarising action of ACh through mAChRs in the presence of *d*-TC. In normal ganglia the threshold concentration of ACh for muscarinic depolarisation was about 10 times higher than for nicotinic depolarisation. The maximum muscarinic depolarisation was about 40% of the maximum nicotinic depolarisation (obtained in the presence of atropine). Chronic denervation shifted the dose-response curve for muscarinic depolarisation to the left by a factor of 10 and almost doubled the maximum obtainable depolarisation. In the same experiments, denervation markedly reduced the nicotinic depolarisation of ACh, measured in the presence of atropine. Since the same authors (DUN et al., 1976 b) did not find changes in the passive and active membrane properties of ganglion cells after denervation, and since the affinity of ACh to its receptors appeared to be the same in innervated and denervated ganglia, the effect of denervation was ascribed to a decrease in the number of nAChRs and an increase in the number of mAChRs.

There appears to be general agreement that the slow EPSP (LN wave) and the late atropine-sensitive depolarisation by ACh are not due to an increase of the membrane ionic conductance, but rather to a decrease, if any change occurs (KOBAYASHI and LIBET, 1968, 1970, 1974; LIBET and KOBAYASHI, 1969; NISHI et al., 1969; WEIGHT and VOTAVA, 1970).

Several ionic mechanisms have been proposed to explain the late muscarinic depolarisation. WEIGHT and VOTAVA (1970) and WEIGHT (1974) provided evidence for a decrease of the K^+ conductance during the LN wave of frog ganglia blocked by high concentrations of nicotine. This view has been criticised by KOBAYASHI and LIBET (1974), who pointed to the not too surprising possibility that the late muscarinic depolarisation may not be identical in the presence and absence of nicotine. Studying the effect of hyperpolarising and depolarising currents on the slow EPSP, they concluded that the behaviour of an early phase of the slow EPSP was compatible with a decrease in the K^+ conductance, but only in ganglia blocked by nicotine. This phase was not observed in unblocked ganglia or ganglia incubated in d-TC; the slow EPSP in the latter condition did not respond to artificial polarisation changes as would be expected if the underlying mechanism was a decrement of the K^+ conductance. KUBA and KOKETSU (1974), working on "nicotinised" frog ganglia, considered the slow EPSP to be generated by increases in the conductances for Na^+ and Ca^{2++} and a simultaneous decrease of the conductance for K^+. The electrogenesis of the muscarinic depolarisation remains, therefore, to be clarified. It is of interest that the long latency of the muscarinic response to ACh is not restricted to autonomic ganglion cells but was also observed in smooth muscle cells (PURVES, 1974).

2. Muscarine

The first systematic study of the ganglionic actions of highly purified natural muscarine (Fig. 1) was probably that of AMBACHE et al. (1956). Working with the *in situ perfused superior cervical ganglion of the cat*, they found a variable stimulating effect of muscarine as deduced from contractions of the nictitating membrane. They estimated muscarine to be roughly 100 times as potent a stimulant as ACh and noted even then that the response to muscarine developed more slowly than that to the (nicotinic) action of ACh. In chronically denervated ganglia, muscarine produced more regular ganglion-stimulating effects. Atropine in small doses, which had little effect on the response to ACh, abolished the response to muscarine. However, C_6 was also found to block the stimulant effect of muscarine on the innervated ganglion, but was ineffective in chronically denervated ganglia. Essentially identical results were obtained by KONZETT and WASER (1956) under comparable experimental conditions with crystalline natural muscarine. The conclusion of both groups of investigators was that muscarine had "nicotinic" actions in the ganglion.

Whereas in the *inferior mesenteric ganglion* of the atropinised cat (HERR and GYERMEK, 1960) and in the atropinised pelvic nerve-bladder preparation of dog (GYERMEK and UNNA, 1960) natural and dl-muscarine, respectively, were devoid of any stimulant action, GYERMEK et al. (1963) observed an atropine-sensitive ganglion-stimulating effect of natural muscarine in the cat inferior mesenteric ganglion in situ. The racemic form was less potent, and the $d(-)$muscarine inactive. GYERMEK et al. (1963) appear to have been the first to realize that muscarine acted through mAChRs, and that ACh stimulated the ganglion through the two types of AChRs.

Synthetic dl-muscarine stimulated about 70% of *cat superior cervical ganglia in situ* in a study by SANGHVI et al. (1963). The compound produced a long-lasting contraction of the nictitating membrane, which occurred after a characteristic delay. Whereas repetitive injections of dl-muscarine into the blood supply of the nictitating membrane elicited contractions without any decline of sensitivity, ganglionic stimulation by the alkaloid was subject to tachyphylaxis. Sub-threshold doses of dl-muscarine facilitated ganglionic transmission. The discharges induced by dl-muscarine in the postganglionic nerve were of very low amplitude, especially compared with those elicited by the nicotinic stimulant, DMPP. The stimulant effect was readily blocked by low doses of atropine and cocaine, but not by C_6. SANGHVI et al. (1963) associated the receptor involved in the ganglionic action of dl-muscarine with that mediating the late negative (LN) wave of a curarised ganglion in response to tetanic preganglionic stimulation (ECCLES, R.M. and LIBET, 1961). JONES (1963) made very similar observations with dl-muscarine in the cat superior cervical ganglion in situ. She also found that about 70% of the non-sensitised innervated ganglia, but all the chronically denervated ones, were responsive to the compound. During the early phase of nicotine-induced ganglionic blockade ("depolarisation block") the effect of dl-muscarine was abolished, but it reappeared later on, at a time when nicotine and DMPP were still ineffective. In addition to atropine and cocaine, morphine and methadone also selectively blocked the muscarine response. In contrast, preceding preganglionic stimulation potentiated the effect of dl-muscarine.

The ganglionic surface potential and the postganglionic nerve activity of the cat superior cervical ganglion in situ in response to dl-muscarine were studied by BROWN, D.A. (1966b) and JARAMILLO and VOLLE (1967a). Their findings can be summarised as follows. After a delay of several seconds, muscarine induced an initial transient hyperpolarisation of the ganglion, which was followed by a small depolarisation of 5–10 min duration. Coinciding with the delayed depolarisation, asynchronous firing occurred in the postganglionic nerve. When injected at intervals of 15–30 min, muscarine produced regular identical responses. The compound also transiently depressed ganglionic transmission during the initial hyperpolarising phase. "Synaptic potentials" (N waves) induced by preganglionic volleys in a ganglion blocked by C_6 were depressed during both the hyperpolarising and the depolarising phase of the muscarine action. Whereas both phases were blocked by small doses of atropine, they were augmented by d-TC and by isoprenaline.

In the *isolated kitten superior cervical ganglion*, dl-muscarine induced a small depolarisation with no clear dose–effect relationship (BROWN, D.A., 1966a). The depolarisation was resistant to C_6, but was prevented by hyoscine.

The ganglionic response to muscarine, in summary, consists of an initial transient hyperpolarisation (in the cat superior cervical ganglion in situ), followed by a long-lasting low-amplitude depolarisation accompanied by an asynchronous postganglionic discharge. Except for the duration, mainly of the second phase, the bi-phasic effect of dl-muscarine is similar to that of ACh, methacholine, and oxotremorine. The compound is devoid of nicotinic actions, but activates both inhibitory and excitatory mAChRs in ganglia. Reports on the effect of muscarine on parasympathetic ganglia are lacking.

3. Methacholine (Acetyl-β-Methylcholine)

In the *cat superior cervical ganglion in situ*, methacholine (Fig. 1) produced a characteristic bi-phasic response (PAPPANO and VOLLE, 1962; TAKESHIGE et al., 1963; TAKESHIGE and VOLLE, 1964c). After a latency of several seconds, the ganglion was briefly hyperpolarised; this transient hyperpolarisation was followed by a longer-lasting low-amplitude depolarisation accompanied by a weak asynchronous discharge. Methacholine was considerably less potent than ACh. An effect was seen in only about 50% of non-sensitised ganglia (HAEFELY, unpublished). Repetitive pregan-glionic stimulation and anticholinesterase agents markedly enhanced the ganglionic firing in response to methacholine (TAKESHIGE and VOLLE, 1964c), whereas the initial hyperpolarisation remained unchanged or was slightly enhanced and the late depo-larisation was reduced. During ganglionic stimulation by pilocarpine, the hyperpo-larising effect of methacholine was markedly enhanced, while the late depolarisation and firing were depressed or abolished (TAKESHIGE and VOLLE, 1964c). The gan-glionic effects of methacholine were resistant to C_6 and abolished by small doses of atropine.

Besides having ganglion-stimulating properties, methacholine depressed gan-glionic transmission. VOLLE (1967) found a reduction of the synaptic potentials (N waves after blockade of action potentials by C_6) during both hyperpolarisation and depolarisation induced by methacholine. The depressant action of methacholine on ganglionic transmission was blocked by atropine; its independence from gan-glionic polarisation makes a presynaptic site of action very probable.

In the *isolated kitten superior cervical ganglion*, concentrations of methacholine below 10^{-4} g/ml produced hyperpolarisation (BROWN, D.A., 1966a). While higher concentrations were able to depolarise the ganglion, the maximum depolarisation was only 3–25% that obtained in the same preparations with carbachol. The effects of methacholine were resistant to C_6, but readily abolished by hyoscine.

In the *isolated rabbit superior cervical ganglion*, intracellular recording revealed a dose-dependent depolarising effect of methacholine that was virtually identical with that of ACh in the presence of *d*-TC (DUN et al., 1976a). Denervation shifted the dose-response curve for methacholine to the left by a factor of 10 and doubled the maximum depolarisation obtainable.

Isolated hypogastric ganglia of the guinea-pig and the rat were unresponsive to methacholine up to 100 µg/ml, even in the presence of eserine (BENTLEY, 1972). In 3 of 15 preparations, the only effect of methacholine was a marked facilitation of ganglionic transmission. In one-third of *perfused guinea-pig hypogastric ganglia*, methacholine caused a small contraction of the vas deferens, which amounted on average to 18.6% of the response to nerve stimulation. No effect of methacholine was observed in the isolated rat hypogastric ganglion.

In the *isolated frog paravertebral sympathetic ganglia*, GINSBORG (1965), using intracellular recording, observed a transient depolarisation with methacholine in concentrations above 10^{-3} M. Bursts of action potentials were induced at the onset of depolarisation. The depolarising action of methacholine was abolished by both C_6 and atropine in concentrations that nonetheless blocked ganglionic transmission. Methacholine depressed ganglionic transmission, usually even in non-depolarising concentrations.

In the *parasympathetic ciliary ganglion of the cat in situ*, methacholine was devoid of any ganglionic action (SCHAFFNER, 1973; SCHAFFNER and HAEFELY, 1974).

Methacholine can be described as a purely muscarinic ganglionic agent in mam-malian sympathetic ganglia. Ganglionic stimulation is not regularly observed in the cat superior cervical ganglion without sensitising procedures, and even in sensitised ganglia its stimulant effects are weak. The affinity of methacholine for inhibitory and excitatory mAChRs appears to be almost the same. In the parasympathetic ganglia investigated so far, methacholine had no action. The blockade of the stimulant action of methacholine in frog sympathetic ganglia by C_6 is a puzzling finding that requires further studies.

4. Pilocarpine

A stimulating action of pilocarpine (Fig. 1) on the *cat superior cervical ganglion* was observed by DALE and LAIDLAW (1912) after i.v. injections and after painting of the ganglion surface. In the subsequent four decades several reports, mostly concerned with the late pressor effect of pilocarpine, similarly indicated a stimulant action of the alkaloid on sympathetic ganglia (for this older literature see TRENDELENBURG, 1967), although the techniques and the pharmacological methods of analysis used were not always convincing. A re-examination by TRENDELENBURG (1954, 1955, 1957) clearly established that pilocarpine stimulated the superior cervical ganglion (in 60% of cats) and other sympathetic ganglia of cat. He found that the response of the sympathetically innervated organ taken as an indicator of ganglionic activity had a delayed onset compared with the response to nicotine and ACh, and also that it was of longer duration. Tachyphylaxis to pilocarpine was marked. Non-stimulating doses of the alkaloid facilitated transmission through the superior cervical ganglion. Both stimulation and facilitation were abolished by atropine and cocaine in doses that did not affect transmission. Ganglionic stimulation by pilocarpine was resistant to C_6; it was abolished shortly after an injection of nicotine, but enhanced during the later phase of transmission block induced by repeated injections of nicotine. The sensitivity of the cat superior cervical ganglion perfused in situ with Locke or Tyrode solution to the facilitatory action of pilocarpine was 1–10% that of the blood-perfused ganglion; only 25% of the artificially perfused ganglia were stimulated by the drug (TRENDELENBURG, 1956 b). It potentiated the ganglionic excitation produced by ACh, nicotine, carbachol, choline, and KCl. In contrast, the ganglionic stimulation by histamine and 5-hydroxytryptamine was reduced or abolished shortly after pilocarpine, as was that by pilocarpine after 5-hydroxytryptamine and histamine. A quantitative study of the effects of pilocarpine in the cat superior cervical ganglion in situ was performed by IORIO and McISAAC (1966). The drug induced dose-dependent contractions of the nictitating membrane in doses between 3 and 10 µg i.a. The maximum effect was about 30% of the maximum amplitude obtained with nicotine (1 µg). After repetitive preganglionic nerve stimulation the dose-response curve of pilocarpine was shifted to the left and the maximum almost doubled. Atropine shifted the dose-response curve of pilocarpine in sensitised ganglia to the right without affecting the maximum; C_6 did not significantly alter the effect of pilocarpine. An electrophysiological study by TAKESHIGE and VOLLE (1964 c) in the cat superior cervical ganglion revealed that pilocarpine produced a low-amplitude depolarisation, occurring 4–6 s after the close arterial injection and lasting 20–30 min after a dose of 10–40 µg. Asynchronous postganglionic firing was observed during the first 5–10 min of depolarisation. In contrast to ACh and methacholine, no hyperpolarising phase was present in the response to pilocarpine (Fig. 3). Identical findings were reported by ROSZKOWSKI et al. (1971). During the action of pilocarpine, the early (nicotinic) and the late (muscarinic) depolarisations of ACh were diminished, as was the depolarisation by methacholine. The hyperpolarising phases of the ACh and metacholine effects were either unmasked or, if already present before pilocarpine, markedly accentuated. In very similar experimental conditions, HAEFELY (1974c) confirmed the long-lasting ganglionic depolarisation and firing produced by pilocarpine. During the effect of pilocarpine in a ganglion blocked by C_6, short tetanic preganglionic trains of stimulation were applied. The resulting N and LN waves were reduced, the firing occurring during the N wave unaltered, the firing usually seen during the LN wave abolished, and the P wave markedly accentuated. The pilocarpine-induced postganglionic firing was depressed during the P waves. The findings of TAKESHIGE and VOLLE (1964c) and HAEFELY (1974c) show that during the stimulation of excitatory mAChRs by pilocarpine, the nicotinic effects are affected only slightly if at all, the stimulation of mAChRs is blocked, and the activation of inhibitory mAChRs is enhanced. These conclusions are further supported by the findings of ROSZKOWSKI et al. (1971). In anaesthetised cats, the nictitating membrane contractions and the rise of arterial blood pressure in response to the muscarinic ganglion stimulant McN-A-343 were blocked after a high dose of pilocarpine, whereas responses of the nictitating membrane and the pressor response to nicotinic stimulants were unaltered or increased. Similar interactions between pilocarpine and NcN-A-343 were observed on mAChRs of the smooth muscle of guinea-pig ileum.

The *rat superior cervical ganglion* was found by SCHNEYER and HALL (1966) to be stimulated by pilocarpine given i.p. and to mediate the increase of the amylase content of the saliva.

In *cat stellate ganglion*, pilocarpine also produced a long-lasting stimulation assessed by tachycardia (FLACKE and FLEISCH, 1970). The onset was delayed compared with nicotinic effects. In contrast to findings in cat superior cervical ganglion, the authors observed no tachyphylaxis in response to pilocarpine. The maximum tachycardic effect of pilocarpine was about 80% that obtained with nicotinic stimulants. Whereas nicotinic antagonists increased the maximum response to pilocarpine, the ED_{50} was unaltered. Atropine shifted the dose-response curve of pilocarpine to the right, and at higher doses depressed the maximum, the dose-ratio plot being compatible with a competitive antagonism up to a dose ratio of 100.

Results quite different from those in mammalian sympathetic and parasympathetic ganglia were reported by GINSBORG (1965). In *isolated frog paravertebral ganglia*, pilocarpine produced neither depolarisation nor ganglionic discharges. The only effect of pilocarpine in concentrations above $2 \times 10^{-4} M$ was a block of ganglionic transmission. The possibility remains that the apparent absence of muscarinic stimulation by pilocarpine (and McM-A-343) in the experiments of GINSBORG (1965) was due to the high concentrations used and to the in vitro conditions.

In *cat parasympathetic ciliary ganglion in situ*, pilocarpine was devoid of stimulating and blocking actions (SCHAFFNER, 1973; SCHAFFNER and HAEFELY, 1974).

In summary, pilocarpine is a rather potent stimulant of mammalian sympathetic ganglia through mAChRs. Interestingly, the drug has no effect on inhibitory mAChRs. In the parasympathetic ciliary ganglion of the cat, pilocarpine is inactive. In isolated frog sympathetic ganglia, the only effect of pilocarpine is to block transmission. The long-lasting effect of pilocarpine might be related to its being a tertiary amine, in contrast to other muscarinic stimulants, thus permitting an intracellular accumulation of the drug with a subsequent slow disappearance.

5. Carbachol (Carbaminoylcholine)

The main action of carbachol (carbamoylcholine) (Fig. 1) is undoubtedly on the nAChR. However, a muscarinic component is also present in its ganglion-stimulating action.

In experiments with *cat superior cervical ganglion in situ*, injections of carbachol in doses of 1 and 3 µg into the carotid artery induced a simple depolarisation of the ganglion (BROWN, D.A., 1966 a). After higher doses, the ganglionic negativity was usually increased; however, in some ganglia di- and tri-phasic changes of the ganglionic surface potential were observed. Either an initial depolarisation was separated from a late one by a transient hyperpolarisation, or a simple depolarisation wave was preceded by a short hyperpolarisation. Carbachol initiated asynchronous discharges in the postganglionic nerve. C_6 reduced, but never abolished the ganglionic depolarisation and the postganglionic discharge. Carbachol-induced ganglionic hyperpolarisation was never diminished, but rather enhanced by C_6. In contrast, hyoscine always increased the carbachol-induced depolarisation and abolished any hyperpolarisation. The effect of hyoscine on the postganglionic discharge was mainly to shorten it. The combination of C_6 and hyoscine depressed postganglionic firing more completely than either of the two compounds given alone. Nictitating membrane contractions induced by i.a. injection of carbachol (5 µg) were markedly reduced in size and duration by atropine and abolished by C_6 (BRIMBLE and WALLIS, 1974). It follows that carbachol stimulates both nAChRs and excitatory mAChRs and, in addition, it seems very likely that the drug also activates inhibitory mAChRs. Since most nicotinic stimulants produce a secondary hyperpolarisation as a consequence of depolarisation (HAEFELY, 1974 a, b), a re-investigation of the nature of the various carbachol-induced polarisation changes is obviously necessary.

In *isolated superior cervical ganglia of kitten and rats*, BROWN, D.A. (1966 b) confirmed the complexity of the carbachol-induced changes of ganglionic polarisation that were measured by the fluid electrode technique. Although C_6 substantially (55–75%) diminished carbachol-induced depolarisation, the antagonism was incomplete. However, the C_6-resistant depolarisation was readily abolished by hyoscine. On the other hand, hyoscine reduced (by 30%) but did not abolish carbachol-induced depolarisation. In low concentrations, carbachol sometimes produced a slight hyperpolarisation.

In the *isolated rabbit superior cervical ganglion*, intracellular recording showed carbachol to be somewhat less potent as a muscarinic depolarising compound and slightly more potent as a nicotinic stimulant than ACh (DUN et al., 1976 a). However, as for ACh, denervation markedly reduced the nicotinic effect and increased the muscarinic effect of carbachol.

The results of BROWN, D.A. (1966 a, b) and of DUN et al. (1976 a) clearly indicate that carbachol is a mixed nicotinic and muscarinic ganglion-stimulating agent. It probably also acts on inhibitory mAChRs (see HAEFELY, 1972). Carbachol is therefore not the ideal compound to use as a reference nicotinic stimulant, as it frequently is.

6. Arecoline

FELDBERG and VARTIAINEN (1934) observed contractions of the nictitating membrane when 50 µg or more of arecoline (Fig. 1) was injected into the fluid perfusing the *cat superior cervical ganglion in situ*. This effect of arecoline was at that time considered to represent a "nicotine-like" action. The injection of arecoline (75 µg) into the blood supply of cat superior cervical ganglion produced a contraction of the nictitating membrane that lasted about 1 min (BRIMBLE and WALLIS, 1974). This response was abolished by atropine but only immaterially reduced in size and duration by C_6. The surprisingly few studies performed with arecoline in sympathetic ganglia indicate that its stimulant action is predominantly, if not entirely, on mAChRs. This is in line with the effects of arecoline in the central nervous system, which are also blocked by atropine.

7. Choline

In *cat superior cervical ganglion in situ*, GEBBER and VOLLE (1965) found choline to have one-third to one-quarter the potency as a ganglion-stimulating agent as ACh. In non-sensitised ganglia, depolarisation and postganglionic firing induced by choline were abolished by C_6. In ganglia sensitised by AChE inhibitors, preganglionic stimulation, and isoprenaline, large doses of choline produced a late atropine-sensitive firing. The authors concluded that choline was a much less potent stimulant of mAChRs in the ganglion, which is in line with its weak muscarinic effect on autonomic effector organs.

8. Oxotremorine [1-(2-oxopyrrolidino)-4-pyrrolidino butyne-2]

In *cat superior cervical ganglion in situ*, whether normally innervated or chronically denervated, oxotremorine (Fig. 1) induced a slowly developing, low-amplitude firing (De GROAT and VOLLE, 1963). This effect was enhanced by prior conditioning orthodromic stimulation at 30/s for 30 s, and also by isoprenaline (DE GROAT and VOLLE, 1966). It was enhanced and prolonged by d-TC, unaffected by C_6, and abolished by atropine. Very similar results were obtained by BRIMBLE and WALLIS (1974), except that these authors obtained a small reduction by C_6 in the size and the duration of the contraction of the nictitating membrane in response to an i.a. injection of 20 µg oxotremorine. The compound induced a bi-phasic change of the ganglionic surface potential (JARAMILLO and VOLLE, 1967a). An initial transient hyperpolarisation was followed by a long-lasting low-amplitude depolarisation, as observed with methacholine (TAKESHIGE and VOLLE, 1964c). The biphasic changes of the ganglionic polarisation were abolished by atropine. Surprisingly, the ganglionic depolarisation was obtained only once in a given ganglion. Upon repeated administration of oxotremorine at suitable intervals, the evoked postganglionic firing increased in spite of the absence of depolarisation. Oxotremorine depressed orthodromic transmission only on the first application. The resistance to oxotremorine-induced ganglionic inhibition and depolarisation was explained by JARAMILLO and VOLLE (1967a) by the persistence of ganglionic depolarisation, which is indicated by the reduction of the after-negativity of orthodromic ganglionic action potentials.

In *cat ciliary ganglion in situ*, oxotremorine failed to produce any trace of polarisation changes and ganglionic firing, even after sensitisation by preganglionic stimulation and by isoprenaline (SCHAFFNER, 1973; SCHAFFNER and HAEFELY, 1974).

Oxotremorine can, therefore, be regarded as a powerful stimulant of the cat superior cervical ganglion producing a long-lasting depolarisation and firing. On the parasympathetic ciliary ganglion of cat, however, oxotremorine is devoid of any stimulant effect.

9. Furtrethonium (Furfuryltrimethylammonium) and Aceclidine

The structure formulae of these compounds are shown in Fig. 1.

In the *cat superior cervical ganglion in situ*, JARAMILLO and VOLLE (1967b) found furtrethonium and McN-A-343 to possess identical activities and similar potencies. Furtrethonium in lower doses produced a monophasic, low-amplitude depolarisation accompanied by asynchronous firing in the postganglionic nerves. This firing, which occurred with a latency of several seconds, was abolished by atropine. At higher doses, a biphasic depolarisation composed of the delayed ganglionic negativity also seen with low doses occurred, and, in addition, a transient, more marked depolarisation 2–3 s after the injection, which was accompanied by a brisk high-amplitude discharge. This early ganglionic depolarisation was insensitive to both atropine and C_6, as was the early firing. The only difference between McN-A-343 and furtrethonium was the sensitivity to trimethaphan of the early firing produced by furtrethonium. Furtrethonium also depressed ganglionic transmission during the late depolarisation; this could not be antagonised by atropine.

The 5-methyl derivative of furtrethonium had actions essentially identical with those of its parent compound, but was approximately ten times more potent, corresponding to its more potent muscarinic action on various non-neuronal target cells (ING et al., 1952). LUKOMSKAYA (1969) observed a 100- to 200-fold increase of the sensitivity to methylfurmethide and aceclidine of the cat superior cervical ganglion after chronic denervation.

10. 4-(m-Chlorophenylcarbamoyloxy)-2-Butynyl-Trimethylammonium Chloride (McN-A-343)

ROSZKOWSKI (1961) discovered the unusual pharmacological profile of the synthetic compound 4-(*m*-chlorophenylcarbamoyloxy)-2-butynyltrimethylammonium chloride (McN-A-343) (Fig. 1). It is characterised, after an i.v. injection of as little as 8 µg/kg, by a small initial depressor effect followed by a large, protracted increase in the arterial blood pressure. In a careful analysis, ROSZKOWSKI (1961) and LEVY and AHLQUIST (1962) arrived at the conclusion that McN-A-343 affected autonomic parameters predominantly by a stimulation of sympathetic ganglia. This stimulant effect was enhanced rather than depressed by C_6; however, it was readily abolished by atropine. The unique feature of this compound is its relatively weak muscarinic action outside sympathetic ganglia, as for example in the isolated heart and on intestinal smooth muscle. ROSZKOWSKI'S (1961) report stimulated many investigations on the muscarinic mechanisms in autonomic ganglia.

In *cat superior cervical ganglion in situ*, McN-A-343 produced a stimulation, as shown by contractions of the nictitating membrane (ROSZKOWSKI, 1961; JONES, 1963; MURAYAMA and UNNA, 1963); the effect resembled that of pilocarpine. Tachyphylaxis was evident when repeated injections were made at intervals of less than 30 min. Small doses of atropine, cocaine and morphine blocked the effect of McN-A-343, whereas C_6, TEA and mepyramine were without effect. McN-A-343 facilitated ganglionic transmission of submaximal preganglionic stimuli and potentiated the ganglion-stimulating effect of KCl. Most remarkably, McN-A-343 did not contract the nictitating membrane when injected into its blood supply. Very similar results were described by JONES (1963), who stated that in contrast to muscarine, McN-A-343 stimulated all the superior cervical ganglia studied. Chronic denervation markedly enhanced the effects of McN-A-343 (see, however, GREEN, 1969; BREZENOFF and GERTNER, 1969), as did both nicotine during its late "non-depolarising phase" of ganglionic blockade and the maximal preganglionic stimulation. JONES (1963) drew attention to the structural similarities between *l*-muscarine, pilocarpine, AHR-602, and McN-A-343. In their important investigation of the alteration of ganglionic sensitivity to various agents by preganglionic stimulation, TRENDELENBURG and JONES (1965) described many details of this interesting phenomenon in connection with the ganglionic action of McN-A-343. SMITH (1966 b) observed cross-tachyphylaxis between McN-A-343 and histamine and also 5-hydroxytryptamine. The ganglionic effects of McN-A-343 were absent after the administration of pilocarpine (ROSZKOWSKI et al., 1971). In addition to procaine and $CaCl_2$, the anticholinesterases, physostigmine and neostigmine, selectively depressed responses of the superior cervical ganglion to McN-A-343, histamine, and 5-hydroxytryptamine, but not to DMPP and preganglionic volleys. Conversely, during slow perfusion of the ganglion with a calcium-free Ringer solution, the responses to McN-A-343 and the other non-nicotinic stimulants were enhanced, whereas those to DMPP were not. In a study of denervation supersensitivity of the cat superior cervical ganglion in situ, VICKERSON and VARMA (1969) found a higher maximum of nictitating membrane contraction in response to McN-A-343 after chronic denervation. CHINN and WEBER (1974) achieved selective block of the ganglionic response to McN-A-343 by methylphenidate and pheniprazine. No explanation can be offered for these effects.

The electrical events occurring in cat superior cervical ganglion under the action of McN-A-343 were studied by JARAMILLO and VOLLE (1967 a, b). After a latency of 6–8 s, the compound induced a low-amplitude postganglionic firing, which persisted for one to several minutes. Higher doses of McN-A-343 elicited a distinctly bimodal discharge. A first component had a rapid onset (2–4 s) and a large amplitude, and lasted only about 10 s. Thereafter, low-amplitude firing was present exactly as after low doses. The smallest dose producing the early discharge was 5–10 times higher than that required for the induction of the low-amplitude firing. Atropine selectively depressed the latter component, leaving the early and brisk response unaltered. Doses of C_6 and trimethaphan that blocked ganglionic transmission did not affect the early and late response. The late, but not the early firing induced by McN-A-343 was enhanced by isoprenaline. The ganglionic discharges in response to McN-A-343 coincided with a moderate ganglionic depolarisation. Interestingly, the amplitude of depolarisation decreased after higher doses, although the postganglionic discharges, especially the early ones, increased with increasing doses. The ganglionic polarisation changes were unaffected by C_6 and clearly enhanced by atropine, despite its reduction of the late firing. Small doses of McN-A-343 facilitated ganglionic transmission. With higher doses, transmission was enhanced initially (during the early firing) and subsequently depressed. Atropine did not affect the depression of ganglionic transmission. At the time of maximum depression of ganglionic transmission, McN-A-343 enhanced the firing but reduced the depolarisation induced by KCl, ACh, and TMA. This enhancement by McN-A-343 was unaffected by atropine. The atropine-sensitive ganglionic firing produced by McN-A-343 was blocked by a nitrogen mustard analogue of C_6 (HANCOCK and VOLLE, 1968). Preliminary findings by KOSS and RIEGER (1975) indicate that McN-A-343 has a much more powerful stimulating effect on ganglion cells innervating the nictitating membrane than on those mediating pupillary dilation.

In the *isolated rat superior cervical ganglion*, McN-A-343 produced dose-dependent depolarisation, the maximum being about 60% of the carbachol ceiling effect (WATSON, 1970).

In *cat stellate ganglion in situ*, AIKEN and REIT (1969) produced strong evidence for a selective muscarinic stimulant effect of McN-A-343 on adrenergic ganglion cells. In cardiac ganglia of the spinal dog, McN-A 343 produced a very strong, dose-dependent stimulation (FLACKE and FLEISCH, 1970). Atropine shifted the dose-response curve for cardiac acceleration by McN-A-343 to the right and beyond 30 µg/kg also depressed the maximum.

Both the *perfused and the isolated hypogastric ganglion* of the guinea-pig in situ were completely insensitive to McN-A-343, whereas the perfused, but not the isolated hypogastric ganglion of the rat was excited in about 60% of the preparations.

In the *isolated paravertebral ganglia of the frog*, McN-A-343 (in concentrations higher than 10^{-5} M) produced neither depolarisation nor firing, but depressed ganglionic transmission (GINSBORG, 1965). In the *inferior mesenteric ganglion of the cat in situ*, McN-A-343 induced atropine-sensitive discharges for about 10 min (MURAYAMA and UNNA, 1963).

In the *isolated rat intestine*, SMITH (1966a) found no evidence for a stimulant effect of McN-A-343 on parasympathetic ganglia. In the *cat ciliary ganglion in situ*, McN-A-343 showed no excitatory action, but depressed ganglionic transmission (SCHAFFNER, 1973; SCHAFFNER and HAEFELY, 1974). Atropine and hyoscine partially antagonised this depressant effect. The absence of ciliary ganglion stimulation with McN-A-343 was also observed by KOSS and RIEGER (1974). Several structural analogues of McN-A-343 were studied for their ganglionic actions by ROSZKOWSKI and YELNOSKY (1967).

In summary, McN-A-343, which has very weak muscarinic actions on smooth muscles, strongly stimulates various mammalian sympathetic ganglia through mAChRs. Inhibitory mAChRs are not activated by the compound. On the whole, therefore, the ganglionic actions of McN-A-343 most closely resemble those of pilocarpine. It must be stressed, however, that the ganglionic effects of McN-A-343 contain an important non-muscarinic component. Thus, in contrast to that with pilocarpine, the depolarisation brought about by McN-A-343 is unaffected by both C_6 and atropine, and these two antagonists also do not block the early firing induced by higher doses of McN-A-343. The depression of ganglionic transmission was also resistant to atropine. Apparently McN-A-343 does not stimulate parasympathetic ganglia.

11. n-Benzyl-3-Pyrrolidyl Acetate Methobromide (AHR-602)

AHR-602 shows close structural similarities to methacholine (Fig. 1). Pharmacologically, the compound resembles McN-A-343 insofar as when given by i.v. injection it produces a small initial depressor effect followed by a significant prolonged rise of the arterial blood pressure, which was recognised as being due to the stimulation of sympathetic ganglia (FRANKO et al., 1963). The effect of AHR-602 was resistant to C_6, but readily abolished by small doses of atropine. Like McN-A-343, AHR-602 has only insignificant muscarinic effects on smooth muscle preparations (its potency on intestinal smooth muscle being about 0.1% that of ACh and methacholine) and on the heart (FRANKO et al., 1963). JONES et al. (1963) and DREW and LEACH (1974) arrived at the same conclusion when analysing the pressor effect of AHR-602 in spinal cats, the pressor effect being abolished by adrenergic neuron blockers, atropine, cocaine, morphine, and methadone, but not by C_6. Furthermore, nicotine during the initial depolarising phase abolished, while nicotine during the late nondepolarising phase of ganglionic block potentiated the pressor effect of AHR-602. The adrenal medulla seems to make little contribution to the effect of AHR-602 on blood pressure.

AHR-602 stimulated all *cat superior cervical ganglia studied in situ* (JONES, 1963). Chronic denervation increased the sensitivity of the ganglion. The onset of nictitating membrane contractions was delayed by about 6 s. The resistance of the ganglionic action of AHR-602 to C_6, its blockade by atropine, cocaine, morphine, methadone, and by nicotinic depolarisation went parallel with the resistance and blockade of the pressor effect.

The findings on AHR-602 presented so far suggest a close similarity of its ganglionic actions to e.g., those of muscarine. However, JARAMILLO and VOLLE (1967a) observed one property peculiar to AHR-602. In cat superior cervical ganglion in situ, this compound, in contrast to muscarine, produced a monophasic depolarisation with no trace of initial hyperpolarisation. Although the asynchronous postganglionic firing in response to AHR-602 was enhanced by isoprenaline, blocked by small doses of atropine, and resistant to C_6, the depolarisation could not be abolished by atropine, though it could by high doses of C_6. Similarly, the depression of ganglionic transmission that occurred during depolarisation was increased rather than reversed by atropine. Moreover, during the depression of ganglionic transmission, AHR-602 enhanced the ganglion-stimulating effect of TMA.

Using the *urinary bladder of cats and dogs in situ*, SAXENA (1972) observed bladder contractions in response to high doses of AHR-602 injected into the abdominal aorta. He concluded that the compound was acting by stimulation of mAChRs in the parasympathetic ganglion cells in the bladder wall, because its action was abolished by atropine, by nicotine, and by destruction of the ganglion cells (painting of the bladder surface with a phenol solution). The contractile effect of AHR-602 was resistant to cocaine and morphine.

In *cat parasympathetic ciliary ganglion in situ*, AHR-602 had no effect even after drugs and procedures that usually increase the ganglionic sensitivity to muscarinic agents (SCHAFFNER, 1973; SCHAFFNER and HAEFELY, 1974).

It is difficult, at present, to characterise AHR-602 with respect to its ganglionic actions. Although the action potentials it elicits in the cat superior cervical ganglion were blocked by atropine, the depolarisation was resistant to antimuscarinic drugs. It is very interesting that the direct stimulating effect of AHR-602 on smooth muscles is very weak (SAXENA, 1972) and that the compound apparently does not activate inhibitory mAChRs. Hence, in almost all respects AHR-602 acts very similarly to McN-A-343.

12. Quaternary Amino-Acid Esters

Four quaternary amino-acid esters (ethyl β-dimethylaminopropionate methiodide, methyl β-dimethylaminopropionate methiodide, methyl β-dimethylaminobutyrate methiodide, ethyl β-dimethylaminobutyrate methiodide) injected in doses of between 2 and 10 µg into the arterial supply of the cat superior cervical ganglion induced contractions of the nictitating membrane and postganglionic firing lasting about 1 min (BRIMBLECOMBE and SUTTON, 1968). These effects were blocked by C_6 but also markedly reduced by atropine, suggesting a mixed stimulant action on both nAChRs and mAChRs.

13. Benzyltrimethylammonium and Pyridylmethyltrimethylammonium

HAMILTON and RUBINSTEIN (1968) studied the nicotinic and muscarinic actions of benzyltrimethylammonium and of d-, β-, and γ-substituted pyridylmethyltrimethylammonium by giving i.a. injections into the blood supply of the cat superior cervical ganglion and recording the responses of the nictitating membrane. The nAChRs were blocked by 20 mg/kg C_6 i.v. and the mAChRs by 2 mg/kg atropine i.v., while the nicotinic stimulating potencies varied up to several hundred times amongst these compounds and the muscarinic stimulating actions were almost identical.

14. Cholinesterase Inhibitors

VOLLE and KOELLE (1961) and VOLLE (1962) consistently obtained firing in the acutely denervated superior cervical ganglion of the cat in situ after injections of about 3 µmol *diisopropylphosphofluoride (DFP)* into the arterial supply. This dose blocked ganglionic AChE by at least 99%. The ganglionic asynchronous discharges started 5–10 min after the injections and persisted for the duration of the experiment (up to 4 h). They were abolished by atropine. In chronically denervated ganglia, even ten times the doses effective in innervated ganglia failed to produce firing. The DFP-induced discharges in acutely denervated ganglia were readily blocked for 1–2 min by an injection of $CaCl_2$ in doses that did not alter the size of orthodromic action potentials or the postganglionic discharge induced by ACh injected i.v. but did reduce the ganglion-stimulant effects of KCl (KOMALAHIRANYA and VOLLE, 1962). The doses of $MgCl_2$ required to block the DFP firing also blocked ganglionic transmission and ACh-induced firing. Similar effects were seen with $CdCl_2$. DFP did not alter the KCl-induced firing. d-TC and mecamylamine in doses that completely blocked ganglionic transmission increased the DFP-induced firing (VOLLE, 1962), but TEA, atropine, and procaine depressed it and C_6 was without effect. DFP-induced firing was persistently enhanced after repetitive preganglionic stimulation at a rate of 30/s for 2 min (VOLLE, 1962).

Eserine had an effect similar to that of DFP in the acutely denervated cat superior cervical ganglion, although the spontaneous asynchronous discharge induced by this reversible AChE inhibitor lasted only for 30–50 min (TAKESHIGE and VOLLE, 1962). Prior conditioning of the ganglia with repetitive preganglionic stimulation reduced the dose of eserine required for the induction of firing in the resting ganglion by a factor of about 10. As with DFP, the eserine-induced firing was enhanced by d-TC and mecamylamine and blocked by small doses of atropine. Eserine did not evoke discharges from the chronically denervated ganglion. TEA enhanced eserine-induced firing in small doses and blocked it in large doses. In the presence of very low doses of eserine and of a dose of d-TC that blocked ganglionic transmission, repetitive stimulation of the preganglionic nerve at 15/s produced an asynchronous firing that was blocked by atropine. Similarly, 10-s trains of preganglionic volleys at 60/s induced an atropine-sensitive asynchronous firing. TAKESHIGE and VOLLE (1962) concluded that the asynchronous firing induced by eserine and by repetitive stimulation resulted from ACh released at presynaptic endings and that eserine and the repetitive stimulation were acting on a cholinoceptive site not involved in normal transmission. The involvement of mAChRs in the generation of eserine-induced firing was further supported by its sensitivity to tetrakis-(2-chlorethyl-1,6-hexandiamine, a nitrogen mustard analogue of C_6, which also blocked the ganglionic stimulant effect of McN-A-343 (HANCOCK and VOLLE, 1968).

Neostigmine was reported by MASON (1962a) to cause a contraction of the nictitating membrane when injected in high amounts i.v. into the blood supply of the acutely or chronically denervated cat superior cervical ganglion. The contraction occurred rapidly and lasted for 2–4 min. The responses to neostigmine declined on repeated injections but were resistant to atropine as well as to d-TC and C_6. Eserine never caused contractions of the nictitating membrane, as neostigmine did. Blockade of ganglionic transmission by C_6 was rapidly reversed by neostigmine, but not by eserine. This reversal by neostigmine was seen even after both atropine and DFP. MASON (1962b) reported a depolarising effect of neostigmine on isolated normal and chronically denervated isolated superior cervical ganglia of rat and kitten in a study with the fluid electrode technique, thereby confirming previous findings of PASCOE (1956) in the isolated rat ganglion. The concentrations required were 10^{-5}–10^{-4} g/ml. C_6 prevented depolarisation by neostigmine. A depolarisation also occurred rapidly in the cat superior cervical ganglion in situ after injection of neostigmine into the arterial blood supply. It was still obtained after large doses of eserine.

TAKESHIGE and VOLLE (1963b) observed the occurrence of asynchronous postganglionic discharges appearing 10–20 s after the injection of neostigmine (20–100 μg) into the carotid artery, the firing persisting for 4–15 min. Doses two–five times higher were required to induce discharges in the chronically denervated cat superior cervical ganglion. Similar results were reported by KOSTOWSKI and GUMULKA (1966). d-TC enhanced and atropine blocked the firing induced by neostigmine; d-TC evoked postganglionic firing after the discharges induced by neostigmine had dissipated (TAKESHIGE and VOLLE, 1963b). Also after the dissipation of neostigmine-induced firing, preganglionic stimulation during the action of *d*-TC induced an asynchronous firing during and after the end of the stimulation period which could be blocked by atropine.

In the dog given C_6 or chlorisondamine to block ganglionic transmission, neostigmine evoked a pressure response and restored the carotid occlusion reflex (FENNER and HILTON, 1963). Transmission through the superior cervical ganglion was not restored to normal by neostigmine as judged by nictitating membrane responses. The restoration of the carotid occlusion reflex by neostigmine was blocked by atropine.

An induction of atropine-sensitive asynchronous postganglionic discharges in the cat superior cervical ganglion in situ has also been found with another irreversible anticholinesterase, *2-diethoxyphosphenylthio-ethyldimethylamine acid oxalate (217 AO)* (DE GROAT and VOLLE, 1966; DE GROAT, 1970). The effect of this agent was very similar to that of DFP. Parasympathetic postganglionic fibres to the cat urinary bladder were also excited by 217 AO (SAUM and DE GROAT, 1973).

Ambenonium restored the stimulant action of ACh on the cat superior cervical ganglion blocked by C_6 or mecamylamine together with atropine (BOISSIER et al., 1974). It was concluded that the stimulant effect of ACh after ambenonium occurred at mAChRs in the ganglion.

From the various studies it becomes clear that several cholinesterase inhibitors have ganglionic actions unrelated to the inhibition of this enzyme. They are able to induce action potentials in ganglion cells in the absence of preganglionic ACh, and this stimulation most probably involves mAChRs. Neostigmine has a complex action, producing ganglionic depolarisation that is blocked by C_6 and asynchronous discharges that are sensitive to blockade by atropine.

Besides stimulating mAChRs in ganglia directly, the anticholinesterases greatly enhance the reactivity of mAChRs to stimulation. There is, at present, no explanation for this phenomenon.

II. Possible Involvement of a Second Messenger in Muscarinic Excitation of Autonomic Ganglia

It has been clearly established that changes of neuronal activity in various parts of the nervous system are associated with altered levels of cyclic nucleotides (GREENGARD, 1975). Orthodromic stimulation of frog sympathetic ganglia resulted in increased levels of cyclic adenosine 3′,5′-monophosphate (cAMP) and cyclic guanosine 3′,5′-monophosphate (cGMP) (WEIGHT et al., 1974). Blockade of nAChR did not affect these changes. However, atropine blocked the increase of cGMP. Neither nucleotide was elevated when the release of ACh from preganglionic nerve endings was abolished in high-magnesium, low-calcium Ringer solution. Incubation of slices of bovine superior cervical ganglion with ACh or bethanechol substantially increased the level of cGMP and raised that of cAMP slightly (KEBABIAN et al., 1975a, b). The effect of the two agents on both nucleotides was blocked by atropine but not by C_6. The pure nicotinic stimulant, DMPP, did not alter the levels of the nucleotides. It was therefore proposed that the activation of excitatory mAChRs results in depolarisation and excitation through a primary increase of cGMP. A model was presented, according to which activation of mAChRs would activate a membrane-bound guanylate cyclase. GMP formed in this way might stimulate a cGMP-dependent protein kinase that phosphorylates a specific membrane protein, thereby altering its conductance for specific ions and the membrane potential (CAS-NELLIS AND GREENGARD, 1974). Interestingly, muscarinic agents increased the level of cGMP also in slices of rabbit cerebral cortex, in the rat heart ventricle, and in the guinea-pig ileum, suggesting that activation of muscarinic receptors in various organs increases cGMP and might mediate the muscarinic effects (LEE et al., 1972). This attractive hypothesis requires confirmation by some critical experiments. For instance, it is imperative to clarify the cause–effect relationship between ganglionic membrane potential change and cGMP increase. According to the available information, the latter could be a phenomenon completely independent of the slow EPSP. The effect of specifically preventing the rise of the nucleotide level, or of increasing it by another mechanism than activation of mAChRs, on muscarinic ganglionic transmission, remains to be investigated.

C. 5-Hydroxytryptamine (5-HT) and Related Indolealkylamines

A stimulant effect of 5-HT on the perfused *cat superior cervical ganglion* was first mentioned by ROBERTSON (1954). About 70% of ganglia with normal blood supply were excited by i.a. injections of 5-HT (1–100 µ) (TRENDELENBURG, 1956a). This stimulation was unaffected by C_6, atropine, and mepyramine, but reduced by cocaine. A very marked tachyphylaxis occurred after 5-HT. Nictitating membrane responses to submaximal preganglionic stimuli were enhanced by the amine (TRENDELENBURG, 1956a, 1957; WEINSTOCK and SCHECHTER, 1975). Injections of 5-HT into the perfused ganglion enhanced the responses to ACh, nicotine, carbachol, choline, and KCl (TRENDELENBURG, 1956b). The sensitivity of the perfused ganglion was lower (stimulation of only 25% of the ganglia) than that of the ganglion with an intact blood supply. Cross-tachyphylaxis occurred among 5-HT, histamine, and pilocarpine. During the depression of ganglionic transmission by hydralazine, the facilitating action of 5-HT was converted into a depressant one (GERTNER and ROMANO, 1962). Nictitating membrane contractions elicited by i.a. injections of 5-HT were selectively and surmountably reduced by low doses (0.5–10 g) of *dl*-propranolol and its *l* isomer, but not by the *d* isomer, which is devoid of β-blocking activity (WEINSTOCK and SCHECHTER, 1975). In higher doses, both isomers and the racemic propranolol produced an unsurmountable block of the stimulant effect of 5-HT, most probably due to their local anaesthetic action. These findings raise the interesting possibility that β-adrenergic blocking agents may be able to selectively block neuronal excitation by 5-HT.

The use of electrophysiological methods has revealed the complexity of the effects of 5-HT in cat superior cervical ganglion (DE GROAT and VOLLE, 1966; JARAMILLO and VOLLE, 1968; MACHOVÁ and BOŠKA, 1969; HAEFELY, 1971, 1972, 1974d; DE GROAT and LALLEY, 1973). The immediate effect of a bolus injection of 5-HT into the blood supply of the ganglion is a brief ganglionic depolarisation lasting 5–10 s, with accompanying discharges. Increasing doses produce increments of depolarisation only over a very narrow range. Above a maximally depolarising dose only a slight prolongation of the effect can be obtained. The maximum depolarisation is only a small fraction of that observed with nicotinic stimulants. The brief initial depolarisation is usually followed by a slight hyperpolarisation, which may be followed, after high doses, by a secondary late depolarisation. This is of longer duration than the first one and is accompanied by a low-amplitude discharge. The delayed depolarisation and firing were seen most clearly after sensitisation of the ganglion by repetitive preganglionic stimulation and after an injection of isoprenaline. Picrotoxin in doses that had no effect on the responses to ACh and KCl preferentially depressed the early firing and, usually incompletely, the early depolarisation produced by 5-HT. The late effects of 5-HT were depressed selectively by bicuculline. The stimulant effect of 5-HT was resistant to the 5-HT antagonist methysergide, to C_6, TEA, atropine, and morphine, when these were given in doses that did not affect ganglionic transmission, but was sensitive to cocaine. LSD in doses too low to depress ganglionic transmission did not diminish the stimulant effect of 5-HT. Depolarisation and firing induced by 5-HT were, however, selectively reduced or abolished for 10–15 min after a preceding injection of 5-HT, 5-hydroxy-α-methyltryptamine, tryptamine, α-methyltryptamine, and – less effectively – of bufotenine and psilocybin. During the initial depolarisation, ganglionic transmission was transiently facilitated, while the late depolarisation was accompanied by depression. The stimulant effects of 5-HT were masked in part by a primary depressant action of the compound.

Bufotenine produced a longer depolarisation and firing than 5-HT (HAEFELY, 1974 d). However, the main part of the stimulation could be blocked by C_6. The small and brief depolarisation and firing that were resistant to C_6 resembled those produced by 5-HT.

Tryptamine produced a C_6-resistant ganglionic depolarisation, which was, however, accompanied by postganglionic firing only in a few exceptional cases (HAEFELY, 1974 d).

5-Hydroxy-α-methyltryptamine produced more marked and prolonged depolarisation and firing than 5-HT, but C_6 abolished all effects of 5 hydroxy-α-methyltryptamine except its prevention of 5-HT-induced stimulation (HAEFELY, 1974 d).

The effects of 5-HT on other sympathetic ganglia have been studied less systematically. In the *isolated rat superior cervical ganglion* incubated with 5-HT, no stimulation was observed by DE KALBERMATTEN (1962) or JÉQUIER (1965), whereas WATSON (1970) found peak depolarisations amounting to 20–25% of the maximum depolarisation produced by carbachol.

The *isolated rabbit superior cervical ganglion* was depolarised by 5-HT in concentrations of $10^{-5} M$ and higher (WALLIS and WOODWARD, 1973–1975). Prolonged tachyphylaxis occurred. Depolarisations induced by injections of 5-HT into the perfusing medium were followed by ouabain-sensitive hyperpolarisation. The depolarising effect of 5-HT was reduced by picrotoxin, BOL-148, morphine, and phenylbiguamide, and less effectively by LSD and methysergide. The amplitude of 5-HT-induced depolarisation was markedly reduced in a Na^+-deficient solution and the persisting effect abolished by the additional omission of Ca^{2+} (WALLIS and WOODWARD, 1975). C_6 enhanced the amplitude and duration of depolarisation. Recording by the sucrose-gap method allowed WALLIS and WOODWARD (1973) to detect a depolarising effect of 5-HT on preganglionic terminals. Also in the rabbit isolated superior cervical ganglion, WALLIS and WOODWARD (1974) observed a depressant effect of 5-HT on isolated orthodromic responses, while the early facilitation of ganglionic transmission, which is greatest 40–75 ms after a conditioning stimulus, was markedly enhanced by the amine. The inhibition of a test orthodromic response by a conditioning impulse 100–300 ms before was reduced or abolished by 5-HT. Late facilitation, occurring 700–2000 ms after a conditioning volley, was increased by 5-HT, although less markedly than was the early facilitation. These findings indicate that the overall effect of 5-HT on ganglionic transmission might vary considerably, depending on the rate of preganglionic stimulation, and may provide the clue to the fact that investigators taking the nictitating membrane responses as the parameter of ganglionic output consistently observed facilitation by 5-HT, whereas most of those looking at postganglionic action potentials found a depression.

In *rat stellate ganglia*, whether isolated or in situ, HERTZLER (1961) observed a facilitatory effect of 5-HT.

In *cat stellate ganglion in situ*, AIKEN and REIT (1969) found 5-HT to be a more potent and effective stimulant of cholinergic neurones mediating sweat secretion in the front foot pads than of the noradrenergic neurones responsible for tachycardia.

In the *cat superior mesenteric ganglion* in situ, 5-HT induced postganglionic discharges that were resistant to C_6 and atropine but selectively blocked by morphine, though not by cocaine (GYERMEK and BINDLER, 1962a). In a series of derivatives of tryptamine, all compounds had a weaker ganglion-stimulating action than 5-HT. A blockade of the stimulating action of 5-HT was observed with tryptamine, 3-indoleacetamidine, 5-hydroxy-α-methyltryptamine and 5- and 7-benzyloxygramine.

In the *cat inferior mesenteric ganglion* in situ, SAUM and DE GROAT (1973) observed a brief (2–6 s) burst of postganglionic discharges after close-arterial injection of 5–50 µg 5-HT, thus confirming earlier observations of GYERMEK and BINDLER (1962). After sensitisation of the ganglion by repetitive preganglionic stimulation, this early discharge was followed by a late one, which lasted for 0.5–2 min. Transmission through the inferior mesenteric ganglion was depressed for 0.5–3 min after low (0.01–1 µg) doses of 5-HT. After higher doses, this inhibition was preceded in most experiments by a facilitation. Both facilitation and inhibition were reversibly antagonised by picrotoxin.

In *isolated paravertebral sympathetic ganglia of the bullfrog*, 5-HT produced a consistent depolarisation, which was converted into hyperpolarisation after soaking of the ganglion in nicotine 0.12 mM for 40 min (WATANABE and KOKETSU, 1973).

In *dog small intestine*, BURKS (1973) provided evidence that 5-HT excited intraneural cholinergic nerve elements, since the intestinal contracting effect of 5-HT was blocked by tetrodotoxin, nicotinic depolarisation, and atropine, but not by TEA. Early findings of ROBERTSON (1953) in the guinea-pig and rabbit ileum had pointed in the same direction. Recent studies provide evidence for the stimulant effect of 5-HT on parasympathetic ganglion cells of the intestine. HIRST and SILINSKY (1975) applied 5-HT by microelectrophoresis to neurones of the submucous plexus of the guinea-pig small intestine. All neurones were depolarised and, if the amount of depolarisation by 5-HT was sufficient, action potentials were initiated. The effect of 5-HT was depressed by *d*-TC, but remained unaffected by methysergide.

The *cat parasympathetic ciliary ganglion* (SCHAFFNER, 1973; SCHAFFNER and HAEFELY, 1974) was affected by 5-HT in a much simpler way than was the superior cervical ganglion (HAEFELY, 1974d). The only effect observed was a low-amplitude depolarisation accompanied by discharges. Depolarisation coincided with facilitation after lower doses and with depression of ganglionic transmission after higher doses. Sensitising the ciliary ganglion with repetitive preganglionic stimulation or isoprenaline had virtually no effect on the response to 5-HT.

Parasympathetic ganglia in the wall of the cat urinary bladder in situ were stimulated by close-arterial injections of 5-HT via the inferior mesenteric artery (SAUM and DE GROAT, 1973). A brisk discharge lasting 2–3 s in postganglionic pelvic nerve fibres led to a short-lasting contraction of the urinary bladder. Both responses were depressed by picrotoxin which, however, also diminished the effect of nicotine. The effect of 5-HT was resistant to C_6 and atropine. Interestingly, a late discharge, as seen in sympathetic ganglia, could never be obtained in pelvic nerves, even after conditioning repetitive preganglionic stimulation. Transmission through the pelvic ganglia was depressed for 0.5–5 min in a dose-dependent manner by 5-HT; after 20 μg 5-HT, transmission was blocked. In about one-third of the preparations, the depression of transmission was preceded by a facilitation lasting 2–8 s. Depression of the responses to preganglionic stimulation was only seen at low rates of stimulation. The inhibitory effect of 5-HT was also observed on postganglionic discharges reflexly induced by distention of the urinary bladder (DE GROAT and RYALL, 1969). 5-HT also transiently abolished the muscarinic asynchronous firing induced in postganglionic pelvic nerve fibres by the anticholinesterase 217 AO, following repetitive preganglionic stimulation (SAUM and DE GROAT, 1973).

Early findings of ROBERTSON (1953) indicated that 5-HT was able to produce contractions of the guinea-pig and rabbit ileum by an action on nervous structures. Cholinergic ganglion cells of the *myenteric plexus* of the *guinea-pig ileum* in vitro were neither depolarised nor hyperpolarised by 5-HT (HENDERSON and NORTH, 1975); the amine did, however, reduce the amplitude of EPSPs in most cells, probably by reducing the release of ACh from presynaptic terminals. Interestingly, every ganglion cell of the *submucous plexus of the guinea-pig ileum* was depolarised by iontophoretically applied 5-HT; with sufficiently intense iontophoretic currents, the cells discharged action potentials (HIRST and SILINSKY, 1975).

5-HT has very complex actions in autonomic, especially sympathetic, ganglia. Besides significant inhibitory effects that were not seen in the cat ciliary ganglion, the indolalkylamine stimulated sympathetic as well as parasympathetic ganglion cells. The receptors mediating this stimulation are clearly different from cholinergic ones and from receptors involved in the action of histamine and polypeptides. In sympathetic ganglia, tachyphylaxis to the stimulant effect of 5-HT is very marked.

Besides an immediate depolarisation and discharge, 5-HT in higher doses and after sensitisation also produced a delayed stimulation. Picrotoxin rather selectively and surmountably depresses the early stimulation. The electrogenesis of the early depolarisation produced by 5-HT is probably similar to that underlying the nicotinic depolarisation, since it was often followed by a poststimulation hyperpolarisation, and since it was markedly reduced in the absence of extracellular Na^+.

D. Histamine

After the failure to observe a stimulant action of histamine in the perfused *cat superior cervical ganglion* by FELDBERG and VARTIAINEN (1934) and the finding of only very inconsistent stimulation by KONZETT (1952), TRENDELENBURG (1954) was able to stimulate about 80% of blood-perfused cat superior cervical ganglia with intra-arterial injections of histamine (2–55 μg) as seen by contractions of the nictitating membrane. The effect was short and disappeared upon repeated administration.

It was not blocked by C_6 and atropine but was abolished during the depolarising phase of nicotine block and following mepyramine and cocaine. Doses of histamine about one-hundredth those resulting in contraction of the nictitating membranes facilitated ganglionic transmission. This effect was also abolished by mepyramine and cocaine, but remained unaffected by atropine (TRENDELENBURG, 1955). The secondary rise in blood pressure observed after i.v. injections of histamine was found to result mainly from stimulation of the adrenal medulla and only to a minor extent from a stimulation of adrenergic vasomotor neurones. TRENDELENBURG (1956b) confirmed the early findings of a very low sensitivity of the perfused ganglion to histamine and the absence of any stimulation in about three-quarters of the cats. However, histamine regularly facilitated responses of the nictitating membrane to submaximal preganglionic stimuli (see also TRENDELENBURG, 1957) and to injections of ACh, nicotine, carbachol, choline, and KCl. A reciprocal blocking action (cross-tachyphylaxis) of the stimulant effects was observed with pilocarpine, histamine, and 5-HT. During the late phase of ganglion block produced by repeated injections of nicotine, the stimulant effect of histamine was still present, although in contrast to that of 5-HT, it was not potentiated (TRENDELENBURG, 1959). GERTNER and KOHN (1959), using the perfused cat superior cervical ganglion in situ, considered the depression of ganglionic transmission by histamine to be a more consistent response than facilitation and excitation. The doses used by these authors were considerably higher (100 µg and more) than those studied by earlier investigators. The stimulant effects of histamine on the cat superior cervical ganglion in situ were found to be enhanced by prior repetitive preganglionic stimulation (TRENDELENBURG and JONES, 1965). Neither atropine or C_6 alone nor their combination abolished the facilitatory effect of preganglionic stimulation. During the slow infusion of the ganglion with calcium-free Ringer's solution, the stimulant effect of histamine was enhanced (SMITH, 1966b). This author also found a cross-desensitisation between histamine and McN-A-343. The stimulant effect of histamine was depressed by procaine, isotonic $CaCl_2$, eserine and neostigmine. After tachyphylaxis to histamine, the stimulant effect of angiotensin was depressed, whereas histamine was still active after tachyphylaxis to angiotensin had been induced (LEWIS and REIT, 1965). In the superior cervical ganglion of pithed cats sensitised by repetitive preganglionic stimulation, histamine produced a dose-dependent stimulation assessed by the contraction of the nictitating membrane (IORIO and MCISAAC, 1966). The maximum contraction obtainable by histamine was somewhat less than 50% of the maximum response to nicotine, while it amounted to only 10% in non-sensitised ganglia. The dose-response curve was flatter than that of pilocarpine, and especially than that of nicotine. Mepyramine resulted in a parallel shift of the histamine dose-response curve to the right. According to BREZENOFF and GERTNER (1969), chronic denervation of the ganglion did not result in a hypersensitivity to histamine.

In the *cat stellate ganglion*, histamine was found to stimulate noradrenergic ganglion cells preferentially over cholinergic neurones (AIKEN and REIT, 1969).

In the isolated *rat superior cervical ganglions*, depolarisation by histamine was weak or absent. When present, it disappeared with repeated exposure, but could not be prevented by mepyramine (WATSON, 1970).

In the *rabbit isolated superior cervical ganglion*, BRIMBLE and WALLIS (1973) presented evidence for the existence of both H_1- and H_2-type histamine receptors.

Histamine in concentrations of 0.33–33 μM regularly reduced the amplitude of the postganglionic action potentials in response to isolated single preganglionic stimuli. If preganglionic stimulation was repetitive (2/s), depression was virtually absent and often replaced by facilitation. The histamine H_1 blocker, mepyramine, accentuated the histamine-induced depression and changed facilitation into depression. In contrast, the histamine H_2 blocker, burimamide, blocked the depressant effect of histamine and accentuated the facilitating action. Localisation of the facilitatory H_1 receptor and of the inhibitory H_2 receptor (presynaptically or postsynaptically) is not yet possible.

In the *cat parasympathetic ciliary ganglion* in situ, i.a. injections of histamine induced a very weak depolarisation and, after a latency of several seconds, an asynchronous firing in the postganglionic ciliary nerves (SCHAFFNER, 1973; SCHAFFNER and HAEFELY, 1974). The amplitude and duration of this discharge increased dose-dependently. Prior repetitive stimulation of the preganglionic nerve or injections of isoprenaline increased the sensitivity of the ganglion, as well as the maximum amplitude and duration of discharges. The ganglion-stimulating effect of histamine was blocked by mepyramine. In the lower dose range, histamine facilitated ganglionic transmission, whereas after doses of over 1 μmol a weak depression occurred.

Both sympathetic and parasympathetic ganglia of the cat possess histamine H_1 receptors that mediate ganglionic depolarisation and discharge. Normal ganglia are rather insensitive to the amine and a consistent effect is only seen after sensitising procedures such as repetitive preganglionic stimulation or depolarisation by isoprenaline. As with most of the non-nicotinic ganglion-stimulating agents, the effect of histamine was very sensitive to blockade by cocaine, $CaCl_2$ and morphine. The superior cervical ganglion perfused with artificial solutions could only exceptionally be stimulated by histamine, whereas the facilitation of ganglionic transmission appeared to be a regular finding in sympathetic and parasympathetic ganglia.

E. Polypeptides

I. Angiotensin II

Angiotensin II was first found by LEWIS and REIT (1965) to stimulate the *cat superior cervical ganglion* in situ. Their findings were confirmed and expanded in this particular ganglion (LEWIS and REIT, 1966; TRENDELENBURG, 1966a; HAEFELY et al., 1966; MACHOVÁ and BOŠKA, 1967a, b). Angiotensin II has the following characteristic effects in the cat superior cervical ganglion:

The *individual sensitivity of ganglia* to the peptide varies enormously (HAEFELY et al., 1966; MACHOVÁ and BOŠKA, 1967a; HAEFELY, 1970), although this is not apparent from most papers dealing with angiotensin II. The unpredictability of the response of a given ganglion to angiotensin II is most obvious when it is compared with that of the threshold dose of a nicotinic stimulant, e.g., DMPP.

The *responsiveness to angiotensin II* can be markedly enhanced by various sensitising procedures capable of increasing the effects of muscarinic stimulants, such as preganglionic stimulation (LEWIS and REIT, 1966; TRENDELENBURG, 1967; HAEFELY, 1970), strong nicotinic stimulation with consequent desensitisation of the nAChR (LEWIS and REIT, 1966; TRENDELENBURG, 1967), and isoprenaline (HAEFELY, 1970).

In sensitised ganglia, based on the threshold molar amount, angiotensin II is one of the most potent nicotinic ganglion-stimulating agents (HAEFELY, 1970).

Ganglionic depolarisation is very small or absent, even in the presence of a marked postganglionic discharge induced by angiotensin II (HAEFELY, 1970).

Postganglionic discharges appear after a delay of several seconds, reach their maximum very slowly, and last 30–60 s (HAEFELY, 1970).

Angiotensin II produces *marked tachyphylaxis* (LEWIS and REIT, 1966). Cross-tachyphylaxis to bradykinin, histamine, 5-hydroxytryptamine, and oxytocin does not occur after angiotensin II. However, during tachyphylaxis to histamine, the effect of angiotensin II is reduced (LEWIS and REIT, 1966).

While *the effect of angiotensin II is resistant* to blockers of the nAChR and to atropine, it was found to be reduced by the antihistamine, mepyramine (LEWIS and REIT, 1966; see, however, MACHOVÁ and BOŠKA, 1967a,b). Morphine (0.1 mg/kg/i.v.) and cocaine (1 mg/kg/i.v.) markedly depressed the response to angiotensin II (LEWIS and REIT, 1966; TRENDELENBURG, 1967).

Angiotensin II facilitated orthodromic transmission in all ganglia tested, even those in which the same dose of angiotensin II failed to evoke postganglionic action potentials (HAEFELY et al., 1966; MACHOVÁ and BOŠKA, 1967a,b; HAEFELY, 1970).

The *ganglion perfused with Locke's solution* appeared to be at least as sensitive as the blood-perfused ganglion to the action of angiotensin II (LEWIS and REIT, 1966).

Very recently, DUN and NISHI (1975) reported that angiotensin II produced a depolarisation of single cells of cat isolated superior cervical ganglion; in many cells the peptide induced a repetitive activity that was independent of the availability of the preganglionic transmitter. The depolarisation was due to an increased permeability of the membrane to sodium ions.

Ganglion-stimulating effects of angiotensin II were also observed in the *cat stellate ganglion in situ* by AIKEN and REIT (1968). They injected the peptide into the arterial supply of the ganglion in spinal cats and used the increase of the heart rate as an index of ganglionic stimulation. Angiotensin II produced tachycardia after a considerably longer latency than nicotine. In the same preparation, AIKEN and REIT (1969) analysed the effect of angiotensin II on adrenergic ganglion cells innervating the heart (and producing tachycardia) and on cholinergic ganglion cells innervating the front foot pads (and producing sweat secretion). The peptide stimulated the adrenergic neurones, but not the cholinergic ones.

FARR and GRUPP (1967) ascribed the angiotensin II-induced cardio-acceleration and increased contractile force upon systemic administration in dog to stimulation of cells in the *caudal cervical ganglion*. In the chloralosed, atropinised dog, angiotensin II reduced the pressor effect of ACh (MALMEJAC et al., 1968). This was taken as evidence for a depressant effect of small angiotensin II doses on the nicotinic ganglion-stimulating effect of ACh.

WATSON (1970) determined the depolarising effect of various agents on the *isolated rat superior cervical ganglion* by means of the fluid electrode technique. Angiotension II evoked depolarisations amounting to 17–32% of the maximum depolarization obtained with carbachol, and thus was more effective than bradykinin, 5-HT, and histamine. In the plasma-perfused cat superior cervical ganglion, PANISSET (1967) found that angiotensin II increased the amount of ACh released per stimulus from preganglionic endings. Facilitation of ganglionic transmission, which was a regular finding with angiotensin II in contrast to the stimulant effect (HAEFELY, 1970), might, therefore, have an important preganglionic component.

In the *cat parasympathetic ciliary ganglion in situ*, angiotensin II was devoid of any effect (SCHAFFNER, 1973; SCHAFFNER and HAEFELY, 1974). Cells of the isolated cat ciliary ganglion were not depolarised by angiotensin II (DUN and NISHI, 1975).

In the four sympathetic ganglia studied, angiotensin II was found to have stimulant actions. Sensitising procedures were usually required before angiotensin II had any noticeable effects. Specific receptors mediate the effect of angiotensin II. Cholinergic ganglion cells in the sympathetic stellate ganglion and in the parasympathetic ciliary of the cat are not affected by the peptide. The ionic mechanisms underlying the stimulant effect of angiotensin II are unknown.

II. Bradykinin

Bradykinin seems to be the only kinin whose ganglionic actions have been studied.

In the *cat superior cervical ganglion in situ*, the effects of bradykinin are almost identical with those of angiotensin II (LEWIS and REIT, 1966; HAEFELY et al., 1966; TRENDELENBURG, 1967; HAEFELY, 1970). They are, therefore, not discussed in detail. Only differences in the action of the two peptides will be mentioned.

Most importantly, there is no cross-tachyphylaxis between the two peptides (LEWIS and REIT, 1965), and it follows that the receptive sites for the two polypeptides must be different. In contrast to angiotensin II, LEWIS and REIT (1965) found the effect of bradykinin to be resistant to the antihistamine mepyramine, and still present during tachyphylaxis to histamine. During the late "non-depolarising" phase of the ganglionic block induced by one or repeated doses of nicotine, the effect of angiotensin II injected into the cat superior cervical ganglion was enhanced while that of bradykinin was reduced (TRENDELENBURG, 1967). C_6 removed the facilitating and inhibiting effects, respectively.

In the *isolated rat superior cervical ganglion*, the maximum depolarisation produced by bradykinin and recorded with a fluid electrode amounted to only 10% of the maximum depolarisation obtained with carbachol (WATSON, 1970). Hence, under these conditions, bradykinin was a less effective depolarising agent than angiotensin II.

In the *isolated rabbit superior cervical ganglion*, bradykinin increased the amplitude of the postganglionic compound action potential in response to isolated single preganglionic stimuli and reduced the early facilitation of a test response that occurs 40–75 ms after a conditioning stimulus (WALLIS and WOODWARD, 1974). The effect of bradykinin was thus the reverse of that of 5-HT. Bradykinin, also in contrast to 5-HT, produced an inconsistent small depolarisation.

Like angiotensin, bradykinin had no effect on the *cat parasympathetic ciliary ganglion* in situ (SCHAFFNER, 1973; SCHAFFNER and HAEFELY, 1974).

On the whole, bradykinin resembles angiotensin II very closely in its action on autonomic ganglia. The stimulating effect becomes prominent only after sensitising procedures and, as far as can be judged from the few studies now available, is restricted to adrenergic ganglion cells, being absent in cholinergic postganglionic neurones.

III. Various Peptides

1. Posterior Pituitary Hormones

In the cat superior cervical ganglion in situ *oxytocin* had a stimulant effect as assessed by the contraction of the nictitating membrane (LEWIS and REIT, 1966). Oxytocin was at least as potent as angiotensin II. Profound long-lasting tachyphylaxis precluded a more detailed analysis of the oxytocin effect. Tachyphylaxis to oxytocin did not affect the responsiveness of the ganglion to angiotensin II and bradykinin.

Vasopressin had no ganglion-stimulating effect on the cat superior cervical ganglion (LEWIS and REIT, 1966).

2. Eledoisin and Physalaemin

LEWIS and REIT (1966) found eledoisin devoid of any stimulant action on the cat superior cervical ganglion in situ, since the nictitating membrane did not contract after i.a. injection towards the ganglion. In the same ganglion, HAEFELY (1970) observed a very brief, just visible postganglionic discharge in response to eledoisin and physalaemin, provided the ganglion had been sensitised by prior preganglionic tetanisation. The two peptides failed to facilitate ganglionic transmission.

3. Substance P

A crude preparation of substance P from horse intestine failed to stimulate the cat superior cervical ganglion in situ in experiments of LEWIS and REIT (1966). HAEFELY (unpublished results) observed no effects of synthetic substance P on the same ganglion.

F. Cardiac Glycosides

KONZETT and CARPI (1956) studied the effects of several cardiac glycosides on the *cat superior cervical ganglion in situ*. When they infused scillaren A into the carotid artery for 8–15 min, a marked and sustained contraction of the ipsilateral nictitating membrane and a dilatation of the ipsilateral pupil developed in most cats after a latency of 1–2 min. The peak contraction was obtained 5 min after the start of the infusion; thereafter, the nictitating membrane slowly and partially relaxed despite continuous infusion of the glycoside. After termination of the infusion, full relaxation took about 25 min. A similar ganglionic stimulation was observed with k-strophanthoside and digitoxin. Once a response to the glycoside had been obtained in a cat, no nictitating membrane contraction could be obtained upon a second infusion. The effect of the glycosides was unaffected by C_6, d-TC, and TEA given before or during the infusion. However, the nictitating membrane rapidly relaxed when procaine was injected into the carotid artery during the glycoside-induced contraction.

A similar depression of the ganglion-stimulating effect of the cardiac glycosides was observed with calcium. When the ganglion-stimulating effect of a first glycoside infusion was prevented or interrupted by calcium, a second infusion was able to elicit the nictitating membrane contraction usually seen as the response to a first exposure of the ganglion to the drug. Ganglionic transmission was affected variably by the infusion of a glycoside; both facilitation and depression of nictitating responses to preganglionic stimuli were observed. Facilitation was regularly seen in those cats in which the infusion produced no contraction of the membrane. However, the most consistent effect of the glycosides at the end of an infusion was a block of ortho-dromic transmission, which did not recover for the rest of the experiment. During this block of transmission, the responses of the nictitating membrane to stimulation of the postganglionic trunk were normal.

These findings differ in several points from those of earlier studies performed by KONZETT and ROTHLIN (1952), where perfusion of the cat superior cervical ganglion with Locke solution was used. Single injections of 1–30 μg digitoxin, lanatoside C, k-strophanthoside, or scillaren A enhanced the nictitating membrane contractions in response to preganglionic stimulation and to injections of ACh, choline, and KCl. The glycosides produced no ganglionic stimulation by themselves. After higher doses, the initial facilitating effect on ganglionic stimulants was sometimes converted into a depression. The facilitatory effect of glycosides on the ganglionic response to chemical stimulants was also observed in chronically denervated ganglia. The relative facilitatory potencies of the glycosides corresponded to their positive inotropic potencies, scillaren A being more potent than k-strophanthoside and the equipotent lanatoside C and digitoxin.

In the eviscerated atropinised cat, the cardiac glycosides named above transiently enhanced the pressor effect of intra-aortic injections of ACh (KONZETT and CARPI, 1956). The authors concluded that the glycosides facilitated the nicotinic stimulation of sympathetic ganglia giving rise to vasoconstrictor fibres as well as the adrenal medulla.

In the *isolated rat superior cervical ganglion* incubated with ouabain 5–10 $^4 M$, DE RIBAUPIERRE et al. (1968) observed a spontaneous asynchronous activity in the postganglionic nerve, which could be blocked by d-TC. During the appearance of postganglionic discharges, ganglionic transmission was depressed. The effects of ouabain were reversible upon washing and no ultramorphological changes were observed. Ouabain diminished the amplitudes of the N wave (sum of the individual EPSPs recorded from the ganglionic surface) and of the intraganglionic presynaptic spikes recorded from the ganglionic surface (DUNANT, 1969). DE RIBAUPIERRE et al. (1968) explained their findings by the depolarising effect of ouabain on the preganglionic terminals, which would result in a release of ACh responsible for the spontaneous firing, and also in a reduction of the transmitter release by a preganglionic spike, thus leading to a depression of ganglionic transmission. The authors did not consider postsynaptic effects of ouabain in the ganglion.

In experiments that were not directed towards investigation of the ganglionic effect of ouabain, the glycoside was used to inhibit the Na^+ and K^+ pump in cells of the cat superior cervical ganglion in situ (HAEFELY, 1974a). It was found that the sensitivity to ouabain varied widely from one animal to another. A given dose could result in a sudden marked depolarisation with block of transmission or in a slowly developing slight depolarisation with initial facilitation of transmission. Both types of responses were usually accompanied by an initial spontaneous low-amplitude discharge in postganglionic nerves (HAEFELY, unpublished results).

The few studies conducted on the ganglionic effects of cardiac glycosides reveal the complex changes and sites of action. As one would expect, the glycosides reduce the membrane potential of presynaptic endings and of ganglion cells by inhibiting the active extrusion of sodium. At presynaptic terminals, this results in a release of ACh in the absence of action potentials and in a decreased release of the transmitter by action potentials. Ganglion cells are depolarised; at a certain level of depolarisation, action potentials will be generated until further depolarisation impedes the generation of spikes. Recently, sympathetic ganglia have been proposed as the primary site of digoxin-induced arrhythmias (WEAVER et al., 1976).

G. Veratrum Alkaloids

Several purified alkaloids (protoveratrine A and B, veratridine, germerine) and two alkaloid mixtures (veratrine, protoveratrine) induced contractions of the ipsilateral nictitating membrane upon i.a. injection towards the cat superior cervical ganglion perfused with Locke solution (KONZETT and ROTHLIN, 1955). Effective doses varied between 0.5 and 100 μg. Small doses regularly enhanced the ganglion-stimulating effects of ACh and KCl, while higher doses depressed them. The effects of veratrum alkaloids were similar in innervated and chronically denervated ganglia, and veratridine appeared to be the most potent of the alkaloids named.

KOMALAHIRANYA and VOLLE (1962) made observations on the *cat superior cervical ganglion in situ* with normal blood supply that are at variance with those reported by KONZETT and ROTHLIN (1955). Intra-arterial injections of veratrine failed to induce action potentials in the acutely and chronically denervated ganglion. The alkaloid mixture (25–100 μg i.a.), however, increased the amplitude and duration of postganglionic action potentials evoked by single preganglionic stimuli. With the higher doses, veratrine produced a complete but transient block of transmission. The enhancement of discharges induced by ACh was not very pronounced. In contrast, veratrine markedly enhanced the persistent asynchronous postganglionic firing induced in acutely denervated ganglia by the AChE inhibitor, diisopropyl-phosphorofluoridate (DFP). Larger doses of veratrine (100 μg) blocked the DFP-induced discharges after a transient facilitation. Ganglionic polarisation was not recorded by KOMALAHIRANYA and VOLLE (1962).

In the *frog isolated sympathetic paravertebral ganglion*, germine-3-acetate induced stimulus-bound repetitive activity (LOWNDES and HAMILTON, 1973). The threshold concentration for stimulus-bound repetition in response to an orthodromic stimulus was lower (1 μg/ml) than that required for the induction of repetitive activity after an antidromic action potential (5–20 μg/ml). Stimulus-bound repetition induced by germine-3-acetate was not blocked by *d*-TC, in contrast to that elicited by anticholinesterases (RIKER and KOSAY, 1970).

Veratridine (50 μg) abolished the after-positivity of the ganglionic action potential of the cat superior cervical ganglion in situ and greatly increased and prolonged the after-negativity (TAKESHIGE and VOLLE, 1964a). Furthermore, it enhanced the depolarising action of KCl and methacholine and increased the bimodal depolarisation that occurs after ACh. Both the early (nicotinic) and the late (muscarinic) firing induced by ACh were also enhanced. The action of veratridine persisted for several hours.

The mechanism of action of veratrum alkaloids in autonomic ganglia is not well established. Both pre- and postganglionic sites appear to be involved. While the effect of the alkaloids seems to be negligible in the resting ganglion, on-going ganglionic activity is markedly affected. It seems reasonable to assume that veratrum alkaloids affect ganglia and other neuronal structures in a similar way, namely by increasing the membrane permeability for sodium and by decelerating the inactivation of the sodium-carrying system (ULBRICHT, 1969).

H. Batrachotoxin

In the rabbit superior cervical ganglion in situ, small doses of batrachotoxin (0.3 μg i.a.)facilitated the second spike (S_2), representing a group of slowly conducting fibres in a postganglionic nerve in response to a single preganglionic stimulus (KAYAALP et al., 1970). Higher doses blocked ganglionic transmission and depolarised the ganglion. The effect of batrachotoxin was explained by its effect on the membrane conductance. It is known that the toxin increases the Na^+ permeability of the squid axon by persistent opening of Na^+ channels (NARAHASHI et al., 1971).

J. Inorganic Cations

I. Potassium

It seems that FELDBERG and VARTIAINEN (1934) were the first to study KCl on a ganglion in searching for a non-specific ganglion-stimulating agent. They added KCl to the fluid perfusing the cat superior cervical ganglion in situ and observed dose-dependent contractions of the nictitating membrane. Non-stimulating doses of KCl transiently enhanced the responses to preganglionic stimuli and to injected ACh, whereas high doses blocked transmission. That KCl acted on both pre- and postsynaptic sites was demonstrated by BROWN and FELDBERG (1936). They found that KCl caused the release of ACh in the normally innervated ganglion; this liberation was blocked by calcium. They also showed that both innervated and chronically denervated ganglion cells were excited by KCl. Moreover, the block of transmission occurring after high doses of KCl was ascribed to a postsynaptic action, since preganglionic stimulation still released ACh.

In contrast to nicotinic and especially to non-nicotinic agents, the ganglion-stimulating effect of KCl was not enhanced by prior tetanic preganglionic stimulation (TRENDELENBURG and JONES, 1965). However, histamine, pilocarpine, and 5-HT potentiated the stimulant effect of KCl in the perfused cat superior cervical ganglion (TRENDELENBURG, 1959b), as did McN-A-343 (MURAYAMA and UNNA, 1963). The stimulant effect of KCl in the cat superior cervical ganglion was not altered by chronic denervation (BROWN, D.A., 1969). In contrast to $BaCl_2$ (TAKESHIGE and VOLLE, 1964b), the stimulant effect of KCl was not reduced by C_6 and atropine (BROWN, D.A., 1966b). KCl produced a monophasic depolarisation of the cat superior cervical ganglion in situ (BROWN, D.A., 1966b; HAEFELY, 1974a). The ganglionic depolarisation was dose-dependent, a maximum being obtained by the infusion of isotonic KCl into the blood supply of the ganglion (HAEFELY, 1974a). The dose–response ratio for depolarisation is much steeper than that for nicotinic ganglion-stimulant agents.

HAEFELY (1974a) used short-lasting perfusions with isotonic KCl to assess zero membrane potential in the cat superior cervical ganglion in situ. This maximum depolarisation was almost twice the maximum depolarisation obtained with nicotinic agents (HAEFELY, 1974b). Intracellular recordings are required to decide whether the larger depolarisation observed with isotonic KCl than with maximal doses of nicotinic agents is due to the fact that KCl depolarises satellite cells in addition to the ganglionic cells. While tetrodotoxin, which blocks the electrically operated sodium channel responsible for the spike potential, abolished the ganglionic firing produced by KCl, it did not affect KCl-induced depolarisation (HAEFELY, 1974a). During depolarisation induced by nicotinic agents, KCl produced the same absolute depolarisation as before the nicotinic stimulant, but the KCl-induced ganglionic discharges were abolished. Similar findings were obtained with KCl during the late hyperpolarising phase of the effect of nicotine or DMPP (HAEFELY, 1974a). While ganglionic depolarisation increased with incremental doses of KCl, the postganglionic discharges became extremely short after higher doses, because the level of depolarisation at which discharges cease was reached in a very short time.

After moderate doses of KCl, discharges occurred during the ascending phase of depolarisation, ceased at the peak of depolarisation, and reappeared, although less intensely, during repolarisation (HAEFELY, unpublished). The level of depolarisation, at which ganglionic transmission is blocked is lower in the ascending phase of the KCl depolarisation than in the repolarising phase, i.e., transmission reappears at a level of depolarisation at which complete block is present in the ascending phase.

KCl-induced depolarisation was unaltered when the cat superior cervical ganglion was perfused with a solution in which sodium was replaced by lithium, whereas the discharge normally generated during the depolarisation was abolished (PAPPANO and VOLLE, 1967). Since lithium was unable to support ganglionic action potentials, the above findings illustrate the independence of potassium-induced depolarisation from other monovalent cations and, at the same time, the dependence of action potentials on sodium.

Depolarisation by KCl is the least specific means of stimulating autonomic ganglion cells. KCl reduces the potassium concentration gradient between both sides of the ganglion cell membrane. The advantage of using KCl for ganglionic excitation is the independence of its depolarising action from specific pharmacological receptors. Drawbacks are the massive changes of the extracellular electrolytes produced and the likelihood that all cellular elements of a ganglion (ganglion cells, satellite cells, vascular smooth muscle cells, preganglionic fibres) are affected alike.

II. Caesium

BROWN and FELDBERG (1936) observed a ganglion-stimulant action of caesium in the perfused cat superior cervical ganglion. The contractions of the nictitating membrane induced by CsCl were longer-lasting than those seen after KCl. When the ganglion was perfused with a medium containing caesium instead of potassium, a spontaneous ganglionic firing appeared after a rather long latency (10–90 min, depending on the concentration), which was suppressed by C_6, but not by atropine (HANCOCK and VOLLE, 1969). The firing was absent or extremely small in chronically denervated ganglia. The shape of orthodromic ganglionic action potentials was altered in a complex sequence during the infusion of caesium. Initially, the spike amplitude and the after-positivity were increased, while in later phases the spike height decreased and its duration was prolonged, whereas the after-positivity was replaced by a large after-negativity. HANCOCK and VOLLE (1969) concluded that caesium in some way caused the release of ACh from presynaptic nerve endings.

In bullfrog sympathetic paravertebral ganglia incubated for about 1 h in caesium-containing Ringer solution (3 mM), single preganglionic stimuli, but not direct or antidromic stimuli, induced repetitive firing (RIKER et al., 1973). Cells that did not show repetitive firing had EPSPs of greater amplitude and duration than normal. It has been suggested that the effect of caesium was due to the uptake of the cation into preganglionic nerve terminals, where it would prolong the action potential and thereby enhance the release of ACh. It appears that caesium acts predominantly on preganglionic excitation.

III. Barium

$BaCl_2$ (0.5–500 µg) induced sustained depolarisation and firing in the cat superior cervical ganglion in situ (TAKESHIGE and VOLLE, 1964 b; VOLLE, 1967). Threshold doses for the induction of depolarisation were about 20 times higher in chronically denervated ganglia than in normally innervated ones. In chronically denervated ganglia, firing was induced only exceptionally by $BaCl_2$, and only in extremely high doses. The effect of $BaCl_2$ was readily abolished by C_6 or mecamylamine. When ACh was injected into innervated or denervated ganglia 1 min after $BaCl_2$, both the early (nicotinic) and the late (muscarinic) firing were markedly enhanced, whereas the ACh-induced depolarisations were unaffected by low doses of $BaCl_2$ and reduced by higher doses. $BaCl_2$ blocked depolarisation and discharge by KCl. On the other hand, depolarisation and firing by $BaCl_2$ were absent up to 15 min after the effect of KCl had subsided. TAKESHIGE and VOLLE (1964 b) considered three possible mechanisms for the ganglionic actions of barium. $BaCl_2$ might release ACh from presynaptic terminals, as it has been shown to do in cholinergic motor nerves. The marked dependence of the stimulant action of $BaCl_2$ on endogenous ACh could also be explained by a penetration of the divalent cation into the ganglion cells with a consequent decrease of the negativity of the cell interior, whereby the penetration would occur under the synaptic action of ACh. Finally, barium was considered to be able to decrease the permeability of the ganglion cell membrane for K^+.

IV. Calcium

The actions of $CaCl_2$ in the cat superior cervical ganglion in situ were found to be very complex (TAKESHIGE and VOLLE, 1964 a; VOLLE, 1967). It caused a dose-dependent depolarisation (0.2–5 mg) lasting up to 1 min, which was prevented by C_6. Although the depolarisation was large enough, postganglionic discharges were never elicited. The sensitivity of the ganglion to the depolarising effect of $CaCl_2$ was greatly reduced after chronic denervation, but still antagonised by C_6. In medium doses, $CaCl_2$ inconsistently enhanced the early (nicotinic) firing and regularly depressed the late (muscarinic) discharge induced by ACh. Higher doses of $CaCl_2$ depressed both phases of ACh-induced firing. The effects of calcium on the ganglion cannot yet be explained with certainty. TAKESHIGE and VOLLE (1964a) discussed the possibilities that the cation increased the release of ACh by entering the preganglionic terminals or that it moved into ganglion cells under the postsynaptic effect of ACh. The absence of discharges after $CaCl_2$ in spite of sufficient depolarisation might indicate a simultaneous "labilising" and "stabilising" effect of the membrane at different sites, i.e., an inhibition of spike generation in spite of a decrease of the membrane potential. This view is consistent with the findings of rhythmic discharges of ganglion cells and a failure of transmission with lowered calcium (LARRABEE et al., 1939; HARVEY and McINTOSH, 1940), and with the occurrence of repetitive after-discharges following each preganglionic volley during the early stage of calcium deprivation (BRONK et al., 1938).

K. Conclusions

All autonomic ganglion cells of mammals and amphibia are synaptically excited by ACh through the interaction with nAChRs. This "nicotinic pathway" is probably the only one by which orthodromic action potentials are generated under physiological conditions. Under special circumstances, certain autonomic ganglion cells are also stimulated by endogenous as well as exogenous ACh through mAChRs. ACh shares this muscarinic ganglion-stimulating action with other cholinomimetics of the "muscarine type", e.g., muscarine, methacholine, bethanechol, pilocarpine, oxotremorine, furtrethonium, McN-A-343, and AHR-602. The sensitivity to muscarinic stimulation of the different autonomic ganglia varies enormously, from dog and cat stellate ganglia, which apparently contain a large number of mAChRs, and the cat ciliary ganglion, which does not seem to be equipped with mAChRs at all, an intermediate position being taken by the cat superior cervical ganglion. Muscarinic stimulation differs in many respects from nicotinic stimulation.

1. The *sensitivity of ganglia to muscarinic stimulants* is usually rather low, but is markedly enhanced by various procedures and agents, which rarely potentiate nicotinic stimulation, such as tetanic preganglionic stimulation, chronic denervation, several depolarising compounds (KCl, isoprenaline), and calcium deprivation. Probably the most effective unmasking and enhancement of the muscarinic responses are obtained during the late non-competitive phase of ganglionic blockade by nicotine.

2. *Muscarinic excitation* (depolarisation and discharge) has a characteristic delayed onset. This latency probably does not reflect a lower accessibility of the nAChRs (although a different localisation of nicotinic and muscarinic AChRs is in no way ruled out), but is rather due to the underlying molecular mechanisms.

3. Although the *ionic mechanism of muscarinic excitation* is not yet clear, a decrease of the membrane conductance, rather than the increase underlying nicotinic stimulation, is, however, involved. Muscarinic stimulation is accompanied by an increase of the level of cGMP in ganglion cells. If this biochemical effect turned out to be causally related to muscarinic stimulation, it might explain its latency.

4. *Muscarinic stimulation* is easily depressed by non-specific stabilising agents such as procaine, calcium, and morphine.

Autonomic ganglia can also be stimulated by endogenous mediators that are present in the circulating blood. All autonomic ganglia studied so far are stimulated by 5-HT and, to a more varying degree, by histamine. The receptors mediating stimulation by 5-HT are not specifically blocked by the 5-HT antagonists so far known, but with some selectivity by picrotoxin and propranolol. The stimulant effect of histamine is blocked by histamine H_1 blockers. The polypeptides angiotensin II, bradykinin, and oxytocin have a weak stimulant action on mammalian sympathetic ganglia, but apparently not on parasympathetic ganglia. The significance of the presence of specific receptors in all or some autonomic ganglia for the blood-borne mediators is obscure. A physiological role of these mediators in the modulation of ganglionic transmission is not very likely. Autonomic ganglia are not stimulated by all endogenous mediators or putative neurotransmitters; e.g., autonomic ganglia are a notable exception in not being stimulated by glutamate, in contrast to all neuronal elements of the central nervous system studied so far.

Autonomic ganglia are stimulated by cardiac glycosides and veratrum alkaloids, the former resulting in depolarisation by inhibiting the $Na^+ + K^+$-stimulated ATP-ase, the latter by increasing the sodium permeability and by decelerating the inactivation of the electrically operated sodium ionophor. Both groups of compounds act on presynaptic terminals as well as on ganglion cells.

The least specific chemical stimulus of autonomic ganglia is potassium. Barium, calcium, and caesium act in a complex way on pre- and postganglionic sites.

References

Aiken, J.W., Reit, E.: Stimulation of the cat stellate ganglion by angiotensin. J. Pharmacol. Exp. Ther. *159*, 107–114 (1968)

Aiken, J.W., Reit, E.: A comparison of the sensitivity to chemical stimuli of adrenergic and cholinergic neurons in the cat stellate ganglion. J. Pharmacol. Exp. Ther. *169*, 211–223 (1969)

Ambache, N., Perry, W.L.M., Robertson, P.A.: The effect of muscarine on perfused superior cervical ganglia of cats. Br. J. Pharmacol. *11*, 442–448 (1956)

Bentley, G.A.: Pharmacological studies on the hypogastric ganglion of the rat and guinea-pig. Br. J. Pharmacol. *44*, 492–509 (1972)

Boissier, J.-R., Renier, E., Renier-Cornec, A., Hazard, R.: Récepteurs et cholinestérases impliqués dans les effets ganglionnaires de l'acétylcholine après gang</nplégiques puis anticholinestéra-siques. J. Pharmacol. (Paris) *5*, 363–374 (1974)

Brezenoff, H.E., Gertner, S.B.: A study of ganglionic denervation supersensitivity using McN-A-343 and histamine as ganglion stimulating agents. Proc. Soc. Exp. Biol. *130*, 1229–1233 (1969)

Brimble, M.J., Wallis, D.I.: Histamine H_1 and H_2-receptors at a ganglionic synapse. Nature *246*, 156–158 (1973)

Brimble, M.J., Wallis, D.I.: The role of muscarinic receptors in synaptic transmission and its modulation in the rabbit superior cervical ganglion. Eur. J. Pharmacol. *29*, 117–132 (1974)

Brimblecombe, R.W., Sutton, J.V.: The ganglion-stimulating effects of some amino-acid esters. Br. J. Pharmacol. *34*, 358–369 (1968)

Bronk, D.W., Larrabee, M.G., Gaylor, J.B., Brink, F.: The influence of altered chemical environment on the activity of ganglion cells. Am. J. Physiol. *123*, 24–25 (1938)

Brown, A.M.: Cardiac sympathetic adrenergic pathways in which synaptic transmission is blocked by atropine sulphate. J. Physiol. (Lond.) *191*, 271–288 (1967)

Brown, D.A.: Effects of hexamethonium and hyoscine on the drug-induced depolarisation of isolated superior cervical ganglia. Br. J. Pharmacol. *26*, 521–537 (1966a)

Brown, D.A.: Electrical responses of cat superior cervical ganglia in vivo to some stimulant drugs and their modification by hexamethonium and hyoscine. Br. J. Pharmacol. *26*, 538–551 (1966b)

Brown, D.A.: Responses of normal and denervated cat superior cervical ganglia to some stimulant compounds. J. Physiol. (Lond.) *201*, 225–236 (1969)

Brown, G.L., Feldberg, W.: The action of potassium on the superior cervical ganglion of the cat. J. Physiol. (Lond.) *86*, 290–305 (1936)

Burks, T.F.: Mediation by 5-hydroxytryptamine of morphine stimulant actions in dog intestine. J. Pharmacol. Exp. Ther. *185*, 530–539 (1973)

Casnelli, J.E., Greengard, P.: Guanosin 3′,5′-cyclic monophosphate-dependent phosphorylation of endogenous substrate proteins in mammalian smooth muscle membranes. Proc. Natl. Acad. Sci. USA *71*, 1891–1895 (1974)

Chinn, C., Weber, L.J.: The actions of several psychoactive agents upon the muscarinic mechanisms in the superior cervical ganglion of the cat. Neuropharmacology *13*, 39–52 (1974)

Dale, H.H., Laidlaw, P.P.: The significance of the suprarenal capsules in the action of certain alkaloids. J. Physiol. (Lond.) *45*, 1–26 (1912)

De Groat, W.C.: The actions of γ-aminobutyric acid and related amino acids on mammalian autonomic ganglia. J. Pharmacol. Exp. Ther. *172*, 384–396 (1970)

De Groat, W.C., Lalley, P.M.: Interaction between picrotoxin and 5-hydroxytryptamine in the superior cervical ganglion of the cat. Br. J. Pharmacol. *48*, 233–244 (1973)

De Groat, W.C., Ryall, R.W.: Reflexes to sacral parasympathetic neurones concerned with micturition in the cat. J. Physiol. (Lond.) *200*, 87–108 (1969)

De Groat, W.C., Volle, R.L.: Ganglionic actions of oxotremorine. Life Sci. *2*, 618–623 (1963)

De Groat, W.C., Volle, R.L.: Interactions between the catecholamines and ganglionic stimulating agents in sympathetic ganglia. J. Pharmacol. Exp. Ther. *154*, 200–215 (1966)

Dolivo, M., Koelle, G.B.: Properties of nicotinic and muscarinic receptors of isolated rat ganglion. Experientia *26*, 679 (1970)

Drew, G.M., Leach, G.D.H.: The effects of anticholinesterases on synaptic transmission through nicotinic and muscarinic receptors in rat sympathetic ganglia in vivo. Br. J. Pharmacol. *52*, 51–59 (1974)

Dun, N., Nishi, S.: Action of angiotensin II on mammalian ganglion cells. Pharmacologist *17*, 223 (1975)

Dun, N., Nishi, S., Karczmar, A.G.: Alteration in nicotinic and muscarinic responses of rabbit superior cervical ganglion cells after chronic preganglionic denervation. Neuropharmacology *15*, 211–218 (1976 a)

Dun, N., Nishi, S., Karczmar, A.G.: Electrical properties of the membrane of denervated mammalian sympathetic ganglion cells. Neuropharmacology *15*, 219–223 (1976 b)

Dunant, Y.: Presynaptic spike and excitatory postsynaptic potential in sympathetic ganglion. Their modifications by pharmacological agents. Prog. Brain Res. *31*, 131–139 (1969)

Dunant, Y., Dolivo, M.: Relations entre les potentiels synaptiques lents et l'excitabilité du ganglion sympathique chez le rat. J. Physiol. (Paris) *59*, 281–294 (1967)

Eccles, R.M., Libet, B.: Origin and blockade of the synaptic responses of curarized sympathetic ganglia. J. Physiol. (Lond.) *157*, 484–503 (1961)

Farr, W.C., Grupp, G.: The mechanism of the positive inotropic and chronotropic effects of angiotensin. Fed. Proc. *26*, 465 (1967)

Feldberg, W., Vartiainen, A.: Further observations on the physiology and pharmacology of a sympathetic ganglion. J. Physiol. (Lond.) *83*, 103–128 (1934)

Fenner, P.A., Hilton, J.G.: The effects of neostigmine upon ganglionic responses after administration of blocking drugs. Br. J. Pharmacol. *21*, 323–330 (1963)

Flacke, W., Fleisch, J.H.: The effect of ganglionic agonists and antagonists on the cardiac sympathetic ganglia of the dog. J. Pharmacol. Exp. Ther. *174*, 45–55 (1970)

Flacke, W., Gillis, R.A.: Impulse transmission via nicotinic and muscarinic pathways in the stellate ganglion of the dog. J. Pharmacol. Exp. Ther. *163*, 266–276 (1968)

Fleisch, J.H., Flacke, W., Gillis, R.A.: Nicotinic and muscarinic receptors in the cardiac sympathetic ganglia of the dog. J. Pharmacol. Exp. Ther. *168*, 106–115 (1969)

Franko, B.V., Ward, J.W., Alphin, R.S.: Pharmacological studies of N-benzyl-3-pyrrolidyl acetate methobromide (AHR-602), a ganglion stimulating agent. J. Pharmacol. Exp. Ther. *139*, 25–30 (1963)

Gebber, G.L., Snyder, D.W.: Observations on drug-induced activation of cholinoceptive sites in a sympathetic ganglion. J. Pharmacol. Exp. Ther. *163*, 64–74 (1968)

Gebber, G.L., Volle, R.L.: Ganglionic stimulating properties of aliphatic esters of choline and thiocholine. J. Pharmacol. Exp. Ther. *150*, 67–74 (1965)

Gertner, S.B., Kohn, R.: Effect of histamine on ganglionic transmission. Br. J. Pharmacol. *14*, 179–182 (1959)

Gertner, S.B., Romano, A.: The effect of hydralazine on ganglionic transmission. J. Pharmacol. Exp. Ther. *138*, 309–314 (1962)

Gillis, R.A., Flacke, W., Garfield, J.M., Alper, M.H.: Actions of anticholinesterase agents upon ganglionic transmission in the dog. J. Pharmacol. Exp. Ther. *163*, 277–286 (1968)

Ginsborg, B.L.: The actions of McN-A-343, pilocarpine and acetyl-β-methylcholine on sympathetic ganglion cells of the frog. J. Pharmacol. Exp. Ther. *150*, 216–219 (1965)

Green, R.D.: The effect of denervation on the sensitivity of the superior cervical ganglion of the pithed cat. J. Pharmacol. Exp. Ther. *167*, 143–150 (1969)

Greengard, P.: Cyclic nucleotides, protein phosphorylation, and neuronal function. Adv. Cyclic Nucleotide Res. *5*, 585–601 (1975)

Gyermek, L., Bindler, E.: Blockade of the ganglionic stimulant action of 5-hydroxytryptamine. J. Pharmacol. Exp. Ther. *135*, 344–348 (1962a)

Gyermek, L., Bindler, E.: Action of indole alkylamines and amidines on the inferior mesenteric ganglion of the cat. J. Pharmacol. Exp. Ther. *138*, 159–164 (1962b)

Gyermek, L., Unna, K.R.: Pharmacological comparison of muscarine and muscarone with their dehydro derivatives. J. Pharmacol. Exp. Ther. *128*, 37–40 (1960)

Gyermek, L., Sigg, E.B., Bindler, E.: Ganglionic stimulant action of muscarine. Am. J. Physiol. *204*, 68–70 (1963)

Haefely, W.: Some actions of bradykinin and related peptides on autonomic ganglion cells. In: Bradykinin and related kinins. Sicuteri, F., Rocha e Silva, M., Black, N. (eds.), pp. 591–599. New York: Plenum Press 1970

Haefely, W.: Effects of serotonin (5-HT) and some related indole compounds in a mammalian sympathetic ganglion. Experientia *27*, 1112 (1971)

Haefely, W.: Electrophysiology of the adrenergic neuron. In: Handbook of experimental pharmacology. Blaschko, H., Muscholl, E. (eds.), Vol. XXXIII, pp. 661–725. Berlin, Heidelberg, New York: Springer 1972

Haefely, W.: The effects of 1,1-dimethyl-4-phenyl-piperazinium (DMPP) in the cat superior cervical ganglion in situ. Naunyn Schmiedebergs Arch. Pharmacol. *281*, 57–91 (1974a)

Haefely, W.: The effects of various "nicotine-like" agents in the cat superior cervical ganglion in situ. Naunyn Schmiedebergs Arch. Pharmacol. *281*, 93–117 (1974b)

Haefely, W.: Muscarinic postsynaptic events in the cat superior cervical ganglion in situ. Naunyn Schmiedebergs Arch. Pharmacol. *281*, 119–143 (1974c)

Haefely, W.: The effects of 5-hydroxytryptamine and some related compounds on the cat superior cervical ganglion in situ. Naunyn Schmiedebergs Arch. Pharmacol. *281*, 145–165 (1974d)

Haefely, W., Huerlimann, A., Thoenen, H.: The effect of bradykinin and angiotensin on ganglionic transmission. In: Hypotensive polypeptides. Erdös, E.G., Back, N., Sicuteri, F., Wilde, A.F. (eds.), pp. 314–327. Berlin, Heidelberg, New York: Springer 1966

Hamilton, J.T., Rubinstein, H.M.: Nicotinic and muscarinic activity of benzyltrimethylammonium and its α-, β-, and γ-substituted pyridyl-methyltrimethylammonium analogs. J. Pharmacol. Exp. Ther. *160*, 112–123 (1968)

Hancock, J.C., Volle, R.L.: Ganglionic blockade by a nitrogen mustard analog of hexamethonium. Arch. Int. Pharmacodyn. *175*, 295–303 (1968)

Hancock, J.C., Volle, R.L.: Enhancement by caesium ions of ganglionic hyperpolarisation induced by dimethylphenylpiperazinium (DMPP) and repetitive preganglionic stimulation. J. Pharmacol. Exp. Ther. *169*, 201–210 (1969)

Hancock, J.C., Kosersky, D.S., Volle, R.L.: Cholinoceptive sites in the rat superior cervical ganglion. Pharmacologist *11*, 286 (1969)

Harvey, A.M., MacIntosh, F.C.: Calcium and synaptic transmission in a sympathetic ganglion. J. Physiol. (Lond.) *97*, 408–416 (1940)

Henderson, G., North, R.A.: Presynaptic action of 5-hydroxytryptamine in the myenteric plexus the guinea-pig ileum. Br. J. Pharmacol. *54*, 265 P (1975)

Herr, F., Gyermek, L.: Action of cholinergic stimulants on the inferior mesenteric ganglion of the cat. J. Pharmacol. Exp. Ther. *129*, 338–342 (1960)

Hertzler, E.C.: 5-Hydroxytryptamine and transmission in sympathetic ganglia. Br. J. Pharmacol. *17*, 406–413 (1961)

Hirst, G.D.S., Silinsky, E.M.: Some effects of 5-hydroxytryptamine, dopamine and noradrenaline on neurones in the submucous plexus of guinea-pig small intestine. J. Physiol. (Lond.) *251*, 817–832 (1975)

Ing, H.R., Kordik, P., Tudor Williams, D.P.H.: Studies on the structure-action relationships of the choline group. Br. J. Pharmacol. *7*, 103–116 (1952)

Iorio, L.C., McIsaac, R.J.: Comparison of the stimulating effects of nicotine, pilocarpine, and histamine on the superior cervical ganglion of the cat. J. Pharmacol. Exp. Ther. *151*, 430–437 (1966)

Jaramillo, J., Volle, R.L.: Ganglion blockade by muscarine, oxotremorine and AHR-602. J. Pharmacol. Exp. Ther. *158*, 80–88 (1967a)

Jaramillo, J., Volle, R.L.: Nonmuscarinic stimulation and block of a sympathetic ganglion by 4-(m-chlorophenylcarbamoyloxy)-2-butynyltrimethylammonium chloride (McN-A-343). J. Pharmacol. Exp. Ther. *157*, 337–345 (1967b)

Jaramillo, J., Volle, R.L.: A comparison of the ganglionic stimulating and blocking properties of some nicotinic drugs. Arch. Int. Pharmacodyn. *174*, 88–97 (1968)

Jéquier, E.: Effet de la sérotonine sur la transmission synaptique dans le ganglion sympathique cervical isolé du rat. Helv. Physiol. Acta *23*, 163–179 (1965)

Jones, A.: Ganglionic actions of muscarinic substances. J. Pharmacol. Exp. Ther. *141*, 195–205 (1963)

Jones, A., Gomez Alonso de la Sierra, B., Trendelenburg, U.: The pressor response of the spinal cat to different groups of ganglion-stimulating agents. J. Pharmacol. Exp. Ther. *139*, 312–320 (1963)

de Kalbermatten, J.P.: Effet de la sérotonine sur l'hypersensibilité de dénervation du ganglion sympathique cervicale isolé du rat. Helv. Physiol. Acta *20*, 294–315 (1962)

Kayaalp, S.O., Albuquerque, E.X., Warnick, J.E.: Ganglionic and cardiac actions of batracho-toxin. Eur. J. Pharmacol. *12*, 10–18 (1970)

Kebabian, J.W., Bloom, F.E., Steiner, A.L., Greengard, P.: Neurotransmitters increase cyclic nucleotides in postganglionic neurons: immunocytochemical demonstration. Science *190*, 157–159 (1975a)

Kebabian, J.W., Steiner, A.L., Greengard, P.: Muscarinic cholinergic regulation of cyclic guanosine 3',5'-monophosphate in autonomic ganglia: possible role in synaptic transmission. J. Pharmacol. Exp. Ther. *193*, 474–488 (1975b)

Kharkevich, D.A.: Ganglion-blocking and ganglion-stimulating agents. Oxford: Pergamon Press 1967

Kobayashi, H., Libet, B.: Generation of slow postsynaptic potentials without increases in ionic conductance. Proc. Natl. Acad. Sci. USA *60*, 1304–1311 (1968)

Kobayashi, H., Libet, B.: Actions of noradrenaline and acetylcholine on sympathetic ganglion cells. J. Physiol. (Lond.) *208*, 353–372 (1970)

Kobayashi, H., Libet, B.: Is inactivation of potassium conductance involved in slow postsynaptic excitation of sympathetic ganglion cells? Effects of nicotine. Life Sci. *14*, 1871–1883 (1974)

Koketsu, K.: Cholinergic synaptic potentials and the underlying ionic mechanism. Fed. Proc. *28*, 101–112 (1969)

Koketsu, K., Nishi, S., Noda, Y.: Effects of physostigmine on the afterdischarge and slow post-synaptic potentials of bullfrog sympathetic ganglia. Br. J. Pharmacol. *34*, 177–188 (1968a)

Koketsu, K., Nishi, S., Soeda, H.: Acetylcholine-potential of sympathetic ganglion cell membrane. Life Sci. *7*, 741–749 (1968b)

Komalahiranya, A., Volle, R.L.: Actions of inorganic ions and veratrine on asynchronous post-ganglionic discharge in sympathetic ganglia treated with diisopropyl phosphorofluoridate (DFP). J. Pharmacol. Exp. Ther. *138*, 57–65 (1962)

Konzett, H.: The effect of histamine on an isolated sympathetic ganglion. J. Mt. Sinai Hosp. *19*, 149–153 (1952)

Konzett, H., Carpi, A.: Weitere Untersuchungen zur ganglionären Wirkung von herzwirksamen Glykosiden. Helv. Physiol. Acta *14*, 235–250 (1956)

Konzett, H., Rothlin, E.: Effect of cardioactive glycosides on a sympathetic ganglion. Arch. Int. Pharmacodyn. *89*, 343–352 (1952)

Konzett, H., Rothlin, E.: Die Wirkung von Veratrum-Alkaloiden auf ein sympathisches Ganglion. Naunyn Schmiedebergs Arch. Exp. Pathol. Pharmakol. *225*, 101–103 (1955)

Konzett, H., Waser, P.G.: Zur ganglionären Wirkung von Muscarin. Helv. Physiol. Acta *14*, 202–206 (1956)

Koss, M.C., Rieger, J.A.: Analysis of nicotinic and muscarinic transmission in the cat ciliary ganglion. Pharmacologist *16*, 311 (1974)

Koss, M.C., Rieger, J.A.: Muscarinic transmission in the superior cervical ganglion of the cat. Pharmacologist *17*, 272 (1975)

Kostowski, W., Gumulka, W.: Actions of neostigmine and physostigmine on sympathetic ganglia in the cat. Int. J. Neuropharmacol. *5*, 193–198 (1966)

Kuba, K., Koketsu, K.: Ionic mechanism of the slow excitatory postsynaptic potential in bullfrog sympathetic ganglion cells. Brain Res. *81*, 338–342 (1974)

Larrabee, M.G., Brink, F., Bronk, D.W.: The effect of chemical agents on the excitability of ganglion cells. Am. J. Physiol. *126*, 561 *P* (1930)

Lee, T.-P., Kuo, J.F., Greengard, P.: Tole of muscarinic receptors in regulation of guanosine 3′:5′-cyclic monophosphate content in mammalian brain, heart muscle, and intestinal smooth muscle. Proc. Natl. Acad. Sci. USA *69*, 3287–3291 (1972)

Levy, B., Ahlquist, R.P.: A study of sympathetic ganglionic stimulants. J. Pharmacol. Exp. Ther. *137*, 219–228 (1962)

Lewis, G.P., Reit, E.: The action of angiotensin and bradykinin on the superior cervical ganglion of the cat. J. Physiol. (Lond.) *179*, 538–553 (1965)

Lewis, G.P., Reit, E.: Further studies on the actions of peptides on the superior cervical ganglion and suprarenal medulla. Br. J. Pharmacol. *26*, 444–460 (1966)

Libet, B.: Long latent periods and further analysis of slow synaptic responses in sympathetic ganglia. J. Neurophysiol. *30*, 494–514 (1967)

Libet, B., Kobayashi, H.: Generation of adrenergic and cholinergic potentials in sympathetic ganglion cells. Science *164*, 1530–1532 (1969)

Libet, B., Chichibu, S., Tosaka, T.: Slow synaptic responses and excitability in sympathetic ganglia of the bullfrog. J. Neurophysiol. *31*, 383–395 (1968)

Lowndes, H.E., Hamilton, J.T.: Induction of stimulus-bound repetition in sympathetic ganglia by germine-monoacetate. Eur. J. Pharmacol. *23*, 293–296 (1973)

Lukomskaya, N.Ya.: Changes in cholinoreception of the superior cervical sympathetic ganglion of cat after denervation. Evolutsionnaya Biochimiya i Fiziologiya *1*, 65–72 (1969) (Russ.)

Machová, J., Boška, D.: A study of the action of angiotensin on the superior cervical ganglion in comparison with other ganglion stimulating agents. Eur. J. Pharmacol. *1*, 233–239 (1967a).

Machová, J., Boška, D.: L'action des gangliostimulants sur la transmission synaptique. Thérapie *22*, 1337–1342 (1967b)

Machová, J., Boška, D.: The effect of 5-hydroxytryptamine, dimethylphenylpiperazinium and acetylcholine on transmission and surface potential in the cat sympathetic ganglion. Eur. J. Pharmacol. *7*, 152–158 (1969)

Malmejac, J., Riev, M., Clostre, F., Schlotterer, M.: Action ganglionnaire de l'angiotensine. C.R. Acad. Sci. [D] (Paris) *266*, 1153–1155 (1968)

Mason, D.F.J.: A ganglion stimulating action of neostigmine. Br. J. Pharmacol. *18*, 76–86 (1962a)

Mason, D.F.J.: Depolarising action of neostigmine at an autonomic ganglion. Br. J. Pharmacol. *18*, 572–587 (1962b)

Murayama, S., Unna, K.R.: Stimulant action of 4-m(chlorophenylcarbamoyloxy)-2-butynyltrimethylammonium chloride, (McN-A-343) on sympathetic ganglia. Fed. Proc. *21*, 322 (1962)

Murayama, S., Unna, K.R.: Stimulant action of 4-(m-chlorophenylcarbamoyloxy)-2-butynyltrimethylammonium chloride (McN-A-343) on sympathetic ganglia. J. Pharmacol. Exp. Ther. *140*, 183–192 (1963)

Narahashi, T., Deguchi, T., Albuquerque, E.X.: Effects of batrachotoxin on nerve membrane potential and conductances. Nature [New Biol.] *229*, 221–222 (1971)

Nilwises, N., Schmidt, G.: Wirkungen von Atropinverbindungen auf die synaptische Übertragung im isolierten Cervicalganglion der Ratte. Naunyn Schmiedebergs Arch. Exp. Pathol. Pharmakol. *251*, 335–343 (1965)

Nishi, S., Soeda, H., Koketsu, K.: Unusual nature of ganglionic slow EPSP studied by a voltage-clamp method. Life Sci. *8*, 33–42 (1969)

Panisset, J.-C.: Effect of angiotensin on the release of acetylcholine from preganglionic and postganglionic nerve endings. Can. J. Physiol. Pharmacol. 45, 313–317 (1967)

Pappano, A.J., Volle, R.L.: The reversal by atropine of ganglionic blockade produced by acetylcholine. Life Sci. 12, 677–682 (1962)

Pappano, A.J., Volle, R.L.: Actions of lithium ions in mammalian sympathetic ganglia. J. Pharmacol. Exp. Ther. 157, 346–355 (1967)

Pascoe, J.E.: The effects of acetylcholine and other drugs on the isolated superior cervical ganglion. J. Physiol. (Lond.) 132, 242–255 (1956)

Purves, R.D.: Muscarinic excitation: A microelectrophoretic study on cultured smooth muscle cells. Br. J. Pharmacol. 52, 77–86 (1974)

De Ribaupierre, F., Dunant, Y., Dolivo, M., Forogloukerameus, C.: L'action présynaptique de l'ouabaïne sur le ganglion sympathique. J. Physiol. (Paris) 60, 531–532 (1968)

Riker, W.K., Kosay, S.: Drug induction and suppression of stimulus-bound repetition in sympathetic ganglia. J. Pharmacol. Exp. Ther. 173, 284–292 (1970)

Riker, W.K., Russell, N.J., Stoll, S.: Cesium: postjunctional repetitive firing in sympathetic ganglion. Life Sci. 13, 1069–1075 (1973)

Robertson, P.A.: An antagonism of 5-hydroxytryptamine by atropine. J. Physiol. (Lond.) 121, 54 P–55 P (1953)

Robertson, P.A.: Potentiation of 5-hydroxytryptamine by the true cholinesterase inhibitor 284 C 51. J. Physiol. (Lond.) 125, 37 P-38 P (1954)

Roszkowski, A.P.: An unusual type of sympathetic ganglionic stimulant. J. Pharmacol. Exp. Ther. 132, 156–170 (1961)

Roszkowski, A.P., Yelnosky, J.: Structure-activity relationships among a series of acetylenic carbamates related to McN-A-343. J. Pharmacol. Exp. Ther. 156, 238–245 (1967)

Roszkowski, A.P., Misekova, D., Volle, R.L., Hancock, J.C., Richards, R.K.: Antagonism of the ganglion stimulating and parasympathetic actions of McN-A-343 by pilocarpine. Arch. Int. Pharmacodyn. 193, 124–133 (1971)

Sanghvi, I., Murayama, S., Smith, C.M., Unna, K.R.: Action of muscarine on the superior cervical ganglion of the cat. J. Pharmacol. Exp. Ther. 142, 192–199 (1963)

Saum, W.R., De Groat, W.C.: The action of 5-hydroxytryptamine on the urinary bladder and on vesical autonomic ganglia in the cat. J. Pharmacol. Exp. Ther. 185, 70–83 (1973)

Saxena, P.R.: Contraction of the urinary bladder by muscarinic ganglionic stimulants: possible existence of muscarinic receptor sites on its parasympathetic ganglia. Arch. Int. Pharmacodyn. 199, 16–28 (1972)

Schaffner, R.: Morphologie, Physiologie und Pharmakologie des Ganglion ciliare der Katze. Ph.D. Thesis, University of Basle 1973

Schaffner, R., Haefely, W.: The ciliary ganglion of the cat: pharmacological aspects. Naunyn Schmiedebergs Arch. Pharmacol. 282, Suppl., R 83 (1974)

Schneyer, D.A., Hall, H.D.: Autonomic pathways involved in a sympathetic-like action of pilocarpine on salivary composition. Proc. Soc. Exp. Biol. 121, 96–100 (1966)

Smith, J.C.: Observations on the selectivity of stimulant action of 4-(m-chlorophenylcarbamoyl)-2-butynyltrimethylammonium chloride on sympathetic ganglia. J. Pharmacol. Exp. Ther. 153, 266–275 (1966a)

Smith, J.C.: Pharmacological interactions with 4-(m-chlorophenylcarbamoyloxy)-2-butynyltrimethylammonium chloride, a sympathetic ganglion stimulant. J. Pharmacol. Exp. Ther. 153, 276–284 (1966b)

Takeshige, C., Volle, R.L.: Bimodal response of sympathetic ganglia to acetylcholine following eserine or repetitive preganglionic stimulation. J. Pharmacol. Exp. Ther. 138, 68–73 (1962)

Takeshige, C., Volle, R.L.: Cholinoceptive sites in denervated sympathetic ganglia. J. Pharmacol. Exp. Ther. 141, 206–213 (1963a)

Takeshige, C., Volle, R.L.: Asynchronous postganglionic firing from the cat superior cervical sympathetic ganglion treated with neostigmine. Br. J. Pharmacol. 20, 214–220 (1963b)

Takeshige, C., Volle, R.L.: Similarities in the ganglionic actions of calcium ions and atropine. J. Pharmacol. Exp. Ther. 145, 173–180 (1964a)

Takeshige, C., Volle, R.L.: The effects of barium and other inorganic cations on sympathetic ganglia. J. Pharmacol. Exp. Ther. 146, 327–334 (1964b)

Takeshige, C., Volle, R.L.: Modification of ganglionic responses to cholinomimetic drugs following preganglionic stimulation, anticholinesterase agents and pilocarpine. J. Pharmacol. Exp. Ther. 146, 335–343 (1964c)

Takeshige, C., Pappano, A.J., De Groat, W.C., Volle, R.L.: Ganglionic blockade produced in sympathetic ganglia by cholinomimetic drugs. J. Pharmacol. Exp. Ther. *141*, 333–342 (1963)

Trendelenburg, U.: The action of histamine and pilocarpine on the superior cervical ganglion and the adrenal glands of the cat. Br. J. Pharmacol. *9*, 481–487 (1954)

Trendelenburg, U.: The potentiation of ganglionic transmission by histamine and pilocarpine. J. Physiol. (Lond.) *129*, 337–351 (1955)

Trendelenburg, U.: The action of 5-hydroxytryptamine on the nictitating membrane and on the superior cervical ganglion of the cat. Br. J. Pharmacol. *11*, 74–80 (1956 a)

Trendelenburg, U.: Modification of transmission through the superior cervical ganglion of the cat. J. Physiol. (Lond.) *132*, 529–541 (1956 b)

Trendelenburg, U.: The action of histamine, pilocarpine, and 5-hydroxytryptamine on transmission through the superior cervical ganglion. J. Physiol. (Lond.) *135*, 66–72 (1957)

Trendelenburg, U.: Non-nicotinic ganglion-stimulating substances. Fed. Proc. *18*, 1001–1005 (1959)

Trendelenburg, U.: Observations on the ganglion-stimulating action of angiotensin and bradykinin. J. Pharmacol. Exp. Ther. *154*, 418–425 (1966 a)

Trendelenburg, U.: Transmission of preganglionic impulses through the muscarinic receptors of the superior cervical ganglion of the cat. J. Pharmacol. Exp. Ther. *154*, 426–440 (1966 b)

Trendelenburg, U.: Some aspects of the pharmacology of autonomic ganglion cells. Ergeb. Physiol. Biol. Chem. Exp. Pharmakol. *59*, 1–85 (1967)

Trendelenburg, U., Jones, A.: Facilitation of ganglionic responses after a period of preganglionic stimulation. J. Pharmacol. Exp. Ther. *147*, 330–335 (1965)

Ulbricht, W.: The effect of veratridine on excitable membranes of nerve and muscle. Ergeb. Physlol. *61*, 18–71 (1969)

Vickerson, F.H.L., Varma, D.R.: Effects of denervation on the sensitivity of the superior cervical ganglion of the cat to acetylcholine and McN-A-343. Can. J. Physiol. Pharmacol. *47*, 255–259 (1969)

Volle, R.L.: The actions of several ganglion blocking agents on the postganglionic discharge induced by diisopropylphosphorofluoridate (DFP) in sympathetic ganglia. J. Pharmacol. Exp. Ther. *135*, 45–53 (1962)

Volle, R.L.: Muscarinic and nicotinic stimulant actions at autonomic ganglia. International encyclopedia of pharmacology and therapeutics, Sect. 12, Vol. 1. Pergamon Press 1966 a

Volle, R.L.: Modification by drugs of synaptic mechanisms in autonomic ganglia. Pharmacol. Rev. *18*, 839–869 (1966 b)

Volle, R.L.: Similarities in the actions of potassium and calcium ions on ganglionic afterpotentials. J. Pharmacol. Exp. Ther. *158*, 253–263 (1967)

Volle, R.L., Koelle, G.B.: The physiological role of acetylcholinesterase (AChE) in sympathetic ganglia. J. Pharmacol. Exp. Ther. *133*, 223–240 (1961)

Wallis, D.I., Woodward, B.: The depolarising action of 5-hydroxytryptamine on sympathetic ganglion cells. Br. J. Pharmacol. *49*, 168 P (1973)

Wallis, D.I., Woodward, B.: The facilitatory actions of 5-hydroxytryptamine and bradykinin in the superior cervical ganglion of the rabbit. Br. J. Pharmacol. *51*, 521–531 (1974)

Wallis, D.I., Woodward, B.: Membrane potential changes induced by 5-hydroxytryptamine in the rabbit superior cervical ganglion. Br. J. Pharmacol. *55*, 199–212 (1975)

Watanabe, S., Koketsu, K.: 5-HT hyperpolarisation of bullfrog sympathetic ganglion cell membrane. Experientia *29*, 1370–1372 (1973)

Watson, P.J.: Drug receptor sites in the isolated superior cervical ganglion of the rat. Eur. J. Pharmacol. *12*, 183–193 (1970)

Weaver, L.C., Akera, T., Brody, T.M.: Digoxin toxicity: primary sites of drug action on the sympathetic nervous system. J. Pharmacol. Exp. Ther. *197*, 1–9 (1976)

Weight, F.F.: Synaptic potentials resulting from conductance decreases. In: Synaptic transmission and neuronal interaction, pp. 141–152. New York: Raven Press 1974

Weight, F.F., Votava, J.: Slow synaptic excitation in sympathetic ganglion cells: evidence for synaptic inactivation of potassium conductance. Science *170*, 755–758 (1970)

Weight, F.F., Petzold, G., Greengard, P.: Guanosine 3',5'-monophosphate in sympathetic ganglia: increase associated with synaptic transmission. Science *186*, 942–944 (1974)

Weinstock, M., Schechter, Y.: Antagonism by propranolol of the ganglion stimulant action of 5-hydroxytryptamine. Eur. J. Pharmacol. *32*, 293–301 (1975)

CHAPTER 11

Ganglion Activity
of Centrally Acting Neurotropic Agents

A. Nistri and J.P. Quilliam

A. Introduction

There are at least two compelling reasons for considering the effects of centrally acting drugs on peripheral autonomic ganglia. The first is that these ganglia serve as convenient and readily accessible models for investigation of the general features of the physiology of neurotransmission. Such studies in turn might contribute to the understanding of synaptic transmission in the brain, where technical difficulties often hamper direct and conclusive investigation. There are functional analogies in synaptic transmission at ganglionic and central levels. For example, acetylcholine (ACh) and catecholamines seem to have transmitter roles in some areas of the brain as well as in peripheral ganglia. Therefore studies of the action of neurotropic drugs on ganglionic function may not only shed light on the mode of action of these compounds at the cellular level, but also assist in the understanding of their central effects in animals and in man. Further, these drugs may be used as pharmacological tools in research on general aspects of synaptic neurophysiology.

The second reason is that, although it is always hoped theoretically that the effects of centrally acting drugs will be confined to the central nervous system, in practice the administration of these agents clinically may also give rise to some actions at autonomic ganglia (among other peripheral sites), which may explain unwanted side-effects or form the basis for specific and required therapeutic actions.

In this chapter, it is our main intention to present evidence of the interaction of some centrally acting drugs with the function of vertebrate sympathetic ganglia, since the bulk of available research has been carried out upon them. We shall not attempt to review the effects of such drugs on invertebrate ganglia, although it is recognised that studies on such preparations as squid, snail, or sea-hare ganglia have contributed to the understanding of synaptic transmission; the reader is referred to the work of others, such as CHALAZONITIS (1967), GERSCHENFELD (1973), BARKER (1975), and NISTRI et al. (1975).

B. Methods

Advances in neuroscience disciplines now allow investigators to study the effects of drugs on ganglia be several different techniques. First, the morphological approach, using histological or more recently electron-microscopical techniques reveals the normal structural arrangements at synapses and the changes in these following electrical stimulation or drug action. The electron-microscopical study of the transmitter-storing particles, namely the synaptic vesicles, before and after drug adminis-

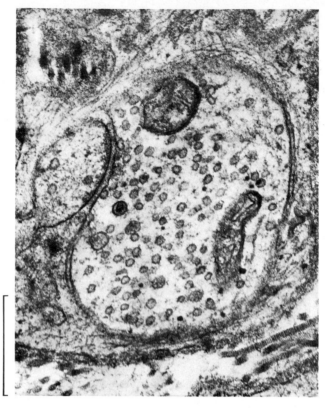

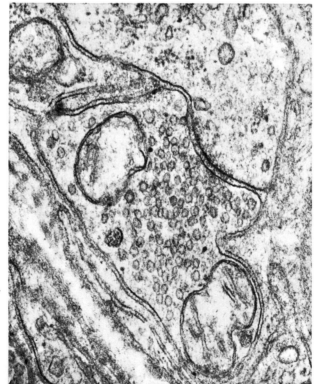

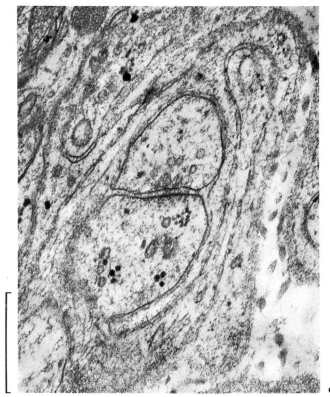

Fig. 1 a–c. Effects of chlorpromazine (CPZ) on vesicle populations of rat superior cervical ganglia. Ganglia were maintained in vitro at 35 °C without stimulation in control-modified McEwan's (1956) solution (Quilliam and Tamarind, 1973 a) for the first 30 min of the experimental period and this was replaced for a second (final) 30 min by fresh control solution **(a)** or by fresh solution containing 0.0314 mM CPZ **(b)**. **(c)** for the first 30 min the ganglion was maintained in control McEwan's solution, for the second 30 min in Ca^{2+}-free solution containing 1 mM ethylene-diamine-tetra-acetate (EDTA), and for a final 30 min in normal Ca^{2+} solution with 0.0314 mM CPZ (Tamarind, 1974). Vesicle counts were made in the 0.25-μm zone adjacent to the presynaptic membrane, these values being termed the "local vesicle population" and expressed as vesicles/μm². Note the much greater packing density of vesicles in **b** than in **a** and **c**. Calibration bar = 0.5 μm.

tration provides an interesting structural commentary on the subcellular actions of drugs, an approach which has been used in our laboratory.

Quilliam and Tamarind (1970, 1973 a) and Tamarind (1974) examined the effects of some centrally active drugs on synaptic local vesicle populations (LVP) in the rat superior cervical ganglion in vitro (Fig. 1). They found that the LVP varied so markedly between individual synaptic profiles even within a single preparation that subjective impressions of difference between preparations were usually misleading and statistical analysis of results was essential. Their pooled controls (Quilliam and Tamarind, 1973 b) from 284 synapses in 12 ganglia yielded a mean of 124 ± 3.2 (s.e.) vesicles/μm², which was very similar to the finding of Perri et al. (1972). Electrical stimulation at 10 Hz for 3 min before fixing of the ganglion gave a rise lasting for

20 min and peaking in 1 min to a LVP value of 165 ± 6.0 (s.e.), a response that can be modified by drugs (QUILLIAM and TAMARIND, 1973 a).

Histochemical data can add another dimension to the subcellular picture, as has the pioneering work of KOELLE and FRIEDENWALD (1949), KOELLE (1950), and KOELLE and KOELLE (1959), which visualised, by an indirect technique, the synaptic locus of acetylcholinesterase, the enzyme responsible for the inactivation of the transmitter, ACh. Unfortunately, we still lack a reliable, direct histochemical method of staining acetylcholine, but developments in staining for choline acetyltransferase offer much of interest (BURT, 1971; KASA, 1971).

By employing the Flack-Hillarp method of fluorescing catecholamines in UV light (FALCK et al., 1962), catecholamine-containing neurones in ganglia can be rendered visible under the microscope (ERANKO, 1967) and their response to drug treatment followed.

A second type of approach is electrophysiological, relying on extracellular or intracellular recordings from ganglionic neurones in the presence or absence of drugs. Thirdly, there are sensitive neurochemical methods of measuring concentrations of neurotransmitters, their precursors and their metabolites in small tissue samples, such as ganglia. The activity of the enzymes involved in transmitter metabolism can also be estimated. Thus the acute or chronic effects of drugs may be expressed in quantitative chemical terms. Obviously investigations that embody a multidisciplinary approach will probably offer special rewards.

On the basis of methods such as those outlined above, the site and mode of action of centrally acting drugs at ganglionic level may be defined. For example, it is important to know whether a ganglion-blocking compound produces its effects by inducing failure of axonal conduction or of synaptic transmission or of both. If there is failure of synaptic transmission, the next step will be to clarify whether this is due to a presynaptic action of the drug on synthesis, storage, or release of the natural transmitter or to a postsynaptic action on the receptors or more generally upon the membrane properties and characteristics of the ganglionic neurone.

C. Volatile Anaesthetics

The considerable interest in the effects of general anaesthetic agents on ganglionic transmission stems from the possibility that the changes in blood pressure, heart rate, pupillary size, etc. produced by them may be due partly to an action of these drugs on ganglia. A pioneer electrophysiological approach to this topic was that of LARRABEE and BRONK (1947). LARRABEE and POSTERNAK (1952) recorded the electrical activity from the cat stellate ganglion and observed a depression of ganglionic transmission after administration of many general anaesthetics. These findings stimulated questions such as:

1) Did anaesthetic drugs depress axonal conduction?

2) Did they block only synaptic transmission?

3) If so, was the block due to effects on the pre- or postsynaptic membrane of the synapse or upon both?

4) Did anaesthetics depress ganglionic "metabolism" in a general biochemical sense?

LARRABEE and his associates undertook a detailed electrophysiological and pharmacological study to answer some of these questions. First, they found that chloretone, ether, and chloroform all failed to slow down the oxygen consumption of ganglia in vitro in doses capable of inducing ganglionic blockade (LARRABEE et al., 1952) so that a metabolic effect of these drugs seemed unlikely. Secondly, LARRABEE and POSTERNAK (1952) showed that the concentrations of these agents blocking axonal conduction were several times higher than those required to block ganglionic transmission. Therefore, the site of action of these compounds appeared to be synaptic. The depression of in vivo synaptic transmission by ether or chloroform during surgical anaesthesia was subsequently confirmed by LARRABEE and HOLADAY (1952).

The outstanding exception to the above-mentioned results is urethane, which can anaesthetise the laboratory animal without evident blockade of ganglionic transmission. Indeed, in high dosage, urethane blocks first axonal conduction and then synaptic transmission (LARRABEE and POSTERNAK, 1952). This unusual and convenient feature makes urethane the general anaesthetic agent of choice for administration to animals in experimental studies on ganglionic transmission.

As the studies of LARRABEE and his colleagues showed that the action of some anaesthetics was synaptic, it fell to NORMANN and LÖFSTROM (1955) to quantitate the contribution a postsynaptic effect might make to ganglionic block. They found that the blocking effect of tubocurarine in the cat in situ stellate ganglion preparation was additive to that of ether or chloroform, suggesting a mode of action similar to that of tubocurarine. At the time of its introduction, RAVENTOS (1956) suggested that ganglionic blockade was a feature of the cardiovascular action of halothane, but this was not confirmed by SEVERINGHANS and CULLEN (1958) in human beings. In this confused field, MILLAR and BISCOE (1966), working with rabbit ganglia, suggested that halothane and ether produce their cardiovascular effects mainly by a direct action on the vascular smooth muscle, and they offered evidence for this. BISCOE and MILLAR (1966) did, however, find some evidence of depression of ganglionic transmission by ether, halothane or cyclopropane, and to explain this "paradox", they postulated that only some of the ganglionic synapses had stopped operating during anaesthesia and that those remaining unaffected produced enough amplification to account for an increased total postganglionic discharge. In contrast to these findings, a mainly synaptic action of ether and halothane was proposed by GARFIELD et al. (1968), who thought that presynaptic reduction of transmitter release could be the basis of the ganglionic blockade. Ganglionic transmission was depressed most powerfully by ether and halothane, while cyclopropane was less active and nitrous oxide exerted little or no blocking effect. Similar ganglion-blocking potencies were found by PRICE and PRICE (1967). In dog, ALPER et al. (1969) showed that these drugs blocked synaptic transmission by binding with nicotinic postsynaptic receptors while ganglionic muscarinic receptors were relatively unaffected. A similar selective action of methoxyflurane on nicotinic ganglionic receptors was found by PILON et al. (1973). BISCOE (1969) discussed the lack of consistency of these results and MILLAR et al. (1969) subsequently confirmed that halothane increased sympathetic *post*ganglionic discharges in rabbit whereas depression of *pre*ganglionic discharges was observed in dog and cat. The critical studies of SKOVSTED et al. (1969) led them to conclude that in cat, halothane lowers blood pressure mainly through a reduction in central sympathetic activity, except when high doses are used which also block ganglionic synapses and peripheral junctions (PISKO et al., 1970).

However, Christ (1977) found that when given in doses similar to those used in clinical anaesthesia, halothane blocked the nicotinic receptors of the in vitro stellate ganglion of the hamster without apparent interaction with muscarinic receptors, and suggested that blockade by halothane of ganglionic discharges evoked by high-frequency stimulation might be due to presynaptic depression of ACh release.

When dealing with the action of general anaesthetics, it is often assumed implicitly that these agents have a general depressant action on synaptic transmission at multiple levels in the nervous system and that the activity of almost all excitable cells is thus reduced. Such a widespread action could be taken as an example of drug actions not involving *specific* receptors (Wenke, 1971). However, the observations by Alper et al. (1969) suggest that, at least with transmission in cardiac sympathetic ganglia, selectivity of drug action exists. The idea of such a selectivity in some types of ganglia is supported by the intracellular studies of Nicoll (1978) on amphibian ganglia, which showed that general anaesthetics depressed excitatory postsynaptic potentials selectively; this author proposed that general anaesthetics might interact with postsynaptic Na^+ channels, as suggested by Baker (1975) in invertebrate preparations and by Adams (1976) for the frog neuromuscular junction. Recent experimental findings are in keeping with the view that general anaesthetics and neurodepressants (including tranquillizers) might interfere with synaptic Na^+ channels in the central nervous system (Constanti and Nistri, 1976; Smaje, 1976; Nistri and Constanti, 1978). Moreover, general anaesthetics produce a block of synaptic transmission more easily than a block of axonal conduction when certain frequencies of stimulation are used or when specific postsynaptic receptors, such as the nicotinic ones, are involved. It is interesting to note that urethane and some barbiturate compounds (see below) do not act by interfering with ganglionic transmission. Studies on single neurones of molluscan ganglia also indicate a degree of selectivity of action (Chalazonitis, 1967).

In conclusion, volatile general anaesthetic agents appear to exert a degree of selectivity at the ganglionic site. While this degree of selectivity of action may not be high and does not exclude other sites of action, it may be enough to account for the changes in function of vascular smooth muscle and of other autonomically innervated organs during general anaesthesia.

D. Central Nervous System Depressants

The actions of barbiturate compounds on ganglionic function have long attracted interest. Early observations seemed to indicate that pentobarbitone anaesthesia did not change the electrical activity of ganglionic preparations (Eccles, 1935; Lloyd, 1937; Whitteridge, 1937). However, these reports were not confirmed by subsequent electrophysiological studies after World War II, when Larrabee and his associates reported that pentobarbitone blocked synaptic transmission in cat and rat sympathetic ganglia in vitro and that this effect was produced by barbiturate concentrations similar to those expected in blood during pentobarbitone anaesthesia and ten times smaller than those needed to block axonal conduction (Larrabee and Posternak, 1952). Such an action of pentobarbitone was not associated with a decrease in ganglionic oxygen consumption (Larrabee et al., 1952), so demonstrating direct depression of synaptic ganglionic transmission in vitro. MILLAR and BISCOE (1965, 1966) confirmed this finding in in vivo studies. Thiopentone also blocks synaptic transmission in vivo but less potently than volatile anaesthetics (LARRABEE and HOLADAY, 1952).

A detailed investigation into the action of several barbiturate agents on in vivo ganglionic activity was provided by EXLEY (1954), who showed that amylobarbitone blocked synaptic transmission without significantly affecting the conduction of nerve impulses along the fibres. Using rat in vitro ganglia under controlled conditions, QUILLIAM and SHAND (1964) observed that amylobarbitone in concentrations able to block transmission also produced a modest block of nerve conduction. However, such a block could account only in part for the reduction in ganglionic transmission, which must be largely attributed to the more specific depression of synaptic function. This led these authors to classify amylobarbitone as a "moderately selective blocking drug" in the rat sympathetic ganglia (Table 2). From the same school, ELLIOTT (1965) found that the blocking effect of this drug was relatively independent of the frequency of presynaptic stimulation. According to EXLEY (1954), the blocking potency of amylobarbitone was about one-quarter that of a typical ganglion-blocking agent, such as tetraethylammonium. By using a quantitative method to describe the relative potencies of barbiturate drugs on ganglionic transmission, he found that amylobarbitone and butobarbitone were the most active barbiturate compounds tested, while the potency of pentobarbitone was about 40% and the corresponding values for phenobarbitone and thiopentone were 15 and 13%, respectively, of amylobarbitone. A similar range of potencies was also found by BROWN and QUILLIAM (1964a), although these authors obtained lower relative potency values for mephobarbitone, phenobarbitone, and barbitone than those of EXLEY (1954). EXLEY (1954) also measured the ACh release from the perfused ganglion and found no significant effect of a single injection of an "anaesthetic dose" of amylobarbitone. Only if very high doses were used was a reduction in the ACh release seen. This contrasts strongly with the potent depression of ACh release by barbiturates from central or postganglionic nerve terminals (PEPEU and NISTRI, 1973).

While the bulk of available evidence from very early studies led to the concept of a postsynaptic action of barbiturate drugs, the subsequent work employing a different method for the assay of ACh and of drug administration through the perfusion fluid revealed quite a different perspective. For example, MATTHEWS and QUILLIAM (1964) found that doses of amylobarbitone as low as $50 \mu M$ reduced both ACh release and ganglionic transmission and that the addition of choline to the ganglion perfusing fluid partly counteracted the reduction of ACh release but left the depression of ganglionic transmission unchanged. QUILLIAM and TAMARIND (1970) reported that amylobarbitone raised the LVP to 179 ± 7.3 (s.e.) synaptic vesicles/μm^2, a finding in keeping with a reduced ACh release if it is accepted that an accumulation of synaptic vesicles reflects a diminished discharge of transmitter into the synaptic cleft. On the basis of quantitative experiments on rabbit isolated sympathetic ganglia, ELLIOTT and QUILLIAM (1964) proposed a classification of centrally acting drugs into three groups, based upon the site and mode of the ganglionic action of each.

Table 1 shows amylobarbitone in the category with little preganglionic depressant activity, for its main site of action is synaptic and not axonal. The in vivo studies performed on cat sympathetic ganglia by BROWN and QUILLIAM (1964a) showed that

Table 1. Centrally acting drugs affecting synaptic transmission through rabbit superior cervical ganglia

Group I	
Drugs with little or no preganglionic depressant action	Hexamethonium
	Meprobamate
	Paraldehyde
	Amylobarbitone
	Methylpentynol
Group II	
Drugs with moderate preganglionic depressant action	Prochlorperazine
	Methylpentynol carbamate
	Promethazine
	Perphenazine
	Procaine
Group III	
Drugs with strong preganglionic depressant action	Chlorprothixene
	Promazine
	Dihydrochlorprothixene
	Chlorpromazine

Modified from ELLIOTT and QUILLIAM (1964).

many barbiturate compounds, when administered by close *intra-arterial* injections through the lingual artery, blocked ganglionic transmission in doses clearly higher than those expected in human blood after sedative doses. However, anaesthetic doses of pentobarbitone, which is commonly used as a general anaesthetic agent for laboratory animals, can induce ganglionic depression and hence hypotension. Similarly, the noticeable ganglion blocking property of amylobarbitone shown by EXLEY (1954) and by BROWN and QUILLIAM (1964 a) may contribute to the blood pressure-lowering effect of this drug in man.

While the synaptic blocking action of barbiturate drugs had been firmly established, the precise nature of the postsynaptic action of these compounds and its relative importance in the ensuing reduction in ganglionic transmission was investigated by BROWN and QUILLIAM (1964 b). They made a quantitative study of the antagonistic action of several drugs, including amylobarbitone and pentobarbitone, on the stimulant effect of ACh, carbachol, and KCl. By plotting log dose-response curves in the presence or in the absence of the antagonist substance, they showed that tetraethylammonium, hexamethonium, amylobarbitone, and pentobarbitone were relatively specific and competitive blockers of carbachol- or ACh-induced depolarizations. Interestingly enough, the greater ganglionic blocking action of amylobarbitone over pentobarbitone was paralleled by a greater anti-ACh effect of the former over the latter. It may be concluded that the binding of amylobarbitone and pentobarbitone to specific postsynaptic cholinergic receptors represents an important and probably dominant contribution to the development of ganglionic blockade following the administration of these two drugs (BROWN and QUILLIAM, 1964 b; SHAND, 1965).

In addition to a strong depression of excitatory postsynaptic potentials and of responses to carbachol in frog ganglia by pentobarbitone, NICOLL (1978) made the unexpected observation that the drug also specifically potentiated the responses to GABA. He had previously reported such a potentiation in frog motor neurones (NICOLL, 1975a) and in frog primary afferent fibres (NICOLL, 1975b); these findings might explain the reversal by pentobarbitone of bicuculline-induced depression of GABA effects on ganglia (BOWERY and DRAY, 1976). In this connexion, it is interesting to note that benzodiazepine drugs potentiate the action of GABA on central neurones (CHOI et al., 1977; NISTRI and CONSTANTI, 1978).

The actions of two non-barbiturate hypnotic agents, chloral hydrate and paraldehyde, on the ganglionic function have been also studied. BROWN (1962) found that when given by intra-arterial injection, chloral hydrate potentiated both ganglionic transmission and the effect of exogenous ACh by an eserine-like action. However, chloral hydrate, when administered through the fluid perfusing a ganglion, reduced ACh release (MATTHEWS and QUILLIAM, 1964), which might account for the ganglionic block that sometimes occurs after perfusion with this drug. In passing, it may be noted that the metabolite of chloral hydrate, trichloroethanol, appears to be more active than the parent compound in the perfused ganglion.

Using the perfused cat superior cervical ganglion preparation, QUILLIAM (1959) reported that paraldehyde seemed to produce ganglionic block by synaptic action. The relatively slight depressant effect of paraldehyde on ganglionic ACh output cannot contribute materially to ganglion block, according to the findings of MATTHEWS and QUILLIAM (1964). BROWN and QUILLIAM (1964b) showed that paraldehyde had a mainly postsynaptic action, which is not that of a specific cholinergic antagonist since this drug also blocks the postsynaptic stimulant action of intra-arterial KCl. The potency of paraldehyde as a ganglionic blocker is weak compared with that of typical ganglion-blocking agents such as hexamethonium and tetraethylammonium or with that of the most potent barbiturate, amylobarbitone (QUILLIAM and SHAND, 1964). ELLIOTT (1965) showed that the frequency of stimulation of the preganglionic trunk modified the effect of paraldehyde only slightly. Thus the ganglionic block induced by paraldehyde is the result of several effects: the major non-specific postsynaptic action, combined with minor contributions from a modest decrease in presynaptic ACh output and some axonal block (QUILLIAM and SHAND, 1964; SHAND, 1965). In the light of these observations, paraldehyde was allocated to the category of moderately selective ganglionic blockers, but its position in this group is the lowest and is thus close to QUILLIAM and SHAND's (1964) category of non-selective drugs (see Table 2).

In addition, hypnotic doses of paraldehyde would not be expected to exert any significant effect on autonomic ganglia (BROWN and QUILLIAM, 1964a). Therefore, the ganglionic action of paraldehyde probably has little clinical significance.

GALLAGHER et al. (1976) investigated the action of ketamine (a so-called "dissociative" anaesthetic agent) on synaptic transmission in frog sympathetic ganglia. They found that the magnitude of the compound action potential evoked by stimulation of B fibres was decreased. There was an anti-nicotinic effect, as shown by a decrease in the size of the miniature excitatory postsynaptic potentials and of the responses to iontophoretically applied ACh. In addition, there was a late anti-muscarinic effect. In high doses, ketamine reduced the K^+ permeability of ganglion cells. The authors suggested that the ganglionic action of ketamine might explain the peripheral effects of this agent following clinical administration.

Table 2. Ganglionic-blocking properties of drugs on the
rat superior cervical ganglia in vitro

Drugs highly selective for synaptic transmission	Nicotine Hexamethonium Tetraethylammonium Tubocurarine
Drugs moderately selective for synaptic transmission (some drugs may affect action potentials)	Atropine Amylobarbitone Paraldehyde
Drugs non selective for synaptic transmission (i.e., able to produce block of nerve conduction)	Procaine Methylpentynol Methylpentynol carbamate Mephenesin Benactizine

Modified from Quilliam and Shand (1964).

A number of less commonly used central nervous system depressants can produce ganglionic block in in vivo or in vitro sympathetic ganglia. Among these
compounds are benactyzine, hydroxyzine, azacyclonal, promazine, methylpentynol,
and its carbamate derivative. Usually these compounds had effects that were not
clearly specific to one or other of the steps in ganglionic synaptic transmission, i.e.,
ACh release or axonal conduction. Their mode of action can therefore be classed as
non-selective and may depend on the local anaesthetic, atropine-like, or anti-adrenergic properties each of these drugs may possess to differing extents (Quilliam, 1959;
Marley and Paton, 1959; Matthews and Quilliam, 1964; Brown and Quilliam,
1964; Quilliam and Shand, 1964; Elliott, 1965; Shand, 1965).

Methylpentynol carbamate appears to have stimulant effects on cat sympathetic
ganglia in vivo (Marley and Paton, 1959) but depressant actions of the rat isolated
ganglia (Shand, 1965), and this inconsistency remains to be elucidated.

The local vesicle population in ganglia exposed to methylpentynol carbamate
was elevated to 152 ± 4.9 (s.e.) vesicles/μm^2, as against the control value of 124 ± 3.2
(s.e.) vesicles/μm^2 (Quilliam and Tamarind, 1970).

E. Neuroleptics

I. Phenothiazines

Although early pharmacological observations led to a suggestion that chlorpromazine (CPZ) might be a possible ganglion-blocking agent (Courvoisier et al., 1952),
subsequent studies showed that the inhibition of the contraction of the cat nictitating
membrane was due very largely to a peripheral effect of CPZ (Reuse, 1954). As CPZ
antagonized the contraction elicited by intravenous injections of adrenaline, the
antiadrenergic effect of CPZ was held generally accountable for the effect on the

nictitating membrane. Among its broad spectrum of activities, CPZ also antagonized the action of parasympathetic stimulation by a peripheral effect (BRADLEY, 1963).

ELLIOTT and QUILLIAM (1964) found that CPZ and other phenothiazines blocked transmission in in vitro sympathetic ganglia by strongly depressing axonal conduction; occasionally these compounds produced a stimulatory or facilitating effect at synapses. Thus phenothiazines may have a dual action on ganglia and are classified in Table 1 in group III according to ELLIOTT and QUILLIAM (1964). In the in vivo experiments of this study, CPZ did not reverse the ganglionic block produced by exogenous adrenaline. The rather non-specific effect of two phenothiazines, perphenazine and pecazine, on cat ganglia was always associated with peripheral effects on neuro-effector organs, as shown by BROWN and QUILLIAM (1964a). When isolated ganglia were exposed to 0.0314 mM CPZ, the local synaptic vesicles population rose to 175 ± 4.9 (s.e.) compared with a control of 124 ± 3.2 (s.e.) vesicles/μm^2 (QUILLIAM and TAMARIND, 1970).

Figure 1 shows such an effect of CPZ on the LVP (B), and also shows that the removal of Ca^{2+} by disodium ethylene-diamine-tetra-acetate (EDTA) prevents (C) the CPZ-induced augmentation of the LVP (QUILLIAM and TAMARIND, 1973a; TAMARIND, 1974). The CPZ-evoked rise in LVP might represent a reduced release of ACh from preganglionic terminals or the initial facilitating synaptic action of CPZ described by ELLIOTT and QUILLIAM (1964).

ELLIOTT (1969) investigated the mechanism by which CPZ lowered systemic blood pressure in cat. He confirmed that CPZ and other phenothiazines produce hypotension mostly by an anti-adrenergic action at the level of the effector organs and partly by an action on the central sympathetic system regulating the blood pressure (i.e., the medullary vasomotor nuclei). Ganglionic block by CPZ did not appear to contribute to this response as might have been predicted from ganglionic studies.

Recent work has shown that neuroleptic drugs are possible antagonists of central dopamine (DA) receptors (ANDEN et al., 1970). At peripheral ganglia, it is suggested that DA modulates synaptic transmission and has an inhibitory effect on the postganglionic membrane (LIBET and TOSAKA, 1970; LIBET and OWMAN, 1974; LIBET et al., 1975). It is interesting to note that CPZ can antagonise the inhibitory effect of injected DA but not that of noradrenaline (NA) on ganglionic transmission (WILLEMS, 1974), which might suggest that DA receptors in the ganglia are similar to those found in the brain. Both groups of receptors might thus produce the postganglionic response through the activation of 3,5-cAMP, the so-called second messenger (GREENGARD and KEBABIAN, 1974; KOBAYASHI et al., 1978).

II. Thioxanthenes

Two representative compounds of this group of drugs, chlorprothixene and dihydrochlorprothixene, are sometimes used in the treatment of psychiatric disorders. Both possess ganglionic blocking properties in rabbit sympathetic ganglia in vitro, according to ELLIOTT and QUILLIAM (1964), and their mode of action is rather unselective. These authors assigned them to their group III of Table 1, which includes drugs with some facilitating effect at synaptic level. Their action thus closely resembles that of CPZ.

III. Rauwolfia Alkaloids

Reserpine is the rauwolfia alkaloid most commonly used for therapeutic purposes. It used to be employed as an antipsychotic agent, but its present use is virtually confined to the treatment of hypertension, since intraneuronal catecholamine stores in central and peripheral nerve endings are readily depleted by this drug. For this reason, only relatively brief consideration will be given to the effects of reserpine on the ganglion.

While reserpine clearly depletes the noradrenaline (NA) content of sympathetic ganglia (MUSCHOLL and VOGT, 1958), its effect on ganglionic transmission has been a matter of controversy. Some authors reported an enhancement of ganglionic transmission after reserpine (GOLDBERG and DA COSTA, 1960; COSTA and BRODIE, 1961; COSTA et al., 1961), while others could not confirm this finding (TRENDELENBURG and GRAVENSTEIN, 1958; REINERT, 1963; WEIR and MCLENNAN, 1963; DE GROAT and VOLLE, 1966). MUSCHOLL and VOGT (1958) pointed out that an almost complete loss of ganglionic NA after reserpine is still compatible with normal synaptic transmission. REINERT (1963) suggested that some technical artefact(s) (such as the progressive dehydration of the experimental animal after injection of reserpine) might be responsible for the apparent enhancement in ganglionic transmission. Histochemical studies have revealed that sympathetic ganglia contain some catecholamine(CA)-containing cells, the CA stores of which are rather resistant to the depleting effect of reserpine (NORBERG et al., 1966; VAN ORDEN et al., 1970). CATTABENI et al. (1972), using a highly sensitive neurochemical method, found that the ganglionic DA content is more resistant than the NA content to the depleting action of reserpine. It seems likely that the intraneuronal catecholamine of these reserpine-resistant cells in DA. Much renewed interest in the action of reserpine on ganglia thus stems from the proposed role of DA as a transmitter involved in the generation of the slow inhibitory postsynaptic potential proposed by LIBET and TOSAKA (1970) and by LIBET and OWMAN (1974). Chronic treatment of rabbits with small doses of reserpine can yield animals whose sympathetic ganglia display abnormally small slow inhibitory potentials (LIBET, 1970). These findings, however, were not consistent and have been explained on the basis of the resistance of DA pools to the effect of reserpine. Other explanations for the variable results with reserpine have been put forward by LIBET (1964).

Reserpine can also stimulate enzymatic activity of sympathetic ganglia of rats and lambs to give a two- to threefold increase in ganglionic tyrosine hydroxylase, which is the rate-limiting step in the biosynthesis of catecholamines (MUELLER et al., 1969; CHEAH et al., 1971). This rise in enzymatic activity is thought to be due to trans-synaptic induction of this enzyme as a consequence of increased preganglionic sympathetic outflow following the loss of postganglionic sympathetic transmission. Therefore, a change in the synthesis of neuronal proteins is an example of a long-term effect of reserpine administration and reveals an interesting regulating mechanism between the pre- and postganglionic neurones. Similar findings were also obtained in other tissues (COSTA et al., 1974).

IV. Butyrophenones

Haloperidol and triperidol are two commonly used drugs of this group. It has been stated by several investigators that haloperidol in the therapeutic dose range has minimal effects on ganglionic function and the peripheral sympathetic system (JANSSEN, 1967; EDMONDS-SEAL and PRYS-ROBERTS, 1970). Neither haloperidol nor pimozide, a recently introduced antipsychotic agent, modifies synaptic transmission in the in situ paravertebral ganglia of the dog (WILLEMS, 1974). However, these compounds block the inhibitory action of DA and of apomorphine (a DA agonist) but not the effects of other catecholamines (WILLEMS, 1974). It is interesting to note that haloperidol, which is considered to be a DA antagonist in the central nervous system (VAN ROSSUM, 1966; WOODRUFF, 1971), can also antagonize the ganglionic action of DA. Triperidol (0.02 mM) reduces in vitro ganglionic transmission and ACh release (CASATI et al., 1973).

F. Antidepressants

I. Monoamine Oxidase Inhibitors (MAOI)

In a detailed study on the effects of several MAOIs on ganglionic activity in cat, GERTNER (1961) noted that they blocked synaptic transmission. Harmine was the most powerful of the group; furthermore its action was reversible only on repeated washing. MAOIs did not reduce ganglionic ACh release or postsynaptic responses to injected ACh. Iproniazid, when bath-applied, reduces both pre- and postganglionic action potentials of the rabbit sympathetic ganglia in vitro (ELLIOTT and QUILLIAM, 1964). However, REINERT (1963) showed that chronic treatment with nialamide, iproniazid, or tranylcypromine in rabbits failed to affect ganglionic activity, although the NA content of ganglia was considerably increased. A further confusing finding was that iproniazid increased the number of presynaptic vesicles and that this effect is further stimulated by the administration of L-Dopa, a catecholamine precursor (CLEMENTI et al., 1966). Although MAOIs effectively block monoamine oxidase (MAO) activity in sympathetic ganglia after systemic administration (LEVINE, 1962), there is no evident dose or time relationship between the enzymatic inhibition and the blockade of ganglionic transmission, a finding confirmed by HENDERSON (1971), who studied both MAO activity and synaptic potentials of rabbit ganglia in vitro. He also found that pargyline inhibited *irreversibly* the enzyme activity and depressed all the components of the multiphasic postsynaptic potential. However, repeated washing of the preparation led to the recovery of synaptic transmission but not, of course, to a return of enzyme activity. Therefore, it seems that MAOIs can block ganglionic function non-specifically by an action little related to their ability to inhibit MAO, and that such a block is observable only after acute administration of these drugs. It is important to note that the activity of these compounds on ganglia may explain, at least in part, the noticeable orthostatic hypotension often observed after their administration to man.

II. Tricyclic Antidepressants

The effects of imipramine, the prototype of this group of drugs, on ganglionic function were first explored by OSBORNE and SIGG (1960), who found a small reduction of ganglionic transmission. SIGG et al. (1963) were unable to confirm it shortly afterwards, when using the contraction of the cat nictitating membrane. The peripheral effects of imipramine probably overshadow the ganglionic ones so markedly that contradictory ganglionic findings are inevitable. Different techniques showed a mild depressant action of tricyclic compounds, such as imipramine or nortryptiline, on ganglionic synaptic transmission in studies by CAIRNCROSS et al. (1967) and by KADZIELAWA et al. (1968). Doxepin, a substance pharmacologically related to tricyclic antidepressants, also produced ganglionic block (TEHRANI et al., 1975). Tricyclic antidepressants were particularly effective in enhancing the inhibitory action of exogenous NA. No effect was observed when animals were pretreated with reserpine (CAIRNCROSS et al., 1967), and little or no potentiation toward injected DA and adrenaline was present (KADZIELAWA et al., 1968). Further investigations (MALSEED et al., 1972) showed that a selective potentiation of the effects of injected DA was given by protryptiline, compared with potentiation of NA. The action of adrenaline could be enhanced by desipramine, protryptiline or nortryptiline. Nevertheless, the attempts to block the ganglionic re-uptake of DA selectively through the use of desmethylimipramine (desipramine), diphenylpyramine, chlorpheniramine, or cocaine were unsuccessful owing to the noticeable ganglionic blockade produced by these drugs in an unspecific, local-anaesthetic manner (LIBET and OWMAN, 1974). Tricyclic antidepressants increased the disappearance of NA from electrically stimulated ganglia, although no change was seen in the NA stores of resting ganglia (BHATNAGAR and MOORE, 1971). It should be borne in mind that as NA is located mostly in the postsynaptic neurones (GIACOBINI, 1969), the effects of tricyclic antidepressants on synaptic transmission of sympathetic ganglia may tend to be rather non-specific, and are further complicated by their additional anti-muscarinic properties. In fact, an atropine-like action of desipramine on sympathetic ganglia was shown by CHINN and WEBER (1974).

G. Anti-Manic Drugs

Lithium salts have been used for several years in attempts to suppress manic attacks (GERSHON and SHOPSIN, 1973; JOHNSON, 1975). Lithium ions, which possess larger hydrated radius than sodium ions, have been also used by electrophysiologists to investigate ionic species involved in ganglionic synaptic potentials. The effects of ionic substitution with lithium or other substances have been discussed by PAPPANO and VOLLE (1967); KOKETSU (1969); VOLLE and HANCOCK (1970), and KOKETSU and YAMAMOTO (1974). Since it is speculated that lithium may exert its therapeutic action in man by altering the function of brain endogenous catecholamines (GERSON and SHOPSIN, 1973; JOHNSON, 1975), the effects of lithium and NA on the sympathetic ganglion in situ were investigated by TEHRANI et al. (1974) on the assumption that such a preparation might be considered to be a suitable synaptic model for central neurones. They reported a ganglion-depressant action of lithium which also enhanced the inhibitory effect of exogenous NA, and suggested that lithium might block ganglionic NA uptake.

Conversely, rubidium, an ion claimed to have antidepressant properties in man (PLATMAN, 1971; FIEVE et al., 1973), reduced ganglionic transmission by a proposed stimulation of NA release (TEHRANI et al., 1974). DAWES and VIZI (1973) claimed that lithium ions stimulated ACh release from rabbit ganglia in vivo. On the other hand, KOKETSU and YAMAMOTO (1974), working on amphibian ganglia, concluded that lithium ions may reduce synaptic transmission by impairing ACh release from pre-ganglionic fibres. Therefore the action of lithium on ACh release varies, probably being dependent on the animal species and/or the experimental techniques used. The significance of these findings to the mode of action of lithium and rubidium on the brain remains to be established.

H. Narcotic Analgesics

The superior cervical ganglion is less sensitive to the effects of morphine than some other neuro-effector systems. Ganglionic transmission is only slightly affected by low doses of this opiate, for only high doses induce ganglionic blockade (HEBB and KONZETT, 1949). Nonetheless, studies of the action of morphine on ganglia have been carried out for two main reasons: 1) to establish the site of its synaptic actions on a preparation in which both pre- and postsynaptic events can be recorded concurrently, and 2) to investigate the effect of morphine on the actions of naturally occurring substances such as histamine, 5-hydroxytryptamine (5-HT, serotonin); the role of these two last substances in ganglionic function is a matter of debate.

In vivo studies by TRENDELENBURG (1957) have shown that morphine blocks the contraction of the cat nictitating membrane, possibly by reducing the release of postganglionic NA. However, KOSTERLITZ and WALLIS (1966), in in vitro studies on rabbit cervical ganglia treated with small doses of hexamethonium to reduce ganglionic transmission and consequently to reduce the synaptic "safety factor", demonstrated that morphine decreased the height of the synaptic potential, an effect that was antagonised by nalorphine. Again, relatively large doses of morphine were needed to produce this effect, and the significance of these findings in relation to the mode of action of morphine is an open question. However, it is worth noting that the concentrations of ACh necessary to stimulate the ganglionic cells are also relatively higher than those needed to stimulate intestinal smooth muscle, a tissue in which the anticholinergic actions of morphine are easily demonstrable. Therefore, for reasons such as access of drugs to the receptor sites and drug receptor kinetics, the effect of morphine on ganglionic potentials, while small, is of importance as an example of narcotic drug interaction with a synaptic mechanism. As KOSTERLITZ and WALLIS (1964, 1966) reported that there is no block of axonal conduction by morphine in the concentrations used, it is of great interest to establish whether the effects of morphine involve an action at specific synaptic receptor sites. TRENDELENBURG (1957) showed that morphine antagonised neither the stimulant action of nicotinic compounds nor the non-specific depolarization induced by potassium ions, but the stimulant effects of histamine or 5-HT were decreased. Muscarinic receptors in the ganglion are also easily blocked by morphine (TRENDELENBURG, 1966b). Ganglionic stimulation by the two naturally occurring peptides, angiotensin and bradykinin, is reduced by morphine (TRENDELENBURG, 1966a). A similar antagonism between morphine and 5-HT has been found in the cat inferior mesenteric ganglion (GYERMEK and BINDLER, 1962a) and between morphine and histamine in the cat adrenal medulla (TRENDELENBURG, 1961). It seems, therefore, that the synaptic actions of morphine at receptor level have limited specificity, since, whereas nicotinic or potassium stimulation are not antagonised, the actions of muscarinic agents or of several endogenously occurring substances are clearly blocked. As the physiological role of histamine or 5-HT in ganglionic function is not known, the significance of these reactions remains puzzling. It should be noted that cocaine shares many of the effects of morphine on ganglia (Trendelenburg, 1967), while methadone, a less strongly addictive narcotic agent, similarly mimics morphine (Trendelenburg, 1961). Quilliam and Tamarind (1973a) observed that morphine SO_4 (30 μM) did not change the local synaptic vesicle populations in resting ganglia from the control counts, but significantly lowered the LVP in ganglia following preganglionic electrical stimulation. Out of all the experimental procedures employed by these authors, an increase in the total length of contact between pre- and postsynaptic components followed only electrical stimulation in the presence of morphine. The significance of this finding with morphine to its mode of action and to the vesicle hypothesis was discussed by these workers.

J. Central Nervous System-Stimulant Drugs

Among this heterogeneous group, four substances, amphetamine, lysergic acid diethylamide (LSD), psilocybin, and mescaline, all of which have hallucinogenic properties in man, will be discussed first. Kewitz and Reinert (1954) described a dual action of amphetamine on autonomic ganglia, which initially stimulated and then depressed, as does nicotine. Several mechanisms of action of amphetamine on ganglia have been proposed. Reinert (1960), working on cat superior cervical ganglia in vivo, suggested that it depolarized ganglion cells by acting on postsynaptic nicotinic receptors, and stressed the difference between the action of amphetamine and that of tyramine, ephedrine, or phenylethylamine. A different hypothesis of action was offered by Downing (1972), who found a decreased ganglionic transmission with amphetamine when the rat in vitro preparation was stimulated preganglionically at a frequency of 0.1 Hz. On the other hand, with increasingly faster stimulation rates, he observed a progressive decrease of transmission, which could be partly reversed by amphetamine, adrenaline, or noradrenaline. The effects of these three sympathomimetic substances were abolished by α-blockers but remained unaffected by pretreatment with reserpine. No direct postsynaptic action of amphetamine was seen. Downing (1972) suggested that amphetamine acted upon α-adrenoreceptors located on presynaptic nerve endings whose role was to regulate the release of ACh. By comparing the activity of several sympathomimetic compounds on the in vivo superior cervical ganglia and ciliary ganglia of the cat, Pardo et al. (1963) found that amphetamine was less potent than other adrenergic drugs. They claimed that the ganglionic block produced by amphetamine was unlikely to be due to release of endogenous catecholamines. Watson (1972) also reported that amphetamine was not active on rat in vitro ganglion preparations. Therefore, it seems that these weak ganglionic actions of amphetamine are not mediated by endogenous catecholamines. Nevertheless, most workers have considered mainly the interaction between NA and amphetamine. From more recent studies, DA appears to have a physiological role in ganglia and, furthermore, amphetamine stimulates the release of DA from brain neurones (von Voigtlander and Moore, 1970). Therefore, amphetamine might produce ganglionic depression partly through the release of DA from ganglionic stores. Methylphenidate, a central-stimulant drug with amphetamine-like actions, specifically antagonises muscarinic receptors in the cat superior cervical ganglion in vivo (CHINN and WEBER, 1974).

LSD has little effect on autonomic ganglia. In relatively high doses, it blocks the stimulant action of 5-HT and of nicotinic agents on the inferior mesenteric ganglion of the cat, thus displaying weak specificity (GYERMEK and BINDLER, 1962a). It was suggested by GADDUM and PICARELLI (1957) that there are two different types of receptor involved in mediation of 5-HT responses in the guinea-pig ileum, only one type being sensitive to LSD. It is possible that the 5-HT receptors in autonomic ganglia belong to a category that is not specifically affected by LSD. In keeping with the latter view, it is interesting to note that 5-HT was found by HAEFELY (1974) to have stimulant as well as inhibitory effects on ganglia. LSD in *high* doses blocked only the excitatory effects of 5-HT. LSD or psilocybin can also produce inhibitory actions on ganglionic transmission (HAEFELY, 1974). 2-Bromolysergic acid diethyl-amide (BOL), an LSD analogue devoid of hallucinogenic properties in man, appears to be a more potent and more selective anti-5-HT agent than LSD in autonomic ganglia (GYERMEK and BINDLER, 1962a). Psilocybin has little effect on the 5-HT responses of the same preparation (GYERMEK and BINDLER, 1962b) and blocks only the excitatory actions of 5-HT (HAEFELY, 1974).

In the superior cervical ganglion of the cat, mescaline in high doses (3 mM) produced ganglionic depression, which was not counteracted by chlorpromazine or other ataractic compounds (ELLIOTT and QUILLIAM, 1964). Lower doses tended to produce facilitation of transmission, possibly through depolarization of the postsynaptic membrane. ELLIOTT (1965) noted that the ganglion-blocking action of mescaline (like that of nicotine, adrenaline, or methylpentynol) tended to be reversed by repetitive preganglionic stimulation. He suggested that mescaline might supplement a deficient ACh release in the repetitively stimulated ganglion, either by depolarizing the postsynaptic membrane or by facilitating ACh release.

The three natural alkaloids, strychnine, picrotoxin, and bicuculline, produce generalised convulsions following systemic administration. Much interest in their central actions arose from observations of their antagonism towards the inhibitory effects of some amino acids on brain and spinal neurones (for reviews, see CURTIS and JOHNSTON, 1974; KRNJEVIĆ, 1974). Strychnine appears to be an antagonist of glycine effects, whereas bicuculline and picrotoxin reduce those of γ-aminobutyric acid (GABA). However, these convulsants possess several other actions, so that their specificity as amino-acid antagonists might be questioned.

The autonomic ganglion is an appropriate neuronal model upon which to investigate the mode of action and the specificity of these convulsant agents, since ganglionic blockade and depolarisation are induced by GABA but not by glycine whether recorded extracellularly (DE GROAT, 1970; BOWERY and BROWN, 1974) or intracellularly (KOKETSU et al., 1974; ADAMS and BROWN, 1975). Bicuculline blocks the GABA-induced depolarization but has little action against GABA-induced depression of transmission in the cat superior cervical ganglion (DE GROAT et al., 1971). In addition, this alkaloid shows some anti-muscarinic properties and a weak direct depressant action on ganglionic transmission. Therefore, even if nicotinic or catecholamine responses were relatively unaffected by bicuculline, it would appear that this compound is not an ideal GABA antagonist, as the specificity problems encountered in the work on brain and spinal cord are also present in the peripheral nervous system. The interaction between bicuculline and pentobarbitone has already been discussed in Chap. D.

Like bicuculline, picrotoxin transiently depresses ganglionic transmission (DE GROAT, 1970) and reduces the GABA-evoked responses in the superior cervical ganglion, nodose ganglion, and dorsal root ganglion of the cat (DE GROAT, 1970, 1972; DE GROAT et al., 1972). This antagonism by picrotoxin has also been observed with intracellular recordings from amphibian sympathetic ganglia (KOKETSU et al., 1974). However, picrotoxin also antagonises the initial stimulant effect of 5-HT on the cat superior cervical ganglion (DE GROAT and LALLEY, 1973) and vesical (urinary bladder) autonomic ganglia (SAUM and DE GROAT, 1973), whereas bicuculline only affects the late component of the 5-HT-induced response (DE GROAT and LALLEY, 1973). Therefore, the antagonism of the GABA-evoked responses by picrotoxin in autonomic or sensory ganglia appears to have little specificity.

The classic observations of FELDBERG and VARTIAINEN (1934) and of LANARI and LUCO (1939) revealed that strychnine blocked transmission in the superior cervical ganglion. DE GROAT (quoted by MCKINSTRY and KOELLE, 1967a) found that the cat superior cervical ganglion was quite sensitive to strychnine sulphate, since as little as 2.5–12.5 µg given intra-arterially produced ganglionic block. However, this effect of strychnine seems to have little bearing on the understanding of the nature of strychnine-glycine interactions in the feline spinal cord, since the effects of glycine on autonomic ganglia are virtually negligible. While the ganglionic action of GABA is strychnine-insensitive (DE GROAT, 1970), strychnine sulphate, when perfused through the superior cervical ganglion in a dose range of 1–100 µg/ml, reduces ACh release following electrical stimulation of the preganglionic trunk (MCKINSTRY and KOELLE, 1967a), a finding that contrasts with stimulation by strychnine of the release of brain ACh (BELESLIN et al., 1965; HEMSWORTH and NEAL, 1968). However, in the frog spinal cord, strychnine increases the ACh content (NISTRI and PEPEU, 1974), and this might be explained by a decrease in ACh release since strychnine does not block enzymatic inactivation of ACh (NISTRI et al., 1974). Furthermore, strychnine reduces the ACh release in the olivocochlear bundle (MCKINSTRY and KOELLE, 1967b). This prevention of ACh release by strychnine might explain its ganglion-blocking property, and it is conceivable that this action may also take place at some central cholinergic synapses and may so contribute to the effects of strychnine on brain neurones.

Leptazol is a potent convulsant agent whose mode of action is poorly understood. Among the several hypotheses for its action is the suggestion that leptazol acts by reducing the refractory period of synaptic transmission (ESPLIN and ZABLOCKA-ESPLIN, 1969). Leptazol increases the sympathetic discharges (CAMP, 1928) through an effect that was reputed to be central in origin. The claims of ECKENHOFF (1949) that leptazol increased ganglionic transmission and reversed barbiturate-induced depression were not confirmed in subsequent studies on the in vivo superior cervical ganglion preparation of cat by BROWN and QUILLIAM (1964a), who found that large doses of leptazol depressed ganglionic transmission, a depression that was additive to that produced by barbiturates or troxidone. These authors also reported that bemegride, another CNS-stimulant compound, possessed ganglionic effects similar to those of leptazol.

K. Tranquillizers

Only the benzodiazepine drugs are extensively used as anti-anxiety agents. As they also produce hypotension, several studies have been designed to examine whether this is due to ganglionic block. SCHALLEK and ZABRANSKY (1966) considered that diazepam and chlordiazepoxide reduced blood pressure mainly through a central action. CHAI and WANG (1966) noted that diazepam (2–4 mg/kg IV in cats) produced a small decrease in the contraction of the nictitating membrane following preganglionic stimulation. This effect was believed to result from ganglionic depression. They suggested that following IV diazepam, ganglionic effects were responsible only for the early onset of vasodilation, whereas the sustained later hypotension was attributed to an effect on the hypothalamus. It was then confirmed that diazepam, as well as CPZ, reduced the contral sympathetic outflow as recorded from preganglionic fibres in the cat (SIGG and SIGG, 1969).

Benzodiazepines suppress the post-tetanic potentiation in amphibian in vitro sympathetic ganglia in a dose-dependent manner (SURIA and COSTA, 1973). Diazepam was more potent than chlordiazepoxide, while diazepam metabolites, 3-OH diazepam and N-desmethyldiazepam, were inactive. The block of post-tetanic potentiation had a presynaptic origin and might be caused by a decrease in the synthesis and/or release of ACh. On the other hand, it is known that GABA, an amino acid present in ganglia (BOWERY et al., 1976), blocks ganglionic transmission through a Cl^--mediated action (KOKETSU et al., 1974; ADAMS and BROWN, 1975). It has been claimed recently that in vitro ganglionic effects of diazepam might be due to an increased availability of GABA to postsynaptic receptors (COSTA et al., 1975); see also Chap. D. An alternative hypothesis would be that diazepam increases the synthesis of prostaglandins in sympathetic ganglia (SURIA and COSTA, 1974), and it is known that they have an inhibitory action on transmitter release from several tissue preparations (HEDQVIST, 1970). More convincing experimental evidence needs to be forthcoming before acceptance of the proposal that the modest ganglion-blocking action of diazepam is related in some way to an interference with presynaptic mechanisms, as suggested by the in vitro observations.

L. Anticonvulsant Drugs

The effects of phenobarbitone on ganglionic activity have been considered in the section on central nervous system-depressant agents. Phenytoin (diphenylhydantoin: 30 mg/kg IV) has depressant effects on transmission through the superior cervical ganglion and reduces post-tetanic potentiation (ESPLIN, 1957). This depressant action was confirmed by BROWN and QUILLIAM (1964a), who found a block of the response of the nictitating membrane to preganglionic stimulation. Working on amphibian ganglia in vitro, SURIA and COSTA (1973) noted a suppression of post-tetanic potentiation by phenytoin and the benzodiazepine group. The potency of the former was similar to that of chlordiazepoxide but smaller than that of diazepam.

BROWN and QUILLIAM (1964a) reported that troxidone (trimethadione) had a weak ganglion-blocking effect, was not antagonised by leptazol, and was non-selective, since the responses evoked by cholinergic drugs and by potassium chloride were similarly reduced (BROWN and QUILLIAM, 1964b). Troxidone (5 mM) decreased the

ACh output from cat perfused sympathetic ganglia but, as observed with paraldehyde, there was a dissociation between the degree of synaptic block and the reduction in ACh output, since the latter was always impaired to a greater extent than the
synaptic transmission (Matthews and Quilliam, 1964).

Acknowledgements. The authors are greatly indebted to Dr. D.L. Tamarind for his help and
advice with the preparation of the sections on local vesicle populations and the effects of drugs
thereon.

They gratefully thank Miss C.A. Brown for her enthusiastic help with typing the manuscript.

Professor J.P. Quilliam warmly acknowledges the financial assistance of the following,
which made much of the work carried out in the Department of Pharmacology at St. Bartholomew's Hospital Medical College possible: The Governors of St. Bartholomew's Hospital, The
Medical Research Council of the United Kingdom, The Wellcome Trust, The Peel Trust, United
States Agencies, and The Central Research Fund of the University of London for assistance with
apparatus.

Dr. A. Nistri is grateful to C.N.R. (Rome) for financial support of some of his research
reported here.

The authors are grateful to the Editorial Board of the British Journal of Pharmacology for
permission to reproduce Tables 1 and 2.

References

Adams, P.R.: Drug blockade of open end plate channels. J. Physiol. (Lond.) *260*, 531–552 (1976)
Adams, P.R., Brown, D.A.: Actions of γ-aminobutyric acid on sympathetic ganglion cells. J.
    Physiol. (Lond.) *250*, 85–120 (1975)
Alper, M.H., Fleisch, J.H., Flacke, W.: The effects of halothane on the responses of cardiac
    sympathetic ganglia to various stimulants. Anesthesiology *31*, 429–436 (1969)
Anden, N.E., Butcher, S.G., Corrodi, H., Fuxe, K., Understedt, U.: Receptor-activity and turn-
    over of dopamine and noradrenaline after neuroleptics. Eur. J. Pharmacol. *11*, 303–314 (1970)
Barker, J.L.: C.N.S. depressants: effects on postsynaptic pharmacology. Brain Res. *92*, 35–55
    (1975)
Beleslin, D., Polak, R.L., Sproull, D.H.: The effect of leptazol and strychnine on the acetylcholine
    release from the cat brain. J. Physiol. (Lond.) *181*, 308–316 (1965)
Bhatnagar, R.K., Moore, K.E.: Effects of electrical stimulation, α-methyltyrosine and desmethyl-
    imipramine on the norepinephrine contents of neuronal cell bodies and terminals. J. Phar-
    macol. Exp. Ther. *178*, 450–463 (1971)
Biscoe, T.J.: On understanding anaesthetic effects on the sympathetic nervous system. Anesthe-
    siology *31*, 395–397 (1969)
Biscoe, T.J., Millar, R.A.: The effect of cyclopropane, halothane and ether on sympathetic gan-
    glionic transmission. Br. J. Anaesth. *38*, 3–12 (1966)
Bowery, N.G., Brown, D.A.: Depolarizing actions of γ-aminobutyric acid and related compounds
    on rat superior cervical ganglia in vitro. Br. J. Pharmacol. *50*, 205–218 (1974)
Bowery, N.G., Dray, A.: Barbiturate reversal of amino acid antagonism produced by convulsant
    agents. Nature (Lond.) *264*, 276–278 (1976)
Bowery, N.G., Brown, D.A., Collins, G.G.S., Galvan, M., Marsh, S., Yamini, G.: Indirect effects
    of amino-acids on sympathetic ganglion cells mediated through the release of γ-aminobutyric
    acid from glial cells. Br. J. Pharmacol. *57*, 73–91 (1976)
Bradley, P.B.: Phenothiazine derivatives. In: Physiological pharmacology. Root, W.S., Hofmann,
    F.G. (eds.), Vol. I, pp. 417–477. New York, London: Academic Press 1963
Brown, D.A.: An eserine-like action of chloral hydrate. Br. J. Pharmacol. *19*, 111–119 (1962)
Brown, D.A., Quilliam, J.P.: The effects of some centrally-acting drugs on ganglionic transmission
    in the cat. Br. J. Pharmacol. *23*, 241–256 (1964a)
Brown, D.A., Quilliam, J.P.: Observations on the mode of action of some central depressant
    drugs on transmission through the cat superior cervical ganglion. Br. J. Pharmacol. *23*, 257–
    272 (1964b)

Burt, A.M.: The histochemical localisation of choline acetyltransferase. Prog. Brain Res. *34*, 327–336 (1971)

Cairncross, K.D., McCulloch, M.W., Story, D.F., Trinker, F.: Modification of synaptic transmission in the superior cervical ganglion by epinephrine, norepinephrine and nortryptiline. Int. J. Neuropharmacol. *6*, 293–300 (1967)

Camp, W.J.R.: The pharmacology of cardiazol. J. Pharmacol. Exp. Ther. *33*, 81–92 (1928)

Casati, C., Michalek, H., Paggi, P., Toschi, G.: Effects of triperidol on transmission and on release of acetylcholine in the rat sympathetic ganglion in vitro. Biochem. Pharmacol. *22*, 1165–1169 (1973)

Cattabeni, F., Koslow, S.H., Costa, E.: Gas chromatography–mass fragmentography: a new approach to the estimation of amines and amine turnover. Adv. Biochem. Psychopharmacol. *6*, 37–59 (1972)

Chai, C.Y., Wang, S.C.I.: Cardiovascular action of diazepam in the cat. J. Pharmacol. Exp. Ther. *154*, 271–280 (1966)

Chalazonitis, N.: Selective actions of volatile anaesthetics on synaptic transmission and auto-rhythmicity in single identifiable neurons. Anesthesiology *28*, 111–123 (1967)

Cheah, T.B., Geffen, L.B., Jarrott, B., Ostberg, A.: Action of 6-hydroxydopamine on lamb sympathetic ganglia, vas deferens, and adrenal medulla: a combined histochemical, ultrastructural, and biochemical comparison with the effects of reserpine. Br. J. Pharmacol. *42*, 543–557 (1971)

Chinn, C., Weber, L.J.: The action of several psychoactive agents upon the muscarinic mechanisms in the superior cervical ganglion of the cat. Neuropharmacology *13*, 39–52 (1974)

Choi, D.W., Farb, D.H., Fischbach, G.D.: Chlordiazepoxide selectively augments GABA action in spinal cord cell cultures. Nature (Lond.) *269*, 342–344 (1977)

Christ, D.: Effects of halothane on ganglionic discharges. J. Pharmacol. Exp. Ther. *200*, 336–342 (1977)

Clementi, F., Mantegazza, P., Botturi, M.: A pharmacological and morphologic study on the nature of the dense-core granules present in the presynaptic endings of sympathetic ganglia. Int. J. Neuropharmacol. *5*, 281–285 (1966)

Constanti, A., Nistri, A.: Antagonism by some antihistamines of the amino acid-evoked responses recorded from the lobster muscle fibre and the frog spinal cord. Br. J. Pharmacol. *58*, 583–592 (1976)

Costa, E., Brodie, B.B.: A role for norepinephrine in ganglionic transmission. J. Am. Geriatr. Soc. *9*, 419–425 (1961)

Costa, E., Revzin, A.M., Kuntzman, R., Spector, S., Brodie, B.B.: Role for ganglionic norepinephrine in sympathetic synaptic transmission. Science (N.Y.) *133*, 1822–1823 (1961)

Costa, E., Guidotti, A., Zivkovic, B.: Short and long-term regulation of tyrosine hydroxylase. Adv. Biochem. Psychopharmacol. *12*, 161–175 (1974)

Costa, E., Guidotti, A., Mao, C.C., Suria, A.: New concepts on the mechanism of action of benzodiazepines. Life Sci. *17*, 167–186 (1975)

Courvoisier, S., Fournel, J., Ducrot, R., Kolsky, M., Koetschet, P.: Propriétés pharmacodynamiques du chlorhydrate de chloro-3-(diméthylamino-3'-propyl)-10-phénothiazine (4560 R.P.). (1) Etude éxperimentale d'un nouveau corps utilisé dans l'anaesthésie potentialisée et dans l'hibernation artificielle. Arch. Int. Pharmacodyn. Ther. *92*, 305–361 (1952)

Curtis, D.R., Johnston, G.A.R.: Amino acid transmitters in the mammalian central nervous system. Ergeb. Physiol. *69*, 97–188 (1974)

Dawes, P.M., Vizi, E.S.: Acetylcholine release from the rabbit isolated superior cervical ganglion preparation. Br. J. Pharmacol. *48*, 225–232 (1973)

De Groat, W.C.: The actions of γ-aminobutyric acid and related amino acids on mammalian autonomic ganglia. J. Pharmacol. Exp. Ther. *172*, 384–396 (1970)

De Groat, W.C.: GABA-depolarization of a sensory ganglion: antagonism by picrotoxin and bicuculline. Brain Res. *38*, 429–432 (1972)

De Groat, W.C., Lalley, P.M.: Interaction between picrotoxin and 5-hydroxytryptamine in the superior cervical ganglion of the cat. Br. J. Pharmacol. *48*, 233–244 (1973)

De Groat, W.C., Volle, R.L.: The actions of the catecholamines on transmission in the superior cervical ganglion of the cat. J. Pharmacol. Exp. Ther. *154*, 1–13 (1966)

De Groat, W.C., Lalley, P.M., Block, M.: The effects of bicuculline and GABA on the superior cervical ganglion of the cat. Brain Res. *25*, 665–668 (1971)

De Groat, W.C., Lalley, P.M., Saum, W.R.: Depolarisation of dorsal root ganglia in the cat by GABA and related amino acids: antagonism by picrotoxin and bicuculline. Brain Res. *44*, 273–277 (1972)

Downing, O.A.: Effect of amphetamine on the transmission of repetitive impulses through the isolated superior cervical ganglion of the rat. Br. J. Pharmacol. *44*, 71–79 (1972)

Eccles, J.C.: The action potential of the superior cervical ganglion. J. Physiol. (Lond.) *85*, 179–206 (1935)

Eckenhoff, J.E.: Status report on analeptics. J. Am. Med. Assoc. *139*, 780–785 (1949)

Edmonds-Seal, J., Prys-Roberts, C.: Pharmacology of drugs used in neuroleptanalgesia. Br. J. Anaesth. *42*, 207–216 (1970)

Elliott, R.C.: Centrally-active drugs and transmission through the isolated superior cervical ganglion preparation of the rabbit when stimulated repetitively. Br. J. Pharmacol. *24*, 76–88 (1965)

Elliott, R.C.: Centrally-active drugs and the medullary vasopressor response of the cat; a method of distinguishing between drug actions on the central and peripheral parts of the sympathetic nervous system. Neuropharmacology *8*, 117–129 (1969)

Elliott, R.C., Quilliam, J.P.: Some actions of centrally-active and other drugs on the transmission of single nerve impulses through the isolated superior cervical ganglion preparation of the rabbit. Br. J. Pharmacol. *23*, 222–240 (1964)

Eranko, O.: Histochemistry of nervous tissue: catecholamines and cholinesterases. Annu. Rev. Pharmacol. *7*, 203–222 (1967)

Esplin, D.W.: Effects of diphenylhydantoin on synaptic transmission in cat spinal cord and stellate ganglion. J. Pharmacol. Exp. Ther. *120*, 301–323 (1957)

Esplin, D.W., Zablocka-Esplin, B.: Mechanism of action of convulsants. In: Basic mechanisms of the epilepsies. Jasper, H.H., Ward, A.A., Jr., Pope, A. (eds.), pp. 167–193. Boston: Little, Brown, and Co. 1969

Exley, K.A.: Depression of autonomic ganglia by barbiturates. Br. J. Pharmacol. *9*, 170–181 (1954)

Falck, B., Hillarp, N.A., Thieme, G., Torp, A.: Fluorescence of catecholamines and related compounds condensed with formaldehyde. J. Histochem. Cytochem. *10*, 348–354 (1962)

Feldberg, W., Vartiainen, A.: Further observations on the physiology and pharmacology of a sympathetic ganglion. J. Physiol. (Lond.) *83*, 103–128 (1934)

Fieve, R.R., Meltzer, H., Dunner, D.L., Levitt, M., Mendlewics, J., Thomas, A.: Rubidium: biochemical, behavioural and metabolic studies in humans. Am. J. Psychiatry *130*, 55–61 (1973)

Gaddum, J.H., Picarelli, Z.P.: Two kinds of tryptamine receptors. Br. J. Pharmacol. *12*, 323–328 (1957)

Gallagher, J.P., Dun, N., Higashi, H., Nishi, S.: Actions of ketamine on synaptic transmission in frog sympathetic ganglia. Neuropharmacology *15*, 139–143 (1976)

Garfield, J.M., Alper, M.H., Gillis, R.A., Flacke, W.: A pharmacological analysis of ganglionic actions of some general anaesthetics. Anesthesiology *29*, 79–92 (1968)

Gerschenfeld, H.M.: Chemical transmission in invertebrate central nervous systems and neuromuscular junctions. Physiol. Rev. *53*, 1–119 (1973)

Gershon, S., Shopsin, B. (eds.): Lithium. Its role in psychiatric research and treatment, pp. 1–358. New York: Plenum Press 1973

Gertner, S.B.: The effects of monoamine oxidase inhibitors on ganglionic transmission. J. Pharmacol. Exp. Ther. *131*, 223–230 (1961)

Giacobini, E.: Value and limitations of quantitative chemical studies in individual cells. J. Histochem. Cytochem. *17*, 139–155 (1969)

Goldberg, L.I., Da Costa, R.M.: Selective depression of sympathetic transmission by intravenous administration of iproniazid and harmine. Proc. Soc. Exp. Biol. Med. *105*, 223–227 (1960)

Greengard, P., Kebabian, J.W.: Role of cyclic AMP in synaptic transmission in the mammalian peripheral nervous system. Fed. Proc. *33*, 1059–1067 (1974)

Gyermek, L., Bindler, E.: Blockade of the ganglionic stimulant action of 5-hydroxytryptamine. J. Pharmacol. Exp. Ther. *135*, 344–348 (1962a)

Gyermek, L., Bindler, E.: Action of indole alkylamines and amidines on the inferior mesenteric ganglion of the cat. J. Pharmacol. Exp. Ther. *138*, 159–164 (1962b)

Haefely, W.: The effects of 5-hydroxytryptamine and some related compounds on the cat superior cervical ganglion in situ. Naunyn Schmiedebergs Arch. Pharmacol. *281*, 145–165 (1974)

Hebb, C.O., Konzett, H.: The effect of certain analgesic drugs on synaptic transmission as observed in the perfused superior cervical ganglion of the cat. Q. J. Exp. Physiol. *35*, 213–217 (1949)

Hedqvist, P.: Studies on the effect of prostaglandin E_1 and E_2 on the sympathetic neuromuscular transmission in some animal tissues. Acta Physiol. Scand. [suppl.] *345*, 1–40 (1970)

Hemsworth, B.A., Neal, M.J.: The effect of central stimulant drugs on the release of acetylcholine from the cerebral cortex. Br. J. Pharmacol. *32*, 543–550 (1968)

Henderson, G.: Effect of monoamine oxidase (MAO) inhibition upon the N, P, and LN potentials of the rabbit superior cervical ganglia. Br. J. Pharmacol. *43*, 436P (1971)

Janssen, P.A.J.: The pharmacology of haloperidol. Int. J. Neuropsychiatr. [suppl.] *3*, 10–18 (1967)

Johnson, F.N. (ed.): Lithium research and therapy, pp. 1–569. London: Academic Press 1975

Kadzielawa, K., Gawecka, I., Kadzielawa, R.: The potentiating influence of imipramine on ganglionic effects of catecholamines. Int. J. Neuropharmacol. *7*, 517–521 (1968)

Kasa, P.: Ultrastructural localisation of choline acetyltransferase and acetylcholinesterase in central and peripheral nervous tissue. Brain Res. *34*, 337–344 (1971)

Kewitz, H., Reinert, H.: Wirkung verschiedener Sympathomimetica auf die chemisch und elektrisch ausgelöste Erregung des oberen Halsganglions. Naunyn Schmiedebergs Arch. Pharmacol. *222*, 311–314 (1954)

Kobayashi, H., Hashiguchi, T., Ushiyama, N.S.: Postsynaptic modulation of excitatory process in sympathetic ganglia by cyclic AMP. Nature (Lond.) *271*, 268–270 (1978)

Koelle, G.B.: The histochemical differentiation of types of cholinesterases and their localisations in tissues of the cat. J. Pharmacol. Exp. Ther. *100*, 158–179 (1950)

Koelle, G.B., Friedenwald, J.S.: A histochemical method for locating cholinesterase activity. Proc. Soc. Exp. Biol. Med. *70*, 617–622 (1949)

Koelle, W.A., Koelle, G.B.: The localisation of external or functional acetylcholinesterase at the synapses of autonomic ganglia. J. Pharmacol. Exp. Ther. *126*, 1–8 (1959)

Koketsu, K.: Cholinergic synaptic potentials and the underlying ionic mechanism. Fed. Proc. *28*, 101–112 (1969)

Koketsu, K., Yamamoto, K.: Effects of lithium ions on electrical activity in sympathetic ganglia of the bullfrog. Br. J. Pharmacol. *50*, 69–77 (1974)

Koketsu, K., Shoji, T., Yamamoto, K.: Effects of GABA on presynaptic nerve terminals in bullfrogs *(Rana catesbiana)* sympathetic ganglia. Experientia *30*, 382–383 (1974)

Kosterlitz, H.W., Wallis, D.I.: The action of morphine-like drugs on impulse transmission in mammalian nerve fibres. Br. J. Pharmacol. *22*, 499–510 (1964)

Kosterlitz, H.W., Wallis, D.I.: The effects of hexamethonium and morphine on transmission in the superior cervical ganglion of the rabbit. Br. J. Pharmacol. *26*, 334–344 (1966)

Krnjević, K.: Chemical nature of synaptic transmission in vertebrates. Physiol. Rev. *54*, 418–540 (1974)

Lanari, A., Luco, J.V.: The depressant action of strychnine on the superior cervical sympathetic ganglion and on skeletal muscle. Am. J. Physiol. *126*, 277–282 (1939)

Larrabee, M.G., Bronk, D.W.: Prolonged facilitation of synaptic excitation in sympathetic ganglia. J. Neurophysiol. *10*, 139–154 (1947)

Larrabee, M., Holaday, D.A.: Depression of transmission through sympathetic ganglia during general anaesthesia. J. Pharmacol. Exp. Ther. *105*, 400–408 (1952)

Larrabee, M.G., Posternak, J.M.: Selective action of anaesthetics on synapses and axons in mammalian sympathetic ganglia. J. Neurophysiol. *15*, 91–114 (1952)

Larrabee, M.G., Ramos, J.G., Bülbring, E.: Effect of anaesthetics on oxygen consumption and on synaptic transmission in sympathetic ganglia. J. Cell. Comp. Physiol. *40*, 461–494 (1952)

Levine, R.J.: Inhibition of monoamine oxidase activity in sympathetic ganglia of the cat. Biochem. Pharmacol. *11*, 395–396 (1962)

Libet, B.: Slow synaptic responses and excitatory changes in sympathetic ganglia. J. Physiol. (Lond.) *174*, 1–25 (1964)

Libet, B.: Generation of slow inhibitory and excitatory postsynaptic potentials. Fed. Proc. *29*, 1945–1956 (1970)

Libet, B., Owman, C.: Concomitant changes in formaldehyde-induced fluorescence of dopamine interneurones and in slow inhibitory post-synaptic potentials of the rabbit superior cervical ganglion, induced by stimulation of the preganglionic nerve or by a muscarinic agent. J. Physiol. (Lond.) *237*, 635–662 (1974)

Libet, B., Tosaka, T.: Dopamine as a synaptic transmitter and modulator in sympathetic ganglia: a different mode of synaptic action. Proc. Natl. Acad. Sci. USA *67*, 667–673 (1970)

Libet, B., Kobayashi, H., Tanaka, T.: Synaptic coupling into the production and storage of a neuronal memory trace. Nature (Lond.) *258*, 155–157 (1975)

Lloyd, D.P.C.: The transmission of impulses through the inferior mesenteric ganglia. J. Physiol. (Lond.) *91*, 296–313 (1937)

Malseed, R.T., Rossi, G.V., Goldstein, F.J.: Potentiation of monoaminergic activity in peripheral ganglia by tricyclic antidepressants. Eur. J. Pharmacol. *20*, 34–39 (1972)

Marley, E., Paton, W.D.M.: The effect of methylpentynol and methylpentynol carbamate on the perfused superior cervical ganglion of the cat. Br. J. Pharmacol. *14*, 303–306 (1959)

Matthews, E.K., Quilliam, J.P.: Effects of central depressant drugs upon acetylcholine release. Br. J. Pharmacol. *22*, 415–440 (1964)

McEwan, L.M.: The effect on the isolated rabbit heart of vagal stimulation and its modification by cocaine, hexamethonium, and ouabaine. J. Physiol. (Lond.) *131*, 678–689 (1956)

McKinstry, D.N., Koelle, G.B.: Effects of drugs on acetylcholine release from the cat superior cervical ganglion by carbachol and by preganglionic stimulation. J. Pharmacol. Exp. Ther. *157*, 328–336 (1967a)

McKinstry, D.N., Koelle, G.B.: Inhibition of release of acetylcholine by strychnine and its implications regarding transmission by the olivocochlear bundle. Nature (Lond.) *213*, 505–506 (1967b)

Millar, R.A., Biscoe, T.J.: Preganglionic sympathetic activity and the effects of inhalation anaesthetics. Br. J. Anaesth. *37*, 804–832 (1965)

Millar, R.A., Biscoe, T.J.: Postganglionic sympathetic discharge and the effect of inhalation anaesthetics. Br. J. Anaesth. *38*, 92–114 (1966)

Millar, R.A., Warden, J.C., Cooperman, L.H., Price, H.L.: Central sympathetic discharge and mean arterial pressure during halothane anaesthesia. Br. J. Anaesth. *41*, 918–928 (1969)

Mueller, R.A., Thoenen, H., Axelrod, J.: Increase in tyrosine hydroxylase activity after reserpine administration. J. Pharmacol. Exp. Ther. *169*, 74–79 (1969)

Muscholl, E., Vogt, M.: The action of reserpine on the peripheral sympathetic system. J. Physiol. (Lond.) *141*, 132–155 (1958)

Nicoll, R.A.: Pentobarbital: action on frog motoneurons. Brain Res. *96*, 119–123 (1975a)

Nicoll, R.A.: Presynaptic action of barbiturates in frog spinal cord. Proc. Natl. Acad. Sci. USA *72*, 1460–1463 (1975b)

Nicoll, R.A.: Pentobarbital: differential postsynaptic actions on sympathetic ganglion cells. Science *199*, 451–452 (1978)

Nistri, A., Constanti, A.: Effects of flurazepam on amino acid-evoked responses recorded from the lobster muscle and the frog spinal cord. Neuropharmacology *17*, 127–135 (1978)

Nistri, A., Pepeu, G.: Acetylcholine levels in the frog spinal cord following the administration of different convulsants. Eur. J. Pharmacol. *27*, 281–287 (1974)

Nistri, A., De Bellis, A.M., Cammelli, E., Pepeu, G.: Effect of bicuculline, leptazol, and strychnine on the acetylcholinesterase activity of the frog spinal cord in vivo. J. Neurochem. *23*, 453–454 (1974)

Nistri, A., De Bellis, A.M., Cammelli, E.: Drug-induced changes in behaviour and ganglionic acetylcholine concentration of the leech. Neuropharmacology *14*, 565–569 (1975)

Norberg, K.A., Ritzen, M., Ungerstedt, V.: Histochemical studies on a special catecholamine containing cell type in sympathetic ganglia. Acta Physiol. Scand. *67*, 260–270 (1966)

Normann, N., Löfstrom, B.: Interaction of D-tubocurarine, ether, cyclopropane, and thiopental on ganglionic transmission. J. Pharmacol. Exp. Ther. *114*, 231–239 (1955)

Osborne, M., Sigg, E.B.: Effects of imipramine on the peripheral autonomic system. Arch. Int. Pharmacodyn. Ther. *129*, 273–289 (1960)

Pappano, A.J., Volle, R.L.: Actions of lithium ions in mammalian sympathetic ganglia. J. Pharmacol. Exp. Ther. *157*, 346–355 (1967)

Pardo, E., Gato, J., Gijon, E., De Florida, F.A.: Influence of several adrenergic drugs on synaptic transmission through the superior cervical and the ciliary ganglia of the cat. J. Pharmacol. Exp. Ther. *139*, 296–303 (1963)

Pepeu, G., Nistri, A.: Effects of drugs on the regional distribution and release of acetylcholine: functional significance of cholinergic neurones. In: Psychopharmacology, sexual disorders, and drug abuse. Ban, T.A., Boissier, J.R., Gessa, G.J., Heinmann, H., Hollister, L., Lehmann, H.E., Munkvad, I., Steinberg, H., Sulser, F., Sundwall, A., Vinar, O. (eds.), pp. 563–574. Amsterdam: North-Holland 1973

Perri, V., Sacchi, O., Raviola, E., Raviola, G.: Evaluation of the number and distribution of synaptic vesicles at cholinergic nerve endings after sustained stimulation. Brain Res. 39, 526–529 (1972)

Pilon, R.N., Alper, M.H., Flacka, W.: The effects of methoxyflurane on sympathetic ganglionic transmission. Anesthesiology 39, 302–307 (1973)

Pisko, E., Weinger, F., De Groat, W.C.: The effect of halothane on preganglionic and postganglionic sympathetic activity in the cat. Brain Res. 20, 330–334 (1970)

Platman, S.R.: Lithium and rubidium: a role in the affective disorders. Dis. Nerv. Syst. 32, 604–606 (1971)

Price, H.L., Price, M.L.: Relative ganglion-blocking potencies of cyclopropane, halothane, and nitrous oxide, and the interaction of nitrous oxide with halothane. Anesthesiology 28, 349–353 (1967)

Quilliam, J.P.: Paraldehyde and methylpentynol and ganglionic transmission. Br. J. Pharmacol. 14, 277–283 (1959)

Quilliam, J.P., Shand, D.G.: The selectivity of drugs blocking ganglionic transmission in the rat. Br. J. Pharmacol. 23, 273–284 (1964)

Quilliam, J.P., Tamarind, D.L.: The vesicle population of rat ganglionic synapses and the effects of some drugs. Br. J. Pharmacol. 39, 244–245P (1970)

Quilliam, J.P., Tamarind, D.L.: Local vesicle population in rat superior cervical ganglia and the vesicle hypothesis. J. Neurocytol. 2, 59–75 (1973a)

Quilliam, J.P., Tamarind, D.L.: Some effects of preganglionic nerve stimulation on synaptic vesicle populations in the rat superior cervical ganglion. J. Physiol. (Lond.) 235, 317–331 (1973b)

Raventos, J.: The action of fluothane: a new volatile anaesthetic. Br. J. Pharmacol. 11, 394–410 (1956)

Reinert, H.: The depolarizing and blocking action of amphetamine in the cat's superior cervical ganglion. In: Ciba foundation symposium on adrenergic mechanisms. Vane, J.R., Wolstenholme, G.E.W., O'Connor, M. (eds.), pp. 373–379. London: Churchill 1960

Reinert, H.: Role and origin of noradrenaline in the superior cervical ganglion. J. Physiol. (Lond.) 167, 18–29 (1963)

Reuse, J.J.: Some pharmacological properties of 3-chloro-10-(3'-dimethylamino-propyl)-phenothiazine (chlorpromazine). C. R. Soc. Biol. (Paris) 148, 192–193 (1954)

Saum, W.R., De Groat, W.C.: The actions of 5-hydroxytryptamine on the urinary bladder and on vesical autonomic ganglia in the cat. J. Pharmacol. Exp. Ther. 185, 70–83 (1973)

Shallek, W., Zabransky, F.: Effects of psychotropic drugs on pressor responses to central and peripheral stimulation in cat. Arch. Int. Pharmacodyn. Ther. 161, 126–131 (1966)

Severinghans, J.W., Cullen, S.C.: Depression of myocardium and body oxygen consumption with fluothane in man. Anesthesiology 19, 165–177 (1958)

Shand, D.G.: The mode of action of drugs blocking ganglionic transmission in the rat. Br. J. Pharmacol. 24, 89–97 (1965)

Sigg, E.B., Sigg, T.D.: Hypothalamic stimulation of preganglionic autonomic activity and its modification by chlorpromazine, diazepam, and pentobarbital. Int. J. Neuropharmacol. 8, 567–572 (1969)

Sigg, E.B., Soffer, L., Gyermek, L.: Influence of imipramine and related psychoactive agents on the effects of 5-hydroxytryptamine and catecholamines on the cat nictitating membrane. J. Pharmacol. Exp. Ther. 142, 13–20 (1963)

Skovsted, P., Price, M.L., Price, H.L.: The effects of halothane on arterial pressure, preganglionic sympathetic activity, and barostatic reflexes. Anesthesiology 31, 507–514 (1969)

Smaje, J.C.: General anaesthetics and the acetylcholine-sensitivity of cortical neurones. Br. J. Pharmacol. 58, 359–366 (1976)

Suria, A., Costa, E.: Benzodiazepines and post-tetanic potentiation in sympathetic ganglia of the bullfrog. Brain Res. 50, 235–239 (1973)

Suria, A., Costa, E.: Diazepam inhibition of post-tetanic potentiation in bullfrog sympathetic ganglia: possible role of prostaglandins. J. Pharmacol. Exp. Ther. 189, 690–696 (1974)

Tamarind, D.L.: Electronmicroscopic structure of rat ganglionic synapses and its modification by ions and drugs. Ph.D.Thesis University of London 1974

Tehrani, J.B., Rossi, V.G., Goldstein, F.J.: Effect of lithium and rubidium on the ganglionic inhibitory action of norepinephrine. Life Sci. *15*, 525–535 (1974)

Tehrani, J.B., Rossi, G.V., Goldstein, F.J.: Doxepin and imipramine: effect on catecholamine inhibition of ganglionic transmission. Life Sci. *17*, 257–262 (1975)

Trendelenburg, V.: The action of morphine on the superior cervical ganglion and on the nictitating membrane of the cat. Br. J. Pharmacol. *12*, 79–85 (1957)

Trendelenburg, V.: The pressor response of the cat to histamine and pilocarpine. J. Pharmacol. Exp. Ther. *131*, 65–72 (1961)

Trendelenburg, V.: Observations on the ganglion-stimulating action of angiotensin and bradykinin. J. Pharmacol. Exp. Ther. *154*, 418–425 (1966a)

Trendelenburg, V.: Transmission of preganglionic impulses through the muscarinic receptors of the superior cervical ganglion of the cat. J. Pharmacol. Exp. Ther. *154*, 426–440 (1966b)

Trendelenburg, V.: Some aspects of the pharmacology of autonomic ganglion cells. Ergeb. Physiol. *59*, 1–85 (1967)

Trendelenburg, V., Gravenstein, J.S.: Effect of reserpine pretreatment on stimulation of the accelerans nerve of the dog. Science (N.Y.) *128*, 901–903 (1958)

Van Orden, L.S., III, Burke, J.P., Geyer, M., Lodoen, F.V.: Localisation of depletion-sensitive and depletion-resistant norepinephrine storage sites in autonomic ganglia. J. Pharmacol. Exp. Ther. *174*, 56–71 (1970)

Van Rossum, J.M.: The significance of dopamine-receptor blockade for the mechanism of action of neuroleptic drugs. Arch. Int. Pharmacodyn. Ther. *160*, 492–494 (1966)

Volle, R.L., Hancock, J.C.: Transmission in sympathetic ganglia. Fed. Proc. *29*, 1913–1918 (1970)

Von Voigtlander, P.F., Moore, K.E.: Involvement of nigrostriatal neurones in the in vivo release of dopamine by amphetamine, amantadine and tyramine. J. Pharmacol. Exp. Ther. *184*, 542–552 (1970)

Watson, P.J.: The triphasic response of the isolated superior cervical ganglion of the rat to cholinergic stimulants. Eur. J. Pharmacol. *20*, 60–70 (1972)

Weir, M.C.L., McLennan, H.: The action of catecholamines in sympathetic ganglia. Can. J. Biochem. Physiol. *41*, 2627–2636 (1963)

Wenke, M.: Drug-receptor interactions. In: Fundamentals of biochemical pharmacology. Bacq, Z.M. (ed.), pp. 367–410. Oxford: Pergamon Press 1971

Whitteridge, D.: The transmission of impulses through the ciliary ganglion. J. Physiol. (Lond.) *89*, 99–111 (1937)

Willems, J.L.: Dopamine-induced inhibition of synaptic transmission in lumbar paravertebral ganglia of the dog. Naunyn Schmiedebergs Arch. Pharmacol. *281*, 145–165 (1974)

Woodruff, G.N.: Dopamine receptors: a review. Comp. Gen. Pharmacol. *2*, 439–455 (1971)

Note Added in Proof

Three recent reports are of special relevance to the status of dopamine as a ganglionic transmitter. N.A. Busis, F.F. Weight and P.A. Smith (Science (N.Y.), 200, 1079–1081 (1978) and D.A. Brown, M. Caulfield and P.J. Kirby (in "Recent advances in the pharmacology of adrenoceptors", E. Szabadi, C.M. Bradshaw and P. Bevan, Eds., pp. 325–326, Amsterdam: Elsevier/North-Holland 1978) were unable to show a specific involvement of 3,5-cAMP on the generation of synaptic potentials in sympathetic ganglia. D.A. Brown and M.P. Caulfield (Br. J. Pharmacol. 65, 435–445 (1979)) could find no evidence for specific dopamine receptors in the rat superior cervical ganglion and they noted that dopamine was a hyperpolarizing agent weaker in its effects than NA.

Thus the identity of the inhibitory transmitter in sympathetic ganglia and the mechanism of generation of the inhibitory postsynaptic potential must await further study.

CHAPTER 12

Ganglionic Actions of Anticholinesterase Agents, Catecholamines, Neuro-Muscular Blocking Agents, and Local Anaesthetics

R. L. VOLLE

A. Anticholinesterase Agents

The demonstration by FELDBERG and GADDUM (1934) that acetylcholine is the transmitter in sympathetic ganglia was a milestone in the development of the concept of chemical transmission. Clearly, the isolation of acetylcholine from the fluid perfusing the ganglia constitutes an important part of the evidence supporting the concept that chemical substances mediate synaptic transmission. It should be noted, however, that the recovery of acetylcholine from the perfusion stream is not possible unless an anticholinesterase agent is present in the perfusion fluid. In the absence of the enzyme inhibitor, choline appears in the perfusion fluid as a consequence of the hydrolysis of acetylcholine. Thus, the acetylcholinesterase enzymes destroy acetylcholine and, therefore, can serve to limit the biological life of the transmitter. KOELLE (1963) and ZAIMIS (1963) give complete accounts of the earlier studies of the effects of anticholinesterase agents on ganglionic transmission and are useful reference sources for the period between the 1930s and 1960s.

The anticholinesterase agents affect several aspects of ganglionic transmission. They are known to alter the metabolism of acetylcholine in the presynaptic nerve terminals and to modify both the nicotinic and the muscarinic forms of ganglionic transmission. Some of these topics are reviewed by VOLLE (1966, 1975).

There are marked differences among autonomic ganglia in the distribution of the acetylcholinesterase enzymes (KOELLE, 1963; KOELLE et al., 1975). It appears that all preganglionic cholinergic fibres contain the enzyme, where the role of the enzyme in the nerve terminals may be to regulate the cytoplasmic level of acetylcholine or to participate in the recovery of choline for the synthetic process (vide infra). In the presynaptic terminals, the enzyme is found at both internal and external sites. By contrast, not all ganglion cells contain the enzyme. Whereas parasympathetic ganglion cells contain large amounts of the acetylcholinesterase enzyme, sympathetic ganglia contain varying amounts of the enzyme. KOELLE et al. (1975) suggest that the presynaptic nerve terminals exert a trophic influence on postsynaptic acetylcholinesterase. The functional role of the postjunctional enzyme in ganglionic transmission is not understood (KOELLE et al., 1975).

Inasmuch as synaptic contacts in autonomic ganglia differ markedly from species to species, the cholinesterase enzymes may or may not be of critical importance in transmission. In amphibia ganglia, the synaptic arrangements include axo-axonic junctions with a presynaptic contact on the axon-hillock and axo-somatic junctions with the cell soma. Thus, both sympathetic and parasympathetic amphibian ganglion cells exist primarily as unipolar cells devoid of dendritic processes. Most of the cells receive only a single preganglionic fibre and have synaptic contacts that cover only 3–10% of the cell surface. An average of 9–12 synapses are found on the soma. On the other hand, autonomic ganglia in mammals contain large numbers of axo-dendritic synapses (ELFVIN, 1971a–c). It appears that the activation of 8–10 synapses is required for transmission to be effective in mammalian sympathetic ganglia (BLACKMAN and PURVES, 1969; SACCHI and PERRI, 1971)

It may be for these reasons (differences in acetylcholinesterase distribution and in synaptic arrangements) that contradictory or discordant data concerning the effects of anticholinesterase agents on ganglionic transmission are obtained. There is universal agreement, however, that the effects of anticholinesterase agents on ganglionic transmission are much less pronounced than those on the neuromuscular junction.

I. Effects on Acetylcholine Metabolism

Because of the limited effects of anticholinesterase agents on ganglionic transmission (ECCLES, 1944), it has been suggested that diffusion alone is adequate to account for the termination of transmitter activity in autonomic ganglia (OGSTON, 1955). However,there is some evidence to show that acetylcholinesterase limits intraganglionic diffusion of acetylcholine (BENNETT and MCLACHLAN, 1972a; Fig.1). Repetitive preganglionic stimulation in the presence of physostigmine results in depolarisation of ganglionic cells remote from those being stimulated and unaffected directly by preganglionic stimulation. The decline in depolarisation shown in Fig.1 is due to the presence of hemicholinium-3 in the bathing solution. Since hemicholinium-3 is known to interfere with acetylcholine synthesis, it can be expected to cause a time-dependent reduction in the depolarisation produced by preganglionic stimulation. The demonstration of acetylcholine diffusion in ganglia treated with anticholines-terase agents is probably easier to accomplish when ganglia are isolated and sus-

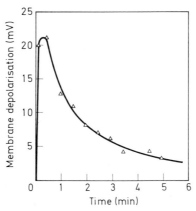

Fig.1. Depolarisation of a ganglion cell by acetylcholine released at synapses of other cells. The monitored cell did not show an EPSP during preganglionic stimulation. The preganglionic nerve was stimulated at the rate of 20 Hz in the presence of physostigmine (8×10^{-6} M) and hemicholinium-3 (2×10^{-5} M). The fade of the depolarisation was due to decreased release of acetylcholine during continued stimulation in the presence of hemicholinium-3 (BENNETT and MCLACHLAN, 1972a)

pended in a bathing solution than when ganglia are studied in situ (VOLLE and KOELLE, 1961), where the turnover of extracellular fluid is more brisk.

In view of the existence in sympathetic ganglia of both nicotinic and muscarinic receptors, and, particularly because the muscarinic responses have a long latency, it would be of interest to know whether the intraganglionic diffusion of acetylcholine results in the heterosynaptic activation of muscarinic receptors. The anticholinesterase agents enhance muscarinic transmission and, under some circumstances, provide an alternate pathway for transmission to occur (vide infra).

Some concepts of the subcellular distribution of acetylcholine and the availability of acetylcholine for release emerge from the study of drugs that interfere with acetylcholine synthesis or with the hydrolysis of acetylcholine. Ganglia perfused with solutions lacking choline or containing hemicholinium-3 are unable to maintain their content of acetylcholine during activity. Under these conditions, the ganglia lose about 85% of their acetylcholine content, a fraction that agrees favourably with the acetylcholine content known to have a relatively rapid rate of turnover. This component of ganglionic acetylcholine is termed the "depot" form and is regarded to be the component available for release by the nerve terminal action potential. The component remaining after treatment of the ganglia with hemicholinium-3 is termed "stationary" and is unavailable for release by the nerve impulse (BIRKS and MACINTOSH, 1961). The stationary pool is probably located at neuronal sites quite remote from the nerve terminals.

The newly formed acetylcholine is either packaged into a form ready for release (the depot pool) or hydrolysed rapidly by acetylcholinesterase enzymes. KOELLE and KOELLE (1959) have shown that the acetylcholinesterase enzymes are present in sympathetic ganglionic nerve terminals both at sites inaccessible to inhibition by quaternary ammonium anticholinesterase agents and at sites readily accessible to such inhibitors. The extracellularly located enzyme is regarded as the functional form and the intracellularly located enzyme as a reserve form. Whether or not such designations describe the function of ganglionic cholinesterase is difficult to establish; however, it is possible that cytoplasmic acetylcholinesterase serves to regulate the cytoplasmic content of acetylcholine and the external enzyme serves to provide choline for the synthesis of acetylcholine.

It can be shown with penetrating anticholinesterase agents that the inhibition of intracellular acetylcholinesterase gives rise to the build-up of high concentrations of acetylcholine within sympathetic ganglia (BIRKS and MACINTOSH, 1961; BROWN et al., 1970; COLLIER and KATZ, 1971, 1974). That the build-up of acetylcholine does not occur in denervated ganglia indicates that the acetylcholine accumulating under these conditions is stored primarily in the preganglionic nerve terminals. Treatment of cat superior cervical ganglia with physostigmine or tetraethylpyrosphosphate results in a two- to four-fold increase in the ganglionic content of acetylcholine but, interestingly, has no effect on transmitter output during nerve stimulation. Since the newly formed acetylcholine of ganglia treated with anticholinesterase drugs is not released by the nerve impulse, it is termed "surplus" acetylcholine.

It is noteworthy that while nerve stimulation has no effect on release from the surplus pool of acetylcholine, elevation of the concentration of extracellular potassium causes acetylcholine release from both the surplus and depot pools of transmitter (COLLIER and KATZ, 1971, 1974). It is likely that the surplus pool of acetylcholine is located in the cytoplasm of the preganglionic nerve terminals in nonvesicular form. This would account for the failure of nerve stimulation to release acetylcholine from the surplus pool. There is no direct evidence on this point. What has not yet been explained, however, is the mechanism whereby acetylcholine is released from the surplus pool by elevated extracellular potassium. As noted elsewhere is this volume, acetylcholine, nicotine, and pilocarpine cause acetylcholine release from the surplus pool of transmitter (MCKINSTRY et al., 1963; MCKINSTRY and KOELLE, 1967; COLLIER and KATZ, 1971, 1974) by a process that is not understood.

As noted before, a primary function for ganglionic acetylcholinesterase may be to provide choline for acetylcholine synthesis in the presynaptic nerve terminals (PERRY, 1953). It is now known that approximately half the acetylcholine released during nerve stimulation is recaptured by the nerve terminals as choline (COLLIER and MACINTOSH, 1969). Transmission failure produced by rapid, repetitive preganglionic stimulation in cat sympathetic ganglia is markedly accelerated by anticholinesterase agents (e.g., VOLLE and KOELLE, 1961). Although the failure may be due to depletion of transmitter stores because of a lack of choline, there is no evidence that choline has any effect on the rate of transmission failure (VOLLE and KOELLE, 1961). It has been shown, however, that choline added to the perfusion stream maintains acetylcholine output during preganglionic stimulation in the presence of physostigmine (MATTHEWS, 1963; Fig. 2). This finding is consistent with the view that the cholinesterase enzymes play a role in making choline available for acetylcholine synthesis. Alternative explanations are also possible. For example, choline may affect the presynaptic nerve terminal action potential so that more transmitter is released per volley or choline may affect the process of transmitter mobilisation so that transmitter depletion does not occur. Tetraethylammonium is known to have such actions.

This question has been re-examined by BENNETT and MCLACHLAN (1972a, b), who used intracellularly recorded postsynaptic potentials as a measure of transmitter release in guinea-pig ganglia. Since a parallel time course exists between transmis-

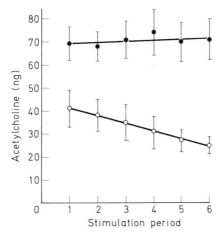

Fig. 2. Recovery of acetylcholine from perfusion stream of ganglia treated with physostigmine (5×10^{-6} g/ml) and perfused with Locke solution containing (●) or not containing (○) choline. The preganglionic nerves were stimulated at a rate of 10 Hz. Each stimulation period was 3 min long (MATTHEWS, 1963)

sion failure due to the inactivation of ganglionic cholinesterases by physostigmine and that due to the choline antagonist hemicholinium-3, they concluded that the effect of physostigmine is to limit the amount of choline available for transport to the nerve terminals and that transmission failure results from an exhaustion of transmitter stores. The critical experiment showing that choline can antagonise transmission failure produced by physostigmine has not been performed and for technical reasons may be difficult to accomplish. However, until such data are obtained, the proposal that ganglionic cholinesterases serve to provide choline for the nerve terminals remains to be established.

II. Nicotinic Ganglionic Transmission

Ganglionic cell responses to injected acetylcholine are enhanced by the anticholinesterase agents (e.g., FELDBERG and GADDUM, 1934; VOLLE and KOELLE, 1961). Similarly, under some circumstances, the anticholinesterase agents can be shown to facilitate ganglionic transmission (HOLADAY et al., 1954), particularly when submaximal preganglionic stimulation is used (McISAAC and KOELLE, 1959; VOLLE, 1962a; Fig. 3). Both these actions of the anticholinesterase agents are due to the elimination of the enzyme and consequently to the preservation of acetylcholine in the ganglia.

Using the inferior mesenteric ganglion of the guinea-pig as a test object, BORNSTEIN (1974) finds that physostigmine prolongs the duration of evoked and spontaneously occurring synaptic potentials significantly (Fig.4). The size of the synaptic potential is also increased by physostigmine. If physostigmine is assumed to have no effect on the membrane properties of the ganglion cells and no direct effect on the receptor-ionophore complex, then it is fair to conclude that the acetylcholinesterase

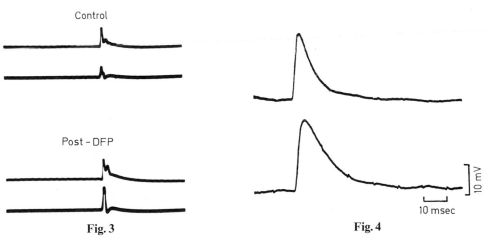

Fig. 3   Fig. 4

Fig. 3. Effect of diisopropylfluorophosphate (1 μmol given by a single injection) on postganglionic action potentials of thyroid (*upper tracing* of pair) and external carotid nerves of cat superior cervical ganglion. Submaximal stimulation at a rate of 1 Hz was used. Action potentials recorded 15 min after injection of the anticholinesterase agents were increased in amplitude (VOLLE, 1962a)

Fig. 4. Synaptic potentials from sympathetic ganglia before *(upper)* and in the presence *(lower)* of physostigmine (BORNSTEIN, 1974)

enzyme affects the synaptic concentration of acetylcholine in sympathetic ganglia. When compared with transmission at the neuromuscular junction, the effect is small.

It is not known whether the anticholinesterase agents have any direct effects on the presynaptic nerve terminals to cause the release of acetylcholine. At the neuromuscular junction, quaternary ammonium anticholinesterase agents cause transmitter release, presumably because of direct actions on the motor nerve terminals (BOYD and MARTIN, 1956; BLABER and CHRIST, 1967; BLABER, 1972). Neostigmine and edrophonium cause an increase in the frequency of miniature end plate potentials. The increase in frequency is slight and occurs only over a limited range of concentrations of the inhibitors.

III. Muscarinic Ganglionic Transmission

Postganglionic discharges are produced when diisopropylfluorophosphate and other anticholinesterase agents are applied to the cat superior cervical ganglia in situ (Fig. 5). The discharges occur after a lag of 10–15 min, although the time of onset can be accelerated by preganglionic stimulation. The anticholinesterase agents have no effect when applied to chronically denervated ganglia, indicating that the presynaptic nerve terminals are the origin of the firing and that the process is trans-synaptic (VOLLE and KOELLE, 1961; VOLLE, 1962b; TAKESHIGE and VOLLE, 1963,b).

Of particular note is the exquisite sensitivity of the anticholinesterase-induced firing to blockade by atropine. Doses of atropine having no discernible effect on transmission cause a prolonged blockade of ganglionic firing either by the anticholinesterase agents or by the muscarinic drugs. The anticholinesterase-induced firing is resistant to blockade by traditional ganglionic blocking substances such as *d*-tubocurarine (Fig. 5). The resistance to blockade by *d*-tubocurarine is more prominent in cat superior cervical ganglia than in rat ganglia (HANCOCK and VOLLE, 1970). In rat ganglia, *d*-tubocurarine causes a partial blockade of the firing produced by anticholinesterase agents. The reason for this species difference is not known.

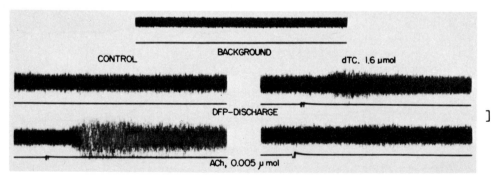

Fig. 5. Postganglionic discharge in cat superior cervical ganglion after the administration of diisopropylfluorophosphate. The *top tracing* shows the background noise level of the recording system. The *tracings on the left* (control) show the postganglionic discharge and the response to acetylcholine superimposed on the discharge. The *tracings on the right* (dTC 1.6 μmol) show the effects of *d*-tubocurarine on the discharge and the response to acetylcholine. The response to acetylcholine, but not the discharge, was blocked (VOLLE, 1962a)

Divalent cations also have a differential blocking effect on the anticholinesterase-induced firing (KOMALAHIRANYA and VOLLE, 1962). Even in amounts having no effect on ganglionic transmission or postganglionic firing by acetylcholine, calcium depresses the discharge produced by the anticholinesterase agents. Unlike atropine, calcium causes only a transient blockade. Cadmium blocks both the response to preganglionic stimulation and the anticholinesterase agents when given in concentrations that have no effect on the ganglionic response to injected acetylcholine. Cadmium is known to have prominent effects on transmitter release (HALASZ et al., 1960; NILSON and VOLLE, 1976), and it may be by this mechanism that cadmium exerts its differential blocking actions on sympathetic ganglia. No such differential blocking action is seen with magnesium. All ganglionic responses to injected acetylcholine or preganglionic stimulation are depressed. Nonetheless, it appears that the ganglionic firing produced by the anticholinesterase agents is more sensitive to blockade by membrane-stabilising substances, including procaine, than is transmission occurring via nicotinic sites (KOMALAHIRANYA and VOLLE, 1962).

The direct effects on ganglia of the anticholinesterase agents to cause muscarinic transmission or to unmask muscarinic receptive sites appear to account for the antagonism by the anticholinesterase agents of hypotension produced in dogs by hexamethonium (HILTON, 1961; LONG and ECKSTEIN, 1961). In these animals, the anticholinesterase agents cause a rise in blood pressure that is prevented by small amounts of atropine. Quaternary ammonium, or non-penetrating, anticholinesterase agents are effective antagonists of hexamethonium, indicating that the vasopressor response is due to actions of the drugs on peripheral tissues. Because the vasopressor response to the anticholinesterase agents is prevented by atropine, it is reasonable to attribute the response to the accumulation of ganglionic acetylcholine at muscarinic, rather than nicotinic sites. This raises the interesting possibility that the muscarinic system in ganglia may act as an alternative pathway by which transmission occurs in blocked ganglia. In many situations both atropine and hexamethonium are required for complete blockade of ganglionic transmission (VOLLE and KOELLE, 1975).

It should be mentioned that neostigmine has direct excitatory actions on ganglionic muscarinic sites (TAKESHIGE and VOLLE, 1963c). Postganglionic firing produced in chronically denervated ganglia of the cat by neostigmine is blocked by atropine and resistant to blockade by hexamethonium. MASON (1962a,b) has also shown that neostigmine, unlike physostigmine, has direct ganglion-stimulating action.

B. Catecholamines

Mammalian sympathetic ganglion cells in vivo contain adrenergic receptors, which can be activated by the application of catecholamines (MARRAZZI, 1939). It is now apparent that both α- and β-adrenergic receptors are present in ganglia (DE GROAT, and VOLLE, 1966a,b; HAEFELY, 1969). Activation of the α receptor leads to ganglionic hyperpolarisation and transmission blockade; both actions are prevented by adrenergic blocking agents such as dihydroergotamine. β-Receptor activation leads to ganglionic depolarisation and facilitation of ganglionic transmission, actions that are prevented by adrenergic blocking agents such as propranolol. Of particular note is

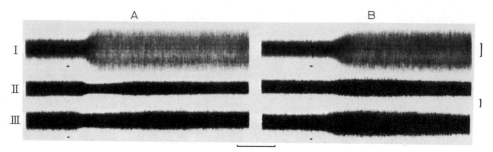

Fig. 6. Effects of isoproterenol (1 μg, IA), norepinephrine (2 μg, IA), and epinephrine (2 μg, IA) on the asynchronous postganglionic discharge evoked by an anticholinesterase agent before and after the administration of dihydroergotamine (50 μg, IA). The responses before and after dihydroergotamine are shown in columns A and B, respectively. *Record I*, the response to isoproterenol. *Record II*, the response to norepinephrine. *Record III*, the response to epinephrine. The records were obtained in three different experiments. The ganglia were conditioned by repetitive preganglionic stimulation (30 Hz for 30 s). Vertical calibrations are each 10 μV. The top vertical calibration applies to record I and the bottom vertical calibrations to records II and III. The horizontal calibration is 10 s. The dot at the bottom of each record indicates drug injections (DE GROAT and VOLLE, 1966 b)

the striking enhancement by β-receptor agonists of the ganglionic firing produced by muscarinic stimulating drugs (DE GROAT and VOLLE, 1966 b). In addition, some of the catecholamines decrease transmitter release from the presynaptic nerve terminals (HAEFELY, 1969; KOBAYASHI and LIBET, 1970; CHRIST and NISHI, 1971 a, b; DUN and NISHI, 1974).

Isoproterenol is known to facilitate transmission in cat superior cervical ganglia (MATTHEWS, 1956; PARDO et al., 1963; DE GROAT and VOLLE, 1966 a; KRSTIC, 1971; but see HAEFELY, 1969). The facilitation of transmission by isoproterenol coincides with ganglionic cellular depolarisation and with changes in the contour of the ganglionic spike that are consistent with depolarisation. There is no postganglionic firing associated with the depolarisation produced by isoproterenol. Whereas isoproterenol has no effect on ganglionic discharges produced by nicotinic ganglion-stimulating agents, it causes a marked enhancement of ganglionic firing produced by muscarinic drugs or trans-synaptic firing by the anticholinesterase agents (DE GROAT and VOLLE, 1966 b; Fig. 6). All of the ganglionic actions of isoproterenol are blocked by β-adrenergic blocking drugs given in amounts that do not affect ganglionic transmission.

Under some circumstances, epinephrine causes a facilitation of transmission (BÜLBRING, 1944; DE GROAT and VOLLE, 1966 a) and under other circumstances it blocks transmission (MARRAZZI, 1939; LUNDBERG, 1952; MATTHEWS, 1956; WEIR and McLENNAN, 1963; DE GROAT and VOLLE, 1966 a; McISAAC, 1966). In ganglia treated with dihydroergotamine, epinephrine activates β-adrenergic receptors and possesses all the ganglionic actions of isoproterenol (DE GROAT and VOLLE, 1966 a, b). In this situation, the ganglionic inhibitory effects of epinephrine are prevented by α-adrenergic blockade, thus permitting full expression of the facilitatory action of epinephrine. The dual actions of epinephrine can explain the discrepancy reported in various studies (e.g., MARRAZZI, 1939; BÜLBRING, 1944).

Table 1. Effects of norepinephrine and isoproterenol on the cat superior cervical ganglion

	Norepinephrine[a]	Isoproterenol[b]
Ganglionic Action Potential		
Spike	↓	↑
Negative wave	↑	↓
Positive wave	↓	↑
Demarcation Potential	↓	↓
Nicotine		
Depolarisation	–	↓
Firing	–	–
Muscarinic induced firing	↓	↑
Anticholinesterase-induced firing	↓	↑

[a] All actions blocked by α-adrenergic blocking drugs.
[b] All actions blocked by β-adrenergic blocking drugs.

In contrast to isoproterenol, the dominant effect of norepinephrine on ganglia is inhibitory. Norepinephrine blocks transmission and reduces ganglionic responses to muscarinic substances. Ganglionic hyperpolarisation is an inconstant finding (LUNDBERG, 1952; DE GROAT and VOLLE, 1966a,b; HAEFELY, 1969; see Sect. B.I, below). When these actions of norepinephrine are prevented by α-adrenergic blockade, a weak stimulating β-receptor activation may be noted.

The differences between norepinephrine and isoproterenol are listed in Table 1. It should be pointed out that the data are derived from extracellular recording systems used to measure changes produced by the catecholamines in the ganglionic demarcation potential and postganglionic firing. Some data have been verified by means of intracellular recording systems, e.g., norepinephrine causes ganglionic hyperpolarisation (KOBAYASHI and LIBET, 1970).

Dopamine causes inhibition of ganglionic transmission (MCISAAC, 1966), but is only about one-tenth as potent as epinephrine. Like that obtained with epinephrine and norepinephrine, blockade by dopamine is antagonised by α-adrenergic blocking drugs. LIBET and TOSAKA (1970), using sucrose-gap recording systems and isolated rabbit sympathetic ganglia, report that dopamine causes hyperpolarisation and a striking facilitation of muscarinic responses. Thus, dopamine appears to resemble epinephrine more closely than norepinephrine. One important difference is the finding that dopamine-induced facilitation of muscarinic responses is prevented by phenoxybenzamine, but not by β-adrenergic blocking drugs (LIBET and TOSAKA, 1970), a result different from that reported by DE GROAT and VOLLE (1966b) for isoproterenol and epinephrine.

I. Catecholamines and the Slow Synaptic Inhibitory Potential

The identity of the substance mediating the slow inhibitory postsynaptic potential (IPSP) in sympathetic ganglia remains to be established. Both the catecholamines (epinephrine in the frog and dopamine in the mammal) and acetylcholine have been suggested as mediators of the IPSP. Clarification awaits the resolution of an equally fundamental question, the nature of the electrogenic mechanism that produces the IPSP. At least three different electrogenic mechanisms have been proposed.

KOSTERLITZ et al. (1968), using rabbit superior cervical ganglia mounted in a sucrose-gap chamber and treated with hexamethonium to unmask the IPSP, concluded that the IPSP was due to an increase in ganglion cellular permeability to potassium. When the concentration of potassium in the solution bathing the ganglion is varied, the amplitude of the IPSP varies inversely with the concentration of potassium. This is an expected finding if the transmitter causes the IPSP by increasing membrane permeability to potassium.

By contrast, there is evidence to show that the electrogenic basis of the IPSP involves a sodium-pump mechanism. Bullfrog sympathetic ganglia treated with nicotine to block the fast EPSP give rise to an IPSP when the preganglionic nerve is stimulated (NISHI and KOKETSU, 1968). The IPSP is diminished by extrinsic depolarising currents and enhanced by hyperpolarising currents. When intense hyperpolarising currents are applied, the IPSP is decreased in amplitude but never reversed in direction. This suggests that the IPSP is independent of the potassium equilibrium potential of the ganglion cells. Moreover, the IPSP is enhanced by raising the sodium content of the bathing solution; lowering potassium nullifies the effects of raising the sodium content (NISHI and KOKETSU, 1968). In an earlier study by NISHI and KOKETSU (1967), it was found that the IPSP was sensitive to blockade by ouabain $(10^{-6} M)$ and low temperature. Thus, the accumulated evidence points toward a metabolically dependent ionic mechanism for the generation of the IPSP.

According to NAKAMURA and KOKETSU (1972), epinephrine applied to bullfrog ganglia in the sucrose-gap system causes ganglionic hyperpolarisation with characteristics identical with those seen for the IPSP. The epinephrine-induced hyperpolarisation occurs when the cell is driven beyond the equilibrium potential for potassium ions. Replacement of sodium ions by lithium ions or the addition of ouabain reduces the hyperpolarising response to epinephrine. In addition, the hyperpolarisation is depressed by reducing the temperature of the ganglion cells. Like the IPSP, the epinephrine-induced hyperpolarisation can be explained by an electrogenic sodium pump system.

Some bullfrog ganglion cells respond to the application of epinephrine with depolarisation (NAKAMURA and KOKETSU, 1972). Depolarisation by epinephrine is unaffected by lithium substitution for sodium, low temperature, or ouabain. Although there is no obvious way to account for this different cellular response to epinephrine, the fact that the depolarisation is unaffected by those changes in the bathing solution that eliminate ganglionic hyperpolarisation argues for a specificity of action for such changes. WEIGHT and PADJEN (1937a) criticise the use of ouabain as a method for evaluating the electrogenic mechanism of the IPSP, and point out the complexities of ouabain actions. However, if ouabain, lithium, or low temperatures cause large changes in ganglionic cellular electrolyte balance, then marked changes should also be expected in the depolarising response to the catecholamines.

It is not easy to demonstrate ganglionic hyperpolarisation by catecholamines in amphibian ganglia (NAKAMURA and KOKETSU, 1972; KOKETSU and MINOTA, 1975). Either no change in resting membrane potential or slight depolarisation (less than 5 mV) is also observed. Similarly, membrane resistance is either unchanged or

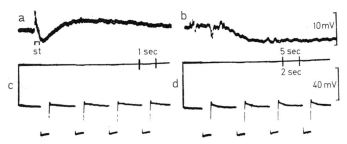

Fig. 7 a–d. Response to norepinephrine in cells of rabbit superior cervical ganglion, with *d*-tubocurarine (15 µg/ml) and harmine (5 µg/ml) present. **a** Response to brief train of stimuli, 40 Hz (see bar st) to preganglionic nerve; note the summated fast EPSPs during stimulation, with superimposed S-IPSP developing during and after train, followed by the longer-lasting S-EPSP. **b** Same cell as in **a**, in resting state, norepinephrine added to chamber (to give 50 µg/ml) as indicated by the mechnical artefacts; prolonged hyperpolarisation develops several seconds later. **c** Another cell, in resting state, with hyperpolarising pulses of constant current to measure resistance, set off from a baseline by the value of the total transmembrane potential. **d** Same cell as in **c**, but taken 4 min after the addition of norepinephrine, which produced a steady hyperpolarising response of about 6 mV in this case. Time calibration in **d** holds for **c** and **d**; voltage calibration in **b** for **a** and **b**, that in **d** for **c** and **d**, downward signifiying negative polarity of intracellular electrode (KOBAYASHI and LIBET, 1970)

slightly increased. The ganglion cell spike produced by antidromic stimulation is altered markedly by epinephrine (0.3 mM). There is a decrease in the amplitude of the post-spike hyperpolarisation and an increase in the duration of the spike, effects that can be attributed to a decrease in potassium conductance. In some cells, there is a prominent decrease in spike amplitude and a decrease in the rate of rise of the spike, effects attributed to a decrease in sodium conductance.

Somewhat different results are obtained with microelectrodes in isolated rabbit superior cervical ganglia (KOBAYASHI and LIBET, 1970). In the presence of harmine, an inhibitor of monoamine oxidase, norepinephrine and epinephrine (1.5×10^{-4} M) cause a long-lasting hyperpolarisation of the ganglion cells (about 4 mV). Like the IPSP (see also NISHI and KOKETSU, 1968), the drug-induced hyperpolarisation is diminished in amplitude by conditioning depolarising currents. There is no change in membrane resistance during the IPSP or during the hyperpolarisation produced by norepinephrine (Fig. 7; KOBAYASHI and LIBET, 1970). Dopamine (LIBET and TOSAKA, 1970; LIBET and KOBAYASHI, 1974) also causes ganglionic hyperpolarisation. The α-adrenergic blocking drugs dibenamine, phenoxybenzamine, and dihydroergotamine prevent these responses to the catecholamines. Conversely, the β-adrenergic blocking drugs, propranolol and pronetholol, are without effect (LIBET and TOSAKA, 1970). LIBET and colleagues conclude from these studies that the IPSP is produced by a catecholamine (dopamine or epinephrine) acting on the ganglion cell. They do not comment about the electrogenic mechanism involved, except to demonstrate the apparent lack of effect of the catecholamines on membrane ionic conductances.

In bullfrog ganglia treated with nicotine to eliminate the excitatory postsynaptic potential (EPSP) (WEIGHT and PADJEN, 1973a, b), the IPSP has properties that indicate that the transmitter causes the IPSP by reducing sodium conductance. In addition, the transmitter appears to be acetylcholine and the IPSP appears to result from

a direct action of acetylcholine on the ganglion cell, no intermediary step of catecholamine transmission being required. The IPSP produced under these conditions differs from the IPSP unmasked by curare-like substances in the following ways. Membrane resistance increases during IPSP or the hyperpolarisation produced by the
application of acetylcholine. The acetylcholine hyperpolarisation is unaffected by the
addition of magnesium ions to the bath to depress synaptic activity. [Ganglionic
hyperpolarisation by muscarinic cholinomimetic agents is eliminated by magnesium,
presumably because the muscarinic drugs act by an indirect mechanism (LIBET and
TOSAKA, 1970; LIBET and KOBAYASHI, 1974).] Replacement of sodium by isosmotic
equivalents of sucrose eliminates the acetylcholine potential. Finally, depolarisation
of the ganglion cells by extrinsic currents causes a parallel decrease in the IPSP and
the antidromic spike, suggesting a decrease in sodium conductance as the basis of the
IPSP.

LIBET and KOBAYASHI (1974) confirm the findings of WEIGHT and PADJEN
(1973,b) that acetylcholine, in ganglia treated with nicotine, but not with curare-like
drugs, causes hyperpolarisation by a direct action on the ganglion cells. Catecholamines cause hyperpolarisation that is sensitive to α-adrenergic blockade in both
types of ganglia. Epinephrine is more effective than norepinephrine and dopamine is
the least effective of the catecholamines. Similarly, methacholine causes hyperpolarisation in both types of ganglia and the hyperpolarisation is prevented by atropine.
However, α-adrenergic blockade by phentolamine prevents the responses to methacholine in the curarised ganglion but not in ganglia treated with nicotine (Fig. 8). In
addition, phentolamine blocks the IPSP in both types of ganglia. LIBET and KOBAY-
ASHI (1974) suggest that the cholinomimetic agents can cause ganglionic hyperpolarisation by two distinct processes, one due to direct actions on the ganglion cell and
one to an indirect action on catecholamine-containing cells. For some unknown

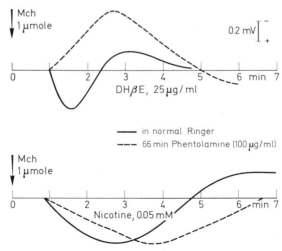

Fig. 8. Effect of phentolamine on ganglionic responses to methacholine. In the first ganglion,
transmission was depressed by dihydro-β-erythroidine; in the second ganglion, by nicotine. The
response to methacholine in Ringer solution is given by the *solid line* and consists of hyperpolarisation followed by depolarisation. The *dashed line* shows the response to methacholine after
phentolamine was used to block α-receptors (LIBET and KOBAYASHI, 1974)

reason, the direct action is expressed only in ganglia treated with nicotine. This is somewhat reminiscent of the findings by TAKESHIGE et al. (1963) that the increased demarcation potential produced by methacholine in untreated cat superior cervical ganglia is unaffected by α-adrenergic blocking compounds given in amounts adequate to block hyperpolarisation by norepinephrine. As noted before (VOLLE, 1966), it is for this reason that a direct action of methacholine on ganglion cells in the cat superior cervical ganglion is postulated.

II. Presynaptic Blockade by Catecholamines

The catecholamines block transmitter release from the presynaptic nerve terminals of rabbit superior cervical ganglia. When applied in amounts that have no direct effect upon the ganglion cells (CHRIST and NISHI, 1971a, b; DUN and NISHI, 1974), epinephrine, norepinephrine, and dopamine depress the EPSP, reduce the frequency of miniature EPSPs, and block impulse transmission. Ganglionic responses to iontophoretically applied acetylcholine are unaffected by the catecholamines (Fig. 9). All the effects of the catecholamines are prevented by phenoxybenzamine and other α-adrenergic blocking agents. The β-adrenergic blocking drugs have no effect.

The mechanism whereby the catecholamines depress transmitter release is not known. There is no evidence of nerve terminal depolarisation by the catecholamines or an impairment of nerve terminal conduction (CHRIST and NISHI, 1971b). Thus, if there is no effect of the catecholamines on the nerve terminal action potential or on the receptor mechanism of the ganglion cell, then the blockade of transmission must be due to an effect on the release process. Support for this possibility is provided by an analysis of the effects of the catecholamine on the quantal parameters of release.

Like that of the neuromuscular junction (DELCASTILLO and KATZ, 1954), transmission in sympathetic ganglia occurs by a quantal process where the quantal content (m) of the EPSP is related directly to the probability (p) that a quantum of transmitter will be released and the size of the pool of quanta (n) available for release (BLACKMAN et al., 1963). If it is assumed that release follows Poisson's law and that values for p do not change during tetanic preganglionic stimulation, then the analytical methodology of ELMQVIST and QUASTEL (1965) can be used to estimate m, p, and n. Under these conditions, m and n, but not p, are decreased by the catecholamines (CHRIST and NISHI, 1971b; DUN and NISHI, 1974). This could mean that the catecholamines depress transmission by reducing the amount of transmitter available for release by the incoming presynaptic volley.

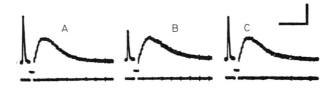

Fig. 9. Blockade by epinephrine ($10^{-5} M$) of ganglionic EPSPs. For each pair of tracings, a ganglionic EPSP precedes the potential produced by the iontophoretic application of acetylcholine. Records A and C are controls; record B was recorded in the presence of epinephrine. The calibrations are 20 mV and 300 ms (CHRIST and NISHI, 1971a)

Several cautionary comments are required. First, there is some reason to think that release in sympathetic ganglia does not follow Poisson's law (KUNO, 1971). Second, the method of rapid repetitive stimulation may not give reliable estimates of the quantal release parameters (CHRISTENSEN and MARTIN, 1970). It is likely that both p and n change in value during the rundown of EPSP amplitudes. For these reasons it may be premature to conclude that the presynaptic inhibitory effects of the catecholamines are due to a decrease in the stores of transmitter available for release.

Uncertainty about the mechanism notwithstanding, catecholamines have prominent presynaptic action. Whether or not the presynaptic action is involved in any putative transmitter role for dopamine (LIBET, 1970) or any other catecholamine is a matter of conjecture. According to HAEFELY (1969), the presynaptic nerve terminals are the primary site of action for the catecholamine and the transmission blockade is best explained by an action at this site.

BIRKS and MACINTOSH (1961) made the curious observation that epinephrine decreases acetylcholine release in cat superior cervical ganglia perfused with a balanced salt solution but increases release when the ganglia are perfused with plasma. In an earlier study, PATON and THOMPSON (1953) describe a blockade by epinephrine of transmitter release. Therefore, there are some, albeit unsettled, neurochemical data to support that obtained with electrophysiological methods.

III. Catecholamines and Ganglionic Cyclic Nucleotides

Preganglionic nerve stimulation (MCAFEE et al., 1971), catecholamines (CRAMER et al., 1973), and muscarinic cholinomimetic agents (KALIX et al., 1974) increase the ganglionic content of cyclic adenosine monophosphate (Table 2). Because of these observations, GREENGARD et al. (1972) proposed that catecholamines function as inhibitory transmitters in sympathetic ganglia and do so by a mechanism involving the ganglionic nucleotides. According to their view, presynaptic activation of muscarinic receptors on catecholamine containing interneurones leads to the release of dopamine, which in turn acts on the ganglion cells to activate the adenylcyclase system to form cyclic adenosine monophosphate. Ganglionic hyperpolarisation and

Table 2. Changes in ganglionic cyclic adenosine monophosphate produced by preganglionic nerve stimulation of isolated rabbit superior cervical ganglia (MCAFEE et al., 1971)

| | Cyclic nucleotide (pmol/mg protein) | |
	Unstimulated	Stimulated
Preganglionic stimulation	17.1 ± 2.5[a]	40.9 ± 3.5
Postganglionic stimulation	14.2 ± 1.4	13.7 ± 1.4
Preganglionic stimulation + ganglionic blockade	17.6 ± 1.4	22.0 ± 1.4

[a] Mean $\pm$ standard error of the mean.

blockade of transmission arises from the accumulation of cyclic adenosine mono-phosphate in the ganglion cells.

This model is based on the following observations. The increase in cyclic adeno-sine monophosphate brought about by either preganglionic stimulation or the appli-cation of muscarinic cholinomimetic agents is prevented by atropine or α-adrenergic blocking drugs (KALIX et al., 1974). Hexamethonium or β-adrenergic blocking agents have no effect. Substances that inhibit the phosphodiesterase enzyme enhance the response to preganglionic nerve stimulation and the cholinomimetic agents. Parallel pharmacological experiments on the dopamine-induced ganglionic hyperpolarisa-tion and on changes in ganglionic cyclic adenosine monophosphate support the suggestion that ganglionic cyclic adenosine monophosphate is the mediator of dopa-mine-induced hyperpolarisation and the ganglionic IPSP (MCAFEE and GREEN-GARD, 1972). For example, theophylline, an inhibitor of phosphodiesterase, enhances both the amplitude of the IPSP and the hyperpolarisation produced by dopamine. Similarly, prostaglandin E_1 depresses both types of ganglionic hyperpolarisation. Finally, monobutyryl cyclic adenosine monophosphate causes ganglionic hyperpo-larisation. Collectively, the experiments from an interesting series of findings to support the contention that cyclic adenosine monophosphate mediates the IPSP and, in general, conform to the model of ganglionic transmission proposed by LIBET (1970).

However, in view of the uncertainties about the electrogenic mechanisms of the IPSP and the role played in the generation of the IPSP by dopamine or the catechol-amines, it may be somewhat early to implicate cyclic adenosine monophosphate in the inhibitory process. In addition, some significant data have not yet been obtained or reported and discrepancies with other findings have not been explained. For example, CRAMER et al. (1973) note that the increase in cyclic adenosine monophos-phate produced by catecholamines is blocked by propranolol, a β-adrenergic block-ing drug. Moreover, they found that isoproterenol (known to cause depolarisation and facilitation of ganglionic transmission) increases the cyclic adenosine mono-phosphate content of rat superior cervical ganglia. In fact, isoproterenol is the most potent and dopamine the least potent of the agents tested. Because dopamine is a weak activator of the adenyl cyclase system and has a long delay in the onset of action, CRAMER et al. (1973) suggest that a metabolite of dopamine, rather than dopamine itself, may be responsible for the stimulatory effect on the adenyl cyclase system.

The precise site of cyclic adenosine monophosphate synthesis in ganglia is not known. In the cow, dopamine causes an increase in the cyclic adenosine monophos-phate content of the ganglion cells (KEBABIAN et al., 1975). There is no increase in the cyclic adenosine monophosphate content of the glial cells. This finding is of interest because KALIX et al. (1974) locate the isoproterenol-induced increase in cyclic adeno-sine nucleotides in non-neural cells, possibly glia. This possibility remains to be established. In view of the convincing evidence of a prejunctional site of action of catecholamines, the question as to whether or not changes in cyclic nucleotide occur in the nerve terminals needs to be assessed.

There is a marked disparity in the response to dopamine among superior cervical ganglia of various species. Dopamine increases ganglionic cyclic adenosine mono-phosphate markedly in bovine ganglia (KEBABIAN and GREENGARD, 1971; KALIX et al., 1974) and not at all in rabbit (KALIX et al., 1974) or rat (CRAMER et al., 1973; OTTEN et al., 1974). In the cat superior cervical ganglion, dopamine causes a moderate increase in the cellular content of cyclic adenosine monophosphate (WILLIAMS et al., 1975). A systematic study to correlate electrophysiological responses to dopamine with changes or lack of changes in cyclic nucleotides needs to be made before a direct involvement of cyclic nucleotides in the ganglionic inhibitory responses to catecholamines can be established. It is curious, for example, that much of the evidence cited by LIBET and his colleagues to establish dopamine as an inhibitory ganglionic transmitter results from studies using the rabbit superior cervical ganglia, a tissue with little or no change in cyclic nucleotides when treated with dopamine.

A better demonstration of parallelism between the hyperpolarisation produced by monobutyryl cyclic adenosine monophosphate and that produced by dopamine (e.g., reversal potential, ionic requirements, etc.) is required before the conclusion that the two occur by the same mechanism is justified. As noted before, there is uncertainty about the electrogenic mechanism that gives rise to the inhibitory effects of dopamine.

Clearly, studies of the link between ganglionic cellular metabolism and synaptic potentials hold great promise, and the results acquired to date are extremely provocative. However, there is only tenuous justification for relating the changes observed in ganglionic cyclic adenosine monophosphate to ganglionic transmission.

IV. Catecholamines as Modulators of Transmission

Several lines of evidence point to dopamine as a candidate for the role of inhibitory transmitter in sympathetic ganglia (LIBET and TOSAKA, 1970). Dopamine is present in some sympathetic ganglia (however, see CROWCROFT, vide infra) and, presumably, in the small, intensely fluorescent cells of the superior cervical ganglia of several species (BJORKLUND et al., 1970). Like epinephrine and norepinephrine, dopamine causes hyperpolarisation of cells in the rabbit superior cervical ganglion. Accordingly, LIBET (1970) proposes that the IPSP is due to an action of dopamine on the ganglion cells and that the dopamine is released from the small intensely fluorescent cells by acetylcholine, which, in turn, is released from preganglionic nerve terminals. This model accounts for the sensitivity of the IPSP to blockade by either atropine or α-adrenergic blocking drugs and for the similarities between the IPSP and ganglionic hyperpolarisation produced by dopamine.

The model has several weaknesses. First, it is obvious that identification of the mediator will not be possible until the question of the electrogenic mechanism of the IPSP is resolved. In some studies membrane conductance is unchanged, while in others it is decreased during the IPSP. Thus, the failure of dopamine or catecholamines to alter membrane conductance during ganglionic hyperpolarisation cannot be interpreted. If a catecholamine is the mediator of the IPSP, then it must be demonstrated that it mimics the effects of the endogenous mediator of the IPSP. Clearly, this cannot be done until the effects of the endogenous mediator are established. The question as to whether the transmitter for the IPSP is dopamine or norepinephrine (or acetylcholine) is unsettled.

It is also important to note that differences in the ganglionic content of dopamine do not correlate well with the presence of the IPSP in sympathetic ganglia (CROW-

CROFT et al., 1971). The inferior mesenteric ganglia of guinea-pig contain many small, intensely fluorescent cells (OSTBERG, 1970) but little or no dopamine. Since evidence of IPSPs is also lacking in these ganglia, the absence of dopamine may be related to a lack of an inhibitory system. However, the dopamine content of the superior cervical ganglion of guinea-pig is approximately the same as that found in rabbit superior cervical ganglia (LAVERTY and SHARMAN, 1965). It is of interest, therefore, that the IPSP has been identified in rabbit, but not in the guinea-pig superior cervical ganglia (CROWCROFT et al., 1971). Whether or not the failure to find IPSPs in guinea-pig ganglia is due to limited sampling of cells remains to be determined. Since the small, intensely fluorescent cells tend to occur in clusters and are limited in number, it is possible that they might be overlooked by the microelectrode.

Alternatively, OSTBERG (1970) differs from MATTHEWS and RAISMAN (1969) and WILLIAMS and PALAY (1969), in that he has not been able to find synaptic contacts between the small granule cells of the inferior mesenteric ganglia and ganglionic cell dendrites. Because of this and because of the tendency of the small cells to cluster around blood vessels, he suggests that the small cells secrete biogenic amines directly into the blood stream after the fashion of the adrenal medullary cells.

Mention must be made of the selectivity of the drugs used to study transmission. The catecholamines have a variety of actions on sympathetic ganglia, including modification of the release of acetylcholine from preganglionic nerve terminals (KO-BAYASHI and LIBET, 1970; CHRIST and NISHI, 1971a,b). Thus, the relative importance of the pre- and postsynaptic actions of the catecholamines is, for the moment, a matter of conjecture. There is clear evidence that the catecholamines have demonstrable actions on both sides of the synapse when applied to the ganglia in adequate concentrations. KOKETSU and MINOTA (1975) find that epinephrine blocks both sodium and potassium conductance in amphibian sympathetic ganglia. However, high concentrations (0.3 mM) are required for these effects to be demonstrable.

The multiple actions of the α-adrenergic blocking drugs must also be recognised. In addition to preventing the ganglionic IPSP, they depress the late EPSP rather severely. While it is possible that this action of dibenamine or phenoxybenzamine reflects a complex interaction between dopamine and muscarinic excitatory receptors (LIBET and TOSAKA, 1970), it is equally possible that the action reflects the well-known atropine-like actions of the drug (BEDDOE et al., 1971). Both α- and β-adrenergic blocking drugs depress ganglionic transmission in rabbit sympathetic ganglia in situ (KAYAALP and MCISAAC, 1969), and the doses required are the same as those required to block α and β receptors on smooth muscle cells. These results do not favour a modulatory role for endogenous catecholamines in sympathetic ganglia.

There is only meagre evidence of a physiological role for adrenergic nerves or interneurones in ganglionic transmission. The morphology suggests that such interactions occur (HAMBERGER and NORBERG, 1965; JACOBOWITZ, 1970). An adrenergic inhibitory mechanism existing in the parasympathetic ganglia of the urinary bladder of cat has been reported (DE GROAT and SAUM, 1972; DE GROAT, 1975). In these ganglia, there is some morphological evidence showing that adrenergic terminals abut with intramural parasympathetic ganglion cells (HAMBERGER and NORBERG, 1965). Activation of the adrenergic terminals by stimulation of the hypogastric nerve reduces transmission in the parasympathetic ganglia. The inhibitory response to hypogastric nerve stimulation occurs with frequencies of stimulation in the range

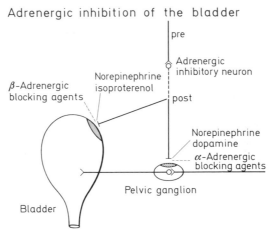

Fig. 10. Diagrammatic representation of receptors mediating adrenergic inhibition in the urinary bladder of the cat. The *dashed line* from the adrenergic inhibitory neurone indicates that the postganglionic axon to the bladder and the pelvic ganglia do not necessarily originate from the same adrenergic inhibitory neurone (DE GROAT, 1975)

found normally in sympathetic ganglia. Transmission is also blocked by epinephrine, norepinephrine, or dopamine and the blockade of transmission produced either by adrenergic nerve stimulation or by the applied catecholamines is prevented by α-adrenergic blocking compounds (Fig. 10). According to this model, adrenergic nerve terminals act directly upon parasympathetic ganglion cells to block transmission.

Transmission in ganglia of the myenteric plexus of guinea-pig is blocked by stimulation of sympathetic nerves. Since stimulation of the sympathetic neurones never causes an IPSP in the ganglion cells and catecholamines have no effect on the sensitivity of the cells to acetylcholine (NISHI and NORTH, 1973), the blockade of transmission is attributed to a presynaptic effect of the adrenergic neurones on transmitter release from the preganglionic fibres (HIRST and MCKIRDY, 1974). This finding is consistent with the well-known ability of norepinephrine to depress transmitter release from preganglionic fibres (vide supra).

Thus, it appears that ganglionic transmission in parasympathetic ganglia can be prevented by stimulation of appropriate sympathetic neurones, because of either pre- or postsynaptic effects of norepinephrine.

C. Neuromuscular Blocking Agents

The prototype of this class of drugs is *d*-tubocurarine, an agent with rather powerful effects on transmission in autonomic ganglia (KHARKEVICH, 1967). The doses of *d*-tubocurarine that are required to block neuromuscular transmission also depress transmission in autonomic ganglia. For reasons that are not understood, transmission in parasympathetic ganglia appears to be more sensitive to blockade by *d*-tubocurarine than is transmission in sympathetic ganglia (GUYTON and REEDER, 1950). Compared with transmission at the gastrocnemius muscle, transmission in ciliary and cardiac vagal ganglia is only slightly less sensitive to d-tubocurarine, whereas transmission in the superior cervical, coeliac and stellate ganglia is five to ten times less sensitive to blockade by d-tubocurarine.

The reasons for the differential sensitivity of ganglia to blockade by d-tubocurarine are not clear. It should be noted, however, that different cell groups within the same ganglion show differences in sensitivity to blockade by d-tubocurarine (VOLLE, 1962a). Whether these results are due to differences in the intraganglionic distribution of the blocking drug or to basic differences in the transmission process is not known.

The blockade of ganglionic transmission by d-tubocurarine parallels that produced by hexamethonium in almost every way. Transmission is blocked at a time when transmitter release is normal, the ganglionic cellular resting membrane potential is normal, and the response to applied acetylcholine is depressed. Like hexamethonium, d-tubocurarine causes a more substantial blockade of transmission during rapid preganglionic stimulation than during low rates of stimulation. For all of these reasons, d-tubocurarine is viewed as acting as a competitive antagonist of the nicotinic acetylcholine receptor of the ganglion cells.

Under some circumstances, d-tubocurarine may actually cause ganglionic stimulation of normal and denervated superior cervical ganglia (BÜLBRING and DEPIERRE, 1949). Similarly, ganglia treated with anticholinesterase agents (VOLLE, 1962b) or N-ethylmaleimide (KOMALAHIRANYA and VOLLE, 1963) are stimulated by d-tubocurarine. In the last two situations, the prior administration of hexamethonium prevents ganglionic stimulation by d-tubocurarine, thus suggesting that stimulation by d-tubocurarine involves activation of the acetylcholine nicotinic receptor.

Drugs related pharmacologically to d-tubocurarine also block ganglionic transmission, but do so with varying degrees of potency (Table 3). RANDALL and JAMPOLSKY (1953) found that dimethyl-d-tubocurarine and benzoquinonium possess the blocking potency of d-tubocurarine. Although their effects have not been well studied with electrophysiological methods, it is assumed that the mechanism of blockade is the same for all these agents. In the case of gallamine, it would be interesting to know whether gallamine would prevent ganglionic transmission through muscarinic sites, since this substance also possesses some atropine-like actions.

Table 3. Relative potencies of neuromuscular blocking agents

	Neuromuscular blockade	Ganglionic blockade	Fall in blood Pressure
d-Tubocurarine	1	1	1
Dimethyl-d-tubocurarine	4	1/5	1/5
Gallamine	1/5	1/100	1/40
Dihydro-β-erythroidine	1/2	1/3	1/2
Benzoquinonium	1	1/9	1/8
Decamethonium	8	1/12	1/16
Succinylcholine	2	1/70	1/100

GROB (1967).

The curare-like drug dihydro-β-erythroidine is often used to unmask ganglionic potentials in isolated mammalian and amphibian ganglia (ECCLES and LIBET, 1961; LIBET and KOBAYASHI, 1974). This substance has no effect on transmitter release, the ganglionic resting membrane potential, or ganglionic muscarinic receptors. The drug does not contain a quaternary nitrogen group and, for that reason, can penetrate into ganglionic regions that are inaccessible to d-tubocurarine. Although thorough comparative studies have not been carried out, dihydro-β-erythroidine appears to act on ganglia in the same way as does d-tubocurarine.

The depolarising neuromuscular blocking compounds have only a very low ganglionic blocking potency (Table 3). Decamethonium has about one-twelfth the activity of d-tubocurarine on sympathetic ganglia (RANDALL and JAMPOLSKY, 1953). In contrast to blockade of neuromuscular transmission, the blockade of ganglionic transmission by decamethonium appears to be of the competitive type (BARLOW and ZOLLER, 1964). Similarly, succinylcholine is almost devoid of effect on sympathetic ganglia (RYBOLOVLEV, 1952; PATON, 1949). Large doses of succinylcholine are required to cause ganglionic depolarisation or blockade.

Finally, the neuromuscular blocking substance α-bungarotoxin (CHANG and LEE, 1963) does not appear to affect ganglionic transmission in mammals. Since α-bungarotoxin is highly specific for nicotinic receptors of the muscle end plate, its failure to affect nicotinic receptors in ganglia points to fundamental differences in the chemical nature of the two nicotinic receptors. The weak ganglionic blocking actions of succinylcholine and decamethonium support this conclusion.

D. Local Anaesthetics

Unlike the blockade of transmission caused by hexamethonium, that produced by procaine has a significant presynaptic component (HARVEY, 1939). In addition to abolishing the ganglionic response to preganglionic stimulation and applied acetylcholine, procaine causes a marked reduction in the output of transmitter from the preganglionic nerve terminals. Moreover, local anaesthetics differ from classic blocking drugs by also suppressing ganglionic responses to non-specific stimulants such as potassium chloride.

A thorough electrophysiological analysis of the effects of procaine on ganglionic transmission has been made by KHARKEVICH (1959, 1960a, b, 1962) and KHARKEVICH and TISHCHENKO (1957). A number of similarities and differences can be demonstrated between procaine and traditional ganglion-blocking drugs. For example, procaine, like hexamethonium, causes a frequency-dependent blockade of transmission, with a more intense blockade occurring at the elevated frequencies of transmission. Both hexamethonium and procaine depress the after-discharge produced by rapid preganglionic stimulation. Unlike hexamethonium, however, procaine blocks the ganglionic action potentials produced by antidromic stimulation of postganglionic neurones. In addition, procaine reduces post-activation facilitation but intensifies post-activation inhibition. Thus, procaine is similar to hexamethonium in its effects on facilitation but not those on inactivation. It appears that the local anaesthetics have prominent actions on all neuronal elements in ganglia, whereas hexamethonium has a prominent effect only on the acetylcholine nicotinic receptor.

It is interesting that parasympathetic ganglia are more sensitive to blockade by local anaesthetics than are sympathetic ganglia (ZIPF and DITTMANN, 1972). As with d-tubocurarine, there is no explanation for this apparent differential sensitivity.

E. Conclusions

Autonomic ganglia possess receptive sites for a wide variety of substances, some of which may subserve a physiological function. For the most part, the anti-cholinesterase agents cause changes in ganglionic transmission because of the preservation of ganglionic acetylcholine in the synapse. Although there is also a build-up of acetylcholine in the presynaptic nerve terminals after anticholin-esterase agents are given, it is not clear whether the build-up causes abnor-mal transmission to occur. The catecholamines mimic many of the actions of the transmitter substance that causes ganglionic IPSPs. There is thus some reason to suspect that catecholamines play a part in ganglionic transmission.

The general impression seems to be emerging that receptor mechanisms in sym-pathetic ganglia are not as well-differentiated as those of other tissues. The end plate of skeletal muscle, for example, has rather restrictive requirements for the activation of the receptor mechanisms. This situation is in marked contrast to ganglia, where many substances cause excitatory or inhibitory effects when administered in rela-tively low doses. The implications for this veritable pharmacological storehouse of receptors are unclear.

References

Barlow, R.B., Zoller, A.: Some effects of long chain polymethylene bisonium salts on junctional transmission in the peripheral nervous system. Br. J. Pharmacol. 23, 131–150 (1964)

Beddoe, F., Nicholls, P.J., Smith, H.J.: Inhibition of muscarinic receptor by dibenamine. Biochem. Pharmacol. 20, 3367–3376 (1971)

Bennett, M.R., McLachlan, E.M.: An electrophysiological analysis of the storage of acetylcholine in preganglionic nerve terminals. J. Physiol. (Lond.) 221, 657–668 (1972a)

Bennett, M.R., McLachlan, E.M.: An electrophysiological analysis of the synthesis of acetylcho-line in preganglionic nerve terminals. J. Physiol. (Lond.) 221, 669–682 (1972b)

Birks, R.I., MacIntosh, F.C.: Acetylcholine metabolism of a sympathetic ganglion. Can. J. Biochem. Physiol. 39, 787–827 (1961)

Bjorklund, A., Cegrell, L., Falck, B., Ritzen, M., Rosengren, E.: Dopamine-containing cells in sympathetic ganglia. Acta Physiol. Scand. 78, 334–338 (1970)

Blaber, L.C.: The mechanism of the facilitatory action of edrophonium in cat skeletal muscle. Br. J. Pharmacol. 46, 498–507 (1972)

Blaber, L.C., Christ, D.D.: The action of facilitatory drugs on the isolated tenuissimus muscle of the cat. Int. J. Neuropharmacol. 6, 473–484 (1967)

Blackman, J.G., Purves, R.D.: Intracellular recordings from ganglia of the thoracic sympathetic chain of the guinea-pig. J. Physiol. (Lond.) 203, 173–178 (1969)

Blackman, J.G., Ginsborg, B.L., Ray, C.: Synaptic transmission in the sympathetic ganglion of the frog. J. Physiol. (Lond.) 167, 355–373 (1963)

Bornstein, J.D.: The effects of physostigmine on synaptic transmission in the inferior mesenteric ganglion of guinea-pig. J. Physiol. (Lond.) 241, 309–325 (1974)

Boyd, I.A., Martin, A.R.: Spontaneous sub-threshold activity at mammalian neuromuscular junctions. J. Physiol. (Lond.) 132, 61–73 (1956)

Brown, D.A., Jones, K.B., Halliwell, J.V., Quilliam, J.P.: Evidence against a presynaptic action of acetylcholine during ganglionic transmission. Nature (Lond.) *226*, 958–959 (1970)

Bülbring, E.: The action of adrenaline on transmission in the superior cervical ganglion. J. Physiol. (Lond.) *103*, 55–67 (1944)

Bülbring, E., Depierre, F.: The action of synthetic curarizing compounds on skeletal muscle and sympathetic ganglia both normal and denervated. Br. J. Pharmacol. *4*, 22–28 (1949)

Chang, C.C., Lee, C.Y.: Isolation of neurotoxins from the venom of *Bungarus mullicinclus* and their modes of neuromuscular blocking action. Arch. Int. Pharmacodyn. Ther. *144*, 241–257 (1963)

Christ, D.D., Nishi, S.: Site of adrenaline blockade in the superior cervical ganglion of the rabbit. J. Physiol. (Lond.) *213*, 107–117 (1971a)

Christ, D.D., Nishi, S.: Effects of adrenaline on nerve terminals in the superior cervical ganglion of the rabbit. Br. J. Pharmacol. *41*, 331–338 (1971b)

Christensen, B.N., Martin, A.R.: Estimates of probability of transmitter release at the mammalian neuromuscular junction. J. Physiol. (Lond.) *210*, 933–945 (1970)

Collier, B., Katz, H.S.: The synthesis, turnover, and release of surplus acetylcholine in a sympathetic ganglion. J. Physiol. (Lond.) *214*, 537–552 (1971)

Collier, B., Katz, H.S.: Acetylcholine synthesis from recaptured choline by a sympathetic ganglion. J. Physiol. (Lond.) *238*, 639–655 (1974)

Collier, B., MacIntosh, F.C.: The source of choline for acetylcholine synthesis in a sympathetic ganglion. Can. J. Physiol. Pharmacol. *47*, 127–135 (1969)

Cramer, H., Johnson, D.G., Hanbauer, I., Silberstein, S.D., Kopin, I.J.: Accumulation of adenosine 3′,5′-monophosphate induced by catecholamines in the rat superior cervical ganglion in vitro. Brain Res. *53*, 97–104 (1973)

Crowcroft, P.J., Jarrott, B., Ostberg, A.: Are there inhibitory mechanisms in mammalian autonomic ganglia? Proc. Aust. Physiol. Pharmacol. Soc. *2*, 31–32 (1971)

de Groat, W.C.: Nervous control of the urinary bladder of the cat. Brain Res. *87*, 201–211 (1975)

de Groat, W.C., Saum, W.R.: Sympathetic inhibition of the urinary bladder and of pelvic ganglionic transmission in the cat. J. Physiol. (Lond.) *220*, 297–314 (1972)

de Groat, W.C., Volle, R.L.: The actions of the catecholamines on the transmission in the superior cervical ganglion of the cat. J. Pharmacol. Exp. Ther. *154*, 1–13 (1966a)

de Groat, W.C., Volle, R.L.: Interactions between the catecholamines and ganglionic stimulating agents in sympathetic ganglia. J. Pharmacol. Exp. Ther. *154*, 200–215 (1966b)

del Castillo, J., Katz, B.: Quantal components of the end plate potential. J. Physiol. (Lond.) *124*, 560–573 (1954)

Dijl, W. van: Neuromuscular blocking agents. In: Side effects of drugs. Meyer, L., Herxheimer, A. (eds.), Vol. VII, pp. 209–223. Amsterdam: Excerpta Medica 1972

Dun, N., Nishi, S.: Effects of dopamine on the superior cervical ganglion of the rabbit. J. Physiol. (Lond.) *239*, 155–164 (1974)

Eccles, J.C.: The nature of synaptic transmission in a sympathetic ganglion. J. Physiol. (Lond.) *103*, 27–54 (1944)

Eccles, R.M., Libet, B.: Origin and blockade of the synaptic responses of curarized sympathetic ganglia. J. Physiol. (Lond.) *157*, 484–503 (1961)

Elfvin, L.-G.: Ultrastructural studies on the synaptology of the inferior mesenteric ganglion of the cat. J. Ultrastruct. Res. *37*, 411–425 (1971a)

Elfvin, L.-G.: Specialized serial neuronal contacts between preganglionic end fibres. J. Ultrastruct. Res. *37*, 426–431 (1971b)

Elfvin, L.-G.: The structure and distribution of the axodendritic and dendrodendritic contacts. J. Ultrastruct. Res. *37*, 432–448 (1971c)

Elmqvist, D., Quastel, D.M.S.: A quantitative study of end plate potentials in isolated human muscle. J. Physiol. (Lond.) *178*, 505–529 (1965)

Feldberg, W., Gaddum, J.H.: The chemical transmitter at synapses in a sympathetic ganglion. J. Physiol. (Lond.) *81*, 305–319 (1934)

Greengard, P., McAfee, D.A., Kebabian, J.W.: On the mechanism of action of cyclic AMP and its role in synaptic transmission. In: Advances in cyclic nucleotide research. Greengard, P., Robinson, G.A. (eds.), pp. 337–355. New York: Raven Press 1972

Grob, D.: Neuromuscular blocking drugs. In: Physiological pharmacology. Root, W.S., Hofman, F.G. (eds.), Vol. III/C, pp. 389–460. New York: Academic Press 1967

Guyton, A.C., Reeder, R.C.: Quantitative studies on the autonomic actions of curare. J. Pharmacol. Exp. Ther. *98*, 188–194 (1950)

Haefely, W.E.: Effects of catecholamines in the cat superior cervical ganglion and their postulated role as physiological modulators of ganglionic transmission. In: Progress in brain research, mechanisms of synaptic transmission. Akert, K., Waser, P.G. (eds.), pp. 61–72. Amsterdam: Elsevier 1969

Halasz, P., Mechler, F., Feher, O., Damjanovich, S.: The effect of SH-inhibitors on ganglionic transmission in the superior cervical ganglion of the cat. Acta Physiol. Hung. *18*, 47–55 (1960)

Hamberger, B., Norberg, K.-A.: Adrenergic synaptic terminals and nerve cells in bladder ganglia of the cat. Int. J. Neuropharmacol. *4*, 41–45 (1965)

Hancock, J.C., Volle, R.L.: Cholinoceptive sites in the rat superior cervical ganglion. Arch. Int. Pharmacodyn. *184*, 111–120 (1970)

Harvey, A.M.: The action of procaine on neuromuscular transmission. Bull. Johns Hopkins Hosp. *65*, 223–238 (1939)

Hilton, J.G.: The pressor response to neostigmine after ganglionic blockade. J. Pharmacol. Exp. Ther. *132*, 23–28 (1961)

Hirst, G.D.S., McKirdy, H.C.: Presynaptic inhibition at mammalian peripheral synapse? Nature (Lond.) *250*, 430–431 (1974)

Holaday, D.A., Kamijo, K., Koelle, G.B.: Facilitation of ganglionic transmission following inhibition of cholinesterase by DFP. J. Pharmacol. Exp. Ther. *111*, 241–254 (1954)

Jacobowitz, D.: Catecholamine fluorescence studies of adrenergic neurons and chromaffin cells in sympathetic ganglia. Fed. Proc. *29*, 1929–1944 (1970)

Kalix, P., McAfee, D.A., Schorderet, M., Greengard, P.: Pharmacological analysis of synaptically mediated increase in cyclic adenosine monophosphate in a rabbit superior cervical ganglion. J. Pharmacol. Exp. Ther. *188*, 676–687 (1974)

Kayaalp, S.O., McIsaac, R.J.: Effects of the adrenergic receptor blocking agents on the ganglionic transmission. Eur. J. Pharmacol. *7*, 264–269 (1969)

Kebabian, J.W., Greengard, P.: Dopamine-sensitive adenyl cyclase: possible role in synaptic transmission. Science *74*, 1346–1349 (1971)

Kebabian, J.W., Bloom, F.E., Steiner, A.L., Greengard, P.: Neurotransmitters increase cyclic nucleotides in postganglionic neurons: immunocytochemical demonstration. Science *190*, 157–159 (1975a)

Kebabian, J.W., Steiner, A.L., Greengard, P.: Muscarinic cholinergic regulation of cyclic guanosine 3′,5′-monophosphate in autonomic ganglia: possible role in synaptic transmission. J. Pharmacol. Exp. Ther. *193*, 474–488 (1975b)

Kharkevich, D.A.: Effects of the ganglion-blocking agents, Barbamyl and novocain on the development of post-activation facilitation in sympathetic ganglia. Farmakol. Toksikol. *β*, 493–499 (1959) (Russ.)

Kharkevich, D.A.: Effects of ganglion-blocking substances on the rate of conduction of nerve excitation in sympathetic ganglia. Byull. Eksp. Biol. Med. *3*, 61–64 (1960a) (Russ.)

Kharkevich, D.A.: Effects of ganglion-blocking substances on the after discharges. Byull. Eksp. Biol. Med. *6*, 62–66 (1960b) (Russ.)

Kharkevich, D.A.: Ganglion-blocking mechanism of novocain. Fiziol. Zh. S.S.S.R. *8*, 960–966 (1962a) (Russ.)

Kharkevich, D.A.: Gánglionic agents. Moskva: Medgiz 1962b (Russ.)

Kharkevich, D.A.: Ganglion-blocking and ganglion-stimulating agents. Oxford: Pergamon Press 1967 (translated from Russian edition, 1962)

Kharkevich, D.A, Tishchenko, M.I.: Effect of novocain on pessimal inhibition in different links of the reflex arc. Byull. Eksp. Biol. Med. *10*, 72–77 (1957) (Russ.)

Kobayashi, H., Libet, B.: Actions of noradrenaline and acetylcholine on sympathetic ganglion cells. J. Physiol. (Lond.) *208*, 353–372 (1970)

Koelle, G.B.: Cytological distributions and physiological functions of cholinesterases. In: Cholinesterases and anticholinesterase agents. Koelle, G.B. (ed.), pp. 187–298. Berlin, Heidelberg, New York: Springer 1963

Koelle, G.B., Davis, R., Koelle, W.A., Smyrl, E.G., Fine, A.V.: The electron microscopic localisation of acetylcholinesterase and pseudocholinesterase in autonomic ganglia. In: Cholinergic mechanisms. Waser, P.G. (ed.), pp. 251–255. New York: Raven Press 1975

Koelle, W.A., Koelle, G.B.: The localisation of external or functional acetylcholinesterase at the synapses of autonomic ganglia. J. Pharmacol. Exp. Ther. 126, 1–8 (1959)

Koketsu, K., Minota, S.: The direct action of adrenaline on the action potentials of bullfrog's (Rana catesbeiana) sympathetic ganglion cells. Experientia 31, 822–823 (1975)

Komalahiranya, A., Volle, R.L.: Actions of inorganic ions and veratrine on asynchronous post-ganglionic discharge in sympathetic ganglia treated with diisopropyl-phosphorofluoridate (DFP). J. Pharmacol. Exp. Ther. 138, 57–65 (1962)

Komalahiranya, A., Volle, R.L.: Alterations of transmission in sympathetic ganglia treated with a sulfhydryl group inhibitor, N-ethyl-maleimide (NEM). J. Pharmacol. Exp. Ther. 139, 304–311 (1963)

Kosterlitz, H.W., Lees, G.M., Wallis, D.I.: Resting and action potentials recorded by the sucrose-gap method in the superior cervical ganglion of the rabbit. J. Physiol. (Lond.) 195, 39–53 (1968)

Krstic, M.K.: The action of isoprenaline on the superior cervical ganglion of the cat. Neuropharmacology 10, 643–647 (1971)

Kuno, M.: Quantum aspects of central and ganglionic synaptic transmission in vertebrates. Physiol. Rev. 51, 647–678 (1971)

Laverty, R., Sharman, D.F.: The estimation of small quantities of 3,4-dihydroxyphen-ylethylamine in tissues. Br. J. Pharmacol. 24, 538–548 (1965)

Libet, B.: Generation of slow inhibitory and excitatory postsynaptic potentials. Fed. Proc. 29, 1945–1956 (1970)

Libet, B., Kobayashi, H.: Adrenergic mediation of slow inhibitory postsynaptic potential in sympathetic ganglia of the frog. J. Neurophysiol. 37, 805–814 (1974)

Libet, B., Tosaka, T.: Dopamine as a synaptic transmitter and modulator in sympathetic ganglia: a different mode of synaptic action. Proc. Natl. Acad. Sci. USA 67, 667–673 (1970)

Long, J.P., Eckstein, J.W.: Ganglionic actions of neostigmine methylsulfate. J. Pharmacol. Exp. Ther. 133, 216–222 (1961)

Lundberg, A.: Adrenaline and transmission in the sympathetic ganglion of the cat. Acta Physiol. Scand. 26, 252–263 (1952)

Marrazzi, A.S.: Electrical studies on the pharmacology of autonomic synapses. II. The action of a sympathomimetic drug (epinephrine) on sympathetic ganglia. J. Pharmacol. 65, 395–404 (1939)

Mason, D.F.J.: A ganglion stimulating action of neostigmine. Br. J. Pharmacol. 18, 76–86 (1962a)

Mason, D.F.J.: Depolarising action of neostigmine at an autonomic ganglion. Br. J. Pharmacol. 18, 572–587 (1962b)

Matthews, E.K.: The effects of choline and other factors on the release of acetylcholine from the stimulated perfused superior cervical ganglion of the cat. Br. J. Pharmacol. 21, 244–249 (1963)

Matthews, M., Raisman, G.: The ultrastructure and somatic efferent synapses of small granule-containing cells in the superior cervical ganglion. J. Anat. 105, 255–282 (1969)

Matthews, R.J.: The effect of epinephrine, levarterenol, and diisoproterenol on transmission in the superior cervical ganglion of the cat. J. Pharmacol. Exp. Ther. 116, 433–443 (1956)

McAfee, D.A., Greengard, P.: Adenosine 3′,5′-monophosphate: electrophysiological evidence for a role in synaptic transmission. Science 178, 310–312 (1972)

McAfee, D.A., Schorderet, M., Greengard, P.: Adenosine 3′,5′-monophosphate in nervous tissue: increase associated with synaptic transmission. Science 171, 1156–1158 (1971)

McIsaac, R.J.: Ganglionic blocking properties of epinephrine and related amines. Int. J. Neuropharmacol. 5, 15–26 (1966)

McIsaac, R.J., Koelle, G.B.: Comparison of the effects of inhibition of external, internal, and total acetylcholinesterase upon ganglionic transmission. J. Pharmacol. Exp. Ther. 126, 8–20 (1959)

McKinstry, D.N., Koelle, G.B.: Acetylcholine release from the cat superior cervical ganglion by carbachol. J. Pharmacol. Exp. Ther. 157, 319–327 (1967)

McKinstry, D.N., Koenig, E., Koelle, W.A., Koelle, G.B.: The release of acetylcholine from a sympathetic ganglion by carbachol. Relationship to the functional significance of the localisation of acetylcholinesterase. Can. J. Biochem. Physiol. 41, 2599–2609 (1963)

Nakamura, M., Koketsu, K.: The effect of adrenaline on sympathetic ganglion cells of bullfrog. Life Sci. *11*, 1165–1173 (1972)

Nilson, R., Volle, R.L.: Blockade by cadmium (Cd^{++}) of transmitter release at the frog neuromuscular junction. Fed. Proc. *35*, 696 (1976)

Nishi, S., Koketsu, K.: Origin of ganglionic inhibitory postsynaptic potential. Life Sci. *6*, 2049–2056 (1967)

Nishi, S., Koketsu, K.: Analysis of slow inhibitory postsynaptic potential of bullfrog sympathetic ganglion. J. Neurophysiol. *31*, 717–728 (1968)

Nishi, S., North, F.A.: Intracellular recording from myenteric plexus of the guinea-pig ileum. J. Physiol. (Lond.) *231*, 471–491 (1973)

Ostberg, A.: Granule-containing cells of the inferior mesenteric ganglion. Proc. Aust. Phys. Pharmacol. Soc. *1*, 1 (1970)

Ogston, A.G.: Removal of acetylcholine from a limited volume by diffusion. J. Physiol. (Lond.) *128*, 222–223 (1955)

Otten, U., Mueller, R.A., Oesch, F., Thoenen, H.: Location of an isoproterenol responsive cyclic AMP pool in adrenergic nerve cell bodies and its relationship to tyrosine 3-monooxygenase induction. Proc. Natl. Acad. Sci. USA *71*, 2217–2221 (1974)

Pardo, E.G., Cato, J., Gigon, E., Alonso-de-Florida, F.: Influence of several adrenergic drugs on synaptic transmission through the superior cervical and the ciliary ganglia of the cat. J. Pharmacol. Exp. Ther. *139*, 296–303 (1963)

Paton, W.D.M.: Pharmacology of curare and curarising substances. J. Pharm. Pharmacol. *1*, 273–286 (1949)

Paton, W.D.M., Thompson, J.W.: The mechanism of action of adrenaline on the superior cervical ganglion of the cat. Abstr. XIX Int. Physiol. Congress 664–665 (1953)

Perry, W.L.M.: Acetylcholine release in the cat's superior cervical ganglion. J. Physiol. (Lond.) *119*, 439–454 (1953)

Randall, L.O., Jampolsky, L.M.: Pharmacology of drugs affecting skeletal muscle. Am. J. Phys. Med. *32*, 102–105 (1953)

Rybolovlev, S.R.: Curare-like action of Ditylin (di-acetylcholine). Farmakol. Toksikol. *6*, 30–38 (1952) (Russ.)

Sacchi, O., Perri, W.: Quantal release of acetylcholine from the nerve endings of the guinea pig superior cervical ganglion. Pflügers Arch. *329*, 207–219 (1971)

Takeshige, C., Volle, R.L.: Cholinoceptive sites in denervated sympathetic ganglia. J. Pharmacol. Exp. Ther. *141*, 206–213 (1963a)

Takeshige, C., Volle, R.L.: Asychronous postganglionic firing from the cat superior cervical sympathetic ganglion treated with neostigmine. Br. J. Pharmacol. *20*, 214–220 (1963b)

Takeshige, C., Volle, R.L.: Bimodal response of sympathetic ganglia to acetylcholine following eserine or repetitive preganglionic stimulation. J. Pharmacol. Exp. Ther. *138*, 66–73 (1963c)

Takeshige, C., Pappano, A.J., de Groat, W.C., Volle, R.L.: Ganglionic blockade produced in sympathetic ganglia by cholinomimetic drugs. J. Pharmacol. Exp. Ther. *141*, 333–342 (1963)

Volle, R.L.: The responses to ganglionic stimulating and blocking drugs of cell groups within a sympathetic ganglion. J. Pharmacol. Exp. Ther. *135*, 54–71 (1962a)

Volle, R.L.: The actions of several ganglion blocking agents on the postganglionic discharge induced by diisopropyl phosphorofluoridate (DFP) in sympathetic ganglia. J. Pharmacol. Exp. Ther. *135*, 45–53 (1962b)

Volle, R.L.: Modification by drugs of synaptic mechanisms in autonomic ganglia. Pharmacol. Rev. *18*, 839–869 (1966)

Volle, R.L.: Cellular pharmacology of autonomic ganglia. In: Cellular pharmacology of excitable tissues. Narahashi, T. (ed.), pp. 89–140. Springfield: Charles C Thomas 1975

Volle, R.L., Koelle, G.B.: The physiological role of AChE in sympathetic ganglia. J. Pharmacol. Exp. Ther. *133*, 223–240 (1961)

Volle, R.L., Koelle, G.B.: Ganglionic stimulating and blocking agents. In: The pharmacological basis of therapeutics, 5th Ed. Goodman, L.S., Gilman, A. (eds.), pp. 565–574. New York: The Macmillan Company 1975

Weight, F.F., Padjen, A.: Slow synaptic inhibition: evidence for synaptic inactivation of sodium conductance in sympathetic ganglion cells. Brain Res. *55*, 219–224 (1973a)

Weight, F.F., Padjen, A.: Acetylcholine and slow synpatic inhibition in frog sympathetic ganglion cells. Brain Res. *55*, 225–228 (1973b)

Weir, M.C.L., McLennan, H.: The action of catecholamines in sympathetic ganglia. Can. J. Biochem. *41*, 2627–2636 (1963)

Williams, T.H., Palay, S.L.: Ultrastructure of the small neurons in the superior cervical ganglion. Brain Res. *15*, 17–34 (1969)

Williams, T.H., Black, jr., A.C., Chiba, T., Bhalla, R.C.: Morphology and biochemistry of small, intensely fluorescent cells of sympathetic ganglia. Nature (Lond.) *256*, 315–317 (1975)

Zaimis, E.: Actions at autonomic ganglia. In: Cholinesterases and anticholinesterase agents. Koelle, G.B. (ed.), pp. 530–569. Berlin, Heidelberg, New York: Springer 1963

Zipf, H.F., Dittmann, E.Ch.: General pharmacological effects of local anaesthetics. In: Local anaesthetics. Lechat, P. (ed.), pp 191–238. Oxford: Pergamon Press 1972

CHAPTER 13

Ganglionic Activity of Cardiovascular Drugs

D.M. Aviado

A. Introduction

Since the major use of ganglion-blocking drugs is in the treatment of cardiovascular disease, it is necessary to discuss the interaction between these blocking drugs and cardiovascular drugs. This section will examine three form of pharmacological actions and interactions: *first*, the effect of cardiovascular drugs on the autonomic ganglia; *second*, the influence of ganglionic blockade on the haemodynamic action of cardiovascular drugs; and *third*, the influence of cardiovascular drugs on the hypotensive action of ganglion-blocking drugs.

This section covers several categories of cardiovascular drugs, specifically *antihypertensives* which includes adrenergic blocking agents and diuretics, *vasoconstrictors* such as angiotensin and norepinephrine, and *cardiotropic drugs*, both cardiotonic and antifibrillatory. The available information is not uniform and may be complete for some drugs, i.e., guanethidine, but incomplete for others, i.e., digitalis and quinidine. It is necessary to examine the ganglionic effects of cardiovascular agents that are widely used in therapeutics.

B. Antihypertensive Drugs

Prior to the introduction of adrenergic neurone-blocking drugs, the ganglion-blocking drugs were widely used for the treatment of essential hypertension. It became apparent that the use of ganglion blockade to produce vasodilatation had to be supplemented with diuretics and this practice has continued into current use of adrenergic neurone blockade.

It is reasonable to question whether the diuretics exert any ganglionic blockade, thus enhancing the vasodilator action of the antihypertensive drugs. There is no information on ganglionic effects of the thiazide diuretics. A less widely used diuretic, amiloride, was observed by Jaramillo and Volle (1969) to block transmission in the superior cervical ganglia of cat. The blockade is of a different nature from that produced by either hexamethonium or atropine, and it is not possible to relate these observations to the question of interaction between diuretics and ganglionic blockade.

I. Reserpine

In 1967, Trendelenburg reviewed the effects of reserpine on ganglionic transmission. On the basis of results obtained by various investigators, he concluded that depletion of ganglionic norepinephrine by reserpine has failed to provide any evidence for a modulatory role of endogenous norepinephrine on ganglionic transmission (see also Chap. 12, this volume).

Investigations of the ganglionic effects of reserpine have taken a new turn during the past decade. Mueller et al. (1970) administered reserpine to rats and observed an increase in tyrosine hydroxylase activity in the superior cervical ganglion and adrenal medulla. The increase in enzyme activity is believed to be caused by a reflex increase in preganglionic activity. Joh and his collaborators (1973) further observed that there was an accumulation of the enzyme protein rather than activation of pre-existing enzyme molecules to explain the increase in tyrosine hydroxylase activity in the sympathetic ganglia and adrenal medulla.

The above observations raise the following question that has been overlooked. Is it possible that the primary action of ganglion-blocking drugs is the interference in the acetylcholine-mediated increase of tyrosine hydroxylase activity? Since this enzyme catalyses the rate-limiting step in the biosynthesis of catecholamines, the end result of ganglion-blocking drugs, as well as of reserpine, is a reduction in norepinephrine in the adrenergic neurone controlling vasomotor tone. Experimental support is needed for this suggestion, and could be obtained by techniques described in the next paragraph. Thus far, Black and Green (1973) have noted a depletion of tyrosine hydroxylase activity in neonatal animals treated with chlorianclamine.

II. Guanethidine

By histochemical, chemical, and neurophysiological techniques, Juul (1973a,b) and his collaborators (Jensen-Holm and Juul, 1970; Downing and Juul, 1973; Juul and McIsaac, 1973; Juul and Sand, 1973) have characterised the effect of chronic administration of guanethidine as depletion of norepinephrine in the superior cervical ganglia. There was inactivation of the majority of the ganglion cells but no complete blockade of impulse transmission.

Complete degeneration of sympathetic ganglia was observed following chronic administration of guanethidine in newborn rats (Eranko and Eranko, 1971a,b; Burnstock et al., 1971), adult rats (Heath et al., 1973), and newborn mice (Angeletti et al., 1972). A cytotoxic action has also been demonstrated following the addition of guanethidine to tissue cultures of newborn rat and chicken embryo sympathetic ganglia (Heath et al., 1973; Hill et al., 1973). These observations are useful in the understanding of chemical sympathectomy. However, there has been no attempt to determine whether degeneration of the ganglia occurs in patients treated continuously with guanethidine. If ganglion-blocking drugs do not cause degeneration, a revival of the use of these drugs might be forthcoming.

C. Vasoconstrictors

When vasoconstrictors are used for the treatment of shock, the rise in blood pressure is modulated by the baroreceptor reflexes. The concurrent use of ganglion-blocking drugs would lead to interference with the baroreceptor reflexes, resulting in an increase in intensity of the hypertensive effect of such vasoconstrictor drugs as norepinephrine and angiotensin. These two examples have opposite effects on the sympathetic ganglia, i.e., blockade by norepinephrine and stimulation by angiotensin (see Chaps. 10 and 12, this volume).

I. Norepinephrine

During continuous infusion of norepinephrine in the treatment of shock, it is not possible to detect any sympathetic ganglionic blockade induced by norepinephrine, because of the intense vasoconstriction. However, the abrupt fall in blood pressure after discontinuation of the infusion may be brought about, in part, by persistence of the ganglionic blockade caused by norepinephrine (AVIADO, 1970). It is difficult to prove that this is the primary mechanism of post-infusion shock, because of the alterations in blood volume, blood acidity, and electrolytes during the infusion norepinephrine.

II. Angiotensin

Although there has been a considerable amount of investigation on the ganglionic effects of angiotensin, opinion is still divided on questions that relate to the clinical use of this vasoconstrictor drug. The role of the ganglionic stimulatory action in achieving the hypertensive effect of angiotensin is variously believed to be a major one (FARR and GRUPP, 1967, 1971) and a minor one (REIT, 1972). Even the interaction between ganglion-blocking drugs and angiotensin has not been established. The importance of the blockade of reflexes has been ignored and instead, abnormality of vessel tone (HAMER and JACKSON, 1969) and plasma level of renin (SAMWER et al., 1974) have been proposed as the mechanism for interaction between ganglion blockade and angiotensin-induced hypertension.

D. Cardiotropic Drugs

There is a limited amount of information on the ganglionic effects of cardiotonic drugs. Although reserpine reduced ouabain toxicity in the dog, chlorisondamine did not influence it. These observations indicate that sympathetic denervation by the use of ganglion-blocking drugs does not influence the cardiac effects of digitalis (BOYASY and NASH, 1966). Other cardiotonic drugs, such as aminophylline and papaverine, cause depression of transmission in the superior cervical ganglion of cat (VARAGIC and ZUGIC, 1973). The last-named investigators interpret their results as consistent with the view that cyclic AMP may have a mediating role in the process of ganglionic transmission, as originally proposed by KEEN and MCLEAN (1972). However, KATO et al. (1974) have failed to demonstrate a release of adenine nucleotide from the isolated cervical ganglion of the cat, so that it is not yet possible to generalise that drugs which influence cyclic AMP in the heart influence ganglionic synapse by a common mechanism.

The effects of quinidine and procainamide on ganglionic transmission have not been elucidated. It is possible that their local anaesthetic action is behind the blockade of transmission if this is revealed by neurophysiological techniques. Another antifibrillatory agent, bretylium, exerts an effect characteristic of adrenergic neurone blockers (Barany and Treister, 1970; Caramia et al., 1972). There is no reason to suspect that cardiac depression, and more especially anti-arrhythmic activity, is characterised by a specific effect on ganglionic transmission. Additional research is needed to characterise the ganglionic effects of widely used cardiotropic drugs.

References

Angeletti, P.U., Levi-Montalcini, R., Caramia, F.: Structural and ultrastructural changes in developing sympathetic ganglia induced by guanethidine. Brain Res. *43*, 515–525 (1972)
Aviado, D.M.: Norepinephrine. In: Sympathomimetic drugs. Springfield: Thomas 1970
Barany, E.H., Treister, G.: Time relations of degeneration mydriasis and degeneration vasocon-striction in the rabbit ear after sympathetic denervation. Effect of bretylium. Acta Physiol. Scand. *80*, 79–92 (1970)
Black, I.B., Geen, S.C.: Trans-synaptic regulation of adrenergic neuron development: inhibition by ganglionic blockade. Brain Res. *63*, 291–302 (1973)
Boyajy, L.D., Nash, C.B.: Alteration of ouabain toxicity by cardiac denervation. Toxicol. Appl. Pharmacol. *9*, 199–208 (1966)
Burnstock, G., Evans, B., Gannon, B.J., Heath, J.W., James, V.: A new method of destroying adrenergic nerves in adult animals using guanethidine. Br. J. Pharmacol. *43*, 295–301 (1971)
Caramia, F., Angeletti, P.U., Levi-Montalcini, R., Carratelli, L.: Mitochondrial lesions of devel-oping sympathetic neurons induced by bretylium tosylate. Brain Res. *40*, 237–246 (1972)
Downing, O.A., Juul, P.: The effect of guanethidine pretreatment on transmission in the superior cervical ganglion. Acta Pharmacol. Toxicol. *32*, 369–381 (1973)
Eranko, L., Eranko, O.: Effect of guanethidine on nerve cells and small intensely fluorescent cells in sympathetic ganglia of newborn and adult rats. Acta Pharmacol. Toxicol. (Kbn) *30*, 403–416 (1971a)
Eranko, O., Eranko, L.: Histochemical evidence of chemical sympathectomy by guanethidine in newborn rats. Histochem. J. *3*, 451–456 (1971b)
Farr, W.C., Grupp, G.: Sympathetically mediated effects of angiotensin on the dog heart in situ. J. Pharmacol. Exp. Ther. *156*, 528–537 (1967)
Farr, W.C., Grupp, G.: Ganglionic stimulation: mechanism of the positive inotropic and chrono-tropic effects of angiotensin. J. Pharmacol. Exp. Ther. *177*, 48–55 (1971)
Hamer, J., Jackson, E.: The effect of ganglionic blockade on the pressor response to angiotensin in systemic hypertension. Cardiovasc. Res. *3*, 411–414 (1969)
Heath, J., Eranko, O., Eranko, L.: Effect of guanethidine on the ultrastructure of the small, granule-containing cells in cultures of rat sympathetic ganglia. Acta Pharmacol. Toxicol. (Kbn.) *33*, 209–218 (1973)
Hill, C.E., Mark, G.E., Eranko, O., Eranko, L., Burnstock, G.: Use of tissue culture to examine the actions of guanethidine and 6-hydroxydopamine. Eur. J. Pharmacol. *23*, 162–174 (1973)
Jaramillo, J., Volle, R.L.: Ganglionic blocking properties of the diuretic agent amiloride hy-drochloride. Arch. Int. Pharmacodyn. Ther. *177*, 298–310 (1969)
Jenson-Holm, J., Juul, P.: The effects of guanethidine, pre- and postganglionic nerve division on the rat superior cervical ganglion: cholinesterases and catecholamines (histochemistry), and histology. Acta Pharmacol. Toxicol. (Kbn.) *28*, 283–298 (1970)
Joh, T.H., Geghman, C., Reis, D.: Immunochemical demonstration of increased accumulation of tyrosine hydroxylase protein in sympathetic ganglia and adrenal medulla elicited by reser-pine. Proc. Natl. Acad. Sci. USA *70*, 2767–2771 (1973)
Juul, P.: Effects of various antihypertensive guanidine derivatives on the adult rat superior cervical ganglion: histology, ultrastructure, and cholinesterase histochemistry. Acta Pharma-col. Toxicol. (Kbn.) *32*, 500–512 (1973a)
Juul, P.: Accumulation of guanethidine by sympathetic ganglia of reserpinized rats. Acta Phar-macol. Toxicol. (Kbh.) *33*, 79–80 (1973b)
Juul, P., McIsaac, R.L.: The effect on guanethidine on the noradrenaline content of the adult rat superior cervical ganglion. Acta Pharmacol. Toxicol. (Kbh.) *32*, 382–389 (1973)

Juul, P., Sand, O.: Determination of guanethidine in sympathetic ganglia. Acta Pharmacol. Toxicol. (Kbh.) *32*, 487–499 (1973)

Kato, A.C., Katz, H.S., Collier, B.: Absence of adenine nucleotide release from autonomic ganglion. Nature *249*, 576–577 (1974)

Keen, P., McLean, W.G.: The effect of N^6, $O^{2'}$-dibutyryl adenosine $3':5'$-cyclic monophosphate on noradrenaline synthesis in isolated superior cervical ganglia. Br. J. Pharmacol. *46*, 529*P*-530*P* (1972)

Mueller, R.A., Thoenen, H., Axelrod, J.: Inhibition of neuronally induced tyrosine hydroxylase by nicotinic receptor blockade. Eur. J. Pharmacol. *10*, 51–56 (1970)

Reit, E.: Actions of angiotensin on the adrenal medulla and autonomic ganglia. Fed. Proc. *31*, 1338–1343 (1972)

Samwer, K.-F., Schreiber, M., Molzahn, M., Oelkers, W.: Pressor effect of angiotensin II in sodium replete and deplete rats. Relationship to plasma renin, plasma sodium, and hematocrit before and after ganglionic blockade. Pflügers Arch. *346*, 307–318 (1974)

Trendelenburg, U.: Some aspects of the pharmacology of autonomic ganglion cells. In: Reviews of physiology, biochemistry, and experimental pharmacology, Vol. 59. Berlin, Heidelberg, New York: Springer 1967

Varagic, V.M., Zugic, M.: The effect of N^6-2'-O-dibutyryl-3',5'-cyclic adenosine monophosphate, imidazole, and aminophylline on ganglionic transmission in the superior cervical ganglion of the cat. Br. J. Pharmacol. *49*, 407–414 (1973)

CHAPTER 14

Ganglion-Blocking Agents in Internal Medicine

E.V. ERINA

A. Introduction

The major therapeutic use of the ganglion-blocking agents is in the management of arterial hypertension. These were the first potent hypotensive drugs to be developed. Initially, tetraethylammonium chloride was used, but later other compounds were synthesised and used: hexamethonium, Pendiomid, pentapyrrolidinium (pentolinium), mecamylamine, chlorisondamine, pentamethylpiperidine (pempidine), pachycarpinum, nanophynum, diochinum, dicolinum, dimecolinum, ganglerone, and others (see KHARKEVICH, p. 1, for the structures and synonyms of Russian agents). Although the ganglion-blocking agents inhibit transmission in all the autonomic ganglia, the sensitivity of various ganglia to ganglion-blocking agents differs. The highest sensitivity is noticed in pathways of the autonomic system that are in a state of increased functional overexertion (PATON and ZAIMIS, 1952). Thus, in hypertension and some peripheral vascular diseases the sympathetic ganglia are the first to react and the vascular tone decreases; in patients with peptic ulcer the most sensitive ganglia are those of the parasympathetic nervous system, which controls the motor and secretory activity of the stomach. Therefore, ganglion-blocking agents are used in the treatment of different diseases connected with the disturbance of nervous regulation, when a decrease in the efferent impulse transmission to the organs may produce an expected therapeutic effect (in increased tone of the vascular and other smooth muscles, renal colic, causalgias, eclampsia, and also in surgery for the creation of controlled hypotension, etc.).

B. Ganglion-Blocking Agents in the Treatment of Hypertension

In the treatment of patients with essential hypertension the most commonly used ganglion-blocking agents (at the time of their wide use) were the bis-quaternary methonium compounds: hexamethonium (bromide, chloride, diiodide and benzosulphonate [benzohexonium]), pentamethonium bromide, Pendiomid (pentamin), pentapyrrolidinium bitartrate (pentolinium, Ansolysen). The last is 6–10 times as potent as hexamethonium and the duration of its action is longer (MAXWELL and CAMPBELL, 1953; SMIRK, 1953, FREIS et al., 1954). These ganglion-blocking agents are the strongest and most rapidly acting hypotensive agents. Their introduction into the treatment of hypertension changed the course of the most severe forms of arterial hypertension and reduced the mortality. After many months of treatment, in most patients (both those with benign and especially those with malignant hypertension) it was possible to decrease or prevent the development of left heart failure, reduce the incidence of uraemia, and generally improve the prognosis (SMIRK, 1952–1957; MORRISON, 1953; DOYLE and KILPATRIK, 1954; ARNOLD, 1965). All ganglion-blocking agents exhibit essentially the same pharmacological activities, the only differences being in the dosage levels required to produce an equivalent blood pressure reduction and different intestinal absorption after oral administration.

I. Haemodynamic Effects

The interruption of transmission in sympathetic ganglia decreases vascular tone (of the arterioles and veins) and results in a fall in blood pressure. A moderate decrease in peripheral vascular resistance is usually associated with a variable reduction of cardiac output as a consequence of diminished venous return (WERKÖ, 1951; GROB and LANGFORD, 1953; FREIS et al., 1953; GILMORE et al., 1952; VETTER, 1954; AVIADO, 1960). A fall in venous pressure (10–60 mm) may precede the reduction in blood pressure. Substantial falls in venous pressure may be noted in congestive heart failure (RESTALL and SMIRK, 1952; KELLEY et al., 1953; SMITH and FOWLER, 1955). The right heart and pulmonary pressures are reduced as a result of a decrease in venous return and marked peripheral pooling of blood in capacity vessels and a decrease in the active blood volume (FREIS et al., 1953; WERKÖ, 1951; REMMER, 1954). The fall in arterial pressure is therefore much influenced by posture, being greatest when the patient is standing, intermediate during sitting, and smallest in the lying position (RESTALL and SMIRK, 1950; SMIRK, 1954).

These changes depend on the interference with the capacity of the sympathetic nervous system to perform normal circulatory reflex functions (compensatory vasoconstriction). Thus, in the upright position the diminished adrenergic venomotor effect is enhanced by the gravitational effect of pooling in the more dependent areas of the body. In patients treated with ganglion-blocking agents an additional fall in blood pressure usually follows meals, presumably due to uncompensated splanchnic dilatation. More intense ganglion blockade is also noted following a haemorrhage, salt depletion, use of diuretics, or ingestion of alcohol, and during hot weather. Orthostatic hypotension persists longer than recumbent hypotension, and is a major problem in ambulatory patients. It is relieved to some extent by muscular activity. The influence of hexamethonium on the pulse rate is inconsistent, but perceptible hypotension is usually accompanied by mild tachycardia.

Haemodynamic investigations in different vascular beds in patients undergoing therapy with ganglion-blocking agents have yielded evidence that parenteral administration of 50–100 mg hexamethonium causes a slight increase in blood flow to the arms, and a marked increase in blood flow to the legs. The difference in the degree of vasodilatation may be due to the greater sympathetic vasoconstrictor tone in the legs than in the arms (SMIRK, 1954). This is followed by an elevation of skin temperature and volume of the extremities (RESTALL and SMIRK, 1952; SCHNAPPER et al., 1951).

Renal blood flow (RBF) and glomerular filtration rate (GFR) are often decreased at the beginning of treatment with ganglion-blocking agents especially in cases where there is a significant decrease of cardiac output and blood pressure. But in patients on long-term treatment with gradual and moderate reduction of blood pressure renal vascular resistance also decreases, while RBF usually increases without any alteration of GFR or tubular excretory capacity. Even in patients with malignant hypertension, improvements in renal function have been reported (SOKO-LOFF and SCHOTTSTAEDT, 1953; FORD et al., 1953; FREIS, 1953; RATNER and VADKOV-SKAYA, 1958; ERINA and MARTYANOVA, 1958). But sometimes the chronic hypotensive action of hexamethonium causes progressive renal insufficiency and uraemia (McQUEEN and TREWIN, 1952; ULLMANN and MENCZEL, 1956).

In hypertensive patients hexamethonium has been shown to reduce cerebrovascular resistance without significant alterations in cerebral blood flow if the blood pressure has fallen by less than 30%; these changes are favourable for cerebral haemodynamics in hypertension (HAFKENSHIEL et al., 1954; CRUMPTON and MUR-PHY, 1955). Changes in coronary blood flow are variable (AVIADO, 1960).

The principles of methonium treatment have been studied precisely and described by many authors, including SMIRK (1952–1957), FREIS et al. (1952–1957), McMICHAEL (1952), ERINA (1954–1965), and ZAMYSLOVA (1958). Reviewing the results of hexamethonium treatment for periods of up to $3\frac{1}{2}$ years in patients with very severe but potentially reversible hypertensive alterations, SMIRK (1952, 1954b, 1957) came to the definite conclusion that adequate though rarely perfect control of the blood pressure (i.e., decrease of blood pressure to a near-normal level for as much of the 24 h day as is practicable) is possible in almost all patients

II. Dosage of Methonium Compounds

The initial doses of methonium compounds (when given by subcutaneous or intramuscular injection), are usually 15–20 mg hexamethonium, 25–50 mg Pendiomid and 2.5–3 mg pentolinium tartrate. The antihypertensive effect develops within 10–30 min and persists for 2–6 h; injections are given three or four times per day. After every injection the patient is advised to stay lying down (or in a half-sitting position) for about 2 h to prevent marked orthostatic hypotension. A moderate degree of postural hypotension should be considered a positive phenomenon rather than a side effect, because it prolongs the action of each injection. But an excessive decrease of blood pressure is occasionally accompanied by dizziness and weakness. Postural faintness is easily overcome by lying down when such symptoms arise.

Repeated administration of parenteral or oral doses of methonium compounds leads to the development of drug tolerance. Accordingly, as much as a tenfold increase in dose may eventually be necessary to obtain the result initially observed. The dose of hexamethonium should be raised daily or every few days by small increments of 5–10 mg until an effective dose is reached (with careful monitoring of the immediate response). We consider it unnecessary to use single doses of more than 100 mg hexamethonium (daily dose up to 400 mg), because it is now used in combination with modern active drugs that make it possible to use minimal doses of ganglion-blocking agents. SMIRK (1953, 1954b) reported the use of doses of over 400 mg hexamethonium three times daily for long periods without trouble. With the development of pentolinium such large doses became unnecessary.

The duration of the reduction in blood pressure is much prolonged when hexamethonium or pentolinium is dissolved in colloid solutions of dextran 20% or polyvinylpyrrolidone 20–25% to which 0.5% ephedrine hydrochloride has been added (Fig. 1) to prolong absorption further by local vasoconstriction (MASINI and

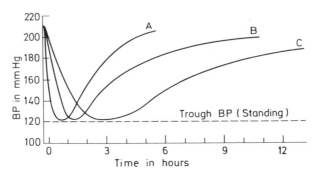

Fig. 1. Influence of ganglion-blocking agents on arterial pressure. *Line A* indicates the approximate course of the blood pressure fall after subcutaneous injections of aqueous solutions of pentamethonium and hexamethonium and after oral doses given on an empty stomach. *Line B* represents the action of hexamethonium dissolved in 20% polyvinylpyrrolidone with the addition of 0.5% ephedrine hydrochloride, or of simple aqueous solution of pentolinium. *Line C* represents the effect of a subcutaneous injection of pentolinium dissolved in 20% polyvinylpyrrolidone or of oral doses of pentolinium (SMIRK, F.H.: Am. J. Med. 1954, *17*, 844)

ROSSI, 1951; SMIRK, 1953). This made it possible to control the blood pressure level by two injections 12-h apart. In the course of treatment marked diurnal variations of blood pressure tend to become less pronounced. They are particularly dangerous in patients with severe hypertension complicated by cerebrovascular, renal, or coronary insufficiency. As shown in Fig. 2, during one initial period of treatment a marked hypotensive response lasted nearly 5 h, while at the end of the second week it was considerably longer; the blood pressure measured in the sitting position is maintained at a normal level throughout the day. The adjustment of dosage is exceedingly important and is best accomplished in a hospital setting. The highest response to a single dose is usually observed in the morning, and the morning dose is therefore sometimes lower than those given at other times. The duration of action of evening doses has been insufficient in some patients, who required an additional injection at night to lower the blood pressure while they were supine. In these cases

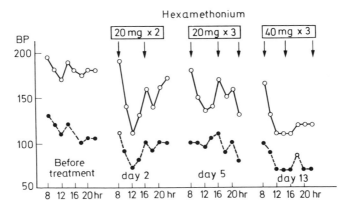

Fig. 2. Daily changes in blood pressure following injections of hexamethonium. *Solid line*, systolic blood pressure; *broken line*, diastolic blood pressure. The arrows indicate the times of injections

the morning orthostatic hypotension was not so extreme (AGREST and HOOBLER, 1955).

In some patients with malignant hypertension hexamethonium was given by continuous intravenous infusion for 6–12 days. An effective reduction of the blood pressure was thus maintained, with levels very near to normal, and papilloedema and retinal changes disappeared much faster than with the intermittent reductions in blood pressure when three subcutaneous injections were administered (SMIRK, 1954 b, 1957 a).

III. Results of Treatment

Effective treatment with hexamethonium (or other ganglion-blocking agents) involving reduction of the blood pressure to normal or individually optimal levels leads to subjective improvement and relief of the main clinical manifestations. Hypertensive headaches are substantially, often completely, relieved and dizziness, dyspnoea, and attacks of cardiac asthma usually disappear within a week (SMIRK, 1953, 1954 a). Electrocardiographic improvement is often present after 2–3 months of treatment and continues for up to one year or longer (DOYLE, 1953). Excessive vasoconstriction of retinal arteries usually disappears. Retinal haemorrhages, oedema, and soft exudates generally clear rapidly. Star-shaped macular figures and papilloedema seldom disappear with less than 3 months of intensive treatment, and may take 12 months. The results were especially striking in patients with malignant hypertension and retinal grades III or IV with encephalopathy. Even short periods of adequate control over blood pressure levels (3–6 months) were beneficial for a substantial majority of patients (especially those with shorter histories of hypertension). Considerable relief from overloading of the cardiovascular system facilitated the disappearance of complications of hypertension and prevented progression of morphological alterations of arterioles thus improving the course and prognosis of the disease (SMIRK and ALSTAD, 1951; SMIRK, 1953966); MORRISON, 1953; DOYLE and KILPATRIK, 1954; ERINA, 1954–1973; DUKHINA, 1963.

Treatment with ganglion-blocking agents is most effective in patients with hypertensive heart failure and cardiac asthma. A decrease in peripheral vascular resistance and right heart pressure resulting from a decrease of venous return facilitates cardiac performance and leads to an improvement in myocardial contractility. In patients with congestive heart failure, ganglionic blockade frequently results in increased cardiac output, without any substantial increase in left vertricular work (FREIS et al., 1953; WILSON and KEELY, 1953; SMITH and FOWLER, 1955; VINOGRADOV and TSIBEKMAKHER, 1966). A direct positive inotropic effect on the myocardium has been demonstrated for hexamethonium, and this may contribute to the increased cardiac output of the decompensated heart (LEE and SHIDEMAN, 1959; VOLLE and KOELLE, 1970). Decreases in heart size may be striking (SMIRK, 1954 a,b). A simultaneous acceleration of blood flow and improvement of external respiration lead to a better oxygen saturation of arterial blood (MALOVA, 1964).

The favourable action of hexamethonium is probably connected with a retention of adrenergic mediators in the tissues, mainly noradrenaline stores in the heart. This is extremely useful in patients with stage II and III hypertension, especially those with atherosclerosis and cardiac insufficiency, in whom the synthesis and metabolism of catecholamines is reduced (KISELEVA, 1968). An increased amount of labelled noradrenaline-H_3 was found by HERTTING et al. (1962) and FRANTSUZOVA (1965) in the heart following hexamethonium administration. This may improve metabolic processes in the myocardium. In patients with congestive heart failure that has persisted during digitalis medication, the addition of ganglion-blocking drugs usually leads to correction of the failure, probably due to the salutary effect of diminished blood pressure. In addition, ganglion-blocking agents prevent negative influences of cardiac glycosides on the excitability of the myocardium (GATSURA and BANDURINA, 1965).

There is evidence that hypertensive patients with coronary insufficiency can experience significant reductions in anginal pain. But excessive falls of blood pressure during the initial period of treatment may occasionally precipitate precordial pain (SMIRK and ALSTAD, 1951; STÜBINGER and KOCH, 1952; DOYLE and KILPATRIK, 1954; SMIRK, 1954a, 1957; ERINA, 1958, 1973; RUBANOVSKY, 1961).

In the treatment of coronary insufficiency, other ganglion-blocking agents have been favoured by some authors – ganglerone[1] and Quateronum[2] (DAVIDOVSKY, 1959; AVAKYAN et al., 1966; MNATSAKANOV et al., 1967). Several observers comment that these drugs (and pentamine) possess not only a vasodilatory but also an anticoagulant effect: they increase the activity of heparin and fibrinolytic activity, and prolong the time of blood coagulation (AGHINA et al., 1954; POSHKUS, 1960).

Ganglerone has been shown to be effective in the treatment of patients with a syndrome of coronary atherosclerosis and cardiac pain complicated by trunkitis and ganglionitis; in these cases it is used intramuscularly (1–2 ml per 1.5% solution twice daily), orally (40 mg three or four times daily), and by means of electrophoresis on the cervical and thoracic vertebral areas (SOROKINA, 1966).

IV. CNS Effects

The methonium ganglion-blocking agents undoubtedly have an influence on the functional state of the central nervous system (CNS) although they do not readily reach the CNS via the blood brain barrier. A sedative effect often occurs soon after injections of Pendiomide and hexamethonium. Electroencephalographic studies yielded evidence of a slowing in the α-rhythms and an increase of their amplitude 10–15 min after intramuscular injections of medium therapeutic doses (50–80 mg) of Pendiomid; 30–45 min later a decrease in the amplitude of ECG waves and further slowing of the α-rhythm was observed (IVANNIKOVA, 1956; ERINA and MARTYANOVA, 1958). Alterations of the functional state of the CNS can be explained not only by a temporary interruption of efferent impulses and changes of afferent neural impulses (from the heart, vessels, and mechanoreceptors), but also by an improvement in cerebral circulation. A number of authors have shown that relief of persistently increased vasoconstriction is usually accompanied by an intensive removal of fluid from the tissues into the intravascular space and an increase in plasma volume. Improvements in metabolic processes in the brain in the presence of insignificant

---

1 γ-Diethylamino-1,2-dimethylpropyl-p-isobutoxybenzoate hydrochloride or α,β-dimethyl-γ-diethylaminopropyl-p-isobutoxybenzoate
2 α,β-Dimethyl-γ-diethylamino-p-butoxybenzoate iodide

increases of cerebral blood flow have been reported (REMMER, 1954; HAFKENSCHIEL, 1954; LEBEDEVA et al., 1965).

Obviously, it is the decrease of cerebral oedema, hypoxia, and dystrophic changes in the brain that enhances a rapid disappearance of hypertensive encephalopathy, regression of papilloedema and retinal oedema, and also a decrease in intraocular pressure in patients with glaucoma (CAMERON, 1951; SMIRK, 1953–1957; ERINA, 1954). Favourable alterations of the psychological status in hypertensive patients with cerebrovascular atherosclerosis and depression have been noted (BOYARIN-TSEVA and MIRONENKO, 1963). Such an effect may be caused by a delay in the release of catecholamines and storage of increased amounts of these substances in the CNS.

It would be a simplification to consider the therapeutic and antihypertensive effects of methonium compounds only as a result of reduction in vascular tone or cardiac output. The action of these drugs must be regarded as a widespread influence on the whole nervous system. Ganglion-blocking agents decrease not only the activity of the sympathetic nervous system, catecholamine biosynthesis in the adrenal medulla, and release of transmitter substances in nerve endings (ZHUKOVA, 1965), but also the activity of the adrenal cortex, mainly the aldosterone secretion (LARAGH, 1960; GERASIMOVA, 1964; MILOSLAVSKY et al., 1971).

One can accept that a long-term treatment leads to a profound inhibition and abolition of numerous reflex neurohumoral reactions and sympathetically mediated vasomotor reflexes involved in the pathological process. Perhaps because of this, in a number of patients with malignant hypertension who received intensive treatment for 2–3 years (later in combination with reserpine), not only a substantial ameliora-tion of hypertension, but even a normalisation of blood pressure persisting after discontinuation of the treatment was noted (Bos et al., 1953; SMIRK, 1954a–1966; ERINA, 1958–1973; ZAMYSLOVA, 1958; PAGE and DUSTAN, 1962; ARNOLD, 1965).

V. Effects on the Endocrine System

Ganglionic blockade and inhibition of adrenergic function result in certain alter-ations of the endocrine system and different aspects of metabolism: they inhibit the function of the thyroid gland, and increase sensitivity to insulin in patients with diabetes mellitus (BRESLAVSKY and VYAZOVSKAYA, 1961). Cases of excessive falls in blood glucose (up to 45–50 mg%) in some elderly patients with essential hyperten-sion have been reported (DRACHEVA, 1965). Experimental studies have shown a temporary increase in the areas of the pancreatic β-cells (VYAZOVSKAYA, 1965).

VI. Undesirable Side Effects

Treatment with ganglion-blocking agents is often accompanied by side effects caused by widespread actions on the autonomic nervous system. Among the mildest unto-ward responses observed to arise from parasympathetic blockade are visual distur-bances (mydriasis, difficulty in accommodation), dry mouth, moderate constipation, occasional diarrhoea, and nausea. These effects tend to become less pronounced when the dosage of drugs is reduced, with regular use of laxatives to produce a daily bowel movement, or following the administration of cholinomimetic (carbachol etc.) or anticholinesterase agents. More severe reactions include marked atonic constipation, paralytic ileus, and urinary retention. They can be relieved by injections of neostigmine.

Excessive sympathetic blockade sometimes causes severe postural hypotension. In some patients syncope may occur without warning symptoms, and collapse may be profound. Several cases of catastrophic falls in blood pressure complicated by coronary thrombosis or cerebral accidents were described when large doses of methonium compounds were injected without adequate monitoring and adjustment of dosage (Locket, 1951; Smirk, 1957). Decreased potency was frequent in male patients. During prolonged methonium treatment of severely hypertensive patients an unexpected pulmonary type of dyspnoea associated with radiological changes in the lungs may occur; the pulmonary lesion (organised fibrinous oedema) is thought to be secondary to attacks of left heart failure, modified by intermittent hypotension (Morrison, 1953; Doniach et al., 1954; Peterson et al., 1959; Volle and Koelle, 1970).

VII. Oral Dosage of Methonium Preparations

Various methonium preparations have been used orally but their hypotensive effect was less constant. Effective control of blood pressure was achieved only in one-quater to one-half the patients (Campbell et al., 1952; Moyer et al., 1953; Smirk, 1954–1957; Freis et al., 1954; Waldman, 1956). This involves serious difficulties in adjustment of the dosage. The absorption of methonium compounds from the intestine is incomplete and irregular (only about 10% of each dose). Absorption can occasionally be considerably increased in patients with delayed gastric emptying, when two or three doses may be retained in the stomach and then suddenly enter the duodenum. Decreased absorption was described in patients with congestive heart failure and intestinal oedema (Milne and Oleesky, 1951; Walker et al., 1954; Volle and Koelle, 1970). The initial oral doses of hexamethonium (100–200 mg) were gradually increased by a titration method to 500–750 mg three or four times daily. In comparison, average daily doses of pentolinium varied from 60 to 600 mg. Undesirable symptoms of parasympathetic blockade are encountered in most patients and they often limit the therapeutic efficacy of ganglion-blocking agents. Therefore, most clinicians prefer parenteral administration of ganglion-blocking agents in situations when a rapid reduction of blood pressure is necessary, although this type of treatment also involves difficulties.

Since 1955, ganglion-blocking agents have been used in combination with rauwolfia preparations and hydralazine. Before the advent of guanethidine and thiazide diuretics this combination was considered the method of choice in the treatment of severe and progressive forms of hypertension (essential and renal). All antihypertensive drugs, by virtue of their additive effects, permit the use of a lower dosage of the ganglion-blocking agents and thereby reduce the untoward responses. Reserpine diminishes constipation due to its augmentation of motor activity of the gastrointestinal tract. Combined treatment allows better control over the blood pressure level with less variation throughout the day.

VIII. Other Ganglion-Blocking Agents for Oral Use

Among other ganglion-blocking agents for oral use, mecamylamine (a secondary amine) and pempidine (a tertiary amine) and its analogue pirilenum[3] are the most effective in reducing blood pressure. A large amount of information concerning the successful treatment of hypertensive patients with these drugs is available (SMIRK and McQUEEN, 1957b; MOYER et al., 1957; HARRINGTON et al., 1958; KITCHIN et al., 1960; LEBEDEV, 1963; NOVIKOVA, 1963; VYSHINSKAYA, 1963; GERMANOV et al., 1963; SAZONOVA, 1965; DRACHEVA et al., 1962–1965; ERINA, 1965, 1973). Their main advantage over methonium compounds is a better gastrointestinal absorption, so that they have a more constant and prolonged hypotensive effect; the development of tolerance to the drug is much less pronounced than with hexamethonium. After oral administration of mean therapeutic doses, 63–76% of the drug is excreted in a day by the kidneys, and when renal function is impaired only 25–37% (HARRINGTON et al., 1958). Pempidine and mecamylamine penetrate the blood-brain barrier and produce inhibiting effects on the central nicotinic receptors (STONE et al., 1956; CORNE and EDGE, 1958; SPINKS et al., 1958; HARRINGTON et al., 1958). Occasionally, tremor and mental confusion have been encountered during long-term treatment with mecamylamine (HARRINGTON and KINCAID-SMITH, 1958; VOLLE and KOELLE, 1970).

The initial dose of pirilenum is usually 2.5 mg, and the average daily doses vary from 7.5 to 60 mg. A decrease in blood pressure usually occurs within 1–2 h after administration of pirilenum and the duration of action is 4–12 h. A more constant hypotensive effect with only minimal side effects was achieved with the combination of pirilenum with reserpine and hypothiazide in patients with severe hypertension (ERINA, 1965).

Unlike those of hexamethonium and even pempidine tartrate, the side effects encountered during treatment with pirilenum are frequently not caused by parasympathetic inhibition, but arise from a relative predominance of parasympathetic activity resulting from a mainly sympathoplegic action of pirilenum when larger doses of pirilenum were used. Abdominal distension in the epigastrium, pylorospasm and increased gastric secretion, occasional vomiting (during the night only), and spastic constipation were observed. At the same time marked bradycardia, orthostatic hypotension and such symptoms as dry mouth and disturbances of vision were noted. The above-mentioned symptoms were abolished by an injection of atropine. Proserine (neostigmine) and carbachol did not relieve them. The milder side effects easily cleared after the omission of one or two doses of pirilenum (ERINA, 1965). Our clinical observations are in agreement with the experimental data reported by pharmacologists who have found that pempidine and pirilenum can cause spastic contractions of the gastric cardia and stimulate intestinal motility (CORNE and EDGE, 1958; SHARAPOV, 1963).

In our experience, pirilenum can be very useful in the treatment of patients with spontaneous marked variations of the blood pressure throughout the day and high levels only in the early evening. These rises of pressure can be lowered by a single dose of pirilenum (2.5–5 mg) given in the afternoon (about 2–4 p.m.). The delayed effect of pirilenum allows its use in patients with cerebral and coronary atherosclero-

---

3 1,2,2,6,6,-Pentamethyl-piperidine-*p*-toluolsulphonate (Pempidine tosylate).

sis (DRACHEVA, 1965; ERINA, 1965). Because of an increased sensitivity to ganglion-blocking agents in older patients, pirilenum needs to be prescribed in very small doses (5–10 mg/day) in such cases. There are several comments on the beneficial use of pirilenum in patients with endarteriitis obliterans and diabetes mellitus; improved peripheral blood flow, favourable changes in blood coagulation, and increased carbohydrate tolerance have been observed (NARGIZYAN and KARAPETYAN, 1965).

IX. Recent Developments

In recent years, with the development of more specific anti-adrenergic agents, the ganglion-blocking agents have become of secondary importance. In most patients with moderate and severe hypertension good blood pressure control can be achieved with the help of modern antihypertensive drugs such as reserpine, methyldopa, guanethidine, clonidine, and the diuretics. But in some cases of progressive and malignant hypertension, when combinations of the above-mentioned drugs are ineffective, ganglion-blocking agents can be highly useful. Because of the rapid onset of the antihypertensive effect ganglion-blocking agents proved to be helpful in the treatment of severe hypertensive emergencies complicated by attacks of cardiac asthma, hypertensive encephalopathy, acute stages of subarachnoid and other forms of cerebral haemorrhage, toxaemia, and eclampsia of pregnancy. In these situations parenteral medication is required (LEBEDEVA et al., 1965; FIALKO and KHORYAKOVA, 1966; ERINA, 1958, 1973; LEVASHOVA, 1971).

Trimetaphan camsylate is now thought to be the most universally effective agent available for the treatment of hypertensive emergencies, especially in cases with acute left ventricular failure and pulmonary oedema or dissecting aortic aneurysm. Trimetaphan is always administered by slow intravenous infusion in a 0.1% concentration in 5% dextrose or saline solution. Its action is very brief, and reliable control of the blood pressure requires constant attention to the rate of administration. The infusion is started at a rate of 30–50 drops/min and sometimes increased to 100 drops. Reduction of blood pressure is immediate (within 3–5 min), and when the infusion is discontinued the return to pretreatment levels is prompt (within 20–25 min). Trimetaphan acts by way of both ganglionic blockade and direct peripheral vasodilatation. Tolerance develops within 48–72 h of continuous infusion. Therefore, when administering this agent to severely hypertensive patients, the physician must initiate careful, more long-acting antihypertensive therapy at the same time, in order to prevent a rise of blood pressure after discontinuation of the infusion. Trimetaphan is one of the few agents that can reduce the blood pressure rapidly and predictably; this can occasionally be advantageous, but it is often dangerous, particularly in patients with severe atherosclerosis (VOLLE and KOELLE, 1970; FROHLICH, 1974). Since it causes the liberation of histamine, trimetaphan should be used with caution in allergic individuals (PAGE and SIDD, 1973).

Pachycarpinum[4], an alkaloid derived from the plant *Sophora pachycarpa*, differs substantially from all the above-mentioned preparations. Like other tertiary amines, pachycarpinum can produce direct central effects resulting in changes of thermoregulation, augmentation of inhibitory processes in the brain cortex, and

---

4 *d*-Sparteine hydroiodide.

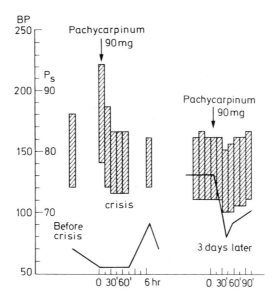

Fig. 3. Changes in blood pressure and heart rate following injections of pachycarpinum in a patient (30 years old) with essential hypertension stage II, during the period of crisis and outside the crisis period. The arrows indicate the time of injections

bradycardia. It is well absorbed from the gastrointestinal tract. Clinical studies yielded evidence that the antihypertensive action of pachycarpinum is very inconsistent. But at the same time, a number of valuable properties of the drug were discovered: it may have a place in the treatment of certain hypertensive crises with pronounced vegetoneurotic and vasomotor irregularities and attacks of paroxysmal supraventricular tachycardia. Intramuscular administration of pachycarpinum (2–3 ml of 3% solution) may result in a reduction in blood pressure within 15–30 min, relief of tachycardia, emotional excitement, migraine and visual disturbances such as scotoma migrans ("migraine ophtalmique"). A distinct antihypertensive effect was evident when pachycarpinum was given at the time of a crisis, even in patients whose blood pressure remained unchanged when it was given at other times (Fig. 3).

Unlike other ganglion-blocking agents, pachycarpinum does not cause orthostatic hypotension. It has occasionally been useful in the treatment of patients with frequent attacks of paroxysmal arrhythmia, which in some cases (Fig. 4) arose during convalescence after myocardial infarction (ERINA, 1957, 1973).

Repeated oral administration of pachycarpinum has been found to be helpful in some types of angioneurotic eczema (ERINA, 1954, 1973), sympathetic trunkitis and ganglionitis, peripheral angiotrophic disorders, endoarteriitis obliterans, and myopathy (GORDON, 1952). The average oral doses are 0.05–0.1 g two or three times a day.

During treatment with pachycarpinum (and to a less extent with a secondary amine nanophinum [5]) of patients with hypertensive disease stages II and III and

---

5 1,2-Dimethyl-piperidine hydrochloride.

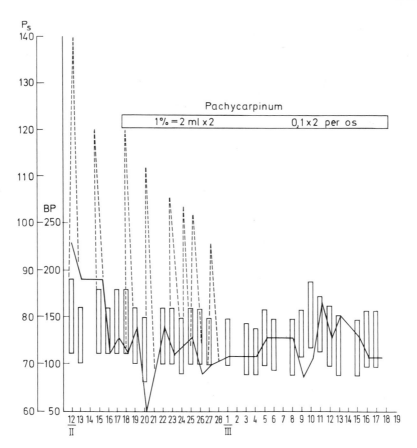

Fig. 4. Effect of pachycarpinum on the blood pressure and heart rate in a patient (54 years old) with moderate hypertension and brief attacks of paroxysmal tachyarrhythmia (10–15/day). The *white columns* indicate the blood pressure; the *broken line* represents the heart rate during attacks of atrial fibrillation; *solid lines* represent the heart rate not during attacks

coronary atherosclerosis, an increase in anginal pain was occasionally observed, and this was not associated with lowering of blood pressure. Exacerbation of precordial pain was usually noted in patients with marked bradycardia. Symptoms of para-sympathetic blockade were never encountered during treatment with pachycar-pinum (Erina, 1958). These observations have been interpreted to mean that pachy-carpinum exerts a marked blocking action on the sympathetic cervical ganglia, with a resulting domination of parasympathetic function and a temporary decrease of coronary blood flow.

Clinical studies have shown that pachycarpinum may be useful in patients with mild forms of hypertension associated with paroxysmal cardiovascular disorders, mainly related to diencephalo-hypothalamic dysfunction. Treatment for about 3–6 weeks (or longer) leads to a reduction in frequency and sometimes to complete relief of the above-mentioned vegetative crises (Erina, 1973).

X. Contraindications

The main contraindication for treatment with ganglion-blocking agents is recent coronary or cerebral thrombosis (less than 2 months before). Extreme caution must be exercised in the use of these drugs in patients older than 60 years, since rapid lowering and fluctuations of pressure may cause ischaemic changes in the heart or brain. In renal insufficiency and impaired excretion of ganglion-blocking agents an unexpected accumulation of the drugs and potentiation of their action can occur (BLAINEY, 1952; WALDMAN, 1956) and this will lead to a deterioration of renal function due to an excessive decrease in systemic arterial pressure. They must not be given for long periods to patients with hypertrophy of the prostate gland.

The use of ganglion-blocking agents is absolutely contraindicated in patients with phaeochromocytoma. Pharmacological denervation enhances the sensitivity of peripheral adrenoreceptors to catecholamines released from the adrenal medulla, and this can produce a dramatic hypertensive crisis (PATON and ZAIMIS, 1952; VITOLINJ, 1961).

C. Ganglion-Blocking Agents in the Treatment of Peptic Ulcer

Ganglion-blocking agents have been tested in clinical trials in the treatment of different gastrointestinal disorders, mainly peptic ulcer.

Clinical studies have shown that intramuscular administration of hexamethonium (60–100 mg) reduces the volume and acidity of gastric secretion and also the tone and motility of the gastrointestinal tract. The stomach is relaxed and dilated, gastric peristalsis nearly ceases for more than 6 h, and the emptying of the stomach is markedly delayed. Propulsive movements of the small intestine may be completely stopped after larger doses of hexamethonium. Changes in the colon are also prominent and the large bowel can be markedly distended with barium (KAY and SMITH, 1950; DOUTHWAITE and THORNE, 1951; ROWLANDS et al., 1952; McGOWAN and STANLEY, 1954; POVALYAEVA, 1956–1969; SHULUTKO, 1959; ELENEVA, 1967a; VOLLE and KOELLE, 1970).

The results of hexamethonium treatment of patients with peptic ulcer and chronic gastritis are highly variable, depending on the initial functional state of the gastroduodenal system and the choice of doses. The use of ganglion-blocking agents seems to be most effective in cases of markedly increased functional activity of the gastrointestinal tract, in fresh ulcers and early recurrences with hypersecretion, which predominates in duodenal ulcers, and expecially in patients with concomitant hypertension. Ganglion-blocking agents exert a greater effect on disturbances of neurohormonal regulation of secretion and motor activity than on locally impaired digestive processes in the stomach and duodenum. Only large doses of hexamethonium affect the humoral component of gastric secretion stimulated by food or histamine (DENISENKO, 1959; GELJFAND and LEVANDOVSKY, 1973; MASEVICH and RYSS, 1973).

Clinical experience has shown that it is not expedient to use large doses of ganglion-blocking agents, taking into account that such medical denervation may cause certain negative dystrophic changes in the gastric mucosa (ANICHKOV and ZAVODSKAYA, 1965). Medium and low doses of ganglion-blocking agents diminish the propagation of excessive nervous impulses both from the central nervous system to the stomach and duodenum and vice versa.

Thus the tissues do not lack nervous control; at the same time various reflectory influences do not manifest themselves in their former exaggerated and destructive character. This provides rest not only for the diseased organ but for the whole body. Most physicians use medium doses of hexamethonium. Since they are more effective against basal than against food-stimulated secretion the medication is given before meals (0.5–1.5 ml of 2.5% solution for subcutaneous administration) three or four times daily, and increased amounts are given at bedtime in an effort to lower the nocturnal gastric secretion. In most of the reports published by BURCHINSKY and co-workers (1968–1975) the use of lower doses of benzohexonium[6] (0.25–0.5 ml of 2.5% solution four times per day) has been emphasised. A favourable action of small doses on both phases of gastric secretion in dogs provided experimental proof for such a scheme of treatment (REINGARD, 1969). Large doses of benzohexonium produce a rapid and profound inhibition of gastric secretion in the complex-reflectory phase, which is followed by an increase of secretion in its neurohumoral phase. Such an effect was never encountered when small doses were used. After single injections of 0.4–1 mg/kg body weight, the secretory activity of the gastric glands remains decreased for a period of 2–3 days, whereas after large doses (5 mg/kg body wt.) it increases at this time.

The course of parenteral treatment varied from 3 to 6 weeks. There was usually a prompt (within the first few days) relief of pain, especially of regular attacks of pain during the night, and also of dyspeptic symptoms; the general condition and sleep improved. Gastrographic investigations revealed a gradual normalisation of peristalsis, particularly in patients with a hyperkinetic type of gastrogram. X-ray examinations showed a rapid disappearance of oedema of the gastric mucosa and pylorospasm. In most cases (67–80% of patients) complete healing of the Haudek's „niches" was obtained within 4 weeks of treatment, perhaps by way of improved gastric circulation (twice as effective as in control groups). There were no recurrences of peptic ulcer for 5–18 months.

The secretion, acidity, and digestive action of the gastric juice decreased significantly if the initial values were high. In patients with normal secretion they usually did not change, and they even increased slightly in cases with initially low levels, mainly when small doses were used (POVALYAEVA, 1959; ANOKHINA, 1968; SHULUTKO, 1959; ELENEVA, 1967a; BURCHINSKY et al., 1975). At the same time, the content of pepsine and pepsinogen decreased and the concentrations of potassium, sodium, and calcium and their ratio in the gastric juice became normal; the content of carbohydrate-protein components (hexoses, bound to proteins and gastromucoproteases) increased significantly, whereas the content of gastromucoproteins decreased (LESHJINSKY et al., 1968–1972). This is consistent with experimental data demonstrating the ability of ganglion-blocking agents to increase the resynthesis of protein, to normalise the content of free amino acids, to decrease the content of total and free histamine, to increase the histaminopectic ability of the gastric mucosa, to intensify

---

6 Hexamethonium dibenzosulphonate or hexamethonium benzenesulphonate.

the excretion of histamine in the gastric juice, and to reduce the amount of histamine in blood (MIRZOYAN and TATEVOSYAN, 1970, 1975). In this connection, hexamethonium appeared to be highly effective in the treatment of reserpine-induced gastric ulcers and prevented their development in animal experiments (ZAVODSKAYA, 1964; KALINICHENKO and BUDANTSEVA, 1973). Treatment with small doses of benzohexonium also reduced pancreatic secretion, increased bicarbonate basicity, and decreased the activity of amylase and lipase. Large doses sometimes intensified the external pancreatic secretion (TRUSOV, 1963; ELENEVA, 1967b; BURCHINSKY and KUSHNIR, 1968). In addition, a normalising effect on some previously disturbed liver functions was observed–the composition of lipids and blood protein fractions, antitoxic function of the liver according to Quick's test, and absorption and excretory function according to data obtained with the radiometric method with ^{131}I-labelled Bengal rose (REJNGARDT et al., 1969).

Within 3–5 weeks of treatment, changes in adrenal cortical functions were observed, namely a decrease of glucocorticoid and androgenic activity in patients with increased initial excretion (mainly in refractory ulcers, frequent recurrences, and ulcer penetration). In cases of decreased initial excretion of corticosteroids, its increase to the normal level was noted. Indices that characterised a simultaneous decrease of mineralocorticoid function also tended to normalisation during treatment (BURCHINSKY et al., 1973). It can be assumed that the favourable influence of benzohexonium on the course of peptic ulcer (first of all, due to prompt relief of the pain syndrome) promotes the cessation of pathological impulse transmission on the adrenal cortex, thus creating conditions for normalisation of its functions and reactivity.

In addition, a positive effect on cholinergic activity has been demonstrated for benzohexonium: it caused a reduction of the initially increased blood concentration of acetylcholine, whereas the high cholinesterase activity remained unaffected (BURCHINSKY et al., 1975).

The use of small doses of ganglion-blocking agents was not accompanied by undesirable reactions of the cardiovascular system. Normalisation of the arterial pressure and a tendency to increased cardiac output and left ventricular work were noted in patients with hypertension and coronary atherosclerosis (BURCHINSKY et al., 1975). To avoid hypotensive reactions patients were recommended to lie down for 1.5–2 h after injections.

Other ganglion-blocking agents besides benzohexonium are used in the treatment of peptic ulcer. Ganglerone acts on both the nicotinic receptors of autonomic ganglia and the synapses of the central nervous system. During the first 10–15 days of treatment it is administered intramuscularly (2 ml per 1.5% solution), and then it is prescribed orally (40 mg three or four times a day for about one month). This drug is free of side effects. MASEVICH and RYSS (1973) consider quateronum as the drug of choice: it acts predominantly on the parasympathetic ganglia and also has a peripheral muscarinolytic effect (MNATSAKANOV, 1966). It is administered orally which is especially important for repeated ambulatory treatment (in an effort to prevent recurrences). Initial doses of 30 mg three or four times a day are gradually increased to 120–240 mg per day. The courses of treatment vary from 1 to 2 months.

Pirilenum (1–2 mg four times a day) has a favourable but slower effect. Prompt relief of ulcer pain may be obtained by subcutaneous administration (0.5–1 ml of 1%

solution) of another ganglion-blocking agent Temechinum[7] which resembles pirilenum in its chemical structure (SHIROKOVA et al., 1972; KRYUKOVA, 1973).

I. Combination of Ganglion-Blocking Agents With Other Preparations

In order to enhance the effectiveness of treatment, ganglion-blocking agents are
combined with anticholinergic agents with peripheral and central actions (atropine,
arpenal[8], methacinum[9], etc.), antacids, sedatives, and vitamin complexes, gastrointestinal irritants are avoided. After disappearance of acute manifestations of the
disease, cholinolytic agents are supplemented with preparations that promote the
stimulation of protein synthesis and rate of regeneration of epithelial cells of the
gastric mucosa. These are derivatives of pyrimidine (methyluracil), anabolic hormones (Nerobol or methandienone), and DOCA, which remove the effects of hormone imbalance and enhance tissue resistance; they are especially indicated in cases
of refractory ulcers combines with diffuse gastritis or duodenitis (LANDA et al., 1971;
LESHJINSKY, et al., 1972; MASEVICH and RYSS, 1975). As follows from the experiments, it is not reasonable to use ganglion-blocking agents for a long time (more
than 6 weeks), since during the reparative period it is essential to avoid the suppression of nervous impulse transmission, which would lead to the recovery of normal
trophic functions of the sympathetic nervous system (ANICHKOV and ZAVODSKAYA,
1965).

However, not all patients experience beneficial effects on gastric secretion. Moreover, it is not always possible to separate the gastrointestinal effects of the ganglion-
blocking agents from their undesirable effects at other sites. Thus, postural hypotension may occur with prolonged use of medium and high doses of ganglion-blocking
agents and be disabling to the patients. This limits their use in many older patients
with arterial hypotension and coronary atherosclerosis. These two factors, undesirable side effects, and variable efficacy (and the difficulties of treatment in ambulatory
conditions) have resulted in the refusal of clinicians in various countries to use
ganglion-blocking agents in the treatment of gastroduodenal ulcers (KIRSNER and
PALMER, 1960; VOLLE and KOELLE, 1970).

Ganglion-blocking agents are contraindicated in scarry stenosis of pylorus and
repeated gastrointestinal haemorrhage.

References

Aghina, A., Bassi, M., de Caro, P.A.: L'azione dei ganglioplegici sulla coagulabilita del sangue.
   Riforma Medica 45, 1244–1247 (1954)
Agrest, A., Hoobler, S.W.: Long-term management of hypertension with pentolinium tartrate
   (ansolysen). J.A.M.A 157, 999–1003 (1955)
Anichkov, S.V., Zavodskaya, I.S.: Pharmacotherapy of peptic ulcer. Leningrad: Medicina 1965
   (Russ.)
Anokhina, L.I.: Changes of gastric functions in patients with peptic ulcer treated with hexonium
   and benzohexonium. Klin. Med. (Mosk.) 46, 2, 79–85 (1968) (Russ.)

---

7 2,2,6,6,-Tetra-methylchinuclidine hydrobromide.
8 N-(3,Diethylaminopropyl)-2,2-diphenylacetamide.
9   6-Dimethylaminoethyl-benzyl-iodmethylate.

Arnold, O.H.: Einfluß der Therapie auf die Prognose der Hochdruckerkrankungen. In: Hochdrucksforschung, pp. 195–201. Stuttgart: Thieme 1965

Avakyan, V.M., Grigoryan, A.M., Arutyunyan, A.S.: Data on the treatment of patients with coronary insufficiency with anticoagulants and quateronum. Ter. Arkh. *38*, 40–43 (1966) (Russ.)

Aviado, D.M.: Hemodynamic effects of ganglion-blocking drugs. Circ. Res. *8*, 304–314 (1960)

Blainey, J.D.: Hexamethonium compounds in the treatment of hypertension. Lancet *1952 CCLXII*, 6718, 993–996

Bos, S.E., Keng, K.L., Velzeboer, C.M.J., de Vries, S.: Essential hypertension in a 12 year old girl treated with hexamethonium compounds. Acta Paediatr. Scand. *42*, 6, 570–575 (1953)

Boyarintseva, S.D., Mironenko, A.I.: Dynamics of psychic state and biochemical changes in patients with hypertension and atherosclerosis during treatment with hexonium. Trudy. I Moskovskogo Meditsynskogo Instituta *25*, 179–189 (1963) (Russ.)

Breslavsky, A.S., Vyazovskaya, R.D.: Effect of benzohexonium on the insular apparatus of the pancreas. Vrach. Delo *11*, 20–24 (1961) (Russ.)

Burchinsky, G.I., Kushnir, V.E.: Some principal problems of the use of ganglion-blocking agents in the treatment of peptic ulcer. Klin. Med. (Mosk.) *46*, 2, 85–89 (1968) (Russ.)

Burchinsky, G.I., Kushnir, V.E.: Ulcer disease. Kiev: Zdorovje 1973 (Russ.)

Burchinsky, G.I., Galetskaya, T.M., Ivanova, E.A., Kaskevich, L.M., Litinskaya, A.V., Reingardt, B.K., Spivak, A.M.: Our experience of employment of cholineblocking agents in the treatment of ulcer disease. Vrach. Delo *2*, 70–76 (1975) (Russ.)

Campbell, A.J.M., Graham, J.G., Maxwell, R.D.H.: Treatment of hypertension by oral methonium compounds. Br. Med. J. *1952 I*, 4752, 251–254

Campbell, A.J.M., Robertson, E.: Treatment of severe hypertension with hexamethonium bromide. Br. Med. J. *1950 II*, 804–808

Cameron, A.J., Burn, R.A.: Hexamethonium and glaucoma. Br. J. Ophthalmol. *36*, 9, 482–491 (1952)

Corne, S.J., Edge, N.D.: Pharmacological properties of pempidine, a new ganglion-blocking compound. Br. J. Pharmacol. Chemother. *13*, 3, 339–349 (1958)

Crumpton, C.W., Murphy, Q.R.: Effects of hexamethonium bromide upon hemodynamics of cerebral and coronary circulation in hypertension. J. Clin. Invest. *31*, 622–625 (1952); Circulation *11*, 106–110 (1955)

Davidovsky, N.M.: Experience in treatment of patients with angina pectoris with a new cholinolytic agent gangleron. Ter. Arkh. *29*, 4, 51–58 (1957) (Russ.)

Denisenko, P.P.: Gangliolytics. Leningrad: Medgiz 1959 (Russ.)

Dennis, E., Ford, R., Herschberger, R., Moyer, J.H.: Pentolinium and hexamethonium combined with Rauwolfia in the treatment of hypertension. N. Engl. J. Med. *253*, 597–600 (1955)

Doniach, J., Morrison, B., Steiner, R.: Lung changes during hexamethonium therapy for hypertension. Br. Heart. J. *16*, 1, 101–108 (1954)

Douthwaite, A.H., Thorne, M.G.: The effects of hexamethonium bromide of the stomach. Br. Med. J. *1951 I*, 4698, 111–114

Doyle, A.E.: Electrocardiographic changes in hypertension treated by methonium compounds. Am. Heart J. *45*, 3, 363–381 (1953)

Doyle, A.E., Kilpatrik, J.A.: Methonium compounds in angina of hypertension. Lancet *1954 CCLXV*, I, 6818, 905–908

Dracheva, Z.N., Kirienko, M.G.: Comparative evaluation of the therapeutic effect of pirilenum and hexonium in treatment of patients with cerebral forms of hypertension. In: Farmakologiya serdechno-sosudistych veshestv. Lugansky, N.I. (ed.), pp. 144–151. Kiev: Zdorovya 1965 (Russ.)

Dukhina, M.A.: Retinal changes in hypertensive patients treated with Rauwolfia and ganglion-blocking agents. Ophthalmol. Zh. *1*, 26–31 (1963) (Russ.)

Eleneva, T.N.: The effect of small doses of benzohexonium on the external secretory function of the pancreas in patients with gastritis. Vrach. Delo *3*, 11–13 (1967a) (Russ.)

Eleneva, T.N., Epstein, B.V., Shlykov, I.A.: Use of benzohexonium in patients with chronic gastritis. Vrach. Delo *2*, 124–125 (1967b) (Russ.)

Erina, E.V.: Treatment of hypertension with ganglion-blocking agents. Ter. Arkh. *26*, 5, 14–24 (1954) (Russ.)

Erina, E.V.: On the effect of pachycarpinum in arrhythmias. Ter. Arkh. 29, 2, 65–69 (1957) (Russ.)

Erina, E.V.: On the effect of ganglion-blocking agents on coronary circulation in hypertensive patients. In: "Gipertoniya", Myasnikov, A.L. (ed.), Vol. V, pp. 174–183. Moskva: Medgiz 1958 (Russ.)

Erina, E.V.: Comparison of the effectiveness of some new ganglion-blocking agents (piperidine derivatives) in the treatment of hypertensive patients. Cardiologiya 3, 29–33 (1965) (Russ.)

Erina, E.V.: Treatment of hypertension. Moskva: Medicina 1973 (Russ.)

Erina, E.V., Martyanova, T.A.: The use of ganglion-blocking agents in the treatment of hypertension. In: Ganglionlitiki i blokatory nervno-myshechnykh sinapsov. Anichkov, S.V. (ed.), pp. 91–86. Leningrad: Medgiz 1958 (Russ.)

Fialko, V.A., Khoryakova, S.Kh.: Emergency treatment of hypertensive crises and pulmonary oedema with pentaminum. In: Gipertoniya bolshogo i malogo kruga krovoobrasheniya. Tez. Dokl. I Vsesoyuznogo syezda kardiologov, pp. 156–157 Moskva: 1966 (Russ.)

Ford, R.W., Moyer, J.H., Spurr, C.L.: Hexamethonium in chronic treatment of hypertension – its effects on renal hemodynamics and on the excretion of water and electrolytes. J. Clin. Invest. 32, 1133–1139 (1953)

Frantsuzova, S.B.: The effect of ganglion-blocking agents on the content of catecholamines in the heart and adrenal glands in rats. In: Neyro-gumoralnaya regulyatsiya v norme i patologii. Uzhgorod Abstr. Prac. Scient. Conference 169–170 (1965) (Russ.)

Freis, E.D., Finnerty, F.A., Schnapper, H.W., Johnson, R.L.: The treatment of hypertension with hexamethonium. Circulation 5, 20–27 (1952)

Freis, E.D., Rose, J.C., Higgins, T.F., Kelley, R.T., Schnapper, H.W., Johnson, R.L.: The haemodynamic effects of hypotensive drugs in man. III. Hexamethonium. J. Clin. Invest. 32, 12, 1285–1293 (1953)

Freis, E.D., Partenope, E.A., Lilienfeld, L.S.: A clinical appraisal of pentapyrrolidinum (M & B 2050) in hypertensive patients. Circulation 9, 4, 450–456 (1954)

Frohlich, E.D.: Inhibition of adrenergic function in the treatment of hypertension. Arch. Intern. Med. 133, 1022–1048 (1974)

Gatsura, V.V., Bandurina, L.I.: Changes of sensitivity to strophantine under the influence of agents which act on the cardiac efferent innervation. Farmakol. Toksikol. 28, 1, 46–47 (1965) (Russ.)

Gerasimova, E.N.: Aldosterone in essential hypertension and secondary renal hypertension. In: Arterialnaya gipertoniya. Myasnikov, A.L., Chazov, E.I. (eds.), pp. 212–221. Moskva: Medgiz 1964 (Russ.)

Germanov, A.I., Guseva, N.I., Yurasova, M.A.: Treatment of hypertensive patients with a new ganglion-blocking agent dimecolinum. Klin. Med. (Mosk.) 41, 5, 23–27 (1963) (Russ.)

Gilmore, H.R., Kopelman, H., McMichael, J., Milne, I.G.: The effect of hexamethonium bromide on the cardiac output and pulmonary circulation. Lancet 1952 II, 288–294

Gordon, Z.L.: Treatment of endarteriitis obliterans with pachycarpinum. Farmakol. Toksikol. 2, 36–40 (1952) (Russ.)

Grob, D., Langford, H.G.: Observations on the effects of autonomic blocking agents in patients with hypertension. Circulation 8, 2, 205–223 (1953a); 8, 3, 352–369 (1953b)

Hafkenschiel, J.H., Friedland, C.K., Zintel, M.A., Crumpton, C.W.: The blood flow and cerebral oxygen consumption in essential hypertension: effect of ganglion-blocking agents and hydrazinophthalazine. J. Clin. Invest. 33, 1, 63–67 (1954)

Harrington, M., Kincaid-Smith, P., Milne, M.D.: Pharmacology and clinical use of pempidine in the treatment of hypertension. Lancet 1958a III, 6–12

Harrington, M., Kincaid-Smith, P.: Psychosis and tremor due to mecamylamine. Lancet 1958b I, 499–501

Herting, G., Axelrod, J., Patrick, R.W.: Actions of bretylium and guanethidine on the uptake and release of (H^3)-noradrenaline. Br. J. Pharmacol. Chemother. 18, 1, 161–166 (1962)

Ivannikova, T.N.: Electroencephalographic study of the changes of the functional state of the central nervous system in hypertensive patients under the influence of different neurotropic agents, Vol. V, pp. 52–70. In: "Gipertoniya". Myasnikov, A.L. (ed.). Moskva: Medgiz 1958 (Russ.)

Ivanova, E.A.: Hemodynamic changes in patients with peptic ulcer during treatment with gangliolytics. Vrach. Delo 6, 21–26 (1971) (Russ.)

Kalinichenko, N.I., Budantseva, S.I.: Comparative evaluation of the effectiveness of the use of benzohexonium, vinilene and the agent "Spedian-2M" in treatment of gastric ulcers induced by reserpine. Farmakol. Toksikol. *36*, 3, 311–314 (1973) (Russ.)

Kay, A.W., Smith, A.N.: Effect of hexamethonium iodide on gastric secretion and motility. Br. Med. J. *1950 I*, 4651, 460–461

Kelley, R.T., Freis, E.D., Higgins, T.F.: The effects of hexamethonium on certain manifestations of congestive heart failure. Circulation 7, 2, 169–174 (1953)

Kilpatrik, J.A., Smirk, F.H.: Comparison of oral and subcutaneous administration of methonium salts in the treatment of high blood pressure. Lancet *1952 CCLXII*, 6697, 8–12

Kirsner, J.B., Palmer, W.L.: Treatment of peptic ulcer. Am. J. Med. *29*, 793–803 (1960)

Kiseleva, Z.M.: On the functional state of the sympathoadrenal system in patients with hypertension and atherosclerosis. In: Vzaimootnoshenije ateroskleroza i arterialnoj gipertonii. Shkhvatsabaya, I.K. (ed.), pp. 67–74. Moskva: Medicina 1968 (Russ.)

Kitchin, A., Lowther, C.P., Turner, R.W.D.: Pempidine – a ganglion-blocking drug for treating hypertension. Lancet *1961 II*, 7164, 143–145

Kryukova, A.Ya.: The use ot temechinum in emergency treatment of patients with peptic ulcer with marked pain syndrome, pp. 169–173. In: Voprosy okazaniya skoroy i neotlozhnoy meditsinskoy pomoshi. Alexejew, U.A. (ed.). Ufa: Bashkir. Med. Institute 1973 (Russ.)

Landa, V.Z., Reingardt, B.K., Starostenko, L.N.: The use of metacinum and dimecolinum in complex therapy of patients with peptic ulcer. Vrach. Delo *3*, 69–72 (1971) (Russ.)

Laragh, J.H., Angers, M., Kelly, W.G., Liebermann, S.: Hypotensive agents and pressor substances. Their effect on the secretory rate of aldosterone in man. J.A.M.A. *174*, 3, 234–240 (1960)

Lebedev, S.V.: The use of pirilenum in treatment of hypertensive patients. Vrach. Delo 7, 21–25 (1963) (Russ.)

Lebedeva, N.V., Gannushkina, I.V., Shaphranova, V.P.: Some data on the effect of ganglion-blocking agents on cerebral circulation (clinical and experimental data). Trudy IV Vsesoyuznogo Syezda nevropatologov i psichiatorov. Banshikov, V.M. (ed.). Vol. I, pp. 444–450. Moskva: Medgiz 1965 (Russ.)

Lee, W.C., Shideman, F.E.: Inotropic actions of quaternary ammonium compounds. J. Pharmacol. Exp. Thcr. *127*, 219–228 (1959)

Leshjinsky, L.A., Pevchikh, V.V., Trusov, V.V.: Comparative study of the effectiveness of nerobol, quateron, and their combination in gastric ulcer. Klin. Med. (Mosk.) *50*, 3, 68–73 (1972) (Russ.)

Levashova, I.I.: The use of ganglion-blocking agents in the delivery complicated by hypertensive syndrome. Akush. Gynecol. (Mosk.) *4*, 34–38 (1971) (Russ.)

Locket, S., Swann, P.G., Grieve, W.S.: Methonium compounds in the treatment of hypertension. Br. Med. J. *1951 I*, 4710, 778–784

Malova, M.N.: Effects of pentamin upon hypertension in the right heart and pulmonary circulation. Proceedings of the XV National Congress of Internal Medicine. Moskva: Medgiz, 434–438 (1964) (Russ.)

Masevich, Ts.G., Ryss, S.M.: Diseases of the digestive organs. Leningrad: Medicina 1975 (Russ.)

Masini, V., Rossi, P.: Preparato di metonia in soluzione ritardante nella cura dell'ipertensione arteriosa. Riforma Med. *65*, 33, 898–900 (1951)

Maxwell, R.D.H., Campbell, A.J.M.: New sympathicolytic agents. Lancet *1953 CCLXIIII*, 6758, 455–457

McGowan, J.A., Stanley, M.: Comparative effects of newer anticholinergic agents (atropine and quaternary ammonium compounds) on human gastric secretion. J. Lab. Clin. Med. *43*, 359–366 (1954)

McMichael, J.: The treatment of hypertension. Brit. Med. J. *4765*, 933–938 (1952)

McQueen, E.G., Trewin, E.: Hexamethonium bromide and kidney function. Med. J. Aust. *1*, 23, 769–771 (1952)

Mirzoyan, S.A., Tatevosyan, A.T. The effects of ganglion-blocking agents on the metabolism of histamine in the gastric mucous membrane. Farmakol. Toksikol. *33*, 4, 415–418 (1970) (Russ.)

Mirzoyan, S.A., Tatevosyan, A.T.: The effect of gangleronum on the content of free aminoacids in the gastric mucous membrane and biological fluids of rats with experimental ulcers. Farmakol. Toksikol. *38*, 2, 198–200 (1975) (Russ.)

Mnatsakanov, T.S.: On the treatment of patients with peptic ulcer with quateronum. In: Kvateron i opyt ego klinicheskogo primeneniya. Mndjoyan, A.L. (ed.). Yerevan: Akad. of Sciences Arm. S.S.R. 1966 (Russ.)

Mnatsakanov, T.S., Barsegyan, B.A.: Acute observations of the action of quateronum on the coronary circulation in hypertensive patients. Zh. Eksp. Klin. Med. 7, 24–26 (1967) (Russ.)

Mnatsakanov, T.S., Mamikonjan, R.S., Tumanyan, A.M.: The use of a new Soviet drug fubromeganum in treatment of peptic ulcer. Klin. Med. (Mosk.) 11, 93–97 (1961) (Russ.)

Morrison, B.: Parenteral hexamethonium in hypertension. Br. Med. J. Vol. I, 4823, 1291–1299 (1953)

Moyer, J.H., Miller, S.J., Ford, R.W.: Orally administered hexamethonium chloride in hypertension. J.A.M.A. 152, 12, 1121–1129 (1953)

Moyer, J., Heider, C., Dennis, E.: Mecamylamine (inversine) in the treatment of hypertension. J.A.M.A. 164, 1879–1886 (1957)

Nargizyan, G.A., Karapetyan, F.V.: On the treatment of hypertensive patients with pirilenum. Vol. II, pp. 11–15. Erevan: Trudy Erevanskogo Instituta Usovershenstvovaniya vrachey 1965 (Russ.)

Novikova, M.N.: Treatment of hypertensive patients with pirilenum. Vrach. Delo 11, 37–41 (1963) (Russ.)

Page, I.H., Dustan, N.P.: Persistance of normal blood pressure after discontinuing treatment in hypertensive patients. Circulation 25, 433–436 (1962)

Page, L.B., Sidd, J.J.: Management of primary hypertension. Boston: Little & Brown 1973

Paton, W.D.H., Zaimis, E.: Paralysis of autonomic ganglia; with special reference to the therapeutic effects of ganglion blocking drugs. Br. Med. J. 1952 I, 4710, 773–778

Peterson, A.G., Dodge, M., Helwig, F.C.: Pulmonary changes associated with hexamethonium therapy. Arch. Intern. Med. 103, 285–288 (1959)

Poshkus, N.B.: The effect of hexonium on the blood coagulation and prothrombin time in dogs, Vol. XVIII, pp. 369–374. Kharkov: Trudy Ukrainskogo Instituta Eksperimentalnoy Endocrinologii 1961 (Russ.)

Povalyaeva, A.D.: On the use of ganglion-blocking agents in peptic ulcer. Klin. Med. (Mosk.) 31, 10, 59–62 (1959) (Russ.)

Ratner, N.A., Vadkovskaya, Yu.D.: The effect of pentaminum and reserpine on the renal functions in hypertension. Ter. Arkh. 30, 12, 25–34 (1958) (Russ.)

Reingardt, B.C., Spivak, A.M., Tsygankov, A.T.: Dynamics of functional state of the liver in patients with peptic ulcer during treatment with benzohexonium. Vrach. Delo 7, 82–85 (1969) (Russ.)

Remmer, H.: Das Verhalten von Kreislauf und Blutvolumen nach Ganglienblockierung mit Pendiomid. Arch. Exp. Pathol. Pharmacol. 222, 1–2, 73–74 (1954)

Restall, P.A., Smirk, F.H.: The treatment of high blood pressure with hexamethonium iodide. N.Z. Med. J. 49, 206–210 (1950)

Restall, P.A., Smirk, F.H.: Regulation of blood pressure levels by hexamethonium bromide and mechanical devices. Br. Heart J. 14, 1, 1–12 (1952)

Rich, C.B., Holubitsky, W.H.: The treatment of hypertension with oral hexamethonium. Can. Med. Assoc. J. 68, 4, 342–347 (1953)

Rowlands, E.N., Wolff, H.H., Atkinson, M.: Clinical assessment of drugs which inhibit gastric secretion with special reference to hexamethonium. Lancet 1952 II, 1154–1158

Rubanovsky B.R.: Treatment of patients with angina pectoris with hexonium. Vrach. Delo 1, 22–25 (1961) (Russ.)

Sazonova, A.I.: Treatment of hypertensive patients with the predominance of cerebral symptoms with dimecolinum. Zh. Nevrol. Psykh. Korsakova 63, 1, 58–60 (1965) (Russ.)

Schnapper, H.W., Johnson, R.L., Tuohy, E.B., Freis, E.D.: The effect of hexamethonium as compared to procaine or metycaine lumbar block on the blood flow to the foot of normal subjects. J. Clin. Invest. 30, 786–791 (1951)

Sharapov, I.M.: Pirilenum. In: Novye lekarstvennye sredstva, Pershin, G.N. (ed.), Vol. V, pp. 110–112. Moskva: Medgiz 1963 (Russ.)

Shirokova, K.I., Yushjenko, N.A., Chistova, S.V.: The effect of temekhinum on secretory, motor and evacuatory functions of the stomach. In: Aktualnye voprosy gastroenterologii, Vasilenko, V.Kh., Loginov, A.S. (ed.), Vol. V, pp. 173–177. Moskva: Medicina 1972 (Russ.)

Shulutko, I.B.: Treatment of patients with peptic ulcer with ganglion-blocking agents. Ter Arkh. *31*, 3, 9–13 (1959) (Russ.)

Smirk, F.H.: Prolongation of action of hypotensive drugs. Lancet *1952 II*, 695–699

Smirk, F.H.: Practical details of the treatment of hypertension by hexamethonium salts and by pentamethylene 1:5-bis-N-(N-methylpyrrolidinum) bitartrate (M & B 2050 A). N. Z. Med. J. *52*, 325–349 (1953)

Smirk, F.H.: Blood pressure reduction in arterial hypertension by hexamethonium and penta-pyrrolidinum salts. Am. J. Med. *17*, 6, 839–850 (1954a)

Smirk, F.H.: Results of methonium treatment of hypertensive patients (based on 250 cases treated for periods up to $3\frac{1}{2}$ years, including 28 with malignant hypertension). Br. Med. J. *1954b*, Vol. I, 4864, 717–723

Smirk, F.H.: High arterial pressure. Oxford: Blackwell Scientific publication 1957a

Smirk, F.H., McQueen, E.G.: Use of mecamylamine in the management of hypertension. Br. Med. J. *1957b I*, 422–425

Smirk, F.H.: Prognosis in retinal grade I and II patient. Antihypertensive therapy. Gross, F. (ed.), pp. 355–369. New York, Berlin: Springer 1966

Smirk, F.H., Alstad, K.S.: Treatment of arterial hypertension with penta- and hexamethonium salts. Br. Med. J. *1951*, Vol. I, 4717, 1217–1220

Smith, K.M., Fowler, P.B.S.: Prevention and treatment of hypertensive heart-failure by ganglion-blocking agents. Lancet *1955 CCLVIII*, 6861, 417–418

Sokoloff, M., Schottstaedt, M.F.: The management of malignant hypertension. Ann. Intern. Med. *38*, 4, 647–665 (1953)

Sorokina, E.I.: The cardiac pain syndrome in patients with coronary atherosclerosis complicated by inflammation of the sympathetic truncus and its treatment. Sov. Med. *29*, 85–90 (1966) (Russ.)

Spinks, H., Young, E.H.P., Farrington, J.A., Dunlop, D.: The pharmacological actions of pempidine. Br. J. Pharmacol. Chemother. *13*, 4–10 (1958)

Stone, C.A., Torchiana, M.L., O'Nell, G., Beyer, K.J.: Ganglionic blocking properties of 3-methylaminoisocamphane hydrochloride (mecamylamine), a secondary amine. J. Pharmacol. Exp. Ther. *116*, 1, 54–55 (1956)

Stübinger, H.G., Koch, B.: Erfahrungen mit einem ganglienblockierenden Präparat (Pendiomide) in der inneren Medizin. Dtsch. Med. Wochenschr. *36*, 1061 1063 (1952)

Trusov, V.V.: The effect of hexonium on the pancreas functions. Kazan. Med. Zh. *3*, 3, 14–21 (1963) (Russ.)

Trusov, V.V.: Clinico-physiological characteristics of fubromeganum in patients with peptic ulcer. Ter. Arkh. *39*, 8, 65–68 (1967) (Russ.)

Ullmann, T.D., Menczel, J.: The effect of a ganglionic blocking agent (hexamethonium) on renal function and on excretion of water and electrolytes in hypertension and in congestive heart failure. Am. Heart J. *52*, 106–120 (1956)

Vakhrushev, Ya.M.: Treatment of patients with ulcer with methyluracil in combination with quateron. Sov. Med. *6*, 140–141 (1973) (Russ.)

Vetter, H., Graner, G., Mizock, H., Steibereither, K.: Herzkatheteruntersuchungen bei massiver Blutdrucksenkung durch Hexamethonium. Klin. Wochenschr. *32*, 5/6, 97–103 (1954)

Vinogradov, A.V., Tsibekmakher, T.D.: Hemodynamic changes in patients with cardiac insufficiency during treatment with hexonium. Kardiologiia 2, 34–38 (1966) (Russ.)

Vitolinj, M., Melzobs, M.: On the mechanism of sensitising influence of ganglion-blocking agents on the effects of adrenaline and noradrenaline. Izv. Akad. Nauk S.S.S.R. [Biol.] 7, 97–101 (1961) (Russ.)

Volle, R.L., Koelle, G.B.: Ganglion stimulating and blocking agents. In: The pharmacological basis on therapeutics. Goodman, L.S., Gilman, A. (eds.), 4th ed. New York: McMillan 1970

Vyazovskaya, R.D.: Some regularities of the endocrine glands reactions on the effect of ganglion-blocking compounds. In: Deystvive farmakologicheskikh veshestv na endokrinnye zhelezy. Genes, S.G., Anichkov, S.V. (ed.), pp. 21–29. Leningrad: Institute Experimental Medicine Acad. Med. Sc. 1965 (Russ.)

Vyshinskaya, T.E.: Treatment of hypertension with dimecolinum. Sov. Med. *11*, 46–51 (1963) (Russ.)

Waldman, S.: Treatment of the ambulatory hypertensive patients with pentolinium tartrate. Am. J. Med. Sci. *231*, 140–150 (1956)

Walker, G., Levy, L., Hyman, A., Romney, R.: Prolonged hypotensive reactions to hexamethonium. J.A.M.A. *154*, 13, 1079–1080 (1954)

Werkö, L., Frisk, A.R., Wade, F.A., Eliasch, H.: Effect of hexamethonium bromide in arterial hypertension. Lancet *1951 CCLXI*, 6681, 170–472

Wilson, V.H., Keely, K.J.: Haemodynamic effects of hexamethonium bromide in patients with pulmonary hypertension and heart failure. S. Afr. J. Med. Sci. *18*, 125–129 (1953)

Zamyslova, K.N.: Combined treatment of hypertensive patients with reserpine and ganglion-blocking agents. Klin. Med. (Mosk.) *8*, 49–54 (1958) (Russ.)

Zhukova, M.N.: On the effect of the new ganglion-blocking agent dimecoline on the excretion of catecholamines and 17-ketosteroids with urine in patients with hypertension, pp. 94–96. In: Gipertonicheskaya bolezn ateroskleroz i koronarnaya nedostatochnost. Mihnev, A.L. (ed.), Kiev: Zdorovya 1965 (Russ.)

CHAPTER 15

Ganglion-Blocking Agents in Anaesthesiology

A.A. BUNATIAN and A.V. MESHCHERJAKOV

A. Introduction

Artificial, or controlled, hypotension was initially introduced into clinical practice as a method of limiting intraoperative bleeding by means of an intentional and measured reduction of arterial pressure. After its introduction in the 1940s, the method attracted attention in a comparatively short time. The introduction of ganglion-blocking agents into medical practice equipped clinicians with a technically simple method of achieving artificial hypotension. The simple technique, although an apparent advantage, resulted, however, in a distinct danger of its unjustifiably wide and insufficiently grounded use. As often happens, specific experimental and clinical studies of the theory behind artificial hypotension lagged behind its wide practical use.

As experience was gained with ganglion-blocking agents and the physiological basis of artificial hypotension was studied, anaesthesiologists developed a more considered way of using it in clinical practice. The range of surgical interventions carried out under controlled hypotension was extending, and, more important, attitudes towards the rationale for using ganglion-blocking agents in certain surgical procedures were gradually changing. While the method was shown to have great advantages in operations on the heart and major vessels it was found that it is less strongly indicated for decreasing bleeding from the tissues during surgery, since most operations can be performed just as well without it. In addition, a deeper knowledge of the haemodynamic principles of artificial hypotension soon proved the danger of combining massive vasodilatation the positions in which the patient must be arranged on the operating table to ensure the needed "dryness" of the surgical field. Ultimately, artificial hypotension found its place in anaesthesiology mainly as a means of reducing the intravascular pressure, and was almost completely abandoned as a method of reducing intraoperative haemorrhage. Thus, artificial hypotension gradually ceased to be a method used for the surgeon's convenience and became a method used when necessary for the patient.

The field of application of ganglionic block in clinical anaesthesiology has recently been extended. For instance, the main consequence of the block of autonomic ganglia – paresis of the smooth-muscle fibres of the vessels – appeared to be a rather valuable means of preserving the peripheral blood flow during open-heart procedures with a cardiopulmonary by-pass, since it is accompanied by peripheral vascu-

---

1 Hygronium resembles (trimetaphan very closely in its pharmacological effect, but is five times less toxic. Chemically, it is a di-iodomethylate of the dimethyl-aminoethyl ester of N-methyl-α-pyrrolidylcarboxylic acid (KHARKEVICH, 1967).

lar spasm and reduction of the peripheral flow. The use of ganglion-blocking agents in such situations improves the blood supply to the peripheral tissues and prevents the development of circulatory hypoxia of a large mass of muscles, subcutaneous cellular tissue, and skin, thus creating the necessary conditions for adequate extra-corporeal circulation. The vasodilating effect of the ganglion-blocking agents proved to be extremely useful in the treatment of acute pulmonary oedema and of some forms of traumatic shock.

Hence, the method of deliberately changing the circulatory conditions with the aid of ganglion-blocking agents is constantly increasing in importance.

Initially only two drugs were used for artificial hypotension: hexamethonium (hexamethonium) and Pendiomid (pentamine). These drugs have distinct ganglion-blocking properties. They proved suitable for inducing controlled hypotension under clinical conditions. However, a disadvantage of these drugs consists in the declining response with repeated doses, which excludes the possibility of their use in the form of a continuous drip infusion. The level of hypotension reached after the administra-tion of ganglion-blocking agents such as hexamethonium and Pendiomid depends almost entirely on the initial dose of the drug, the selection of which is practically impossible on the same basis as the routine anaesthesiological techniques adjusted according to the patient's anthropometric parameters. The response to a single dose of any ganglion-blocking drug varies widely, not only from patient to patient, but even in the same patient with time. Consequently, the main disadvantage of these drugs is that only a poor degree of control of their effect is possible.

The problem of control of artificially reduced arterial pressure was solved to a large extent when drugs appeared that possessed a potent and at the same time very brief ganglion-blocking effect. The almost complete absence of tachyphylaxis and the short duration of effect (5–15 min) permitted the use of these drugs in the form of continuous drip infusions in precisely measured doses. This group of ganglion-blocking agents includes hygronium and trimetaphan (Arfonad) among others. The hypotensive effect of these drugs in ensured not only by the block of the autonomic ganglia and the chromaffin tissue of the adrenal glands, but, in the case of trimeta-phan, also by their direct depressor effect upon the contractile elements of the blood vessels. The degree of ganglionic block can be easily controlled by changes in the rate of infusion. The main haemodynamic shifts developing under the effect of ganglion-blocking agents are presented schematically in Fig. 1.

B. General Characteristics of the Use of Ganglion-Blocking Agents for Artificial Hypotension

I. Indications for the Use of Ganglion-Blocking Agents

Two groups of indications for a ganglionic block can be distinguished.

Indications based on improvement of the peripheral circulation and the *counter-shock action* of the ganglionic block form one group. Such properties are exploited to reduce the patient's response to surgical trauma and prevent centralisation of the circulation, microcirculation disorders, and cardiac rhythm disturbances of an extra-cardiac genesis.

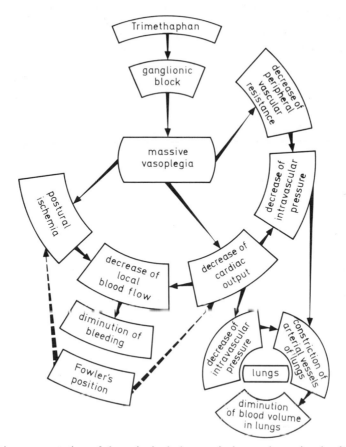

Fig. 1. Schematic representation of the principal changes in haemodynamics developing under the effect of ganglion-blocking agents. (V.P. Osipov, 1973)

When predominantly the *haemodynamic effects* of the ganglion-blocking agents are taken into account, such properties are considered as their ability to decrease the vascular tone in a measured way, to relieve the load on the pulmonary circulation, and to achieve a postural decrease of the blood flow at the incision. The best exsanguinating effect can be achieved in surgical procedures on the head, neck, and chest. In the abdominal and pelvic organs and the lower extremities it is far less distinct.

Hence, the beneficial effects of a ganglionic block can be used both during surgery and during resuscitation and intensive care. Consequently, the indications for the employment of ganglion-blocking agents can be classified into purely surgical, anaesthesiological, and resuscitational (Table 1).

II. Contraindications for the Use of Ganglion-Blocking Agents

In discussion of the contraindications for the use of ganglion-blocking agents those for ganglionic block itself should be distinguished from the contraindications for the

Table 1. Indications for use of ganglion-blocking agents in surgical patients

General nature of indications	Indications based on haemodynamic effects of ganglion-blocking agents			Indication based on inhibition of reflex Pathologic impulse transmission
	To decreasing intravascular pressure	To reduce load on pulmonary circulation	To prevent and decreasing bleeding	
Surgical Indications	1. To facilitate manipulation of major vessels 2. To decrease organ tension (in neurosurgical) procedures, in operations on the eyeball for glaucoma, etc.)	Ligation of common arterial duct complicated by pulmonary hypertension	To decrease tissue bleeding during surgery so as to improve technical conditions for performance of the operation	
Anaesthesiological and resuscitational indications	To normalise elevated blood pressure and prevent hypertensive attacks per- and postoperatively	Pulmonary oedema in cardiac failure	To reduce blood loss during surgery	1. To mitigate patient's response to surgical trauma 2. To eliminate vasospasm and decentralisation of extracorporeal circulation 3. To normalise smooth muscle tone of viscera (bronchial asthma, bronchospasm, spastic ileus, etc.) 4. Heart rhythm disorders of extracardiac aetiology

development of the haemodynamic shifts that result from ganglionic block. The toxicity of the ganglion-blocking agents in routine clinical doses is negligible. Partial and comparatively brief block of the ganglia produce no significant untoward effects.

Consequently, analyses of the possible contraindications for the use of ganglion-blocking agents must place special emphasis on the degree and duration of the haemodynamic changes that accompany the ganglionic block, irrespective of the purpose of its performance in the patient concerned.

First of all it should be taken into consideration that a significant reduction of the blood pressure is inevitably accompanied by a reduction of the cardiac output, which may determine the degree of risk involved in artificial hypotension. Therefore anything that can aggravate the circulation disorders or complicate their compensation should be considered a contraindication for artificial hypotension. This may include the following conditions: circulatory insufficiency, reduction of circulating blood volume of any aetiology, reduction of oxygen capacity of blood (anaemia), and external respiratory insufficiency. Naturally, collapse and existing shock with circulatory disorders prevailing in their clinical pattern are also contraindications for artificial hypotension. This, however, does not exclude the possibility of using ganglionic block for the treatment of shock when measures are taken simultaneously to improve the circulation, such as blood transfusions and monitored infusions of vasopressors ("ganglionic block without hypotension"; VINOGRADOV and DY-ACHENKO, 1961). Circulatory disorders are certainly the cause of functional disorders in the vital organs. Therefore, functional disorders of the liver and kidneys should be considered contraindications for artificial hypotension. This is especially true with patients suffering from disorders of the excretory function of the kidneys, since it is the kidneys that serve as the main route of excretion of the ganglion-blocking agents.

Slowing down of the linear flow rate during artificial hypotension may somewhat stimulate the process of thrombus formation. Therefore ganglion-blocking agents should be used very carefully in patients with such lesions. Finally, pulmonary flow reduction under the effect og ganglion-blocking agents is a contraindication for artificial hypotension in patients with a reduced blood flow in the pulmonary circulation system (the Fallot group of heart diseases).

Definite importance is also attached to the age of the patients. Thus, it was noticed that children under 10–12 years of age tend to display resistance to ganglion-blocking drugs more often than adults. Artificial hypotension is dangerous in patients over 60 years of age because the impairment of the compensatory mechanisms of circulation is more likely to cause ischaemia of the vital organs in this age group than in younger patients. In short, the indications for artificial hypotension must be increasingly strict when the age of the patient falls outside these limits.

It should be mentioned that the above contraindications pertain predominantly to the reduction of blood pressure to subnormal levels (true arterial hypotension). Many of these contraindications can be ignored when the ganglion-blocking agents are used to normalise elevated blood pressure (relative arterial hypotension).

III. Method of Artificial Hypotension

Artificial hypotension is most often used during general anaesthesia, and less often with local anaesthesia. The conditions during general anaesthesia are more suitable for the employment of ganglion-blocking agents, because conscious patients often display a high resistance or even complete insensitivity to them. In addition, it is easier to attain reliable control and prevention of hypoxia under general anaesthesia with artificial pulmonary ventilation.

Artificial hypotension does not require any special premedication, but this should be considered if the patient has been taking sympathomimetic or hypotensive drugs before being prepared for surgery. After sympathomimetics it proves rather difficult to achieve the required hypotensive effect, while after hypotensive agents a persistent state of collapse may develop even with a slight change in the patient's position on the operating table.

Preparations of the phenothiazine group should be used for premedication only with great care, since they may hamper control of the degree of hypotensive effect achieved with the ganglion-blocking agents.

When neuromuscular blocking agents, whether depolarising or non-depolarising, are used during general anaesthesia, their synergism with the ganglion-blocking agents has to be taken into account, since it may result in a prolongation of the myoparalytic effect. In choosing the main anaesthetic agent preference should be given to such drugs as permit the maintenance of a high oxygen concentration in the inhaled gas mixture.

Cyclopropane, although complying with the above-mentioned requirements, is not readily compatible with the ganglion-blocking agents.

Fluothane can produce a hypotensive effect itself, and therefore its combined employment with ganglion-blocking agents is rather useful in some cases. As it increases the effect of the ganglion-blocking agents, Fluothane allows a significant reduction of their dosage for the maintenance of artificial vasodilatation during surgery. But such a combined use of drugs with hypotensive properties demands great care from the anaesthetist.

Adequate pulmonary ventilation is of great importance in anaesthesia with artificial ventilation. Even a slight retention of carbon dioxide in the body may prevent attainment of the necessary level of hypotension, which is why endotracheal intubation and artificial pulmonary ventilation should be considered the most preferable conditions for the use of artificial hypotension.

Monitoring of the level of general anaesthesia under ganglionic block and total myorelaxation is rather difficult, due to the persistent pupillar dilatation and absence of all ocular reflexes. Such indications of the degree of analgesia as reflex changes of pulse rate and blood pressure are lacking. The state of the skin becomes an important criterion. Despite the low arterial pressure, the skin and visible mucosa must remain pink, warm, and dry. The difficulties of controlling anaesthesia maintained under the above conditions necessiate electroencephalographic and electrocardiographic monitoring during surgery. In addition, evaporators of anaesthetics should be used that ensure the most precise and constant dosage of the anaestetic's content in the inhaled mixture.

The administration of any ganglion-blocking agent is started only after the stabilisation of anaesthesia and final positioning of the patient on the operating table. In all cases when the ganglionic block is performed for purposes other than exsanguination of the site of the intervention the position of the patient must be strictly horizontal, while when the ganglionic block is intended to reducing bleeding in the operative field the patient must be placed on the operating table in such a way as to elevate the operative field above the heart. For interventions on the upper half of the body Fowler's position may be used. But the slope of the table should not exceed 10–15°, the patient's head being at the same level as the heart or somewhat lower.

1. Drugs

a) Trimetaphan and Hygronium

The induction of hypotension is started some 5–10 min before the stage of the surgical procedure to be performed under artificial hypotension: Trimetaphan or hygronium is administered with the aid of a separate drip-infusion system. The vial for intravenous administration contains the preprepared 0.1% solution of trimetaphan or hygronium in a 0.5% glucose solution (1 ml of such solution contains 1 mg of the ganglion-blocking agent). Glucose may be substituted by a 0.85–0.9% solution of sodium chloride. The starting rate of infusion of trimetaphan or hygronium is 40–70 drops/min, which corresponds to 2–3 mg dry substance/min.

As soon as 2–3 min after the introduction of the ganglion-blocking agent into the blood stream the arterial pressure begins to fall. The intensity of this fall in response to the initial dose of the drug serves as a criterion of the patient's sensitivity to ganglionic block. Later the rate of infusion is adjusted accordingly, thus maintaining the arterial pressure at the level needed. In the majority of patients the maintenance dose of trimetaphan or hygronium is much lower than the initial dose, being 12–25, and sometimes even 5–8, drops/min.

In a limited number of patients only, the maintenance dose appears to be equal to the initial dose, or even exceed it. In such cases it is preferable to double the concentration of ganglion-blocking agent in the solution, reducing the rate of its infusion accordingly.

The amount of the ganglion-blocking agent used during a surgical operation varies widely – from 20 to 1000 ml and even more, depending on the nature and duration of the operation. The maintenance of hypotension at the required level is achieved by regulating the rate of infusion of the ganglion-blocking agent.

Attempts to achieve deeper artificial hypotension by changing the patient's position on the operating table can be rather risky. They may result in a critical drop in cardiac output, which, in turn, may lead to various complications. To decrease the hypotensive effect, it is sufficient to interrupt the supply of the ganglion-blocking agent to the blood stream. In some 15–20 min the arterial pressure reaches its initial level. Only after that can the patient be taken to the postoperative department, remaining in a horizontal position during transport and for a few hours after surgery. The presence of any residual effect of the ganglionic block can be detected from the degree of mydriasis. Narrowing of the pupils indicates complete cessation of the ganglionic block.

If necessary, the drip infusion of the ganglion-blocking agent can be continued at the bedside after surgery. Here, however, the use hexamethonium or Pendiomid would be preferable, as these ganglion-blocking agents have a prolonged action following intramuscular injection.

When the patient appears to be refractory to hexamethonium or Pendiomid the needed hypotensive effect can be achieved in extreme cases by a combination of these drugs with other ganglion-blocking agents (trimetaphan, hygronium), or drugs of a different spectrum of action (procainamide). This, however, may result in the development of lasting and stable hypotension. In such cases it seems much more reasonable to abandon the idea of conducting the operation under artificial vasodilatation.

b) Hexamethonium and Pendiomid

It is also possible to use hexamethonium and Pendiomid during surgery, but the technique is somewhat different. A 1% hexamethonium solution or a 2% Pendiomid solution is slowly infused intravenously over 2–3 min, some 5–15 min before the stage of the operation that requires artificial hypotension. The initial dose of the drug recommended by most authors is 25 mg hexamethonium or 50 mg Pendiomid. Usually the maximum fall in pressure occurs after 5–15 min, and later the pressure gradually rises to the initial level. The duration of action of the initial dose is approximately the same for hexamethonium and Pendiomid, being 40–60 min on average. The hypotensive effect can be prolonged by repeating the administration of the ganglion-blocking agents. The maintenance dose of hexamethonium and Pendiomid is then selected on the basis of the response to the initial dose of the drug. Generally it is about equal to the initial dose. It should be mentioned that ganglionic block induced by Pendiomid and hexamethonium not easily controlled. It is difficult to balance the dose of the drug, and the degree and duration of its effect.
If it is necessary to neutralise the hypotensive effect of the ganglion-blocking agents, adrenomimetics, ephedrine in particular, can be used reliably. This drug is injected intravenously in fractionated doses of 10–15 mg, which usually proves sufficient to eliminate the state of hypotension (but no the ganglionic block!). Norepinephrine (0.001% solution) can also be used in drip infusion.

The clinical manifestations of artificial hypotension vary with different patients. Common features can also be singled out, however. The arterial pressure is decreased predominantly at the expense of the systolic pressure, which determines the decrease in pulse pressure. The pulse rate changes only slightly. Tachycardia is observed rather seldom. In practically all patients, with only rare exceptions, a submaximal pupillar dilatation develops, and the response to light disappears.

A fall in arterial pressure to 70–60 mm Hg may be followed by a reduction or complete cessation of urine production. The renal function is restored along with the elevation of the blood pressure. When the arterial pressure falls below 90 mm Hg, even if the patient is in a horizontal position, the bleeding of the traumatised tissues is distinctly decreased. This effect depends more on the site of the intervention and the degree of its elevation above the heart than on the level of hypotension. The reduced tissue bleeding is seen most clearly in operations performed on the thoracic organs and neck, and less distinctly in surgery of the abdominal organs and the lower extremities.

The patient's response to trauma is significantly decreased during ganglionic block. Even during the most traumatising procedures the signs of shock are usually absent.

Peroperative use of ganglion-blocking agents has practically no effect upon the duration of action of the main anaesthetics and analgesics. Therefore, the patient wakes after surgery as usual.

2. Degree and Duration of Artificial Hypotension

Controlled hypotension suggests a relatively fast reduction of the blood pressure to the required level and its equally prompt restoration to the normal values. The advantages of artificial hypotension, such as decreased bleeding, easier manipulation of the arteries, begin to manifest themselves when the systolic pressure falls below 90 mm Hg. Hence, it is believed that relative hypotension, with the systolic pressure falling to 90 mm Hg, should be distinguished from true hypotension, with the pressure falling below 90 mm Hg (OSIPOV, 1973).

The safe limits of the depth and duration of hypotension are determined in every case by two factors: the individual characteristics of the patient and his position on the operating table. Accumulated experience indicates that for strong, young patients positioned horizontally and having normal arterial pressure the lower safe limit of artificial hypotension is 60 mm Hg. For patients with elevated blood pressure the limit to which it is believed safe to reduce it is 40–45% of the level considered common in such patients.

In cases in which ganglionic block is combined with positioning of the patient with the heart above most of the rest of the body, the safe level used should be higher, depending on how much his position differs from the horizontal. With the operating table tilted caudally by not more than 15°, this level should be 70 mm Hg.

Anaesthesiologists are agreed that artificial hypotension should be as brief as possible. With good oxygen saturation of the blood fall in arterial pressure by up to 60 mm Hg can be tolerated by a patient without any dangerous sequelae for quite a long time. With hypotension below the level mentioned, the oxygen supply to the brain and myocardium usually appears to be sufficient, while irreversible focal damage of a hypoxic nature may develop in the cells of the liver and kidneys. Deep hypotension, in contrast, even of short duration, is rather dangerous, since it may result in cardiac arrest and signs of hypoxic brain damage even before any pathologic changes appear in the kidneys, liver, and capillaries. A significant deceleration of the blood flow under hypotension predisposes to thrombosis and embolism. The possibility of thrombus formation increases with the depth and duration of hypotension. When the systolic pressure is decreased below 30 mm Hg, capillary stasis develops. In practice, the period of controlled hypotension is determined by the nature of the surgical intervention and the properties of the ganglion-blocking agent used.

In determining the duration of artificial hypotension the following criteria have to be observed: The period of hypotension must be strictly limited to the particular stage of the operation for which it is actually indicated. Usually, true hypotension should not be maintained for over 1–1.5 h. But if there are distinct indications, the systolic pressure can be maintained, with the patient in a horizontal position, 80–60 mm Hg for 2 h or even longer.

The moment and method of interrupting the patient's hypotensive state are of great importance in the prevention of secondary haemorrhage. The incision should be closed only after the systolic pressure has been raised above 90–100 mm Hg and careful haemostasis has been achieved, especially in the case of major operations. Gradual and spontaneous restoration of the arterial pressure is always desirable. If, however, hypotension is eliminated more slowly than needed in the course of the operation, the vascular tone must be restored by means of medication. Norepinephrine (0.001% solution, drip infusion) is the vasoconstricting agent of choice. Ephedrine and phenylephrine (mesathone) can also be used successfully.

When vasopressor agents are used for this purpose it should be borne in mind that the adrenoreceptors of the smooth muscles of the vessels display increased sensitivity to adrenomimetic drugs under the effect of ganglionic block. Therefore, a single intravenous injection of 10–15 mg of ephedrine is usually sufficient. This usually proves enough to eliminate the state of hypotension, although the signs of ganglionic block may persist for some time and disappear much more slowly.

3. Complications

Complications attributable to artificial hypotension were rather common in the early period of its use (HAMPTON and LITTLE, 1953). This was due to the dangerous methods used to decrease the patients' arterial pressure, however, such as arteriotomy and total spinal block. With the introduction of ganglion-blocking agents into anaesthesiological practice the number of complications decreased significantly. KERN (1956) reported only 14 cases with complications among 600 observations, these complications being secondary haemorrhages and haematomas. MESHCHERYAKOV (1960) noted only 3 complications among 250 cases of peroperative ganglionic block. LEBEDEV and FRID (1960) encountered quite innocuous complications in 8 of 230 patients. OSIPOV (1967) mentioned that in 406 cases of ganglionic block complications developed only in 6 patients, taking the form of secondary haemorrhages, lasting hypotension, or delayed waking after general anaesthesia.

Important reviews have appeared in recent years, indicating that complications are very rare in cases of controlled hypotension. Every paper, however, mentions rare cases in which some complications could be directly attributed to the use of controlled hypotension (WAY and CLARKE, 1959; ROLLASON and HOUGH, 1960; ENDERBY, 1961; WARNER et al., 1970; HUGOSSON and HÖGSTRÖM, 1973; PRYS-ROBERTS et al., 1974).

Hence, complications are encountered only rarely with artificial vasodilatation. Nevertheless, it is necessary to know these complications and their causes. Circulatory insufficiency in the vital organs is the most severe, although a rather rare complication. It can be caused either by a fall in the general intensity of the circulation (reduction of cardiac output), or by local circulatory disorders (postural ischaemia). And it should be borne in mind that while signs of cerebral or myocardial ischaemia can be noted immediately, on the operating table, ischaemia of the kidneys and liver manifests itself only in the postoperative period. The leading cause of these complications consists in exceedingly deep and lasting artificial vasoplegy, e.g., a fall in arterial pressure to below 60 mm Hg for a long period of time, incorrect positioning of the patient on the operating table, and inadequate blood replacement against the background of ganglionic block.

Preventive measures must be directed primarily against a sharp reduction of cardiac output. This is provided for by limited tilting of the operation table – caudally not more than 10–15° – so as to prevent orthostatic collapse, and by timely blood replacement.

As soon as signs of cerebral or cardiac circulatory insufficiency develop, the patient must be returned to the horizontal position, and vasodilatation must be interrupted with the aid of very careful administration of vasopressors.

Thromboses of various segments of the vascular bed developing due to the deceleration of the linear flow rate are observed in rare cases in the presence of pathology of the blood coagulation system and vascular wall lesions. Such complications should be prevented by taking careful account of the data recorded at the patient's preoperative clinical examination.

Secondary haemorrhage is a more common complication of artificial vasodilatation, especially when the anaesthetist has not had sufficient experience in using this method during surgery. Its main cause is a premature closing of the incision. Therefore, to avoid this complication the only correct and really effective method is to close the incision only after very careful haemostasis achieved at an arterial pressure of not below 90–100 mm Hg.

If the selected dose of the ganglion-blocking agent or the speed of infusion is incorrect, the patient may develop unusually protracted hypotension. This state can be treated by a repeated, preferably drip, careful infusion of vasopressors and transfusion of blood or blood substitutes. Blood transfusions are especially useful in cases when the administration of vasoconstrictors against the background of a deep ganglionic block proves ineffective. Sometimes operations conducted under artificial vasodilatation may be followed by a transient weakening of intestinal peristalsis and urine retention. This must be due to some residual manifestations of ganglionic block that is accompanied by inhibition of the motility of the gastrointestinal tract and bladder. Such complications usually do not require any special therapy and disappear spontaneously along with the signs of ganglionic block.

A histamine-like reaction in the form of oedema and skin erythema along the veins of the injection site is noted very rarely, and usually disappears spontaneously without any special therapy.

Some patients may develop transient vision disorders after surgery, taking the form of diplopia and impaired accommodation. This, however, may occur in the early hours after the operation, and disappear spontaneously after the signs of the ganglionic block have completely vanished.

C. Use of Artificial Vasodilatation for Various Surgical Interventions and Pulmonary Oedema

I. Coarctation of the Aorta

The haemodynamic features of this malformation are determined by a narrowing of the aortic isthmus to varying degrees, extending in some cases to complete obliteration. This results in a sharp increase of the peripheral vascular resistance, a decrease of the capacity and elasticity of the aortic compensatory chamber, and – in the presence of a normal cardiac output and stroke volume of the left ventricle – a significant increase of the systolic pressure in the aorta and its branches above the site of the narrowing. The presence of a constantly high pressure in the vessels results in a gradual development of sclerosis of their walls. The blood flow in the lower part of the body becomes less, and the blood supply is compensated for at the expense of the development of large collateral arteries.

Surgical correction of this malformation is aimed at restoring normal flow in the aorta (by way of excising the narrowed portion with an ent-to-end anastomosis, isthmoplasty, or by-pass with a vascular prosthesis). Hence, during the operation cross-clamping of the aorta above and below the narrowing for a comparatively prolonged period is mandatory. This results in hypervolaemia and elevated pressure in the vessels above the cross-clamping of the aorta and reduced blood supply to the vital organs of the lower part of the body, including the spinal cord.

Artificial vasodilatation, decreasing the tonicity of the muscle elements of the arteries, provides for an enlargement of the arterial compensatory chamber at the expense of its stretching and of a reduction of the peripheral resistance and arterial pressure, and for a dilatation of the collateral vessels and considerable simplification of the manipulation of the aorta, especially during its mobilisation (ligation of sclerosed intercostal arteries) and during the approximation of the cut ends and construction of the anastomosis.

It usually proves rather difficult to achieve the needed degree of hypotension with the routine doses of trimetaphan or hygronium, which demands an elevation of the total dose of the ganglion-blocking agents.

It must be emphasised that with increasingly distinct aortic stenosis and increasingly rich development of the collateral circulation, the elevation of arterial pressure in the upper part of the body following cross-clamping of the aorta will become less distinct. If there is complete obliteration of the isthmus the application of a clamp may cause no changes in the haemodynamics.

The general scheme of artificial vasodilatation induced during operations for coarctation of the aorta is as follows: Thoracotomy is performed in the conventional way, without vasodilatation. Trimetaphan or hygronium infusion is started only after haemostasis has been achieved. The arterial pressure is reduced to not less than 100–90 mm Hg, bearing in mind its high initial level. Interruption of the infusion of ganglion-blocking agent must be timed in such a qay as to ensure sufficient activity of the circulatory reflexes and contractility of the vessels and to avoid a sharp fall in the arterial pressure at the moment of releasing the clamps on the aorta. The position of the patient on the operating table is horizontal, and there is no need to alter it. If when the surgical procedure is ended the arterial pressure starts to rise, light vasodilatation should be prolonged by intramuscular injection of a long-acting ganglion-blocking agent (Pendiomid, hexamethonium). In some cases such intramuscular injections of Pendiomid or hexamethonium are repeated in small doses (25–50 mg) in the postoperative period. This prevents sharp fluctuations of the arterial pressure after surgery and provides for its stabilisation. Such tactical administration of ganglion-blocking agents is of especial importance when sclerotic changes are rather severe in the walls of the distinctly enlarged and ligated collateral arterial trunks. Stability of haemodynamics in the postoperative period indicates that haemorrhage has been prevented.

II. Patent Arterial Duct

The following haemodynamic changes are typical of this congenital heart disease:

a) increased pulmonary blood flow, since the pulmonary artery receives blood both from the right ventricle, and, in part, from the aorta via the patent arterial duct;

b) increased workload on the heart, since the left atrium receives increased amounts of blood from the pulmonary veins.

Thus, the work of the left ventricle is largely wasted on pumping additional amounts of blood shunted through the patent arterial duct and not actually forming part of the blood supply to the tissues. Cardiac output is increased to compensate for the peripheral blood flow.

Hypervolaemia of the pulmonary circulation system gradually causes persistent pulmonary hypertension and inversion of the blood shunt (from the pulmonary artery into the aorta).

The increased pulmonary resistance may be caused either by the elevated vascular tonicity or by the sclerotic changes (ZARGARLI, 1960) in the vessels. The surgical treatment of the patent arterial duct consists in an interruption of the pathologic communication between the systemic and pulmonary circulation by means of ligating the duct or dividing it between vascular clamps with subsequent suturing of the defects in the aorta and pulmonary artery.

The most critical stage of the intervention is the mobilisation of the major vessels of the arterial duct and its ligation, suturing, or division. A reduction of the intravascular pressure simplifies the mobilisation of the aorta and pulmonary artery, and makes the application of ligatures to the duct less dangerous, especially in adults, in whom the duct walls have often become thin and fragile. An artificial reduction of the arterial pressure can also help to decrease the bleeding and to facilitate haemostasis if the duct is injured during the procedure.

In patients with a patent arterial duct complicated by pulmonary hypertension the operation is associated with an additional risk due to the danger of left ventricular failure developing during the interruption of the communication between the aorta and the pulmonary, which has served hitherto as a safety valve reducing the load on the pulmonary circulation.

Hence, the positive effect of artificial hypotension during such operations does not consist only in simplifying the technical conditions of its performance.

First of all, ganglion-blocking agents, by decreasing the pressure in the systemic circulation to a much higher degree than that in the pulmonary circulation, reduces the pressure gradient between the aorta and the pulmonary artery and, consequently, the amount of the blood shunted (ZARGARLI, 1960; OSIPOV, 1967). In addition, by dilating the vascular bed of the systemic circulation, the ganglionic block results in a smaller return of blood to the heart, thus reducing the blood flow in the lungs and facilitating the work of the left ventricle. This is of great importance in operations on patients with distinct pulmonary hypertension. Even when the elasticity of the pulmonary vessels is significantly reduced, and when intermittent blood shunting from the pulmonary into the systemic circulation is observed, a pulmonary flow reduction under the effect of trimetaphan or hygronium makes the elimination of the "unloading" valve of the right heart, i.e., the arterial duct less dangerous.

Depending on the clinical course of the heart disease and on the conditions of surgery, artificial vasodilatation is used either only during ligation of the duct, or throughout manipulation of the vessels. In some cases the ganglionic block is continued into the postoperative period.

In some patients with the patent arterial duct complicated by pulmonary hypertension ganglion-blocking agents are used predominantly to decrease the cardiac output, and a postural reduction of the blood return to the heart can then be achieved by tilting the caudal end of the operating table down by 10–15° down. In all other cases the horizontal position of the patient on the operating table is preferred.

III. Heart Disease Correction With Extracorporeal Circulation

The replacement of the heart and lungs by corresponding mechanical systems –
pump and oxygenator – that pump the blood retrogradely into the femoral artery or
the aorta and the presence of foreign proteins in the patient's blood as a result of its
dilution with donor blood combine to predetermine pathologic shifts in man and the
functional state of the circulatory system in the first place. During the correction of
complex heart diseases cardiopulmonary by-pass has to be maintained for rather
long periods of time – 2 h or more – and it is then combined with body cooling by
means of so-called hypothermic perfusion. The latter is achieved by cooling the
blood that circulates in a heart-lung machine with a heat exchanger. The resultant
decrease in the tissue oxygen requirement permits a reduction of the volume rate of
perfusion, thus minimising the traumatisation of blood. But it also adds another
component – cooling – to the set of stress factors.

The accumulated clinical and experimental experience with extracorporeal circulation indicates that during clinical perfusion the following main phenomena occur
that ultimately impair the blood supply to and the metabolism of various tissues:
protective redistribution of the flow, centralisation of circulation, and microcirculation disorders (sludging). These changes are characteristic of shock and blood loss,
and are not specific to extracorporeal circulation.

The phenomenon of protective redistribution of the flow arises because the vital
organs are selectively placed in better conditions during the cardiopulmonary by-
pass than are the other organs and tissues. Thus, for example, when the output of the
heart-lung machine is reduced from 2.4 to 0.5 $l/m^2/min$, the share of the cerebral and
coronary flow is doubled. This means that the reduction of the cerebral and coronary
flow and blood supply takes place more slowly than that of the systemic blood flow,
while the flow in the abdominal and pelvic organs and the peripheral tissues falls in
proportion with the general flow reduction, i.e., their share remains practically unchanged (OSIPOV, 1971).

Organ autoregulation of the circulation is considered to be one of the main
mechanisms of the protective flow redistribution. The essence of this mechanism
consists in the ability of the main organs to retain their blood flow on a relatively
constant level, irrespective of the changes in the arterial pressure.

In centralisation of circulation the circulating blood volume is accumulated predominantly in the vicinity of the heart and the major vessels. One of the most
frequent of the mechanisms resulting in this phenomenon consists in an increasing
activity of the sympatho-adrenal system and enhanced sensitivity of small vessels to
vasoactive drugs. This results in blood shunting into the larger vessels, and the
capillary flow decreases significantly, this being especially true of the peripheral
tissues and kidneys. One typical sign of circulation centralisation is impaired thermoregulation, resulting as from of a sharp reduction of blood supply to the skin and
subcutaneous tissues, together with renal function disorders to the degree of complete anuria. Such a centralisation of circulation even prevents body cooling and
rewarming during the perfusion. This results in differences in the intensity of metabolism in various portions and tissues of the body. Such "patchy metabolism" is one of
the sources of metabolic acidosis and of a number of untoward humoral shifts that
occur during cardiopulmonary by-pass in man.

The peripheral circulation disorders manifest themselves clinically in acrocyanosis, mottled skin, and a rising temperature gradient between various parts of the body during the cooling.

The essence of sludging is an intravascular aggregation of erythrocytes, resulting in capillary obstruction. The axiallary movement of the erythrocytes typical of small vessels is distorted. The erythrocytes group in agglomerates, separated from one another by clear zones deprived of erythrocytes. Depending on the stage of its development, the erythrocyte aggregation may be observed in the venules alone (stage 1), in the venules and capillaries (stage 2), and even in the arterioles (stage 3). While the first two stages are not necessarily pathologic, stage 3 sludging, i.e., arteriolar, is a definite sign of a pathologic state (AKOUN, 1965).

The causes of sludging are: reduction of local and general circulation intensity; increase of sympatho-adrenal activity; hypothermia; and metabolic acidosis, hyperlipidaemia, and loss from the erytrocytes of the negative charge that under normal conditions prevents their aggregation and lateral position during their movement along small vessels.

All three above-mentioned phenomena can be manifested to varying degrees during extracorporeal circulation. In any case, they may cause common symptoms. But ultimately they have two main consequences: uneven blood supply to different organs and tissues (from the point of view of the discrepancies between the blood flow and the metabolic requirements of the tissues) and microcirculation disorders.

Hence, summing up, it must be emphasised that during cardiopulmonary by-pass the site of inadequate tissue blood supply, and, consequently, of the source of metabolic acidosis is in the superficial tissues, most especially the skin, the subcutaneous tissues, and a large mass of striated muscles.

The prevention of such complications must include the following measures: perfect anaesthesia during surgery; sufficiently high-volume flow rate; even flow distribution in the body during perfusion; and prevention of microcirculation disorders.

As our experience with cardiopulmonary by-pass has demonstrated over many years, the use of ganglion-blocking agents during the perfusion serves as an effective means of ensuring the above conditions, and also exploits the oxyhaemoglobin level in venous blood as the leading criterion of adequacy of the perfusion, and applies haemodilution. In practice, the most convenient substances are trimetaphan and hygronium.

The use of artificial vasodilatation induced during cardiopulmonary by-pass with trimetaphan or hygronium allows the attainment of decentralisation of the circulation and reduction of the activity of the sympatho-adrenal system. The ganglionic block prevents the development of a protective redistribution of the blood flow during the cardiopulmonary by-pass, thus providing for a more even blood supply to the tissues. Apart from this, its distinct counter-shock action creates optimum conditions for manipulation of the heart, decreasing the response to mechanical injuries.

The positive effects of ganglionic block during cardiopulmonary by-pass are clinically very obvious. The paleness and mottled colouring of the skin are replaced by an intensely pink complexion, the "pale spot" sign disappears, and the tendency to development of metabolic acidosis clearly diminishes, which demonstrates a good blood supply to the peripheral tissues.

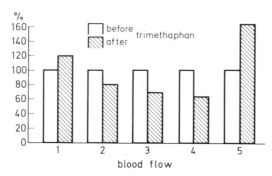

Fig. 2. Blood flow redistribution following trimetaphan during cardiopulmonary by-pass. *1*, superior vena cava flow; *2*, coronary flow; *3*, portal flow; *4*, renal flow; *5*, infrarenal inferior vena cava glow (OSIPOV, 1971)

Experimental studies of the effect of trimetaphan during cardiopulmonary by-pass conducted in our laboratory by OSIPOV (1971) have demonstrated that this effect is in direct contrast to the phenomenon of protective blood flow redistribution. With the volume perfusion rate remaining unchanged, it causes a reduction of the coronary, portal, and renal blood flow, with a simultaneous increase of the blood flow in the system of the superior vena cava and the infrarenal portion of the inferior vena cava (Fig. 2). The peripheral resistance then falls in the three vascular zones, i.e., kidneys and peripheral organs of the upper and lower portions of the body. As a

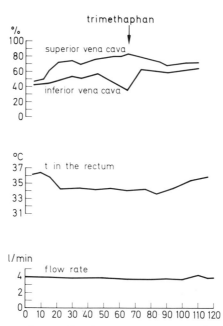

Fig. 3. Reduction of O_2 saturation gradient between superior and inferior venae cavae following trimetaphan during cardiopulmonary by-pass. Surgery: radical correction of tetralogy of Fallot. *Arrows* indicate time of administration of trimetaphan

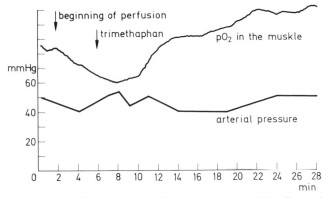

Fig. 4. Effect of trimetaphan on O_2 tension in subcutaneous tissue of the finger during cardiopulmonary by-pass. Surgery: mitral, tricuspid and aortic valve replacement. *Arrows* indicate beginning of perfusion *(left)* and administration of trimetaphan *(right)*

result of this, the extracorporeal circulation becomes easier to control. While prior to the administration of a ganglion-blocking agent the increase of heart-lung machine output results in an increased blood flow predominantly in the viscera, under artificial vasodilatation induced by trophenium an increase of the perfusion volume flow rate is accompanied by an improvement of the blood flow in the peripheral tissues and kidneys as well.

During surgery the more even distribution of the flow following the administration of ganglion-blocking agents is manifested in a distinct reduction of the difference in the oxygen saturation of the blood flowing separately from the inferior and superior venae cavae (Fig. 3). During hypothermic perfusion the evenness of the blood flow in the tissues is manifested in a reduced temperature gradient between different portions of the body during the cooling and rewarming periods.

Data on the beneficial effects of trimetaphan on the microcirculation of the peripheral tissues have been clinically supported. Thus, the studies conducted with the aid of polarography and radioactive clearance indicated that the administration of trimetaphan during the perfusion was invariably accompanied by a growth of O_2 tension in the skin, subcutaneous tissues and muscles. The flow in the muscles increased by 230–290% (Fig. 4).

In our practice of open-heart surgery artificial vasodilatation induced by trimetaphan or hygronium is an indispensible component of anaesthesia, and largely determines the adequacy of the cardiopulmonary by-pass.

1. Technique of Artificial Vasodilatation During Cardiopulmonary By-Pass

When the cardiopulmonary by-pass is to be initiated, the output of the heart-lung machine is gradually increased, the venous return to it being constantly adjusted. Upon attainment of the precalculated level of volume perfusion rate 10–20 mg (0.1%) trimetaphan is added to the heart-lung machine. The degree of ganglionic block achieved is manifested by the degree of mydriasis and the appearance of a pinkish complexion of the skin and visible mucosa. A single injection of trimetaphan

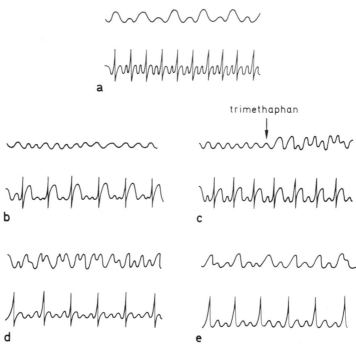

Fig.5, a–e. Dynamics of rheogram from left forearm of patient subjected to heart surgery with cardiopulmonary by-pass. *Arrow* shows moment of the injection of trimetaphan during perfusion. **a** Before perfusion; **b** after beginning of perfusion (temp. 31.5 °C); **c** during perfusion (temp. 32 °C) with infusion of trimetaphan shortly after the beginning; **d** at end of perfusion (temp. 37 °C); **e** after discontinuation of perfusion

is used for 40–60-min perfusions. For longer-lasting hypothermic perfusions trimetaphan is infused by the drip technique (0.1%; 40–60 drops/min). Then, after achievement of the state of a ganglionic block assessed according to the above criteria the infusion rate decreased to 20–25 drops/min. Administration of the drug is terminated before the end of the patient's rewarming, some 10–15 min before termination of the perfusion. The total dose of trimetaphan is 25–50 mg on average. Discontinuation of the extracorporeal circulation should be started with an interruption of venous return to the heart-lung machine, with a simultaneous reduction of the arterial pump output. The blood is pumped into the arterial system of the patient with constant monitoring of the central venous pressure. The arterial pump is arrested only after the venous pressure rise to 160–170 mm H_2O. After a short time, usually some 1–2 min, the venous pressure falls by 30–40 mm H_2O, which serves as a signal for the resumption of blood pumping into the vascular system of the patient, and so on. Such fractionated blood pumping is continued until the central venous pressure stabilises at 160–170 mm H_2O, and the arterial pressure at 80–90 mm Hg. With this method of returning to spontaneous circulation the amount of blood added to the vascular system of the patient can be as much as 30% of the patient's initial blood volume, depending on the degree of artificial vasodilatation. For an adult patient this may amount to 1–1.5.

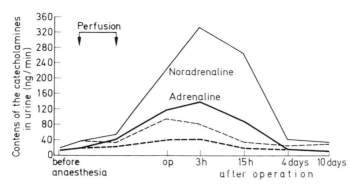

Fig.6. Dynamics of urine catecholamine concentration during and after cardiac surgery with cardiopulmonary by-pass. *Continuous lines* indicate catecholamine concentrations in fast cooling and rewarming of patient during perfusion. *Dotted line* indicates urine concentration of catecholamines during gradual changes of body temperature during perfusion with artificial vasodilatation brought about by means of trimetaphan

    The beneficial clinical effect of the administration of trimetaphan during extracorporeal circulation is very obvious. It becomes especially vivid during hypothermic perfusions. Acrocyanosis and mottled complexion are replaced by a pinkish colouring of the skin, and the pale spot sign disappears, indicating a good blood supply to the peripheral tissues. The clinical impression is also supported by rheovasographic data (Fig. 5).

    In our practice both trimetaphan and hygronium have been used. The dosage, method of administration and clinical effect of hygronium are identical with those of trimetaphan.

    No complications attributable to the employment of ganglionic block during cardiopulmonary by-pass have been encountered in our 2000 operations of this kind. With technically flawless perfusion and artificial vasodilatation, irrespective of the duration of extracorporeal circulation for 2 h or longer, metabolic acidosis never usually develops.

    A comparative study on the state of the sympatho-adrenal system during hypothermic perfusions revealed a considerable reduction of the urine catecholamine level in patients in whom the extracorporeal circulation was conducted against the background of artificial vasodilatation and slow rewarming after hypothermia (Fig.6).

IV. Pulmonary Oedema

In the complex pathogenesis of pulmonary oedema an important role is played by the haemodynamic disorders that ultimately increase the pressure in the pulmonary capillaries and increase the permeability of the alveolar-capillary membrane of the lungs. These disorders are not always the direct cause of pulmonary oedema, but they always favour its development, enhancing the effect of the main causative factor (LAZARIS and SEREBROVSKAYA, 1963). Proceeding from this assumption, one of the most important elements of the treatment of pulmonary oedema consists in eliminating the congestion in the pulmonary circulation.

The following means of affecting the haemodynamics may be used for this purpose:
- Reduction of venous return, and, hence, of cardiac output
- Reduction of pressure in the systemic circulation, thus providing for reflex emptying of the pulmonary vascular depot
- Reduction of the peripheral resistance in the systemic circulation, thus facilitating the work of the left ventricle and reducing the congestion phenomena in the pulmonary circulation
- Reduction of venous pressure in the systemic circulation, thus helping intensive lymph drainage and reversal of pulmonary oedema.

Massive vasodilatation developing in the systemic circulation under the effect of trimetaphan or hygronium produces precisely the haemodynamic shifts that help to eliminate the congestion in the pulmonary circulation and to decrease the pulmonary oedema: reduction of peripheral resistance in the systemic circulation, of systolic arterial and venous pressure; blood depot formation in the distended vessels of the systemic circulation, reduction of blood return to the heart and of cardiac output; reduction in pulmonary blood flow and pulmonary capillary pressure and blood redistribution from the pulmonary into the systemic circulation; and reduction of the mechanical work of both ventricles, especially the left one.

Blood depot formation under the effect of trimetaphan may amount to 30% of the initial circulating blood volume. This so-called bloodless bloodletting has the advantage over the conventional method that it does not provoke reflex vasoconstriction. Upon cessation of the effect of the ganglion-blocking agents the blood from the depot again enters the circulation, which is of special importance in patients subjected to surgery.

The vasoplegic effect of trimetaphan and hygronium depends heavily on the blockade of the chromaffin tissue of the adrenal glands, which results in a decreased secretion of catecholamines. This seems most valuable in the management of pulmonary oedema, the pathogenesis of which is primarily characterised by an increased secretion of catecholamines due to the concomitant hypoxia.

If we add that an important role is played by the reflex mechanism in the development of pulmonary oedema, it will become evident that the ganglionic block induced by trimetaphan or hygronium and the ensuing artificial vasodilatation should be interpreted as an effective measure against this grave complication.

1. Technique of Ganglion Blockade in Pulmonary Oedema

The method of administration of trimetaphan or hygronium for the treatment of pulmonary oedema is in general similar to that described above. The special features include the necessity to induce the ganglionic block on the ward in waking patients with spontaneous respiration. It is recommended that the foot end of the bed be raised during the reduction of arterial pressure, to avoid postural ischaemia of the brain and orthostatic collapse. The cranial end should be gradually elevated as the signs of ganglionic block fade (narrowing of the pupils).

It has to be taken into account that the main purpose of the use of ganglion-blocking agents does not consist in achieving arterial hypotension, but in producing the formation of a depot of a needed amount of circulating blood and in blocking the autonomic ganglia. Therefore there is no need to try to reduce the arterial pressure to the lowest possible level. Experience has demonstrated that a distinct beneficial effect of trimetaphan and hygronium may be observed even without any significant reduction of the arterial pressure.

V. Neurosurgery

Ganglion-blocking agents are used quite widely in neurosurgery. Haemorrhage is known to be the most frequently observed and one of the most severe complications of brain surgery. Therefore the main purpose of controlled hypotension induced by ganglion-blocking agents is to decrease the volume of cerebral blood flow, which greatly diminishes to danger of haemorrhage during the removal of brain tumours, during interventions necessitated by cerebral vascular aneurysms, and in many other surgical interventions (LITTLE, 1955; EGOROV and KANDEL, 1958; ZLOTNIK and LERMAN, 1960; KANDEL et al., 1970; KANDEL and NIKOLAENKO, 1970; McCOMISH and BODLEY, 1971; MANEVICH et al., 1974). It should be emphasised, however, that the advantages of ganglion-blocking agents in neurosurgery are not limited solely to the prevention or significant reduction of haemorrhage. The employment of ganglion-blocking agents both during surgery and postoperatively is considered to be a method of reducing the general reactivity of the organism by blocking the autonomic innervation, which naturally has an important role in the development of the gravest complications of brain surgery – cerebral oedema, surgical shock, multiple intracerebral haemorrhages, pulmonary oedema, etc.

1. Special Features of the Use of Ganglion-Blocking Agents During Brain Surgery

The most important factor in controlled hypotension is not the drug used, but adherence to the principle of ensuring adequate blood flow in the vital organs.

Against the background of a ganglionic block the decisive factor of the organ blood flow is gravity. Most neurosurgical operations are performed with the patient in a position in which the head is above heart level. And this is why the prevention of brain ischaemia during neurosurgical procedures under controlled hypotension is the decisive prerequisite for a favourable outcome of the operation.

The danger of ischaemic injuries is increased by pushing the brain away to facilitate the surgical approach. Vessels with reduced tonicity cannot withstand the pressure and become deflated. In such cases so-called retraction ischaemia may develop. This becomes especially important during brain surgery when controlled hypotension is to be used in the presence of significant disorders of cerebral haemodynamics that manifest themselves in a reduced cerebral blood flow and impaired autoregulation mechanisms.

Opinions differ as to the rationale for controlled hypotension during brain surgery. Many authors believe that this method greatly facilitates the performance and improves its results (MANEVICH et al., 1972, 1974). Others, pointing out the possible ischaemic injury of the brain, caution against extended indications for this method in neurosurgery (GILBERT et al., 1966; BROWN and HORTON, 1966).

The majority, however, believe that if the necessary conditions are fulfilled, controlled hypotension has many advantages than drawbacks in neurosurgery, and that these advantages outweigh the possible hazards and lend support to wide use of this technique in neurosurgery, especially in vascular pathology of the brain.

One essential in neurosurgical operations is a good approach. For this purpose osmotic diuretics are often used. During the first phase of their action hypervolaemia occurs, manifesting itself in a significant elevation of the arterial and central venous pressure and in an increasing heart contraction rate. Hypervolaemia complicates the achievement of controlled hypotension. To achieve the needed level of hypotension during this initial period a high dose of the ganglion-blocking agent being used is required. On the other hand, due to intensive diuresis the patients may develop, or may already have developed, hypovolaemia, so that when the vasoplegic effect of the ganglion-blocking agents is added an excessive reduction in the arterial pressure results. Artificial pulmonary ventilation, anaesthetics, and neuroleptics may also potentiate the effect of the ganglion-blocking agents.

Thus, in neurosurgical procedures account must be taken of a number of factors that can alter the effect of the ganglion-blocking agents over a rather wide range. It is therefore completely wrong to use techniques of artificial vasodilatation that are based on an attempt to reach the needed level of arterial pressure reduction at the expense of changing the dose of the ganglion-blocking agent alone.

Along with an optimum dosage of the ganglion-blocking agent, proper attention should be paid to the effect of the following factors:
- Postural reactions
- Anaesthetics used
- Artificial pulmonary ventilation
- Circulating blood volume.

The last factor is of decisive importance for the prevention of such grave complications as cerebrovascular thrombosis, cerebral infarction, coronary thrombosis, cardiovascular collapse, renal infarction, necrotic nephrosis, oliguria and anuria, vision disorders, and secondary haemorrhages (Little, 1956; Zlotnik, 1965; Osipov, 1967; Manevich et al., 1974).

a) Method of Controlled Hypotension

The choice of the ganglion-blocking agent and its dosage are largely determined by the following factors:
- Intended level of reduction of the arterial pressure
- Position of the patient during surgery
- Type and method of anaesthesia (the effect of the anaesthetics used upon the haemodynamics)
- Initial circulating blood volume and measures aimed at changing this in the course of the procedure (hypervolaemic haemodilution, osmotic diuretics)
- Nature of pathology and particular features of the surgical intervention
- Purpose of using artificial hypotension.

b) Level of Hypotension

If the arterial pressure is reduced to not less than 60 mm Hg for 60 min no signs of brain ischaemia are usually observed. If such hypotension is continued this results in a distinct enhancement of the signs of brain oxygen deficiency (Gribova, 1972).

Taking into consideration the nature of the pathology and the duration of the surgical intervention, it may be concluded that the arterial pressure may be reduced to 60–80 mm Hg within the first hour of the operation for arterial aneurysms, and to 75–80 mm Hg for arteriovenous aneurysms. Throughout the rest of the procedure the arterial pressure should not be reduced below 80 mm Hg.

When controlled hypotension is used during removal of brain tumours, the reduction of the arterial pressure permissible is determined mainly by the initial state of the patient and his position on the operating table.

c) Position of the Patient

Fowler's position (15–25°) and the elevation of the head only at the angle mentioned permit reduction of the dose of the ganglion-blocking agent by almost half. With the patient in a sitting position the dosage of the agents is reduced four- to sixfold. Not infrequently the use of Fluothane or neuroleptanalgesia for anaesthesia makes it possible to dispense with ganglion blockers completely.

With the use of Fluothane, Penthrane or neuroleptanalgesia for anaesthesia the dose of the ganglion-blocking agents is reduced by half (EMELYANOV, 1972; SHUBIN and KORNIENKO, 1972). Artificial pulmonary ventilation applied during a regimen of slight hyperventilation also permits a significant reduction in the dose of the ganglion-blocking agents used for controlled hypotension, as does the use of d-tubocuraine.

d) Circulating Blood Volume

With hypervolaemic haemodilution and during the first phase of the action of osmotic diuretics an elevation of the arterial pressure can be prevented by increasing the dose of the ganglion-blocking agent by half or doubling it. But an increase of this order in the dose of the ganglion-blocking agents may result in the development of a rather persistent, deep hypotension with subsequent increased diuresis and decreased circulating blood volume. To avoid this, postural reactions should be exploited at this stage of the operation to prevent possible elevation of the arterial pressure. By combining Fluothane or neuroleptanalgesia with changes in the patient's position on the operating table (tilting the caudal end downward) it is possible to prevent and to avoid any elevation of the arterial pressure in the presence of hypervolaemia and any excessive reduction of the arterial pressure in case of a circulating blood volume deficit (MANEVICH et al., 1974).

e) Drugs and Techniques of Use

Trimetaphan is infused intravenously by drip infusion (0.1% solution in a 5% glucose solution) at a rate of 60–70 drops/min. After the administration of 20–30 ml of this solution the needed level of the arterial pressure is reached in 3–4 min. After this the drug infusion rate is reduced to 30–40 drops/min (2–4 mg).

Hygronium is also used as 0.1% solution, and is introduced intravenously by the drip technique at the same rats as trimetaphan. A dose of 50–60 mg produces a fall in arterial pressure lasting 18–20 min on average. The required level of hypotension is maintained by means of a drip infusion of the agent (20–30 drops/min).

Pendiomid is given in an initial dose of 10–15 mg by intravenous injection. Later, depending on the patient's tolerance of the drug, 20–50 mg of the ganglion-blocking agents is added. The duration of effect ranges from 30 to 60 min. The administration of the ganglion-blocking agent is started before the stage of the intervention at which haemorrhage can be expected, or before the stage of approaching, examining, and exposing the pathologic formation. In cases of arterial aneurysms administration of the ganglion-blocking agents is started much earlier, especially in cases tending to arterial hypertension, to avoid rupture of the vessels.

In cases of hypervolaemic haemodilution the administration of the ganglion-blocking agents is started simultaneously with the haemodilution itself. After establishment of the absence of any unusual reaction to the test dose of the ganglion-blocking agent the maintenance dose is added.

One very important principle is not to try to overcome the resistance to the drug by increasing the dosage. In such cases it is more reasonable to achieve the needed level of hypotension by way of postural reactions, Fluothane, or droperidol against the background of an adequate circulating blood volume.

f) Indications and Contraindications

Controlled hypotension is indicated for surgical interventions for arterial and arteriovenous aneurysms and for the removal of meningiomas, especially those penetrating the upper sagittal sinus, the falciform process, and the bones of the skull dome.

However, the use of ganglion-blocking agents is different in each particular case. In some cases they are used to decrease the blood filling and tension of the aneurysm so as to facilitate the surgeon's manipulation and to reduce the risk of a rupture of the aneurysm. In other cases, e.g., for removal of meningovascular tumours of the brain, the ganglion-blocking agents are used to reduce venous bleeding. In the postoperative period these drugs are given for the prevention and management of arterial hypertension.

Hence, neurosurgery is a wide field for the use of various ganglion-blocking agents with specific objectives, purposes, and methods of use; knowledge of these permits a significant diminution of the risk encountered in surgery for various cerebral pathology.

References

Akoun, G.: Concept actuel de l'agrégation intravasculaire des érythrocites. "Sludge". Ann. Anesthesiol. Fr. 6, 2 special, 65–88 (1965)

Brown, A.S., Horton, J.M.: Elective hypotension with intracardiac pacemaking in the operative management of ruptured intracranial aneurysms. Acta Anaesthesiol. Scand. [Suppl.] 23, 665–669 (1966), Dyachenko, P.K., Vinogradov, V.M.: Special Anaesthesiology. Leningrad: Medgiz 1962 (Russ.)

Egorov, B.G., Kandel, E.I.: Employment of ganglion-blocking drugs in neurosurgical operations and in the postoperative period. Vopr. Neirokhir. 6, 36 (1958) (Russ.)

Emelyanov, V.K.: Coefficient of anaerobic metabolism as an index of brain oxygen deficit in combined anaesthesia with penthrane in neurosurgical interventions. In: Voprosy anesteziologii i reanimatsii, pp. 54–55. Moskva: Meditsina 1972 (Russ.)

Enderby, G.E.H.: A report on mortality and morbidity following 9, 107 hypotensive anaesthesias. Br. J. Anaesth. 33, 109–114 (1961)

Gilbert, R.G., Brindle, G.E., Galindo, A.: Anesthesia for neurosurgery. London: J.& A. Churchill 1966

Gribova, E.A.: Choice of optimum level of arterial pressure reduction during surgery on cerebral vessels. Avtoref. Diss. Moskva 1972 (Russ.)

Hampton, L.J., Little, D.M.: Results of a questionaire concerning controlled hypotension in anaesthesia. Lancet *1953 I*, 1299–1305

Hugosson, R., Högström, S.: Factors disposing to morbidity in surgery of intracrainal aneurysms with special regard to deep controlled hypotension. J. Neurosurg. *38*, 561–565 (1973)

Kandel, E.I., Nikolaenko, E.M.: Effect of hygronium-induced ganglionic block upon the hemo-dynamics and gas exchange during neurosurgical operations. Id. pp. 228–238 (Russ.)

Kandel, E.I., Nikolaenko, E.M., Salalykin, V.I.: Experience of using hygronium in neurosurgery. In: Novye kurarepodobnye i ganglioblokiruyushie sredstva, pp. 222–228. Moskva: Medit-sina 1970 (Russ.)

Kern, E.: Analise des 600 observations d'hypotension controlée. Anesth. Analg. (Paris) *13*, 440–451 (1956)

Kharkevich, D.A.: Ganglion-blocking and ganglion-stimulating agents. Oxford: Pergamon Press 1967

Lazaris, Ya.A. Serebrovskaya, I.A.: Pulmonary circulation. Moskva: Meditsina 1963 (Russ.)

Lebedev, L.V., Frid, I.A.: Experience of employment of artificial hypotension in surgical clinics. Khirurgiia (Mosk.) 7, 9–12 (1960) (Russ.)

Little, D.M.: Induced hypotension during anesthesia and surgery. Anesthesiology *16*, 320–325 (1955)

Little, D.M.: Controlled hypotension in anesthesia and surgery. Springfield: III. USA 1956 Charles C. Thomas

Manevich, A.Z., Gribova, E.A., Emelyanova, V.K.: Problems of anesthesia in operations on the vessels of the brain. Vestn. Akad. Med. Nauk S.S.S.R. 8, 57–60 (1972) (Russ.)

Manevich, A.Z., Gribova, E.A., Emelyanova, V.K.: Principles of anaesthesia in vascular neuro-surgery. In: Neyrokhirurgicheskaya patologiya tserebralnykh sosudov. pp. 187–190. Moskva: Tzudi instituta nayrokhirzurgii 1974 (Russ.)

McComish, P.B., Bodely, P.O.: Anaesthesia for neurological surgery, pp. 105–116. London: Lloyd-Luke 1971

Meshcherjakov, N.A.: Employment of ganglion-blocking agents in anaesthesiology. Kand. Diss. Leningrad 1960 (Russ.)

Osipov, V.P.: Artificial hypotension. Moskva: Meditsina 1967 (Russ.)

Osipov, V.P.: Pathophysiological and clinical aspects of extracorporeal circulation. Dokt. Diss. Moskva 1971 (Russ.)

Osipov, V.P.: Artificial hypotension. In: Posobie po anesteziologii. Darbinyan, T.M., (ed.), Vol. XX, pp. 347–363. Moskva: Meditsina 1973 (Russ.)

Prys-Roberts, C., Lloyd, J.W., Fisher, A., Kerr, J.H., Patterson, T.J.H.: Deliberate profound hypotension induced with halothane. Brit. J. Anaesth. *46*, 105–109 (1974)

Rollason, W.N., Hough, J.M.: A study of hypotensive anaesthesia in the elderly. Br. J. Anaesth. *32*, 276–281 (1960)

Shubin, V.S., Kornienko, V.N.: Effect of patient's body position on cerebral circulation state. In: Trudy 3-ey Konferentsii neyrokhirurgov Pribaltiyskikh respublik, pp. 217–219. Riga: Medi-cinsky institut 1972 (Russ.)

Vinogradov, V.M., Dyachenko, P.K.: Basis of clinical anaesthesiology. Leningrad: Medgiz 1961 (Russ.)

Warner, W.A., Shumrick, D.A., Caffrey, J.A.: Clinical investigation of prolonged induced hypo-tension in head and neck surgery. Br. J. Anaesth. *42*, 39–44 (1970)

Way, G.L., Clarke, H.L.: An anaesthetic technique for prostaectomy. Lancet *1959 II*, 888–893

Zargarli, F.I.: Some aspects of the clinical course, diagnosis, physiopathology, and surgical management of the patent arterial duct. Kand. Diss. Moskva 1960 (Russ.)

Zlotnik, E.I.: Haemostasis and controlled hypotension in brain surgery. Minsk: Belorusizdat 1965 (Russ.)

Zlotnik, E.I., Lerman, V.I.: Employment of ganglion-blocking agents in neurosurgery. In: Gan-gliolitiki i blockatory neyro-myshechnykh sinapsov, pp. 57–95. Leningrad: Medgiz 1960 (Russ.)

Author Index

Page numbers in *italics* refer to bibliography

Subject Index

The following abbreviations are used, excepting as primary headings, throughout:

Handbook of Experimental Pharmacology

Continuation of "Handbuch der experimentellen Pharmakologie"

Editorial Board:
G. V. R. Born, A. Farah,
H. Herken, A. D. Welch

Springer-Verlag
Berlin
Heidelberg
New York

Handbook of Experimental Pharmacology

Continuation of "Handbuch der experimentellen Pharmakologie"

Editorial Board:
G. V. R. Born, A. Farah,
H. Herken, A. D. Welch

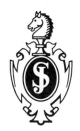

Springer-Verlag
Berlin
Heidelberg
New York

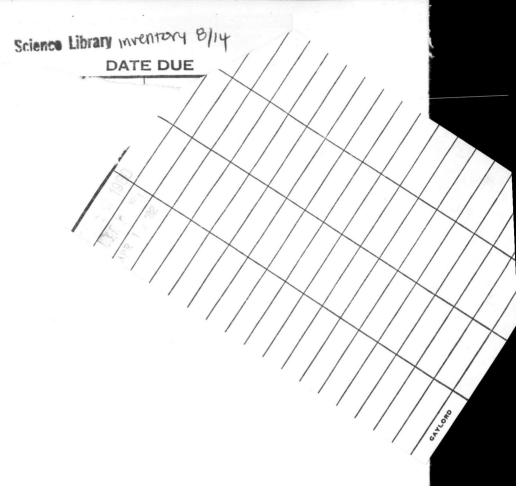